Migration and Migration Status: Key Determinants of Health and Well-Being

Migration and Migration Status: Key Determinants of Health and Well-Being

Guest Editors

Maria De Jesus
Ernesto Castañeda

MDPI

Basel • Beijing • Wuhan • Barcelona • Belgrade • Novi Sad • Cluj • Manchester

Guest Editors
Maria De Jesus
School of International Service
Department of Environment, Development, and Health
Immigration Lab
Center for Latin American and Latino Studies
American University
Washington, DC
USA

Ernesto Castañeda
School of Arts and Sciences
Department of Sociology
Immigration Lab
Center for Latin American and Latino Studies
American University
Washington, DC
USA

Editorial Office
MDPI AG
Grosspeteranlage 5
4052 Basel, Switzerland

This is a reprint of the Special Issue, published open access by the journal *International Journal of Environmental Research and Public Health* (ISSN 1660-4601), freely accessible at: https://www.mdpi.com/journal/ijerph/special_issues/migration__status_key_determinants_health_well_being.

For citation purposes, cite each article independently as indicated on the article page online and as indicated below:

Lastname, A.A.; Lastname, B.B. Article Title. *Journal Name* **Year**, *Volume Number*, Page Range.

ISBN 978-3-7258-4129-5 (Hbk)
ISBN 978-3-7258-4130-1 (PDF)
https://doi.org/10.3390/books978-3-7258-4130-1

Cover image courtesy of Maria De Jesus
Unstably housed migrants set up a tent in front of the Médecins du Monde (Doctors of the World) office building in Lyon, France

Contents

About the Editors ix

Preface xi

Maria De Jesus and Ernesto Castañeda
Social Contexts and Immigration Policies Directly Impact Immigrant Health
Reprinted from: *Int. J. Environ. Res. Public Health* **2025**, *22*, 586,
https://doi.org/10.3390/ijerph22040586 1

Arthur R. Andrews, Kevin Escobar, Sandra Mariely Estrada Gonzalez, Sara Reyes and Laura M. Acosta
Investigating the Potential Double-Edged Score of Immigration-Related Stress, Discrimination, and Mental Health Access
Reprinted from: *Int. J. Environ. Res. Public Health* **2024**, *21*, 373,
https://doi.org/10.3390/ijerph21030373 9

Mario Alberto Viveros Espinoza-Kulick and Jessica P. Cerdeña
"We Need Health for All": Mental Health and Barriers to Care among Latinxs in California and Connecticut
Reprinted from: *Int. J. Environ. Res. Public Health* **2022**, *19*, 12817,
https://doi.org/10.3390/ijerph191912817 20

Yijing Chen, Claudia Rafful, Mercado Mercedes, Lindsey Carte, Sonia Morales-Miranda, Judeline Cheristil and Teresita Rocha-Jiménez
Hoping for a Better Future during COVID-19: How Migration Plans Are Protective of Depressive Symptoms for Haitian Migrants Living in Chile
Reprinted from: *Int. J. Environ. Res. Public Health* **2022**, *19*, 9977,
https://doi.org/10.3390/ijerph19169977 41

Maria De Jesus, Zoubida Moumni, Zara Hassan Sougui, Neeharika Biswas, Raquel Kubicz and Lionel Pourtau
"Living in Confinement, Stopped in Time": Migrant Social Vulnerability, Coping and Health during the COVID-19 Pandemic Lockdown in France
Reprinted from: *Int. J. Environ. Res. Public Health* **2022**, *19*, 10084,
https://doi.org/10.3390/ijerph191610084 56

Cihan Aydiner and Erin L. Rider
Reskilled and Integrated, but How? Navigating Trauma and Temporary Hardships
Reprinted from: *Int. J. Environ. Res. Public Health* **2022**, *19*, 13675,
https://doi.org/10.3390/ijerph192013675 71

Caitlin Bletscher and Sara Spiers
"Step by Step We Were Okay Now": An Exploration of the Impact of Social Connectedness on the Well-Being of Congolese and Iraqi Refugee Women Resettled in the United States
Reprinted from: *Int. J. Environ. Res. Public Health* **2023**, *20*, 5324,
https://doi.org/10.3390/ijerph20075324 89

Nigar G. Khawaja and Robert D. Schweitzer
A Qualitative Study of Adolescents from Refugee Backgrounds Living in Australia: Identity and Resettlement
Reprinted from: *Int. J. Environ. Res. Public Health* **2024**, *21*, 281,
https://doi.org/10.3390/ijerph21030281 116

Liquan Qu, Weidong Xiao and Weidong Gao
Do Resettled People Adapt to Their Current Geographical Environment? Evidence from Poverty-Stricken Areas of Northwest Yunnan Province, China
Reprinted from: *Int. J. Environ. Res. Public Health* **2022**, *20*, 193,
https://doi.org/10.3390/ijerph20010193 . . . . **131**

Emmanuel F. Koku
The Effect of Stigma and Social Networks on Role Expectations among African Immigrants Living with HIV
Reprinted from: *Int. J. Environ. Res. Public Health* **2024**, *21*, 782,
https://doi.org/10.3390/ijerph21060782 . . . . **151**

Wenbin Wang and Yang Cao
Network Diversity and Health Change among International Migrants in China: Evidence from Foreigners in Changchun
Reprinted from: *Int. J. Environ. Res. Public Health* **2022**, *19*, 16227,
https://doi.org/10.3390/ijerph192316227 . . . . **167**

Wentao Si, Chen Jiang and Lin Meng
Leaving the Homestead: Examining the Role of Relative Deprivation, Social Trust, and Urban Integration among Rural Farmers in China
Reprinted from: *Int. J. Environ. Res. Public Health* **2022**, *19*, 12658,
https://doi.org/10.3390/ijerph191912658 . . . . **183**

Chansophal Mak and Elizabeth Wieling
A Systematic Review of Evidence-Based Family Interventions for Trauma-Affected Refugees
Reprinted from: *Int. J. Environ. Res. Public Health* **2022**, *19*, 9361,
https://doi.org/10.3390/ijerph19159361 . . . . **211**

Carina Cione, Emma Vetter, Deziree Jackson, Sarah McCarthy and Ernesto Castañeda
The Implications of Health Disparities: A COVID-19 Risk Assessment of the Hispanic Community in El Paso
Reprinted from: *Int. J. Environ. Res. Public Health* **2023**, *20*, 975,
https://doi.org/10.3390/ijerph20020975 . . . . **229**

Mario Alberto Viveros Espinoza-Kulick
Movement Pandemic Adaptability: Health Inequity and Advocacy among Latinx Immigrant and Indigenous Peoples
Reprinted from: *Int. J. Environ. Res. Public Health* **2022**, *19*, 8981,
https://doi.org/10.3390/ijerph19158981 . . . . **249**

Norma Fuentes-Mayorga and Alfredo Cuecuecha Mendoza
The Most Vulnerable Hispanic Immigrants in New York City: Structural Racism and Gendered Differences in COVID-19 Deaths
Reprinted from: *Int. J. Environ. Res. Public Health* **2023**, *20*, 5838,
https://doi.org/10.3390/ijerph20105838 . . . . **259**

Daile Lynn Rung
COVID-19 and Policy-Induced Inequalities: Exploring How Social and Economic Exclusions Impact 'Temporary' Migrant Men's Health and Wellbeing in Australia
Reprinted from: *Int. J. Environ. Res. Public Health* **2023**, *20*, 6193,
https://doi.org/10.3390/ijerph20136193 . . . . **280**

Rebecca M. Crocker, Karina Duenas, Luis Vázquez, Maia Ingram, Felina M. Cordova-Marks, Emma Torres and Scott Carvajal
"Es Muy Tranquilo Aquí": Perceptions of Safety and Calm among Binationally Mobile Mexican Immigrants in a Rural Border Community
Reprinted from: *Int. J. Environ. Res. Public Health* **2022**, *19*, 8399,
https://doi.org/10.3390/ijerph19148399 . . . . **295**

Carlos Piñones-Rivera, Nanette Liberona, Rodrigo Arancibia and Verónica Jiménez
Indigenous Border Migrants and (Im)Mobility Policies in Chile in Times of COVID-19
Reprinted from: *Int. J. Environ. Res. Public Health* **2022**, *19*, 9728,
https://doi.org/10.3390/ijerph19159728 . . . . **311**

Laurie Cook Heffron, Karin Wachter and Esmeralda J. Rubalcava Hernandez
"Mi Corazón se Partió en Dos": Transnational Motherhood at the Intersection of Migration and Violence
Reprinted from: *Int. J. Environ. Res. Public Health* **2022**, *19*, 13404,
https://doi.org/10.3390/ijerph192013404 . . . . **329**

Andrés Scherman, Nicolle Etchegaray, Isabel Pavez and Daniela Grassau
The Influence of Media Coverage on the Negative Perception of Migrants in Chile
Reprinted from: *Int. J. Environ. Res. Public Health* **2022**, *19*, 8219,
https://doi.org/10.3390/ijerph19138219 . . . . **341**

About the Editors

Maria De Jesus

Dr. Maria De Jesus is a Professor in the Department of Environment, Development, and Health at the School of International Service, the Senior Associate Director of Community-Based Research and Engagement at the Center for Latin American and Latino Studies, and the Faculty Advisor for the M.A. Graduate Certificate in Global Migration at American University in Washington, DC. Her research examines the social determinants of health and the role of culturally responsive and strategic communication in addressing local and global health inequities. Dr. De Jesus' overarching goal is to generate knowledge that can inform health practice and policy, particularly for marginalized populations.

Dr. De Jesus has conducted extensive field research on immigrant health in Central America, Mexico, the U.S., and more recently in France. She collaborates with DC-based non-profit organizations to design research projects and interventions that resonate with the target audience and are tailored to the specific context. She has authored over 60 publications in prestigious journals such as *Global Public Health, AIDS and Behavior, Conflict and Health, Health Education & Behavior,* and *Social Science & Medicine*. Additionally, she contributes to broader public discussions through platforms like *The Conversation* and *The Global Post*. Her work has earned several grants from the National Institutes of Health (NIH), the Department of Health and Human Services, and the DC Center for AIDS Research. Dr. De Jesus is also the recipient of multiple fellowships, including a recent Fulbright U.S. Scholar Fellowship. She has served on several editorial boards, most recently on the *American Journal of Public Health*, and has been an invited guest speaker at numerous health conferences. At American University, she is affiliated with the Center on Health, Risk, and Society, the Metropolitan Policy Center, and the Antiracist Research and Policy Center.

Ernesto Castañeda

Dr. Ernesto Castañeda is Professor of Sociology, Director of the Center for Latin American and Latino Studies, and the Immigration Lab. His research focuses on immigration, borders, Latinx populations, social movements, and health disparities.

Dr. Castañeda is the author of several books, including *Immigration Realities: Challenging Common Misperceptions* (with Carina Cione, Columbia University Press, 2024), *Reunited: Family Reunification and Central American Youth Migration* (with Daniel Jenks, Russell Sage Foundation, 2024), *A Place to Call Home: Immigrant Belonging and Exclusion in New York, Paris, and Barcelona* (Stanford University Press, 2018), *Building Walls: The Exclusion of Latinx People in the U.S.* (Lexington Books, 2019), and *Social Movements 1768–2018* (with Charles Tilly and Lesley Wood, Routledge, 2020). He is also the editor of *Immigration and Categorical Inequality: Migration to the City and the Birth of Race and Ethnicity* (Routledge, 2018) and co-editor (with Cathy L. Schneider) of *Collective Violence, Contentious Politics, and Social Change: A Charles Tilly Reader* (Routledge, 2017). Dr. Castañeda's insights and commentary are frequently featured in public talks, policy discussions, and national and international media outlets.

Preface

The aim of this Reprint is to present empirical evidence, contextual insights, and critical analyses to examine the intersections between migration, migration status, and health and well-being. The authors featured in this issue are affiliated with universities in the United States, Mexico, Chile, Australia, France, Spain, and China. The intended audience spans a wide range of fields, including sociology, psychology, anthropology, geography, political science, international relations, medicine, public health, social work, and Latino and Latin American Studies. Its contributions enhance the understanding of the links between migration, migration status, and health, supporting efforts to advocate for policies and practices that uphold health as a fundamental human right for all. The editors would like to thank the numerous peer reviewers who provided valuable feedback and reviewed the revised versions of the papers submitted to this reprint. Special thanks also to Charlotte DuBois, M.A. student at the School of International Service, American University, for her editorial assistance.

Maria De Jesus and Ernesto Castañeda
Guest Editors

International Journal of
Environmental Research and Public Health

MDPI

Editorial

Social Contexts and Immigration Policies Directly Impact Immigrant Health

Maria De Jesus [1,2,*] and Ernesto Castañeda [1,2,3]

1 Department of Environment, Development, & Health, School of International Service, American University, Washington, DC 20016, USA
2 The Immigration Lab, Center for Latin American and Latino Studies, American University, Washington, DC 20016, USA
3 Department of Sociology, College of Arts and Sciences, American University, Washington, DC 20016, USA
* Correspondence: dejesus@american.edu

At the end of 2023, an estimated 117.3 million people worldwide were forcibly displaced due to persecution, conflict, violence, or human rights violations [1]. This figure translates to 1 in every 69 people worldwide being forcibly displaced or 1.4% of the global population [1]. The figure includes internally displaced persons (68.3 million), refugees under the mandate of the United Nations High Commissioner for Refugees (UNHCR) (31.6 million), asylum seekers (6.9 million), refugees under the mandate of the United Nations Relief and Works Agency for Palestine Refugees in the Near East (6 million), as well as others in need of international protection (5.8 million) [2]. Low- and middle-income countries hosted 75 per cent of the world's refugees and other people in need of international protection [2]. International migration continues to be a major driver of economic growth and a key contributor to these countries' GDPs [2,3].

Global shifts in migration patterns, climate change, rising health and social inequities, and environments that are marked by poverty and violence significantly affect the health of migrants. In these "contexts of vulnerability", migrants often face a range of physical and mental health challenges before, during, and after their migration [4–6]. They are also at heightened risk of isolation, exclusion, discrimination, and insecurity, all of which further harm their well-being [7]. Migrants in irregular or undocumented situations face even greater risks, including exploitation, trafficking, detention, and deportation [8,9]. When evaluating the health and well-being of migrants worldwide, it becomes evident how social determinants of health, social structures, and multi-sectoral policies play a central role [10,11].

The experience of migration and migration status are key social determinants of health and well-being, as they place individuals in circumstances that can significantly affect their health [11,12]. The conditions surrounding migration and its health impacts are shaped by a range of factors that differ across migrant groups and legal statuses [13–15]. The social determinants of health (SDH) framework, highlights the critical role of social, economic, and political factors, along with structural mechanisms, in influencing individual health behaviors and risks (Figure 1) [16].

Key SDHs include migration and migration status, quality childcare and education, employment status, gender equality, income, and access to adequate housing, nutritious foods, and healthcare [17]. The upstream and intermediary determinants help explain why there are differential risks for disease and health outcomes across populations [18,19]. They also create social stratification and health inequities based on migration status, income, education, class, gender, and race/ethnicity [17,20,21].

Received: 8 March 2025
Accepted: 21 March 2025
Published: 9 April 2025

Citation: De Jesus, M.; Castañeda, E. Social Contexts and Immigration Policies Directly Impact Immigrant Health. *Int. J. Environ. Res. Public Health* **2025**, *22*, 586. https://doi.org/10.3390/ijerph22040586

This Special Issue, titled "Migration and Migration Status as Key Determinants of Health", explores five key themes, which are outlined in detail below.

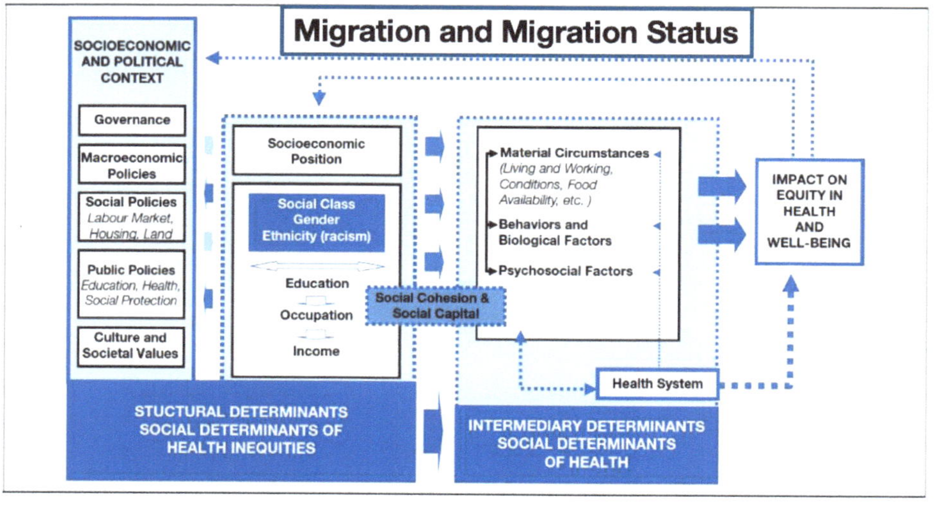

Figure 1. A conceptual framework for the social determinants of health. World Health Organization, 2010.

1. Migration, Mental Health, and Access to Care

The first set of articles share a common focus on how immigration-related stress, discrimination, and systemic barriers contribute to mental health challenges among migrant populations, while also highlighting the complexities of care access and the coping strategies that migrants use to navigate their experiences. In the article "Investigating the Potential Double-Edged Score of Immigration-Related Stress, Discrimination, and Mental Health Access", Andrews et al. explore how discrimination and immigration-related stress lead to post-traumatic stress disorder and depression among Latinx migrants and, in turn, also indirectly encourage help-seeking behaviors, especially for those dealing with trauma. Similarly, Espinoza-Kulick and Cerdeña elucidate the systemic barriers that Latinx migrants face in accessing mental health services in their article titled "We Need Health for All: Mental Health and Barriers to Care among Latinx in California and Connecticut". The authors elucidate the systemic barriers that Latinx migrants face in accessing mental health services. The authors emphasize the need for culturally competent mental health services that account for language barriers, gendered experiences, and the intersecting challenges of immigration status and socioeconomic insecurity.

In the article "Hoping for a Better Future during COVID-19: How Migration Plans are Protective of Depressive Symptoms for Haitian Migrants Living in Chile", Chen et al. demonstrate that Haitian migrants in Chile experienced high levels of depression, exacerbated by changes in migration plans due to the pandemic. Their study reveals that planning to leave Chile was a protective factor against Haitians' depressive symptoms, suggesting that hope and future aspirations can act as crucial coping mechanisms for migrants struggling with mental health, even in the face of discrimination and uncertainty. Similarly, De Jesus et al.'s article, "'Living in Confinement, Stopped in Time': Migrant Social Vulnerability, Coping and Health during the COVID-19 Pandemic Lockdown in France", examines the compounded health, protection, and socioeconomic crises faced by asylum seekers and undocumented migrants during the COVID-19 lockdown in France. The study reveals how lockdown measures exacerbated existing vulnerabilities and emphasizes the need for inclusive health policies that address the root causes of health inequities. The authors advocate for a holistic, migrant-inclusive approach to well-being.

Together, these articles illustrate the significant mental health challenges that are faced by migrants, including discrimination, trauma, and a lack of access to mental healthcare. They underscore the need for policies and services that address these barriers, foster resilience, and support mental health through both practical and emotional coping strategies, while also recognizing the critical role of hope and future planning in the mental well-being of migrant communities.

2. Migrant Integration and Resettlement: Challenges and Nuances

A second theme emerges around the challenges and nuances of migrant integration and resettlement, particularly the impacts of social connection, forming identity, and overcoming barriers to economic and social stability. In the article "Reskilled and Integrated, but How? Navigating Trauma and Temporary Hardships", Aydiner and Rider explore how highly educated Turkish migrants, forced to leave their home country due to political upheaval, face the complex task of transferring their professional credentials and re-establishing their economic status in the United States. While their economic situation eventually improves, the process of re-education and credential recognition remains time-consuming and challenging, affecting both their economic well-being and mental health. In the article titled "'Step by Step We Were Okay Now': An Exploration of the Impact of Social Connectedness on the Well-Being of Congolese and Iraqi Refugee Women Resettled in the United States", Bletscher and Spiers investigate the gendered impacts of resettlement on Congolese and Iraqi refugee women in the U.S. The study highlights how these women struggle with building social networks that provide essential resources and emotional support.

In their article "A Qualitative Study of Adolescents from Refugee Backgrounds Living in Australia: Identity and Resettlement", Khawaja and Schweitzer delve into the identity formation of refugee youth and the challenges of navigating adolescence while integrating into a new cultural environment in Australia. The study highlights the importance of fostering a sense of belonging and the role of school in helping these young people build resilience and a cohesive sense of self, despite the disruptions caused by displacement. In the article "Do Resettled People Adapt to their Current Geographical Environment? Evidence from Poverty-Stricken Areas of Northwest Yunnan Province, China", Qu et al. examine how resettled populations in China adapt to their new environments following poverty alleviation policies. The study finds that while resettlement improves living conditions, barriers to environmental adaptation and the risk of returning to poverty persist. The authors emphasize the need for policies focusing on employment, public services, and social safety nets to better support the long-term integration of resettled populations.

These articles underscore the multifaceted process of the integration and resettlement of migrants, with a focus on the significant challenges that migrants face in terms of economic stability, identity reconstruction, and adapting to new environments. A central takeaway is the critical role of supportive policies in fostering successful resettlement.

3. The Role of Social Networks and Connections in Shaping Migrants' Health and Well-Being

A common thread across the next set of articles is the importance of social networks and connections in shaping the experiences and well-being of migrants. These networks—whether familial, cultural, or community-based—play a significant role in helping migrants navigate challenges relating to identity, health, and integration. In Koku's article, "The Effect of Stigma and Social Networks on Role Expectations among African

Immigrants Living with HIV", we learn how African immigrants living with HIV use their social networks to negotiate stigma and role expectations. The author shows how these social networks, embedded in both home and host countries, influence health outcomes, identity reconstruction, and the ability to cope with migration stressors. Wang and Cao's article, "Network Diversity and Health Change among International Migrants in China: Evidence from Foreigners in Changchun", explores the dual social networks that migrants form—connections to both their home and host country.

In the article "Leaving the Homestead: Examining the Role of Relative Deprivation, Social Trust, and Urban Integration among Rural Farmers in China" by Si, Jiang, and Meng, the authors demonstrate how social networks influence rural-to-urban migration decisions. The authors underscore how social deprivation, economic hardship, and emotional isolation affect the willingness of rural farmers to leave their homesteads, with social trust acting as a crucial factor in this decision-making process. Lastly, in the article "A Systematic Review of Evidence-Based Family Interventions for Trauma-Affected Refugees", Mak and Wieling highlight the centrality of family connections for refugees from collectivistic cultures. The authors suggest that effective interventions for trauma-affected refugee families must take the relational and cultural dynamics within these family networks into account to improve mental health outcomes and ensure long-term well-being.

In summary, these articles demonstrate that social networks—whether family, cultural ties, or community connections—are essential for migrants' well-being. They help migrants cope with health challenges, navigate acculturation stress, and make critical decisions about their lives in both host and home countries. These networks also shape how migrants perceive their identity and role within society, influencing their health outcomes and integration into new environments.

4. The COVID-19 Pandemic: Migration, Health Inequities, and Structural Factors

The COVID-19 pandemic exacerbated existing health inequities among migrant populations, with structural and policy-driven factors significantly impacting their health outcomes. Across the next set of studies, an overarching theme is the disproportionate vulnerability of migrants to both the virus and its social and economic consequences, often compounded by exclusionary policies and systemic inequities. In the article "The Implications of Health Disparities: A COVID-19 Risk Assessment of the Hispanic Community in El Paso", Cione et al. explore how pre-existing inequities, such as high rates of chronic conditions and socioeconomic factors, made Hispanic communities in El Paso more susceptible to severe COVID-19 outcomes. The authors underscore the importance of addressing structural inequality to prevent future health crises and the importance of large-scale surveys, including the collection of social and health data, to have a baseline for evaluating the strengths, challenges, and vulnerabilities of a community's health.

In the article "Movement Pandemic Adaptability: Health Inequity and Advocacy among Latinx Immigrant and Indigenous Peoples", Viveros Espinoza-Kulick highlights how immigrant and Indigenous communities, despite facing systemic barriers such as immigration status and language challenges, have relied on mutual aid and advocacy networks to provide culturally relevant resources. The paper illustrates the importance of community solidarity in mitigating the impact of health inequities during the pandemic.

In the article "The Most Vulnerable Hispanic Immigrants in New York City: Structural Racism and Gendered Differences in COVID-19 Deaths", Fuentes-Mayorga and Cuecuecha Mendoza demonstrate how structural racism and gender disparities shaped the COVID-19 mortality rates among Hispanic immigrants. The study reveals how Hispanic men, especially those working in essential, high-risk jobs, faced higher mortality risks, while gendered experiences and spatial segregation further exacerbated the inequities. Similarly, in the article "COVID-19 and Policy-Induced Inequalities: Exploring How Social and Economic Exclusions Impact 'Temporary' Migrant Men's Health and Wellbeing in Australia", Rung examines how Australia's COVID-19 response policies, which excluded men who had migrated temporarily and their families from economic support, exacerbated the health and well-being challenges for this group. The study reveals the role of "sub-citizenship" status, where temporary migrants face heightened vulnerability to both the virus and the socioeconomic consequences of exclusionary policies.

These articles reveal how migration status, social exclusion, and structural racism intertwine to amplify the impact of the pandemic on migrant communities. They emphasize the urgent need for inclusive policies that address both health inequities and the socioeconomic vulnerabilities that migrants face, while also fostering community-led solutions for resilience.

5. Migrants and Experiences of Violence

A central theme across the next four studies is the complex and violent experiences that are faced by many migrants, shaped by both structural and interpersonal factors. Migrants navigate multiple layers of violence, from the physical dangers of crossing borders to the emotional and physical toll of separation and the psychological impact of hostile media narratives.

In the article by Crocker et al., titled "'Es Muy Tranquilo Aquí': Perceptions of Safety and Calm among Binationally Mobile Mexican Immigrants in a Rural Border Community", Mexican immigrants' perceptions of community safety are contrasted with the violence that they associate with conditions across the border. While some migrants feel safe in their rural communities, they remain deeply aware of the violence in neighboring regions, which informs their overall sense of security and health. In Piñones-Rivera et al.'s article "Indigenous Border Migrants and (Im)Mobility Policies in Chile in Times of COVID-19", the focus shifts to the structural violence that is embedded in immigration and healthcare policies. Indigenous migrants in Chile face violence not only from border closures and healthcare inaccessibility but also from criminalization by state actors. These migrants must navigate dangerous routes for basic healthcare, exposing them to exploitation and abuse.

In the article "'Mi Corazon se Partió en Dos': Transnational Motherhood at the Intersection of Migration and Violence", Cook Heffron, Wachter, and Rubalcava Hernandez delve into how gender-based violence affects Central American women's decisions to migrate, often forcing them to leave their children behind. The violence that they experience, from economic insecurity to sexual violence, shapes their understanding of motherhood and underscores the emotional costs of migration. In the article "The Influence of Media Coverage on the Negative Perception of Migrants in Chile", Scherman et al. demonstrate how the media's portrayal of migrants influences public opinion, fostering xenophobia and discrimination. Negative media coverage exacerbates the social violence that is experienced by migrants, turning public perception against them and heightening the risks that they face in their host country.

Together, these articles highlight how migrants face multiple forms of violence—physical, structural, emotional, and social. These experiences are compounded by migration policies and media portrayals that shape the environments in which migrants live, work, and raise families. The violence that they endure is not just a result of external threats but also deeply intertwined with the social and political systems which they navigate.

6. Conclusions

This volume underlines key themes at the intersections of health, migration, and migration status. Firstly, it examines the significant mental health challenges that are faced by migrants, particularly relating to discrimination, trauma, and limited access to care. Secondly, it underscores the multifaceted process of migrant integration, focusing on the substantial hurdles that migrants encounter in terms of economic stability, identity reconstruction, and adapting to their new environment. Thirdly, it demonstrates how social networks and connectedness influence migrants' perceptions of their identity and role within society, ultimately shaping their health outcomes and integration experiences. Fourthly, it reveals how migration status, social exclusion, and structural racism amplified the impact of the pandemic on migrant communities. Lastly, it explores how migrants' experiences with different forms of violence—physical, structural, emotional, and social—are further exacerbated by migration policies and media portrayals that influence their social contexts.

Migration and migration status are key determinants of health. The 2030 Sustainable Development Agenda, the Global Compact for Safe, Orderly, and Regular Migration and other international frameworks highlight the critical need to monitor health data at the migration–health nexus [22]. These initiatives are essential for tracking progress towards ensuring that no one is left behind, especially in achieving health-related goals and targets that promote equity for all, regardless of migration status. This work calls for a comprehensive, in-depth understanding of the social determinants of health that affect migrants, advocating for inclusive policies and practices that guarantee equitable access to healthcare and protection of migrants' rights, health, and well-being, regardless of their migration status.

Funding: This research received no external funding.

Acknowledgments: The Guest Editors would like to thank the numerous peer reviewers who provided valuable feedback and reviewed the revised versions of the papers that were submitted to this Special Issue.

Conflicts of Interest: The authors declare no conflicts of interest.

List of Contributions

1. Andrews, A.; Escobar, K.; Gonzalez, S.; Reyes, S.; Acosta, L. Investigating the Potential Double-Edged Score of Immigration-Related Stress, Discrimination, and Mental Health Access. *Int. J. Environ. Res. Public Health* **2024**, *21*, 373. https://doi.org/10.3390/ijerph21030373.
2. Espinoza-Kulick, M.; Cerdeña, J. "We Need Health for All": Mental Health and Barriers to Care among Latinxs in California and Connecticut. *Int. J. Environ. Res. Public Health* **2022**, *19*, 12817. https://doi.org/10.3390/ijerph191912817.
3. Chen, Y.; Rafful, C.; Mercado, M.; Carte, L.; Morales-Miranda, S.; Cheristil, J.; Rocha-Jiménez, T. Hoping for a Better Future during COVID-19: How Migration Plans Are Protective of Depressive Symptoms for Haitian Migrants Living in Chile. *Int. J. Environ. Res. Public Health* **2022**, *19*, 9977. https://doi.org/10.3390/ijerph19169977.
4. De Jesus, M.; Moumni, Z.; Sougui, Z.; Biswas, N.; Kubicz, R.; Pourtau, L. "Living in Confinement, Stopped in Time": Migrant Social Vulnerability, Coping and Health during the COVID-19 Pandemic Lockdown in France. *Int. J. Environ. Res. Public Health* **2022**, *19*, 10084. https://doi.org/10.3390/ijerph191610084.
5. Aydiner, C.; Rider, E. Reskilled and Integrated, but How? Navigating Trauma and Temporary Hardships. *Int. J. Environ. Res. Public Health* **2022**, *19*, 13675. https://doi.org/10.3390/ijerph192013675.

6. Bletscher, C.; Spiers, S. "Step by Step We Were Okay Now": An Exploration of the Impact of Social Connectedness on the Well-Being of Congolese and Iraqi Refugee Women Resettled in the United States. *Int. J. Environ. Res. Public Health* **2023**, *20*, 5324. https://doi.org/10.3390/ijerph20075324.
7. Khawaja, N.; Schweitzer, R. A Qualitative Study of Adolescents from Refugee Backgrounds Living in Australia: Identity and Resettlement. *Int. J. Environ. Res. Public Health* **2024**, *21*, 281. https://doi.org/10.3390/ijerph21030281.
8. Qu, L.; Xiao, W.; Gao, W. Do Resettled People Adapt to Their Current Geographical Environment? Evidence from Poverty-Stricken Areas of Northwest Yunnan Province, China. *Int. J. Environ. Res. Public Health* **2023**, *20*, 193. https://doi.org/10.3390/ijerph20010193.
9. Koku, E. The Effect of Stigma and Social Networks on Role Expectations among African Immigrants Living with HIV. *Int. J. Environ. Res. Public Health* **2024**, *21*, 782. https://doi.org/10.3390/ijerph21060782.
10. Wang, W.; Cao, Y. Network Diversity and Health Change among International Migrants in China: Evidence from Foreigners in Changchun. *Int. J. Environ. Res. Public Health* **2022**, *19*, 16227. https://doi.org/10.3390/ijerph192316227.
11. Si, W.; Jiang, C.; Meng, L. Leaving the Homestead: Examining the Role of Relative Deprivation, Social Trust, and Urban Integration among Rural Farmers in China. *Int. J. Environ. Res. Public Health* **2022**, *19*, 12658. https://doi.org/10.3390/ijerph191912658.
12. Mak, C.; Wieling, E. A Systematic Review of Evidence-Based Family Interventions for Trauma-Affected Refugees. *Int. J. Environ. Res. Public Health* **2022**, *19*, 9361. https://doi.org/10.3390/ijerph19159361.
13. Cione, C.; Vetter, E.; Jackson, D.; McCarthy, S.; Castañeda, E. The Implications of Health Disparities: A COVID-19 Risk Assessment of the Hispanic Community in El Paso. *Int. J. Environ. Res. Public Health* **2023**, *20*, 975. https://doi.org/10.3390/ijerph20020975.
14. Espinoza-Kulick, M. Movement Pandemic Adaptability: Health Inequity and Advocacy among Latinx Immigrant and Indigenous Peoples. *Int. J. Environ. Res. Public Health* **2022**, *19*, 8981. https://doi.org/10.3390/ijerph19158981.
15. Fuentes-Mayorga, N.; Cuecuecha Mendoza, A. The Most Vulnerable Hispanic Immigrants in New York City: Structural Racism and Gendered Differences in COVID-19 Deaths. *Int. J. Environ. Res. Public Health* **2023**, *20*, 5838. https://doi.org/10.3390/ijerph20105838.
16. Rung, D. COVID-19 and Policy-Induced Inequalities: Exploring How Social and Economic Exclusions Impact 'Temporary' Migrant Men's Health and Wellbeing in Australia. *Int. J. Environ. Res. Public Health* **2023**, *20*, 6193. https://doi.org/10.3390/ijerph20136193.
17. Crocker, R.; Duenas, K.; Vázquez, L.; Ingram, M.; Cordova-Marks, F.; Torres, E.; Carvajal, S. "Es Muy Tranquilo Aquí": Perceptions of Safety and Calm among Binationally Mobile Mexican Immigrants in a Rural Border Community. *Int. J. Environ. Res. Public Health* **2022**, *19*, 8399. https://doi.org/10.3390/ijerph19148399.
18. Piñones-Rivera, C.; Liberona, N.; Arancibia, R.; Jiménez, V. Indigenous Border Migrants and (Im)Mobility Policies in Chile in Times of COVID-19. *Int. J. Environ. Res. Public Health* **2022**, *19*, 9728. https://doi.org/10.3390/ijerph19159728.
19. Cook Heffron, L.; Wachter, K.; Rubalcava Hernandez, E. "Mi Corazón se Partió en Dos": Transnational Motherhood at the Intersection of Migration and Violence. *Int. J. Environ. Res. Public Health* **2022**, *19*, 13404. https://doi.org/10.3390/ijerph192013404.
20. Scherman, A.; Etchegaray, N.; Pavez, I.; Grassau, D. The Influence of Media Coverage on the Negative Perception of Migrants in Chile. *Int. J. Environ. Res. Public Health* **2022**, *19*, 8219. https://doi.org/10.3390/ijerph19138219.

References

1. UNHCR. Global Trends Forced Displacement in 2023. United Nations High Commission for Refugees. 2023. Available online: https://www.unhcr.org/sites/default/files/2024-06/global-trends-report-2023.pdf (accessed on 28 July 2024).
2. World Migration Report 2024 Reveals Latest Global Trends and Challenges in Human Mobility. World Migration Report. 7 May 2024. Available online: https://worldmigrationreport.iom.int/news/world-migration-report-2024-reveals-latest-global-trends-and-challenges-human-mobility (accessed on 29 December 2024).

3. Castañeda, E.; Aguilar, E.; Turkington, N. *Migration as a Driver of Economic Growth: Increasing Productivity and Filling the Labor Gaps*; Working Paper Series #47; Immigration Lab: Washington, DC, USA; CLALS: Washington, DC, USA, 2024.
4. Voglino, G.; Gualano, M.R.; Moro, G.L.; Forghieri, P.; Caprioli, M.; Elhadidy, H.S.M.A.; Bert, F.; Siliquini, R. Mental health and discrimination among migrants from Africa: An Italian cross-sectional study. *J. Community Psychol.* **2022**, *50*, 601–619. [CrossRef] [PubMed]
5. Nwankwo, E.M.; Govia, I.O. Migration and the Health of Non-migrant Family: Findings from the Jamaica Return(ed) Migrants Study. *J. Immigr. Minor. Health* **2022**, *24*, 689–704. [CrossRef] [PubMed]
6. De Jesus, M.; Ramachandra, S.S.; Jafflin, Z.; Maliti, I.; Daughtery, A.; Shapiro, B.; Howell, W.C.; Jackson, M.C. The environmental and social determinants of health matter in a pandemic: Predictors of covid-19 case and death rates in New York city. *Int. J. Environ. Res. Public Health* **2021**, *18*, 8416. [CrossRef] [PubMed]
7. Castañeda, E. *A Place to Call Home: Immigrant Exclusion and Urban Belonging in New York, Paris, and Barcelona/Ernesto Castañeda*, 1st ed.; Stanford University Press: Redwood City, CA, USA, 2018. [CrossRef]
8. Gimeno-Feliu, L.A.; Pastor-Sanz, M.; Poblador-Plou, B.; Calderón-Larrañaga, A.; Díaz, E.; Prados-Torres, A. Multimorbidity and chronic diseases among undocumented migrants: Evidence to contradict the myths. *Int. J. Equity Health* **2020**, *19*, 113. [CrossRef] [PubMed]
9. Nørredam, M. Migration and health: Exploring the role of migrant status through register-based studies. *Dan. Med. J.* **2015**, *62*, B5068. [PubMed]
10. Marmot, M.; Weil, A.R. Tackling social determinants of health around the globe. *Health Aff.* **2020**, *39*, 1118–1121. [CrossRef]
11. Rami, F.; Searight, H.R.; Morrissey, M.B.; Charvonia, A.; Indart, M.; Brown, L.M.; Holden, K.; Miller, G.E.; Alegría, M.; Wilton, L.; et al. Health Inequities and Social Determinants of Health in Refugee and ImMigrant Communities. *Am. Psychol.* **2023**, *78*, 160–172. [CrossRef] [PubMed]
12. Baah, F.O.; Teitelman, A.M.; Riegel, B. Marginalization: Conceptualizing patient vulnerabilities in the framework of social determinants of health—An integrative review. *Nurs. Inq.* **2019**, *26*, e12268. [CrossRef] [PubMed]
13. Brown, T.H.; Homan, P. The Future of Social Determinants of Health: Looking Upstream to Structural Drivers. *Milbank Q.* **2023**, *101* (Suppl. S1), 36–60. [CrossRef] [PubMed]
14. Wiedmeyer, M.-L.; Goldenberg, S.; Peterson, S.; Wanigaratne, S.; Machado, S.; Tayyar, E.; Braschel, M.; Carrillo, R.; Sierra-Heredia, C.; Tuyisenge, G.; et al. SARS-CoV-2 testing and COVID-19–related primary care use among people with citizenship, permanent residency, and temporary immigration status: An analysis of population-based administrative data in British Columbia. *Can. J. Public Health* **2023**, *114*, 389–403. [CrossRef] [PubMed]
15. Hill, J.; Rodriguez, D.X.; McDaniel, P.N. Immigration status as a health care barrier in the USA during COVID-19. *J. Migr. Health* **2021**, *4*, 100036. [CrossRef]
16. Solar, O.; Irwin, A. A Conceptual Framework for Action on the Social Determinants of Health. In *Social Determinants of Health Discussion Paper 2: Policy and Practice*; World Health Organization: Geneva, Switzerland, 2010.
17. World Health Organization (WHO); Commission on Social Determinants of Health. *Closing the Gap in a Generation: Health Equity Through Action on the Social Determinants of Health: Final Report of the Commission on Social Determinants of Health*; World Health Organization: Geneva, Switzerland, 2008.
18. De Jesus, M.; Williams, D.R. The Care and Prevention in the United States Demonstration Project: A call for more focus on the social determinants of HIV/AIDS. *Public Health Rep.* **2018**, *133* (Suppl. S2), 28S–33S. [CrossRef] [PubMed]
19. Williams, D.R.; Mohammed, S.A.; Leavell, J.; Collins, C. Race, socioeconomic status, and health: Complexities, ongoing challenges, and research opportunities. *Ann. N. Y. Acad. Sci.* **2010**, *1186*, 69–101. [CrossRef] [PubMed]
20. Asad, A.L.; Clair, M. Racialized legal status as a social determinant of health. *Soc. Sci. Med.* **2018**, *199*, 19–28. [CrossRef] [PubMed]
21. Braveman, P.A.; Kumanyika, S.; Fielding, J.; LaVeist, T.; Borrell, L.N.; Manderscheid, R.; Troutman, A. Health disparities and health equity: The issue is justice. *Am. J. Public Health* **2011**, *101*, S149–S155. [CrossRef] [PubMed]
22. NAM Annual Report 2022. National Academy of Medicine. 2022. Available online: https://nam.edu/wp-content/uploads/2023/06/NAM-Annual-Report-2022.pdf (accessed on 10 November 2024).

International Journal of
Environmental Research and Public Health

MDPI

Article

Investigating the Potential Double-Edged Score of Immigration-Related Stress, Discrimination, and Mental Health Access

Arthur R. Andrews [1,2,*], Kevin Escobar [1], Sandra Mariely Estrada Gonzalez [3], Sara Reyes [1] and Laura M. Acosta [1]

1 Department of Psychology, University of Nebraska-Lincoln, Lincoln, NE 68588, USA; kescobar2@huskers.unl.edu (K.E.); laura.acosta@huskers.unl.edu (L.M.A.)
2 Institute for Ethnic Studies, University of Nebraska-Lincoln, Lincoln, NE 68588, USA
3 Department of Psychological Science, University of Texas, Rio Grande Valley, Edinburg, TX 78539, USA
* Correspondence: arthur.andrews@unl.edu

Abstract: Prior work has suggested that discrimination and immigration-related stress may impede mental health care seeking and utilization among Latinx populations. These effects may be more nuanced as both discrimination and immigration-related stress may increase symptomology, particularly post-traumatic stress disorder (PTSD) and depression. Both symptoms may, in turn, prompt attempts to seek care. The current study examined the direct effects of discrimination and immigration-related stress on care access, as well as potentially indirect effects with PTSD and depression symptoms as mediators. Interviews and online surveys were completed with 234 Latinx residents of the Midwest, assessing everyday discrimination, discrimination in healthcare, PTSD symptoms, depression symptoms, current mental health utilization, and previous unsuccessful attempts to seek care. Direct effects of discrimination and immigration-related stress were largely unrelated to care access variables. Discrimination in healthcare settings predicted both unsuccessful attempts to seek care and current use, but this effect was positive. The indirect effect was largely supported, but only for PTSD symptoms and not depression. Results indicate that further investigation is necessary to understand the direct effects of discrimination on care access. Further, discrimination and immigration-related stress may indirectly prompt attempts to seek mental health care.

Keywords: discrimination; immigration stress; depression; PTSD; care access

Citation: Andrews, A.R.; Escobar, K.; Gonzalez, S.M.E.; Reyes, S.; Acosta, L.M. Investigating the Potential Double-Edged Score of Immigration-Related Stress, Discrimination, and Mental Health Access. *Int. J. Environ. Res. Public Health* **2024**, *21*, 373. https://doi.org/10.3390/ijerph21030373

Academic Editors: Maria De Jesus and Ernesto Castañeda

Received: 30 January 2024
Revised: 28 February 2024
Accepted: 12 March 2024
Published: 20 March 2024

1. Investigating the Potential Double-Edged Score of Immigration-Related Stress, Discrimination, and Mental Health Access

Discrimination and immigration-related stress appear to increase mental health symptomology across multiple domains, including depression and PTSD symptoms [1–4]. Despite the increase in symptomology and the potential need for services, both discrimination and immigration-related stress may increase the avoidance of healthcare systems for Latinx populations, especially immigrants and those close to them [5,6]. Based on healthcare utilization models, like the Health Belief Model [7,8], this may place many Latinx populations in a double bind wherein discrimination and immigration-related stress prompt greater need for care but also impede access to that care. The current study will investigate these compounding relationships based on the Health Belief Model in a predominantly immigrant sample of Latinx residents in the Midwest. It also extends prior work as most research examining the effects of discrimination on mental health symptoms, PTSD in particular, focus on African American/Black populations [9,10].

2. The Health Belief Model and the Potential Roles of Discrimination and Immigration Stress

The Health Belief Model is a theoretical model outlining the factors that prompt health behavior change [7]. Much of the Health Belief Model research has focused specifically on healthcare utilization [11,12]. The model overall outlines six factors as necessary for healthcare utilization: (1) perceived susceptibility, (2) perceived severity, (3) perceived benefits, (4) perceived barriers, (5) cue to action, and (6) self-efficacy [7]. According to this model, only perceived barriers would impede attempts to care, while each of the other five would increase care-seeking behaviors. In a mental health utilization context, perceived benefits are defined as including the perceived benefits of seeking treatment and of treatment itself [11]. Said differently, this is the perception that available/accessible treatment will be effective in addressing symptoms. Relatedly, self-efficacy, in this case, would include the perceived ability to access treatment and perform the tasks involved during treatment. Multiple investigations have supported the Health Belief Model in predicting mental health service utilization [13–15]. In particular, these studies often find that perceived benefits to treatment are the strongest predictor of seeking mental health services and that perceived barriers may work in conjunction with perceived benefits (e.g., perceived barriers moderate the effect of perceived benefits) [13–15].

As outlined in more detail elsewhere [16], discrimination may diminish the perceived effectiveness of services and increase perceived barriers to care by increasing the social cost of care. This applies to both discrimination in general, given the lack of representation in healthcare, and discrimination in healthcare settings specifically. Immigration-related stress may operate in a similar fashion in that many factors involved in immigration-related stress may increase multiple perceived barriers, including financial and social costs [5]. From the prior literature, these costs may include fear of deportation and fear of unfair treatment in healthcare settings [5,17]. Both fear of deportation and fear of unfair treatment in healthcare due to immigration status may prompt avoidance of mental health utilization [17]. Although much of this literature has focused on undocumented immigrants, such fear may extend to other Latinx immigrants and those close to them (e.g., fear of deportation of a loved one) [18–20]. Further, due to assumptions surrounding immigration status, many Latinxs born in the U.S. may also experience several immigration-related stressors [18]. Further, the effects of immigration-related stress have less often been examined quantitatively and not within the context of the Health Belief Model.

In contrast to immigration-related stress and discrimination, symptom recognition for both PTSD and depression is, by definition, a necessary component of perceived severity, which would be posited to increase utilization. Thus, self-reporting of symptoms is a direct indicator of perceived severity. Taken together with the extant literature on the effects of discrimination on depression and PTSD [3,9,21–23], this suggests that these symptoms may, therefore, operate as potential mediators of a positive indirect effect of discrimination on seeking mental health care. To date, the potential indirect effect is not well-established. Thus, testing this indirect effect among Latinx populations would represent a novel addition to the research literature and potentially add nuance regarding the conflicting roles of discrimination on care access.

Though examined less frequently, immigration-related stress may operate similarly. Prior work has indicated that immigration-related stress is associated with higher depression symptoms [1,4]. Immigration-related stress may also exacerbate PTSD symptoms, though this has been examined less frequently. Theoretically, immigration-related stress may exacerbate symptoms such as hypervigilance, avoidance, and hyperarousal for Latinx immigrants and those around them. This may result from persistent fears of deportation or challenges fulfilling essential life functions because of immigration status (e.g., transportation because of fear of police interactions).

3. Purpose

The current study sought to quantitatively examine the potential dual roles of discrimination and immigration-related on mental health care seeking. This represents a novel step in examining the potential indirect effects of discrimination and immigration-related stress on mental health care seeking. This is an important step, given prior work indicating that discrimination and immigration-related stress may impede care seeking. Thus, taken together, both discrimination and immigration-related stress may produce conflicting direct and indirect effects on care seeking. To test these hypotheses, the study first examined the direct effects of both factors in potentially reducing care seeking and, subsequently, care utilization. Second, it examined the indirect effects of both factors, with PTSD and depression symptoms as potential mediators. It was hypothesized that both discrimination and immigration-related stress would have negative direct effects on mental health care seeking and care utilization. It was further hypothesized that both discrimination and immigration-related stress would evidence positive indirect effects on care seeking and care utilization with PTSD and depression symptoms as mediators. Specifically, discrimination and immigration-related stress would have positive direct effects on depression and PTSD symptoms. Depression and PTSD symptoms would, in turn, have positive direct effects on care seeking and care utilization.

4. Materials and Methods

4.1. Participants

Participants were 234 Latinx residents of the Midwest from cities and towns of population sizes ranging from approximately 5000 to approximately 300,000. The majority were born outside the U.S. (n = 197; 87.2%) and were cisgender women (n = 165; 70.2%). The largest proportion of participants were born in Mexico (n = 91; 38.7%), followed by Cuba (n = 37; 15.7%), Guatemala (n = 25; 10.1%), Honduras (n = 14; 5.9%), and Colombia (n = 10; 4.2%). Fewer than 10 participants were born in El Salvador, Ecuador, Peru, Venezuela, Nicaragua, and Argentina. The average age was 42.52 years. The majority of participants indicated they completed a high school degree or more (n = 178; 78.1%). Additional background information can be found in Table 1.

Table 1. Demographic and descriptive information.

	n (%)
Gender	
Cisgender women	165 (70.2)
Cisgender men	65 (27.7)
Transgender men	1 (0.4)
Born outside the U.S.	197 (83.8)
Mexico	91 (38.7)
Caribbean	39 (16.6)
Central America	45 (19.1)
South America	23 (9.8)
Education	
Less than high school	50 (21.3)
Completed high school	86 (36.6)
Some college or higher	92 (39.1)
Unsuccessfully sought mental health care	21 (8.9)
Currently receiving care (yes)	21 (8.9)

Table 1. *Cont.*

	n (%)	
	M (SD)	Min-Max
Age	42.52 (14.21)	19–82
Annual household income (in USD)	42,596 (33,963)	0–200,000
PHQ-8 (depression symptoms)	7.12 (5.50)	0–24
Abbreviated PCL-5 (PTSD symptoms)	2.41 (3.11)	0–14
Everyday discrimination	5.26 (4.88)	0–20
Discrimination in healthcare	12.09 (2.98)	4–20
Immigration-related stress	38.15 (9.21)	16–58

4.2. Procedure

Participants were recruited separately through phone and internet surveys. For the phone surveys, participants were recruited through multiple local community agencies that served Latinx populations. Participants were also recruited via respondent-driven sampling, in which existing participants were offered incentives for recruiting additional participants (USD 10 gift card for each participant recruited). Prior participants were not informed as to who completed the survey to preserve the confidentiality of participation. Recruitment for the phone survey occurred from November 2020 to August 2021. Recruitment for the internet survey occurred through a university extension agency, which provides education and resources to the local community. Recruitment for the internet wave occurred from January to April 2022. In both cases, surveys were completed as a larger study focusing on COVID-19, stress exposure, mental health, and healthcare access. In both internet and phone surveys, participants were able to complete the study in either English or Spanish. These procedures were approved by the Institutional Review Board (IRB) at the University of Nebraska-Lincoln

4.3. Measures

4.3.1. Discrimination

Discrimination was measured using two questionnaires. The six-item Everyday Discrimination Scale (EDS) [24] was used to measure general experiences of discrimination in multiple contexts, and the seven-item Discrimination in Medical Settings Scale (DMS) [25] was derived from the EDS such that it represents a context-specific version of the EDS [25]. Both scales have demonstrated good internal consistency and concurrent validity [24–27]. Both have also been used to measure experiences of discrimination in Latinx samples [24]. The EDS demonstrated good internal consistency in the current sample (Cronbach's $\alpha = 0.96$), as did the DMS (Cronbach's $\alpha = 0.94$).

4.3.2. Immigration-Related Stress

Immigration-related stress was measured using the five-item Lack of Legal Immigrant Status subscale from the Stress of Immigration Survey [28]. Only this subscale was used due to brevity. Items assess common fears related to precarious immigration status for the participant, with multiple items also referencing difficulties for family members. Items ask participants "how much stress or worry (they) have experienced" as a result of the fear that they or a family may be deported, not having the correct documents when accessing services, not having a license to drive, difficulties accessing healthcare for the participant or family because of documentation, and difficulties returning to visit their home country. As such, many of these items apply to undocumented and documented immigrants and their families. The scale evidenced strong internal consistency in the current sample (Cronbach's $\alpha = 0.95$).

4.3.3. Post-Traumatic Stress Disorder (PTSD)

PTSD was measured using an abbreviated version of the PTSD Checklist for DSM-5 [29]. The PCL-5 assesses symptoms of PTSD taken directly from the DSM-5 diagnosis and asks participants to rate their frequency from "not at all" (0) to "extremely" (4). The PCL-5 has demonstrated good internal consistency [29]. A Spanish language version has also evidenced good internal consistency with Mexican and Central American samples [30,31]. An abbreviated version was used to accommodate requests for brief surveys from recruitment partners and to minimize the study burden. Five items were initially included (Item B1-Intrusive thoughts, Item B4-Emotional Cue Reactivity, Item C1-Avoidance of external reminders, Item E1-Irritability or anger, and Item E4-Easily startled). However, confirmatory factor analyses indicated that Item E4 had only a moderate loading onto a single item factor ($\lambda = 0.49$), and removing it yielded a good model fit across most indicators, χ^2 (2) = 0.32, CFI = 1.00, RMSEA < 0.001 (90% CI = <0.01–0.07), and SRMR = 0.01. Thus, only four items (B1, B4, C1, and E1) were included in the present analyses.

4.3.4. Depression

Depression symptoms were assessed using a modified version of the nine-item patient health questionnaire (PHQ-9). The PHQ-9 is among the most widely used measures of depression, including in several large international studies of depression [32–35]. The PHQ-9 typically contains nine items, but the final item regarding suicidality was removed so that the study could be more readily administered in an online context. This modification has been used in prior studies where the measure still demonstrates strong internal consistency and concurrent reliability [36]. The Spanish translation of the PHQ-9 has also demonstrated good internal consistency and concurrent validity [34,35]. The eight-item version demonstrated good internal consistency in this sample (Cronbach's $\alpha = 0.91$).

4.3.5. Mental Health Access

Mental health access was measured using two items. The first asked participants if they had sought services since the COVID-19 pandemic began but were unable to receive them. The second asked if participants were currently receiving services. These two items, therefore, represent unsuccessful attempts to receive care and current mental health use, respectively. Participants answered either "yes" or "no", which were then dichotomously coded as "1" and "0", respectively. As part of exploratory follow-up questions, participants who indicated they had been unable to receive services were asked to identify barriers that prevented them from receiving care.

4.3.6. Demographics

Participants also completed items regarding gender, age, U.S. nativity/country of origin, and education.

4.4. Data Analyses

Study hypotheses were tested using two separate path models in which depression and PTSD symptomology were examined as mediators between experiences of discrimination (model 1)/immigration stress (model 2) and the two mental health utilization variables. These models are depicted in Figures 1 and 2, respectively. To test specific hypotheses, the direct effects of discrimination/immigration stress variables on both PTSD and depression were examined, as were the direct effects of PTSD and depression on both mental healthcare access variables and the constituent indirect effects. Additionally, the direct effects of discrimination variables on mental healthcare access variables were also tested. Age, gender, and education were included as covariates in the model. Significance for all effects, including indirect effects, was examined using bootstrapped confidence intervals with 500 sample draws. Because the model includes two dichotomous variables as outcomes and a mediational structure, the Monte Carlo integration was used, and frequently used model fit indices (e.g., CFI) are not available. However, the mediational models were compared against simpler models using log likelihood ratio tests. Specifically, it was compared against two models with no mediational paths in which symptomology was either only outcomes (with only discrimination as predictors) or only predictors (with only healthcare access variables as outcomes. The mediational model was not significantly different from either of the two simpler models (p-values > 0.05). Thus, given the specific hypotheses regarding the indirect role of symptomology, the mediational model was retained and included here.

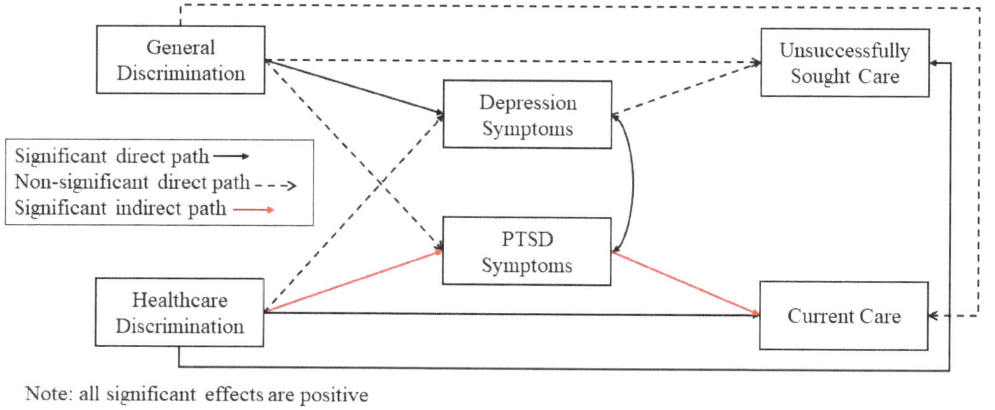

Figure 1. Path model of direct and indirect effects of discrimination on mental health access.

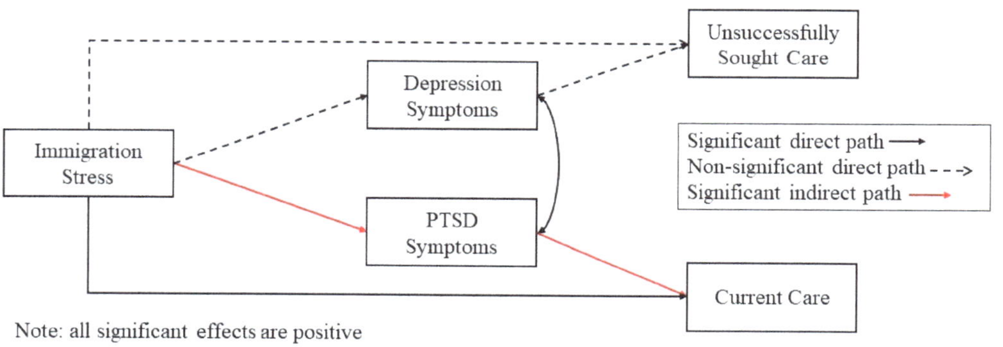

Figure 2. Path model of direct and indirect effects of immigration stress on mental health access.

Prior to completing analyses, analytic assumptions and missing data were assessed. Only items from the EDS evidenced significant missingness (>10% missing). All missing data were estimated using full information maximum likelihood estimation, which has been associated with reduced bias relative to other methods [37]. All other analytic assumptions were met.

5. Results

5.1. Discrimination as a Predictor of PTSD and Depression

In the discrimination model, discrimination in healthcare settings was positively associated with PTSD symptoms, $b = 0.15$, 95% CI = 0.07, 0.25, but was not associated with depression symptoms, $b = 0.10$, 95% CI = −0.01, 0.23. General experiences of discrimination were negatively associated with depression, $b = -0.32$, 95% CI = −0.38, −0.26, but were not associated with PTSD symptoms, $b = -0.03$, 95% CI = −0.08, 0.02. No other variable was associated with depression (i.e., all other confidence intervals included zero). Gender was associated with PTSD symptoms, such that women reported more symptoms than men, $b = 1.23$, 95% CI = 0.28, 2.23. No other variable was associated with PTSD symptoms (i.e., all other confidence intervals included zero). Additional statistical information can be found in Table 2.

Table 2. Predictors of mental health access variables.

Predictor	Dependent Variables	
	Unsuccessfully Seeking Care	Current Care Utilization
	aOR	aOR
Gender	0.85	0.77
Age	0.78	1.10
Everyday discrimination	1.00	1.01
Healthcare discrimination	1.11 *	1.09 *
Depression symptoms (PHQ-8)	0.97	1.08
PTSD symptoms (PCL)	1.16 *	1.18 *
Immigration-related stress	1.03	0.99

Note: * Significance determined using bootstrapped confidence intervals of regression coefficients.

5.2. Immigration Stress as a Predictor of PTSD and Depression

In the immigration stress model, immigration stress positively predicted PTSD symptoms, $b = 0.12$, 95% CI = 0.05, 0.18, but was not associated with depression symptoms, $b = 0.004$, 95% CI = −0.10, 0.10.

5.3. Direct Effects on Mental Health Access Variables

PTSD and Depression Symptoms as Predictors

In the discrimination model, PTSD symptoms were positively associated with having unsuccessfully sought mental health services, aOR = 1.18, $b = 0.16$, 95% CI = 0.03, 0.38, but depression symptoms were not significantly associated with having unsuccessfully sought services, $b = -0.03$, 95% CI = −0.18, 0.09. PTSD symptoms were also positively associated with currently receiving care, aOR = 1.16, $b = 0.15$, 95% CI = 0.01, 0.34. Depression symptoms were not significantly associated with currently receiving mental health services, $b = 0.08$, 95% CI = −0.06, 0.23. These results did not significantly differ in the immigration stress model.

5.4. Discrimination Variables as Predictors of Access Variables

General discrimination was not associated with either unsuccessfully seeking or currently receiving mental health services (confidence intervals include zero). Discrimination in healthcare settings was positively associated with currently receiving mental health services, aOR = 1.11, $b = 0.10$, 95% CI = 0.04, 0.21. Discrimination in healthcare settings was not associated with unsuccessfully seeking mental health services, aOR = 1.09, $b = 0.09$, 95% CI = −0.004, 0.19.

5.5. Immigration Stress as a Predictor of Access Variables

Immigration stress did not predict either currently receiving, aOR = 0.99, $b = -0.01$, 95% CI = −0.08, 0.06, or unsuccessfully seeking mental health services, aOR = 1.03, $b = 0.03$, 95% CI = −0.03, 0.10.

5.6. Indirect Effects with Symptomology as Mediators

Because the direct effects of discrimination on PTSD and PTSD on both mental health service access variables were significant, their resulting indirect effects were tested. A similar pattern was also observed for immigration stress with resulting indirect effects. The indirect effect of discrimination on unsuccessfully seeking care with PTSD as a mediator was significant and positive, $b = 0.02$, 95% CI = 0.01, 0.07. The indirect effect of discrimination on currently receiving care with PTSD as a mediator was also significant and positive, $b = 0.02$, 95% CI = 0.001, 0.05. The indirect effect of immigration stress on unsuccessfully seeking care with PTSD as a mediator was also significant, $b = 0.11$, 95% CI = 0.04, 0.19. The indirect effect on currently receiving care was also significant, $b = 0.09$, 95% CI = 0.02, 0.18.

6. Discussion

The current study examined the potential double-edged sword of discrimination and immigration-related stress. Specifically, the study examined the potential for two opposing effects of discrimination and immigration-related stress on care access: a direct pathway with a lower likelihood of seeking care and an indirect pathway with symptoms as a mediator and a greater likelihood of seeking care. Results testing these hypotheses were mixed. Specifically, general discrimination was only associated with depression symptoms but not PTSD. Conversely, healthcare discrimination and immigration stress were only associated with PTSD, but not depression. Further, discrimination in healthcare settings was associated with currently receiving care, but in the opposite direction than was anticipated. In fact, experiencing discrimination in healthcare settings was associated with *higher* odds of currently receiving care. General discrimination and immigration-related stress were not directly associated with either help-seeking variable.

These results provide novel data supporting only the indirect pathway of discrimination and immigration stress being associated with seeking or receiving mental health services. That is, both immigration-related stress and discrimination were associated with a *greater* likelihood of both attempting to receive care and successfully obtaining it. Further, these effects only occurred via PTSD symptoms and not depression. This fits with other research indicating that experiences of discrimination may uniquely predict PTSD symptoms [9]. However, it differs from prior work in that only discrimination in healthcare settings, but not more broadly, predicted PTSD. It is unclear why general discrimination was not associated with PTSD. It is also unclear why immigration stress was only associated with PTSD. It may be that immigration stress results in significant anxiety and avoidance, specifically.

Other novel findings include that only PTSD and not depression predicted care seeking and access among this Latinx sample. The fact that only PTSD consistently predicted care seeking or access may be explained in multiple ways. First, PTSD may not be treated as successfully as depression, as prior work indicates that those with PTSD often do not receive adequate care, and Latinx populations often experience greater disparities [38]. Thus, depression and PTSD may both prompt service access, but depression may be successfully treated and thus not associated with receiving care. Alternatively, these results may reflect the difficulty in treating PTSD and/or the lack of access to appropriate care for PTSD. This, however, does not explain results in which depression did not predict unsuccessfully seeking care as unsuccessfully seeking care would not be presumed to result in symptom improvement, and depression symptoms would be expected to still correlate with attempts to seek care. Better explaining this pattern of results and linking to the Health Belief Model, depression may result in both greater perceived symptom severity and lower perceived effectiveness of treatment. In other words, they may recognize the symptoms as problematic, which should prompt greater help seeking, but not have confidence that treatment will improve these symptoms, which would prompt less help seeking according to the Health Belief Model. These novel insights regarding the different help-seeking effects of depression and PTSD offer fruitful avenues for future inquiry based on the Health Belief Model.

In addition to novel findings with the indirect effects of discrimination and immigration-related stress via PTSD, the current study did not support the direct effects of discrimination and immigration-related stress on care seeking. In fact, discrimination in healthcare settings was associated with a higher likelihood of having sought care. This directly conflicts with the Health Belief Model, especially given that discrimination in healthcare was associated with greater care access and seeking. One potential reason for the positive effect of healthcare discrimination on currently receiving care may be related to the cross-sectional nature of this study. Specifically, contact with the mental healthcare system or other referring healthcare systems may produce experiences of discrimination. Thus, those who access care may also be more likely to experience discrimination, which may, in turn, lead to worse PTSD symptomology. Longitudinal research is needed to explicate these relations fully. However, the pattern from the current cross-sectional data may reflect an underlying bidirectional relation in which PTSD increases the likelihood of seeking or receiving care, and contact with the healthcare system results in discrimination, which then worsens PTSD symptomology, leading to an increased need for care. Instead of a double-edged sword, healthcare discrimination may place some in a double bind where the system intended to help alleviate symptoms may worsen these symptoms when discrimination is present. These findings offer potential insights for future areas of inquiry, especially as they relate to the longitudinal roles of discrimination and immigration-related stress on care seeking. It further raises questions regarding the timing of such effects.

7. Limitations and Future Directions

The current study should be considered in the context of multiple limitations. First, the lack of longitudinal data makes it difficult to disentangle the effects of discrimination on healthcare access and to test mediation fully. Second, the study's convenience sample may limit generalization to other Latinx populations. While the inclusion of a sample recruited outside of any major metropolitan areas may extend the literature, healthcare systems may differ significantly in these areas, including the extent to which people experience discrimination and other available resources. Relatedly, the sample includes primarily cisgender women, and the sample size was insufficient to test gender differences across the effects examined here. Given gender differences in both symptomology and help seeking, results may differ for cisgender men and trans or gender-diverse populations. However, the current results point to potentially fruitful areas of investigation, including longitudinal examination of discrimination, healthcare access, and help-seeking behavior. Future studies should examine different timescales over which discrimination and immigration-related stress predict help seeking. For example, examining whether experiencing discrimination in healthcare settings results in reduced help-seeking attitudes or behaviors over shorter (e.g., days) and longer (e.g., months or days) time intervals. The current study, combined with prior data, indicates that such investigations may shed important light and nuance onto the role of discrimination for Latinx populations in the U.S. Additionally, these results should be examined in different geographical contexts, as they may differ in contexts depending on how welcoming the community is to immigrants and the availability of services.

8. Conclusions

The current study suggests that discrimination in healthcare settings and immigration-related stress may increase PTSD symptoms, which in turn may prompt attempts to access care. The same effects were not present for depression symptoms. This offers new insights into the unique role of PTSD symptoms as consequences of stressors among Latinx populations and immigrants in particular. This novel and somewhat counterintuitive contribution indicates that both discrimination and immigration-related stress may indirectly increase service seeking because both may increase PTSD symptoms.

Author Contributions: Conceptualization, A.R.A., S.R., S.M.E.G. and L.M.A.; methodology, A.R.A.; validation, A.R.A., K.E. and S.R.; formal analysis, A.R.A.; investigation, A.R.A.; resources, A.R.A.; data curation, S.R., K.E. and A.R.A.; writing—original draft preparation, A.R.A. and K.E.; writing—review and editing, A.R.A. and K.E.; visualization, A.R.A.; supervision, A.R.A.; project administration, S.R., L.M.A. and S.M.E.G.; funding acquisition, A.R.A. All authors have read and agreed to the published version of the manuscript.

Funding: Research was funded by the Office of Research and Economic Development at the University of Nebraska-Lincoln.

Institutional Review Board Statement: The study was conducted in accordance with the Declaration of Helsinki and approved by the Institutional Review Board of the University of Nebraska-Lincoln (protocol number 20553 and initially approved 14 September 2020).

Informed Consent Statement: Informed consent was obtained from all participants involved in the study.

Data Availability Statement: Data are not available for sharing due to privacy concerns of participants. Additional data summaries may be provided upon request.

Acknowledgments: We would like to thank our community partners, El Centro de las Américas, for completing this study.

Conflicts of Interest: The authors declare no conflict of interest.

References

1. Andrews, A.R., III; Haws, J.K.; Acosta, L.M.; Acosta Canchila, M.N.; Carlo, G.; Grant, K.M.; Ramos, A.K. Combinatorial effects of discrimination, legal status fears, adverse childhood experiences, and harsh working conditions among Latino migrant farmworkers: Testing learned helplessness hypotheses. *J. Latinx Psychol.* **2020**, *8*, 179–201. [CrossRef] [PubMed]
2. Bernard, D.L.; Smith, Q.; Lanier, P. Racial discrimination and other adverse childhood experiences as risk factors for internalizing mental health concerns among Black youth. *J. Trauma. Stress.* **2021**, *35*, 473–483. [CrossRef] [PubMed]
3. Budhwani, H.; Hearld, K.R.; Chavez-Yenter, D. Depression in Racial and Ethnic Minorities: The Impact of Nativity and Discrimination. *J. Racial Ethn. Health Disparities* **2015**, *2*, 34–42. [CrossRef] [PubMed]
4. Coffman, M.J.; Norton, C.K. Demands of Immigration, Health Literacy, and Depression in Recent Latino Immigrants. *Home Health Care Manag. Pract.* **2010**, *22*, 116–122. [CrossRef]
5. Dang, B.N.; Giordano, T.P.; Kim, J.H. Sociocultural and structural barriers to care among undocumented Latino immigrants with HIV infection. *J. Immigr. Minor. Health* **2012**, *14*, 124–131. [CrossRef] [PubMed]
6. Ortega, A.N.; Fang, H.; Perez, V.H.; Rizzo, J.A.; Carter-Pokras, O.; Wallace, S.P.; Gelberg, L. Health Care Access, Use of Services, and Experiences Among Undocumented Mexicans and Other Latinos. *Arch. Intern. Med.* **2007**, *167*, 2354–2360. [CrossRef]
7. Abraham, C.; Sheeran, P. *Predicting Health Behaviour: Research and Practice with Social Cognition Models*; Open University Press Berkshire, 2015; pp. 30–55. Available online: https://books.google.com/books?hl=en&lr=&id=pMkvEAAAQBAJ&oi=fnd&pg=PA30&dq=health+belief+model&ots=eXXFA6jrLC&sig=4zFKlDJvM93OJlFAt8xN5Z0RUBc (accessed on 28 January 2024).
8. Champion, V.L.; Skinner, C.S. The health belief model. *Health Behav. Health Educ. Theory Res. Pract.* **2008**, *4*, 45–65.
9. Brooks Holliday, S.; Dubowitz, T.; Haas, A.; Ghosh-Dastidar, B.; DeSantis, A.; Troxel, W.M. The association between discrimination and PTSD in African Americans: Exploring the role of gender. *Ethn. Health* **2020**, *25*, 717–731. [CrossRef]
10. Williams, M.T.; Printz, D.; DeLapp, R.C. Assessing racial trauma with the Trauma Symptoms of Discrimination Scale. *Psychol. Violence* **2018**, *8*, 735. [CrossRef]
11. Henshaw, E.J.; Freedman-Doan, C.R. Conceptualizing mental health care utilization using the health belief model. *Clin. Psychol. Sci. Pract.* **2009**, *16*, 420. [CrossRef]
12. Hunt, J.; Sullivan, G.; Chavira, D.A.; Stein, M.B.; Craske, M.G.; Golinelli, D.; Roy-Byrne, P.P.; Sherbourne, C.D. Race and beliefs about mental health treatment among anxious primary care patients. *J. Nerv. Ment. Dis.* **2013**, *201*, 188–195. [CrossRef]
13. Nobiling, B.D.; Maykrantz, S.A. Exploring Perceptions about and Behaviors Related to Mental Illness and Mental Health Service Utilization among College Students Using the Health Belief Model (HBM). *Am. J. Health Educ.* **2017**, *48*, 306–319. [CrossRef]
14. O'Connor, P.J.; Martin, B.; Weeks, C.S.; Ong, L. Factors that influence young people's mental health help-seeking behaviour: A study based on the Health Belief Model. *J. Adv. Nurs.* **2014**, *70*, 2577–2587. [CrossRef] [PubMed]
15. Langley, E.L.; Wootton, B.M.; Grieve, R. The Utility of the Health Belief Model Variables in Predicting Help-Seeking Intention for Anxiety Disorders. *Aust. Psychol.* **2018**, *53*, 291–301. [CrossRef]
16. Canchila, M.; Reyes, S.; Estrada Gonzalez, S.M.; Dominguez, V.; Acosta, L.M.; Guerra, R.; Pulido, C.; Caicedo, O.; Andrews, A.R. The role of discrimination and vaccine distrust in vaccine uptake among Latines in the Midwest. *Behav. Ther.* **2022**. Available online: https://psycnet.apa.org/record/2023-15394-001 (accessed on 28 January 2024).
17. Hacker, K.; Anies, M.E.; Folb, B.; Zallman, L. Barriers to health care for undocumented immigrants: A literature review. *RMHP* **2015**, *8*, 175–183. [CrossRef] [PubMed]
18. Asad, A.L. Latinos' deportation fears by citizenship and legal status, 2007 to 2018. *Proc. Natl. Acad. Sci. USA* **2020**, *117*, 8836–8844. [CrossRef]
19. Cox, R.B.; Lin, H.; Cartagena, M.J.L.; Greder, K.A.; Larzelere, R.E.; Washburn, I.J.; Sahbaz, S. Validation of the Family Fear of Deportation Scale for youth. *Fam. Relat.* **2023**, *72*, 734–754. [CrossRef]
20. Rayburn, A.D.; McWey, L.M.; Gonzales-Backen, M.A. Living Under the Shadows: Experiences of Latino Immigrant Families at Risk for Deportation. *Fam. Relat.* **2021**, *70*, 359–373. [CrossRef]
21. Brabeck, K.M.; Cardoso, J.B.; Chen, T.; Bjugstad, A.; Capps, R.; Capoverde, E.; Trull, A. Discrimination and PTSD among Latinx immigrant youth: The moderating effects of gender. *Psychol. Trauma: Theory Res. Pract. Policy* **2022**, *14*, 11. [CrossRef]

22. Cobb, C.L.; Xie, D.; Meca, A.; Schwartz, S.J. Acculturation, discrimination, and depression among unauthorized Latinos/as in the United States. *Cult. Divers. Ethn. Minor. Psychol.* **2017**, *23*, 258–268. [CrossRef] [PubMed]
23. Torres, L.; Ong, A.D. A daily diary investigation of Latino ethnic identity, discrimination, and depression. *Cult. Divers. Ethn. Minor. Psychol.* **2010**, *16*, 561. [CrossRef] [PubMed]
24. Pérez, D.J.; Fortuna, L.; Alegría, M. Prevalence and correlates of everyday discrimination among U.S. Latinos. *J. Community Psychol.* **2008**, *36*, 421–433. [CrossRef]
25. Peek, M.E.; Nunez-Smith, M.; Drum, M.; Lewis, T.T. Adapting the Everyday Discrimination Scale to Medical Settings: Reliability and Validity Testing in a Sample of African American Patients. *Ethn. Dis.* **2011**, *21*, 502–509. [PubMed]
26. Stucky, B.D.; Gottfredson, N.C.; Panter, A.T.; Daye, C.E.; Allen, W.R.; Wightman, L.F. An item factor analysis and item response theory-based revision of the Everyday Discrimination Scale. *Cult. Divers. Ethn. Minor. Psychol.* **2011**, *17*, 175. [CrossRef] [PubMed]
27. Taylor, R.J.; Forsythe-Brown, I.; Mouzon, D.M.; Keith, V.M.; Chae, D.H.; Chatters, L.M. Prevalence and correlates of everyday discrimination among black Caribbeans in the United States: The impact of nativity and country of origin. *Ethn. Health* **2019**, *24*, 463–483. [CrossRef] [PubMed]
28. Sternberg, R.M.; Nápoles, A.M.; Gregorich, S.; Paul, S.; Lee, K.A.; Stewart, A.L. Development of the Stress of Immigration Survey (SOIS): A Field Test among Mexican Immigrant Women. *Fam. Community Health* **2016**, *39*, 40–52. [CrossRef]
29. Blevins, C.A.; Weathers, F.W.; Davis, M.T.; Witte, T.K.; Domino, J.L. The Posttraumatic Stress Disorder Checklist for DSM-5 (PCL-5): Development and Initial Psychometric Evaluation. *J. Trauma. Stress.* **2015**, *28*, 489–498. [CrossRef]
30. Miller-Graff, L.E.; Guzman, J.C.; Hare, T. Psychometric Properties of the CES-D, PCL-5, and DERS in a Honduran Adult Sample. *Psychol. Test. Adapt. Dev.* **2023**, *4*, 300–309. [CrossRef]
31. Martínez-Levy, G.A.; Bermúdez-Gómez, J.; Merlín-García, I.; Flores-Torres, R.P.; Nani, A.; Cruz-Fuentes, C.S.; Briones-Velasco, M.; Ortiz-León, S.; Mendoza-Velásquez, J. After a disaster: Validation of PTSD checklist for DSM-5 and the four- and eight-item abbreviated versions in mental health service users. *Psychiatry Res.* **2021**, *305*, 114197. [CrossRef] [PubMed]
32. Kroenke, K.; Spitzer, R.L. The PHQ-9: A new depression diagnostic and severity measure. *Psychiatr. Ann.* **2002**, *32*, 509–515. [CrossRef]
33. Kroenke, K.; Spitzer, R.L.; Williams, J.B. The Phq-9. *J. Gen. Intern. Med.* **2001**, *16*, 606–613. [CrossRef] [PubMed]
34. Wulsin, L.; Somoza, E.; Heck, J. The Feasibility of Using the Spanish PHQ-9 to Screen for Depression in Primary Care in Honduras. *Prim. Care Companion J. Clin. Psychiatry* **2002**, *4*, 191–195. [CrossRef] [PubMed]
35. Zhong, Q.; Gelaye, B.; Fann, J.R.; Sanchez, S.E.; Williams, M.A. Cross-cultural validity of the Spanish version of PHQ-9 among pregnant Peruvian women: A Rasch item response theory analysis. *J. Affect. Disord.* **2014**, *158*, 148–153. [CrossRef] [PubMed]
36. Kroenke, K.; Strine, T.W.; Spitzer, R.L.; Williams, J.B.; Berry, J.T.; Mokdad, A.H. The PHQ-8 as a measure of current depression in the general population. *J. Affect. Disord.* **2009**, *114*, 163–173. [CrossRef]
37. Enders, C.K.; Bandalos, D.L. The relative performance of full information maximum likelihood estimation for missing data in structural equation models. *Struct. Equ. Model.* **2001**, *8*, 430–457. [CrossRef]
38. McClendon, J.; Dean, K.E.; Galovski, T. Addressing Diversity in PTSD Treatment: Disparities in Treatment Engagement and Outcome Among Patients of Color. *Curr. Treat. Options Psych.* **2020**, *7*, 275–290. [CrossRef]

International Journal of
Environmental Research and Public Health

MDPI

Article

"We Need Health for All": Mental Health and Barriers to Care among Latinxs in California and Connecticut

Mario Alberto Viveros Espinoza-Kulick [1,*] and Jessica P. Cerdeña [2,3,4]

1 Ethnic Studies, Cuesta College, San Luis Obispo, CA 93403, USA
2 Yale School of Medicine, Yale University, New Haven, CT 06520, USA
3 Institute for Collaboration on Health, Implementation, and Policy (InCHIP), University of Connecticut, Storrs, CT 06269, USA
4 Department of Anthropology, University of Connecticut, Storrs, CT 06269, USA
* Correspondence: mario_espinozakulick@cuesta.edu; Tel.: +1-805-592-9810

Abstract: Latinx (im)migrant groups remain underserved by existing mental health resources. Past research has illuminated the complex factors contributing to this problem, including migration-related trauma, discrimination, anti-immigrant policies, and structural vulnerability. This paper uses decolonial-inspired methods to present and analyze results from two studies of Latinx (im)migrant communities in central California and southern Connecticut in the United States. Using mixed quantitative and qualitative analysis, we demonstrate the intersectional complexities to be addressed in formulating effective mental health services. Relevant social and structural factors including knowledge of mental health, access to insurance, and experiencing discrimination were significantly associated with anxiety symptoms, based on linear regression analysis. Ethnographic interviews demonstrate how complex trauma informs mental health needs, especially through the gendered experiences of women. Overlapping aspects of gender, language barriers, fear of authorities, and immigration status contoured the lived experiences of Latinx (im)migrants. Thematic analyses of open-ended survey responses also provide recommendations for solutions based on the experiences of those directly affected by these health disparities, particularly relating to healthcare access, affordability, and capacity. Building from these findings and past research, we recommend the adoption of a comprehensive model of mental health service provision for Latinx (im)migrants that takes into account Indigenous language access, structural competency, expanded health insurance, and resources for community health workers.

Keywords: latinxs; migrants; immigration; mental health services; structural vulnerability

Citation: Espinoza-Kulick, M.A.V.; Cerdeña, J.P. "We Need Health for All": Mental Health and Barriers to Care among Latinxs in California and Connecticut. *Int. J. Environ. Res. Public Health* **2022**, *19*, 12817. https://doi.org/10.3390/ijerph191912817

Academic Editors: Maria De Jesus and Ernesto Castañeda

Received: 23 August 2022
Accepted: 3 October 2022
Published: 6 October 2022

Publisher's Note: MDPI stays neutral with regard to jurisdictional claims in published maps and institutional affiliations.

1. Introduction

Latinxs are the largest non-white racial or ethnic group in the United States, numbering 62.1 million and constituting 19% of the population as of 2022 [1]. By 2030, Latinxs are expected to comprise nearly 30% of Americans [2]. Latinxs are also the youngest racial or ethnic group in the U.S.: one-third of the nation's Latinxs are younger than 18 years old [3]. However, a longstanding gap persists in mental health care services that are culturally responsive and effectively implemented among this diverse population [4–7]. This paper builds from existing research documenting influences on mental health among Latinx groups to inform a model for services that addresses the complex overlapping factors of language, cultural relevancy, access, and structural vulnerability.

Latinxs—which is a gender-neutral term for "Latino/as", abbreviated from Latinoamericanos—are a remarkably heterogeneous group. Latinx/o/a is an endonym referring to origin in or heritage from Latin America, including individuals who trace their roots to Central and South America and the Caribbean. Thus, a Quechua-speaking rural Indigenous Ecuadorian, a Spanish-speaking mestizo Costa Rican, a Totonaco-speaking coastal Mexican, a Creyol-speaking Black Haitian, and an Italian-speaking white Argentine may all identify as Latinx in the United States. In addition, many descendants of Spanish settlers in the southwestern U.S.—the *hispanos*, *tejanos*, and *californios*—who became U.S. residents after the Treaty of Guadalupe Hidalgo in 1848, may also identify as Latinx/o/a [8,9]. Responses to the needs of the Latinx community must therefore attend to pluralities in racial identity, language, origin, and migration history [10].

Likely due to this heterogeneity, Latinxs demonstrate variability in the prevalence of mental health disorders. In 2018, 8.6 million Latinx adults had a mental health or substance use disorder [11]. Overall, evidence suggests that Latinx individuals experience lower risk of most mental health disorders compared with non-Latinx white individuals [12]. However, U.S.-born Latinxs report higher rates for most psychiatric disorders compared with Latinx immigrants, and these rates vary when stratified by nativity and disorder and adjusted by demographic and socioeconomic differences [13]. This reflects a pattern of contradictory health disparities that some refer to as the "Latino health paradox". This term identifies that Latinx and immigrant communities experience a distinct mix of risk and protective factors compared to non-Latinx white communities. In particular, recent immigrants tend to have more positive health and resilience, while higher levels of acculturation and longer time living in the United States contribute to a range of health risks [14]. Latinx youth are at particular risk of mental health disorders: among Latinx high school students, 18.9% had seriously considered attempting suicide, 15.7% had made a plan to attempt suicide, 11.3% had attempted suicide, and 4.1% had made a suicide attempt that required medical attention [12,15]. Furthermore, Latinx youth report higher prevalence of illicit substance use and initiation of alcohol or cigarette use in the past year relative to youth belonging to other racial/ethnic groups [16].

Several mutually constitutive and overlapping factors contribute to the development of mental health disorders in Latinxs. First, Latinxs, particularly those who have migrated to the U.S., report high rates of trauma. Migration, or transnational mobility, entails multiple vulnerabilities, including violence and economic precarity in one's country of origin; threats or risks of physical and sexual violence, dehydration, kidnapping, and exploitation during border crossings; family separation; and detention and deportation [17–20]. Experiences are particularly harrowing for women, who may confront rape, forced prostitution, trafficking, and physical violence [21,22]. Reports of trauma exposure are extremely high among Latina migrant women, with prevalence rates around 75% [23–25]. In addition, many Latinxs carry historical trauma relating to the European colonization, enslavement, sexual violence, and genocide of Indigenous peoples of the Americas [26]. Such reproductive and genocidal violence continues with reports of recent coerced hysterectomies on (im)migrant women detained in Georgia [27].

Second, Latinx migrants and their descendants experience discrimination. Both acculturative stress and discrimination have been shown to impact physical health through the mediating effects of anxiety [28]. For example, greater experiences of discrimination moderate the effect of harsh working conditions, increasing symptoms of anxiety and depression among migrant farmworkers in the rural Midwest [29]. Perceived discrimination is also significantly related to substance use behaviors among Latinxs [30]. A recent systematic review found that discrimination, family separation, and fear of deportation exacerbate acculturative stress [31].

Third, restrictive immigration policies and enforcement contribute to psychosocial stress among Latinxs. Increased immigration enforcement is associated with higher mental distress and decreased self-reported health [32]. A systematic review of the impact of immigration policy on mental health identified consistent associations between restrictive immigration policies and outcomes including depression, anxiety, and post-traumatic stress disorder (PTSD) [33]. Self-reports of greater personal and family suffering as a consequence of current immigration policies have a demonstrated association with increased symptoms of depression, anxiety, and psychological distress [34,35]. Citizen children who worry about losing a caregiver suffer from higher rates of depression, anxiety, emotional distress, and hypervigilance [36]. Among pregnant women, fear of deportation and fear of a family member being deported were associated with higher prenatal and postpartum anxiety [37]. Furthermore, following the implementation of 287(g) agreements, which permit cooperation of federal immigration authorities with local police, pregnant Latina women sought prenatal care later and had inadequate care when compared with non-Latina women [38]. One study found that a 1% increase in a state's immigration arrest rate was significantly associated with multiple mental health morbidity outcomes [39]. In the wake of immigration raids and mass deportations, (im)migrants and Latinxs in particular report greater stress and fear and worse health [40,41].

These latter findings are particularly relevant amid intensifying anti-immigrant sentiment and increased deportation in recent years. From 2009 to 2016, five million undocumented (im)migrants were deported [42]. Under the Trump administration, a series of restrictive actions were implemented with serious implications for Latinxs. Within days of his inauguration, former President Trump signed Executive Order 13768 entitled "Enhancing Public Safety in the Interior of the United States", which expanded deportation priorities to effectively include every undocumented (im)migrant, promoted increased use of state and local police to enforce federal immigration law through section 287(g) of the Immigration and Nationality Act (i.e., 287(g) agreements), and directed the hiring of 10,000 Immigration and Customs Enforcement (ICE) officers [43–45]. Following this order, an additional 52 jurisdictions signed 287(g) agreements [46]. In addition, the Trump administration attempted to revoke temporary protected status from individuals who emigrated from Nicaragua, Haiti, and El Salvador; however, this effort was stymied by the Ramos, et al. vs. Nielsen, et al. decision of the U.S. District Court for the Northern District of California [47]. The administration also enacted a "Zero Tolerance Policy" with respect to unauthorized immigration, prosecuting (im)migrants as criminals, detaining them in hieleras or ice-cold cells, and separating children from their parents at the border [44,48]. Since former President Trump's ascendance to political prominence, Latinxs have experienced an uptick in racist and xenophobic violence, with violent hate crimes reaching a 16-year high in 2018 [49]. The Biden administration has begun to counter some of these policies; however, even by their own admission, this is a lengthy political process. Beyond that, the harsh policies enacted by the Trump administration have a lasting impact, even as they are dismantled at the federal level. State and local activists have also continued to mobilize around similar policies, including the building of a border wall in Texas.

Fourth, structural vulnerability—or an individual's "location in their society's multiple overlapping and mutually reinforcing power hierarchies (e.g., socioeconomic, racial, cultural) and institutional and policy-level statuses (e.g., immigration status, labor force participation)" [50]—conditions mental distress and inadequate access to care. Among migrant farmworkers, harsh working conditions significantly predict symptoms of anxiety and depression [29]. Under the Personal Responsibility and Work Opportunity Reconciliation Act of 1996 (PRWORA), permanent residents are ineligible for public assistance during their first five years in the U.S. [51]. Recently, "the public charge rule", a broader interpretation of the Immigration and Nationality Act (INA) § 212(a)(4), which states that individuals are inadmissible to the U.S. if they are "likely at any time to become a public charge", has discouraged noncitizens from pursuing needed benefits prior to regulating their status [52]. Although the Biden administration has repealed the changes made during the Trump administration, fear persists among immigrants who are eligible to access services. In addition, due to their explicit exclusion from the Affordable Care Act, undocumented (im)migrants have almost no access to public health insurance as well as limited options for employer-based or private insurance [53,54].

This structural vulnerability contributes to barriers in accessing mental health care. Nationally, Latinxs have the highest uninsurance rate of any racial/ethnic group, at 29.7% [55]. Only 1 in 10 Latinxs with a mental disorder receive mental health services from a general healthcare provider, and just 1 in 20 receive treatment from a mental health specialist [56]. Latinx youth are half as likely as white youth to receive antidepressant or stimulant treatment for depression and anxiety or attention deficit/hyperactivity disorder (ADHD) and attention deficit disorder (ADD), respectively [57,58]. In addition to fears of deportation, experiences of discrimination and mistrust of the healthcare system contribute to patterns of healthcare avoidance and non-adherence to recommended treatments [59–61]. Furthermore, by June 2020, due to the outbreak of COVID-19 in the U.S., an estimated 41% of Americans had delayed or avoided medical care and this prevalence was 1.5 times higher among Latinxs [62].

Many of the barriers to mental health care are rooted in the same factors that drive disparities in negative health conditions. For instance, immigration policies are often designed to explicitly and systematically exclude immigrant communities, especially undocumented individuals [63]. Further, even when immigrants do access services, they face discrimination that can further activate mental health trauma [35,64]. The provision of services in English only also creates major barriers for communities that speak Spanish [65–68], or any number of non-English and Indigenous languages. Beyond that, Latinx migrant communities are often economically exploited, and therefore face barriers at disparately high rates, including the cost of services themselves, access to childcare, transportation, and the inability to take time off from work [5,6,69–71]. While these barriers are well-documented, more research is needed linking these disparities to potential solutions that can close gaps. In the face of nearly insurmountable odds, many Latinxs cultivate positive mental health and access services when needed. This study utilizes data drawn from decolonial-inspired research to lift up community voices in the articulation of mental health disparities as well as amplifying the effective strategies that resonate with directly affected individuals.

Understanding the complex factors influencing mental health services among Latinxs is necessary to inform effective solutions in policy and practice. Generalized models of mental health care provide insufficient specificity for addressing the complex factors facing Latinx and migrant communities. Our paper aims to answer the following questions: (1) What factors influence mental health among Latinx (im)migrant community members? and (2) How can services be effectively improved to address these factors and reduce these barriers? We draw from two geographically and demographically distinct Latinx populations—multigenerational, majority Mexican/Mexican–Americans in the central coast of California and multi-ethnic, pregnant Latina migrants living in southern Connecticut. Given the diversity of these bicoastal study populations, we capture complexity in experiences and attitudes with respect to mental health and healthcare evident among Latinxs in the United States.

2. Materials and Methods

This paper uses a mixed-methods analytic approach, guided by a decolonial framework [72–75]. Decolonization centers the perspectives of Indigenous peoples throughout research design, interpretation, and dissemination, focusing on the ways in which knowledge production can be directly useful. In the context of Latinx (im)migrant health, this is particularly relevant given the many Indigenous identities, cultures, and languages of Latin American origin [76]. Decolonial-inspired methods are a blueprint for being in active solidarity with the larger struggle of decolonization while working with diverse communities that include Indigenous peoples who are uninvited guests on others' homelands. A decolonial-inspired framework emphasizes practices such as reflexivity to the conditions of settler colonialism, soliciting and valuing advice from community members, and evaluation of embedded research norms.

For this paper, our decolonial-inspired methods focus on research questions that are centered in participants' perspectives, specifically those that are directly useful to improving the conditions under which people live their lives. To compare themes across heterogenous contexts, we draw principally from an ethnographic survey based on the central coast of California with illustrative vignettes from a small-scale ethnographic study based in southern Connecticut. The demographics for both studies are presented in Table 1. Samples from both states were used to reflect the diverse perspectives of Latinx people living in different contexts. In California, 27% of the state population are immigrants, with the majority of immigrants identifying as Latinx and the most common country of origin being Mexico. [77] By contrast, in Connecticut, immigrants comprise about 15% of the population, and the primary sending country is India, followed by Jamaica, the Dominican Republic, and Ecuador [78].

Table 1. Demographic Summary for Each Study Sample.

		Central CA Sample		Southern CT Sample	
Variables	**Response Categories**	*n*	%	*n*	%
Gender	Women	123	82.0	65	100.0
	Men	14	9.3	0	0.0
	Not Listed	13	8.7	0	0.0
Indigeneity	Not Indigenous	125	83.3	59	90.8
	Indigenous	25	16.7	6	9.2
Country of Origin	Belizean	2	1.5	0	0.0
	Brazilian	2	1.6	0	0.0
	Chicana/o/x	5	3.9	0	0.0
	Chilean	2	1.6	1	1.5
	Colombian	0	0.0	1	1.5
	Cuban	1	0.7	0	0.0
	Dominican	1	0.8	7	10.8
	Ecuadorian	0	0.0	18	27.7
	Guatemalan	9	6.6	9	13.8
	Honduran	1	0.7	2	3.1
	Jamaican	0	0.0	1	1.5
	Mexican	91	66.9	15	23.1
	Mexican–American	23	16.9	0	0.0
	Peruvian	2	1.5	2	3.1
	Puerto Rican	0	0.0	7	10.8
	Salvadoran	7	5.1	2	3.1

The California survey assessed health needs and assets, which contained both standard measures and write-in responses. Validity was tested for all items by pilot testing the survey with research experts and local Latinx immigrant and Indigenous community members. Quantitative analyses were conducted on the survey data from this sample. In addition, write-in responses were coded thematically. The Connecticut study included ethnographic interviews and surveys of trauma exposure and symptoms, which were analyzed using qualitative methods. The comparison of themes across sites allowed for the identification of relevant examples that both deepen and broaden the findings available from the survey data. The studies received Institutional Review Board approval from the University of California, Santa Barbara and Yale University.

2.1. Survey Data on Latinx Immigrant Health Needs and Assets

The California study was based on a larger ethnographic project examining Latinx immigrant health and advocacy, which included participant observation in-person and online, a survey of health needs/assets, and interviews and focus groups with Latinx immigrant community members and immigrant health advocates. This larger project allowed for a survey to be developed in collaboration with community representatives and leaders, with findings directly communicated to those stakeholders. Survey data were collected among self-identified Latinx (im)migrant community members and advocates for immigrant health. Respondents were recruited through organizational networks of immigrant and health advocates, community-serving organizations, and key informants identified in the larger ethnographic project. The survey was available in English and Spanish and respondents were encouraged to receive assistance from family members and interpreters as needed to take the survey. These strategies help to ensure the inclusion of hard-to-reach groups who may have limited trust in processes associated with the government, including university-based research. In addition, a random sample of respondents was recruited via Facebook and Instagram posts in English and Spanish.

The survey addressed health holistically and asked about respondents' demographics, experiences of health and healthcare, community-level perceptions, and barriers to health access. In addition to defined-response quantitative measures, open-ended questions were included and analyzed using deductive thematic coding. All measures used for regression analysis are summarized in Table 2.

Table 2. Summary Statistics for Variables used for Regression Analysis.

Categorical Variables	Response Categories	*n*	%
Eligibility criteria	Outside advocate	38	21.5
	Immigrant community members	139	78.5
Language	English	95	53.7
	Spanish	82	46.3
Race	Other Race	22	14.3
	Latina/o/x or Hispanic	132	85.7
Indigeneity	Not Indigenous	125	83.3
	Indigenous	25	16.7
Insurance Coverage	No/Decline to State	34	30.1
	Yes	79	69.9
Continuous Variables		*M*	*SD*
General anxiety disorder symptoms [a]		1.91	0.77
Trust in biomedical healthcare [b]		2.89	0.62
Trust in therapists [b]		2.79	0.76
Mental health knowledge [c]		3.35	1.32
Concern for mental health issues [c]		3.57	1.44
Experiences of discrimination [a]		0.47	0.90

Notes. [a] Range: 0–3, [b] Range: 1–4, [c] Range: 1–5.

2.1.1. Sampling and Eligibility Criteria

To be eligible for the survey, individuals had to be adults and identify as an advocate for immigrant health and/or as an immigrant community member, "i.e., Undocumented, Dreamers, mixed-status family member, resident and/or a naturalized citizen". Advocates for immigrant health were defined on the survey as "individuals that actively participate in social change efforts toward advancing immigrant health equity". Both groups were included for analytic purposes (n = 177). For regression analysis, we controlled for differences between advocates who were not community members (coded "0") with all community members, including those who also identified as advocates (coded "1"). Alternative operationalizations were tested, including the interaction between being a community member and an advocate, but the community member or not variable was the only version significantly associated with anxiety scores in bivariate tests.

2.1.2. Anxiety

Anxiety is one indicator of mental health. General anxiety represents a pattern of experiencing excessive worry and can be caused by many factors. Some external factors that are associated with anxiety include surveillance and isolation, both of which are common to Latinx (im)migrant groups [79,80]. To measure general anxiety, we used the GAD-7 Scale [81]. The GAD-7 asks respondents to indicate the frequency of experiencing seven anxiety symptoms over the past two weeks on a four-point scale (0 = "Not at all", 1 = "Several days", 2 = "Over half the days", 3 = "Nearly every day"; sample item: "Worrying too much about different things"). Among this sample, the measure showed excellent internal reliability, with Cronbach's $\alpha = 0.93$.

2.1.3. Socio-Demographic Factors

To understand aspects of respondents' social position and control for potential group patterns in anxiety symptoms, the survey assessed respondents' primary language spoken, their racial identity, and whether or not they identify as Indigenous. Language was measured by whether they accessed the survey in English (coded "0") or Spanish (coded "1"). These categories were consistent with responses to the question: "What language do you primarily use?", and contained no missing data. Respondents self-identified their race in response to the question: "What race(s) do you primarily identify with?", and were allowed to select all that apply from a list. For this analysis, individuals were divided between those who self-identified as "Latina/o/x or Hispanic" (coded "1") and all other respondents (coded "0"). Finally, respondents were asked: "Do you identify as Indigenous?", and categorized based on their response (0 = No, 1 = Yes). This question was asked separately from race, as the categories "American Indian or Alaskan Native" and "Native Hawaiian or Other Pacific Islander" used for racial classification do not include many Native Americans and Indigenous people who fall outside of these categories [82]. Further, a separate question inquired about tribal affiliation. Sample sizes were too small to perform further disaggregated analyses, as a wide range of affiliations were present among respondents, including tribes with homelands across the Americas.

Respondents were asked to report their age in years. This variable was tested in the regression models, but it was removed for parity as it was not significantly associated with any outcome. However, respondents ranged from 20 to 75 years old and were, on average, 37 years old ($M = 37.52$, $SD = 11.63$). For those immigrant respondents who disclosed the length of time they had lived in the United States ($n = 120$), the time period ranged from 1 year to 75 years, with an average of 22.29 years ($SD = 14.14$).

2.1.4. Mental Health Services Access

Respondents were asked about both general factors of healthcare access as well as domain-specific access points for mental health. First, a four-item scale was constructed to assess trust in biomedical healthcare services. Beginning with the stem: "How much trust do you have in the following types of healthcare providers?", respondents reported on a four-point scale (1 = "Do not trust at all", 2 = "Trust somewhat", 3 = Trust moderately", 4 = "Trust completely") for "general medical doctors (MD, DO)", "Specialty medical doctors (OBGYN, oncologists, etc.)", "Nurses (RN, LVN, CNA, NP)", and "Physicians assistants (PA)". This scale showed strong internal reliability, with Cronbach's $\alpha = 0.84$. A separate measure was used to indicate respondents' trust in "Therapists (psychologists and social workers)", using the same stem and response scale. Health insurance coverage was assessed using the single question: "Do you have health insurance?", with respondents grouped by those who responded affirmatively (coded "1") and those who responded negatively (coded "0"). Having access to insurance coverage increases the likelihood of interactions with biomedical healthcare services. Lastly, the survey inquired about both knowledge and concern for mental health. Knowledge was measured using the question: "On a scale from 1–5, how knowledgeable are you of the following health concerns?", with the item "Mental health" (1 = "No Knowledge" to 5 = "Very Knowledgeable"). Similarly, concern was measured using the question: "On a scale from 1–5, how concerned are you of the following health concerns?", with the item "Mental health" and responses on a five-point scale (1 = "Not Concerned" to 5 = "Very Concerned").

2.1.5. Experiences of Discrimination

The survey provided an opportunity for respondents to share about discrimination within a larger question that asked about personal experiences as well as witnessing and knowing of others' experiences. A three-item scale was constructed by taking the average of dichotomous items (coded "0"/"1"), based on respondents affirming that they had "Experienced this myself", with respect to "Discrimination based on immigration status", "Discrimination based on race or ethnic identity", and "Discrimination based on gender and sexuality". Respondents were allowed to select all that apply, so this does not discount intersectional experiences of discrimination that are on the basis of multiple factors. This scale showed acceptable internal reliability among this sample, with Cronbach's $\alpha = 0.78$. Experiences of discrimination are associated with increased mental health burden, including higher rates of anxiety symptoms [83].

2.1.6. Reported and Perceived Barriers to Mental Health Services

To understand the barriers facing Latinx (im)migrant groups, this survey asked respondents to self-report experienced barriers to healthcare in response to the question: "In the past three months, have you delayed or gone without healthcare for any of the following reasons?" Nineteen response options were provided: "Services are too expensive", "Appointments not available", "Unable to secure childcare", "Unable to get time off of work", "Service providers are too far away", "Didn't realize I had a health problem", "Healthcare providers conflict with my cultural or religious beliefs", "Healthcare providers do not speak my language", "Healthcare providers do not appropriately recognize my gender identity", "Discrimination or hostility when attempting to access healthcare", "Don't have health insurance due to documentation status", "Don't have health insurance for another reason (not related to documentation status)", "My insurance policy didn't cover what I need", "Fearful of police", "Fearful of immigration enforcement (ICE)", "Fearful of getting COVID-19/coronavirus", "Fearful of spreading COVID-19/coronavirus", "Health services closed due to COVID-19/coronavirus", and "Not listed". These options were developed by combining existing measures from health surveys that were relevant to Latinx immigrant and Indigenous communities. General barriers to healthcare create a larger context in which mental health services may be less accessible. A similar question was asked later in the survey with the stem: "On a scale from 1–5, rank how much you perceive the following barriers to prevent this community from accessing healthcare", with the same response categories provided. Both indicators are included to describe the relative prevalence of directly observed as well as perceived barriers to healthcare. Questions about COVID-19 were added during Spring 2020 and are presented with a reduced sample size.

We directly inquired about respondents' perceptions of the community's relationship to mental health through a series of single items. First, respondents were asked: "On a scale from 1–4, please rank how easy or hard it is accessing the following types of resources for this community", including the item "Mental health services" (1 = "Very difficult" to 4 = "Very easy"). These items are supplemented by two open-ended questions that allow for additional interpretation of these findings and how barriers can be overcome: "What are the most pressing health needs for this community?" and "How can society better support immigrant health needs?"

2.2. *Ethnographic Vignettes*

Ethnographic vignettes were derived from seven interviews that are part of a larger project examining intergenerational trauma in the Latin American migrant community of New Haven, Connecticut, based on semi-structured interviews and surveys of trauma experience, adapted from Keller and colleagues [84] and the PTSD Checklist for DSM-5, PCL-5 [85,86]. Although we recognize the impossibility of drawing broad conclusions from a small set of ethnographic vignettes, given the individualistic approach of biomedical treatment, attention to the discrepancies between traumatic histories and diagnostic thresholds is merited. The participants ranged from 19 to 43 years old and, on average, were 30 years old ($SD = 6.60$). All were immigrants, and they had spent between less than 1 and 24 years in the United States ($M = 7.86$, $SD = 7.14$). Participants were recruited from a local women's health clinic, either in-person or through recruitment flyers and follow-up phone calls. Interviews and surveys were conducted in either English or Spanish depending on the participant's preference. Qualitative interviews varied in length between 45 min and 4 h, with an average time around 1.5 h. Interviews and field notes were audio-recorded and transcribed using Trint automated transcription software and reviewed and edited in MAXQDA 2020 [87].

2.3. Analysis

The analytic strategy followed a primarily deductive approach, guided by the research questions motivated in the literature and prompted by the experiences of participants. While existing research has illuminated some of the specific dynamics affecting mental health conditions and strategies for service provision, this paper utilizes multiple data sources to address these questions from the perspective of the individuals directly affected. Expanding culturally competent mental health services was identified as a community need by focus group participants within the California study.

To address the factors that are associated with anxiety among Latinx (im)migrant community members, we used a linear regression model with ordinary least squares (OLS) estimators, including the predictors described above: socio-demographic factors, mental health services access, and experiences of discrimination. All variables were examined for multicollinearity and no issues were detected. Missing data were excluded listwise. No significant differences were found between the analytical sample and the full sample for any of the outcome or predictor variables.

These findings were interpreted using the existing literature as well as relevant vignettes selected from the Connecticut study. Vignettes were constructed after careful review and deductive coding of interview transcripts and field notes, guided by the research questions, with the intent of providing "thick description" of emergent themes [88]. For the Connecticut sample, thematic coding was completed using an inductive, person-centered ethnographic approach. This analysis developed themes using grounded theory methodology focused on inducing categories or typologies from the data. From these, key narratives of the themes of interest to this paper were composed into vignettes from relevant interviews. To understand community-level perceptions of the barriers between (im)migrant groups and mental health services, we utilized summary statistics of survey items as well as additional relevant qualitative themes reflected in ethnographic vignettes. Finally, community-based strategies for bridging gaps in mental health care services were identified using thematic coding of open-ended survey responses. Responses were coded deductively to identify barriers to mental health care as well as suggested solutions. Coded responses were then grouped into three thematic categories based on the relevant emergent patterns: barriers in access, barriers based on cost, and barriers due to low healthcare capacity.

3. Results

3.1. Research Question 1: What Factors Influence Mental Health among Latinx (im)migrant Community Members?

In terms of anxiety, survey respondents indicated on average that they experienced anxiety symptoms "nearly half the days" in the past 2 weeks ($M = 1.91$, $SD = 0.77$, $n = 113$). The summary statistics for all predictor variables are reported in Table 2. When entered together in a linear regression model ($n = 99$), socio-demographic factors, mental health services access, and experiences of discrimination estimated 32.6% of the variance in anxiety scores among respondents ($R^2 = 0.326$) and the model was statistically significant (F (10, 80) = 3.87, $p < 0.001$). The full model is reported in Table 3.

Socio-demographic factors (language, race, and Indigeneity) were not significantly associated with anxiety. The identities individuals hold were not associated with anxiety, but relevant questions of access and discrimination were. Self-reported knowledge of mental health was significantly associated with lower general anxiety scores ($\beta = -0.37$, $p = 0.003$). Those respondents who indicated that they had knowledge about mental health issues, gained through any source, were less likely to report anxiety symptoms over the past two weeks. In contrast, people with insurance reported significantly higher rates of anxiety ($\beta = 0.29$, $p = 0.008$).

Table 3. Factors Associated with General Anxiety Disorder Symptoms among Latinx Immigrant Communities.

Independent Variables	*B*	*SE*	β
Immigrant community member	−0.03	0.19	−0.02
Spanish-speaking	−0.18	0.18	−0.12
Latina/o/x or Hispanic	−0.43	0.24	−0.19
Indigenous	0.29	0.20	−14
Insured	0.47 **	0.17	0.29
Trust in biomedical healthcare	0.11	0.16	0.09
Trust in therapists	0.10	0.14	0.10
Mental health knowledge	−0.21 **	0.07	−0.37
Concern for mental health issues	0.11 *	0.06	0.22
Experiences of discrimination	0.19 *	0.08	0.26
Constant	1.55 ***	0.47	
	Model Summary		
F (10, 80)		3.87 ***	
R^2		0.326	

Note. * $p < 0.05$, ** $p < 0.01$, *** $p \leq 0.001$.

Experiencing discrimination on the basis of immigration status, race, ethnicity, gender, and/or sexuality was significantly and positively associated with anxiety scores among this sample (β = 0.29, p = 0.008). Further, reporting a higher concern of mental health was also associated with a significant increase in symptoms of general anxiety disorder (β = 0.22, p = 0.048). Trust in healthcare providers, both biomedical services and therapists specifically, were not significantly associated with anxiety scores.

Respondents were asked directly to report their own experiences of barriers to healthcare. A high proportion of the sample had reported avoiding healthcare within the past three months for one or more reasons (90.9%). The most commonly reported barriers to healthcare at the individual level were reported by over a quarter of respondents. Two of these were related directly to cost and healthcare capacity: "Appointments are not available" (46%, n = 110) and "Services are too expensive" (38%, n = 110). The remainder were related to the early days of the COVID-19 pandemic: "Fearful of getting COVID-19/coronavirus" (46%, n = 50) and "Health services closed due to COVID-19/coronavirus" (26%, n = 47). Each of these general barriers to healthcare also apply to mental health services. In addition to their own experiences, respondents were asked to rank barriers present within the community overall, on a scale of one to five. The highest-ranked items similarly had to do with COVID-19: "Fearful of getting COVID-19/coronavirus" (M = 4.18, SD = 1.24, n = 50), as well as barriers related to cost and insurance: "Services are too expensive" (M = 4.06, SD = 1.17, n = 96), "Don't have insurance" (M = 3.97, SD = 1.39, n = 94), and "My insurance policy didn't cover what I need" (M = 3.97, SD = 1.26, n = 94). These mirror the findings at the individual level, but further emphasize the lack of insurance coverage in the community, especially adequate insurance that covers preventative care and mental health services. To illustrate some of these dynamics in human terms, Box 1 includes a vignette of migration-related trauma.

The majority of the sample said it was difficult or very difficult to access mental health services for Latinx (im)migrant groups (71%, n = 100). When asked about collective awareness about mental health, the respondents rated the Latinx (im)migrant community as moderately knowledgeable (M = 2.34, SD = 1.08, n = 94) and moderately concerned (M = 2.89, SD = 1.20, n = 88). The substantial variation in these measures highlights the existence of strengths and resources among the community to address mental health, despite persistent gaps in healthcare access. The complex realities that these variables reflect in real life can be seen vividly in the vignetter presented in Box 2.

Box 1. Vignette: Migration-Related Trauma.

Adela is a 19-year-old woman who migrated from Cañar, Ecuador, in the *sierra*, or the Andes mountainous region largely populated by *el pueblo quichua*, or Quechua-speaking Indigenous people. She was the third of five children and her family always struggled financially. When she was 18 years old, her father told her they could no longer support her. This—coupled with rumors and news reports of Venezuelans pouring into the country, killing people—prompted her to leave. Adela departed *calladita*, quietly: she told only her family and close friends as she knew the process of migrating was risky. Her aunt hired a *coyote*, a person to guide her across the border, and after taking a flight into Mexico, she traveled with a group of 18 people over the desert for five days. Adela was picked up by border control and taken to a detention center in Texas. She was placed in a *hielera*, an ice-cold detention cell, with 30 to 40 other migrants. There was one toilet for all of the detainees to use, partially covered by a few bricks for privacy. They were given a few aluminum blankets. Adela suffered near-constant nosebleeds, which she attributes to the freezing conditions. After a week, border patrol released her into Mexico and she attempted to cross again, this time via a more strenuous route through the mountains. She arrived without detection and made her way to Connecticut. Adela describes her neighborhood in Connecticut as "*lindo*" ("nice"), but she admits to experiencing discrimination. Adela endorsed symptoms from each cluster of the DSM-5 criteria for PTSD, with a total PCL-5 score of 14. Adela shared that she avoids unpleasant feelings: she simply tries not to feel anger, sadness, or fear. Her support network is limited, consisting primarily of her partner and her mother whom she occasionally calls when stressed. Adela's narrative demonstrates the confluent influences of migration-related trauma, immigration enforcement, and discrimination, the latter of which strongly parallels findings from the California study.

Box 2. Vignette: "He hit me in a public place."

María Elena is a 27-year-old woman from Cuenca, Ecuador, who came to the U.S. for opportunity. She has a six-year-old daughter whom she left behind in Ecuador. "My father already died. My mother always lived with me. There (in Ecuador), there is little work and it's very hard. Then I got the opportunity to come here (to the U.S.). I came to give (my daughter) a better life ... I took the chance with pain in my soul, leaving my mom and my daughter, but I made the decision so as not to see them suffer." For María Elena, it was not just her family's finances that contributed to her decision to leave: she saw that throughout the country, violence, economic corruption, and drug trafficking were rampant and it was no longer a safe place to raise a child. Fortunately, she was able to secure a visa and came by herself to the States. She met her current partner over Facebook while in Ecuador and connected with him after arriving in Connecticut. Over the first few months, things were "beautiful". However, things then took a turn for the worst. "He was a bit ... like ... his character became possessive, controlling," she explained. Once "he hit me, he hit me in a public place ... and they called the police and took him away." Now, she is expecting a child with him and says that their relationship has improved. María Elena depends on her partner for money. When she was working herself, she could send remittances to Ecuador to support her mother and her daughter, but without work, she is no longer able. Given her partner's involvement in the construction industry, their finances are inconsistent, especially in the colder months. They often run out of money at the end of each month and cannot afford healthcare or medication, so they avoid seeing the doctor or going to the pharmacy. María Elena scored a 19 on the PCL-5, with two symptoms that bother her "very much" and "extremely". In particular, she avoids reminders of the incident in which her partner publicly assaulted her. María Elena's narrative illustrates the particular precarity faced by undocumented women—particularly pregnant women—who depend on their partners for financial support. Her avoidance of healthcare due to insufficient financial resources, attributable to unstable seasonal employment, coupled with her partner's controlling behavior, highlight the need to attend to gender-specific barriers in the design and implementation of mental health interventions.

3.2. Research Question 2: How Can Services Be Effectively Improved to Meet these Factors and Barriers?

At the conclusion of the survey, respondents were provided with the opportunity to write answers to a number of open-ended questions. Relevant to the present analysis on mental health services, the survey asked about the community's most pressing health needs, and collective strategies to support (im)migrant health needs. Thematic coding revealed three categories of barriers that respondents identified and linked to specific health needs and solutions. Each of these categories are interrelated, meaning that addressing one of these barriers effectively necessitates addressing all of them.

Access included a range of factors that prevented individuals who were seeking care from receiving it, or from receiving care that was timely, effective, and useful. The issues that (im)migrants face when accessing healthcare, including fear of driving and public transportation and lack of interpretation/translation services, become known within communities undermining trust with medical services, especially those attached to government institutions. As advocated by one respondent, "Tener mas (*sic*) recurso y confiar en el sistema" (We need more resources and trust in the system). Existing service providers and advocates are responsible for building trusting relationships with underserved communities to expand access to resources that may be underutilized.

The issue of cost was raised both with respect to services themselves and the larger conditions that are affecting communities. Cost was emphasized in terms of the inadequacy of current efforts to provide for low-income individuals, including sliding scale policies and emergency Medi-Cal (California's Medicaid program). Free and low-cost services were identified as a major health need, in part due to the high cost of housing and childcare. Economic marginalization throughout the community has led to the need for "Mas (*sic*) recursos economicos (*sic*) para todos" (More economic resources for all). Beyond the simple financial cost, participants also emphasized the value of services, indicating that many service providers were not considerate and flexible enough to actually solve health problems effectively.

Finally, the survey respondents indicated that health needs grew out of a lack of capacity present within their communities. Mental health service providers, as well as other specialty doctors, were identified as health needs within this community. For undocumented individuals, healthcare resources are especially limited, and this can affect service usage among family members. In addition, COVID-19 was identified as a strain on healthcare capacity itself, and its larger effect on the economy exacerbated ongoing issues of access and cost. Education was offered as one solution to train effective and culturally relevant service providers. These barriers, "Access", "Cost", and "Capacity", are summarized in Table 4.

Table 4. Thematic Analysis of Open-Ended Responses on Barriers to Mental Health Services.

Barriers	Health Needs	Relevant Quotes
Access	Preventative health services Accessibility Transportation Language support Remove fear and stigma Nutrition	"We need health4all. I am undocumented (DACA), and was accessing (student health insurance) but now that I've graduated I will lose coverage". "Necesito más dinero para comida y medicina" [a] "Outreach is essential". "Tener mas [*sic*] recurso y confiar en el sistema". [b]
Cost	Free or low-cost services Affordable sliding scales Insurance coverage Childcare Affordable housing	"Mas recursos economicos [*sic*] para todos" [c] "Recognizing that emergency Medi-Cal and sliding scales are not equitable care." "Ser mas [*sic*] considerados y flexibles ala hora de ayudarlos en cualquier problema ya sea de salud o de algun otro recurso que ocupen para mejorar su estilo de vida" [d]

Table 4. *Cont.*

Barriers	Health Needs	Relevant Quotes
Capacity	High-quality and consistent health services Mental health services Specialty doctors Health promotion and outreach	"More education, more promotion and easier access to services" "Ahora la salud mental no hay ayuda si no tienes papeles ahora la estan ofreciendo solo x lo del COVID-19, si no ni ofrecen ayuda psicológica" [e] "Proveyendo mas (*sic*) servicios y haciendo mas [*sic*] outreach para que la comunidad sepa de ellos, muchas veces si hay servicios pero la gente no esta (*sic*) informada y/o no saben que existen esos servicios" [f]

Note. Quotes are preserved in the language and form written by respondents. All open-ended responses were coded using a deductive thematic strategy. We selected quotes that were clearly written and that summarized patterns repeated in other responses. [a] "I need more money for food and medicine." [b] "We need more resources and trust the system." [c] "More financial resources for all." [d] "Be more considerate and flexible when it comes to helping them with any health problem or any other resource they use to improve their lifestyle." [e] "Now for mental health, there is no help if you do not have papers. Now they are offering it only because of COVID-19; if not, they do not offer psychological help." [f] "Providing more services and doing more outreach so that the community knows about them; many times if there are services but people are not informed and/or do not know that these services exist."

4. Discussion

The findings of this study affirm existing research that links structural factors affecting Latinx migrant communities to mental health outcomes and access to services [4–7,35,64–71]. Our study took a decolonial-inspired approach, motivated by the California respondents who prioritized mental health services as a necessary resource in their communities [89]. We accordingly highlight multiple key findings. First, anxiety and trauma constitute considerable mental health concerns for the Latinxs in our two study populations. Although socio-demographic factors such as language, race, and Indigeneity were not associated with anxiety, experiences of discrimination were positively associated with anxiety. This affirms a link between identity-based violence and various forms of psychological distress, including anxiety, that has been found in many contexts [28–31,35,64]. Our findings further support the widespread nature of these associations. Vignette 1 portrayed the role that trauma—particularly migration-related trauma—can play in the mental health of many Latinxs. Experiences of discrimination were significantly and positively associated with anxiety symptoms in the California sample. Anxiety was higher amongst those individuals who experience multiple forms of discrimination or compounded experiences. Adela's narrative elaborates upon this finding, discussing experiences of discrimination based on her inability to speak English. While some components of migration may be traumatic in and of themselves, the experience of discrimination leads to an undue mental health burden [17–22,26] and may decrease access to existing services. Other relevant forms of discrimination perpetrated against Latinxs can contribute to depression and exacerbate stress [30,31] as well as contributing to physical health symptoms [28].

In addition, particular gender-related concerns may apply to women who depend on their partners financially and thereby for healthcare. The diversity of our two study populations allows us to examine the effects of intersectionality, or the way that lives and identities are shaped by relational power structures in diverse and mutually influencing ways [90]. Although Indigeneity was not associated with anxiety symptoms in the California study survey, Indigenous identity constituted a self-identified risk factor for violence and abuse during Adela's border crossing in Vignette 1. This highlights how race—or phenotype—contributes to trauma risk and attendant vulnerability to mental health disorders. In addition, gender emerged as a particular vulnerability based on results from the Connecticut study. As a woman, Adela feared sexual violence and exploitation by her coyote and the machista, or misogynistic, men who accompanied her during her crossing. In addition, both Adela and María Elena depend on their partners for financial support during their pregnancies. María Elena, who strategically pursued partnership through social media prior to migrating, found herself in an abusive and controlling relationship that escalated to public physical assault requiring police intervention. Their condition as expectant mothers compounds the precariousness of their social and financial positions.

California study participants identified multiple barriers to mental health services, particularly around cost, healthcare capacity, underinsurance, and fears relating to contracting COVID-19. Importantly, participants also named multiple solutions to overcome these barriers to mental health services, which we thematically categorized around cost, access, and capacity. By utilizing a respondent-centered qualitative analysis, our study also identifies solutions that resonate with a diverse range of directly affected individuals. These include support relating to nutrition, transportation, interpreter services, free or sliding-scale care, and health promotion and outreach. Within the California study, the regression results showed a strong significant negative relationship between mental health knowledge and anxiety symptoms. On average, individuals with higher levels of mental health knowledge showed lower rates of anxiety symptoms. Relatedly, concern over mental health issues was associated with higher rates of anxiety symptoms. The results of regression analysis cannot prove causation; however, these findings emphasize opportunities for positive interventions. Existing knowledge of mental health, gained through sources such as health education campaigns, mental health treatment, or traditional knowledge, can be a resource within families and community health programs that develop positive coping skills [91–95]. While mental health education is not a substitute for treatment, it can be a building block for prevention strategies. Knowledge is also a key tool for decreasing concern, even when structural conditions are likely to continue to produce mental health problems and risk factors in the future [7].

Our results further demonstrate a need to attend to structural vulnerability, particularly insurance and documentation status. While insurance may increase opportunities for access to biomedical healthcare, by itself, it is not associated with more favorable outcomes in this case. Having insurance was significantly associated with anxiety symptoms among California participants, contrary to what might be expected. One explanation is that the cost of insurance and related care may cause anxiety [96]. Another possibility is that having insurance reflects a greater level of integration into mainstream U.S. institutions, and therefore a heightened risk for anxiety symptoms related to exclusion and discrimination. Research has found patterns over time where acculturation into U.S. society is linked to multiple forms of psychological distress [97–100].

Although we were unable to conduct quantitative analyses with the Connecticut data due to the small sample size, all but one participant was undocumented and uninsured. Both of these overlapping factors create a harsh structural vulnerability and risk for negative health. Most of the women in the Connecticut study received prenatal care through a privately funded program that covers only prenatal and early pediatric care. This arrangement underscores neoliberal influences on the conditionality of "deservingness" for undocumented migrants [101,102]: women alone do not themselves have a right to healthcare, but women as reproductive agents do. As such, a lack of documentation is a significant contributor to uninsurance and this insurability should be considered when recommending services [103].

Our ethnographic data portray harrowing experiences of migration-related trauma that should be evaluated in migrant populations, particularly those from Central and South America. Threats of violence and rape, and real experiences of inhumane conditions in detention centers, can precipitate psychopathology. Although data suggest that Latinx (im)migrants experience better mental health outcomes relative to their descendants, these migration-related traumas should not be overlooked. Careful screenings—as might be conducted during an intake for political asylum—should be considered in this population to ensure that symptoms of mental health disorders are identified and intervened upon in a prompt manner. These findings highlight the limitations of the use of clinical cutoffs for instruments such as the GAD-7 and PCL-5. In the two vignettes, women reported multiple

PTSD symptoms in each of the DSM-5 clusters yet did not meet the threshold score of 31–33 of probable PTSD. Clinicians should exercise careful judgment when considering the initiation of mental health treatment as even without meeting diagnostic criteria, patients may benefit from early intervention including psychoeducation, community mental health care, or therapy.

Our paper has limitations. First, data for this analysis derive from two separate, independently conducted studies with distinctive aims. Although the authors recognized the advantage of considering how these data informed one another—particularly incorporating mixed quantitative and qualitative methods—the absence of unifying a priori research questions and hypotheses may have informed study designs in ways for which we cannot account post-hoc. Second, our data are limited to two coastal populations that do not fully represent the rich complexity and heterogeneity of the Latinx community. Our sample was largely composed of women, which limited our ability to examine the uniquely gendered experiences of men. In addition, our sample had a high representation of individuals of Mexican origin: although this is consistent with national trends [3], we may not have captured the variety of perspectives of Latinxs of different national origins due to small sampling. We also had low representation of Indigenous-identifying individuals. Notwithstanding Adela's Quechua background in Vignette 1, her experience cannot be considered representative of all Indigenous Latinxs. Our paper also did not address specific concerns of sexual and gender minorities, who face particular challenges with respect to mental health and care [104–106]. Third and relatedly, our sample in the Connecticut study is small, with only 65 participants, and derives from a clinic population, suggesting that even this sample may not reflect the range of health, social, and political–economic experiences of Latinx people in southern Connecticut. Fourth, some of the measures used in the California survey were created or adapted for this population, as consistent with decolonial approaches. Although this offers advantages for data validity and the potential to inform interventions in this community setting, these measures have not been evaluated in other populations and may limit the generalizability of findings. Despite these limitations, however, we believe our paper conveys important findings regarding the variety of contributors to mental distress and impediments to care in a diverse population of Latinxs.

5. Conclusions

Based on our findings, several overlapping factors are relevant to improving mental health care services for Latinx (im)migrants. Based on existing research and the findings of this study, discrimination, structural vulnerability, language barriers, identity, culture, access, and cost were all influences on the mental health needs and service usage of this group [107]. Given the breadth of research that has documented the negative effects of systemic racism, xenophobia, and discrimination, we recommend that scholars and practitioners focus on implementing, testing, and refining models for intervention that are responsive to community needs and adaptable to multiple contexts. Our findings highlighted how structural determinants of negative health outcomes overlap with exclusion from mental health resources, which are crystallized in the experiences of mistrust between communities and healthcare services. This mistrust is evident in the traumatic responses of individuals to experiences of discrimination as well as the patterns of mental health knowledge and concern that contribute to anxiety. Utilizing the World Health Organization Optimal Mix of Services Pyramid [108], we propose a comprehensive model for mental health services for Latinx (im)migrant communities, shown in Figure 1.

This model provides a starting point for providers and evaluators to identify the gaps and next steps in solving the inequities that this study has identified. Fundamental to addressing the mental health needs of the widest group of individuals is to expand public health insurance programs, including undocumented individuals of all ages. Further, additional funding and resources are needed to increase access points for service delivery, which often begins with community health workers. Starting from this point, it is vital to ensure accessibility by providing multilingual interpretation services for individuals seeking care. Increasing capacity for these preventative measures can reduce the strain on general and specialty care providers and provide more effective care for all. However, for those who do need more intensive forms of mental health care, it is necessary that providers be structurally competent, meaning that they can assess how environmental and social factors may be influencing the individual health of their patients. Paid interpreters can ensure multilingual services for individuals who may speak any number of Indigenous languages. Lastly, effective advanced health providers and specialty psychiatric services should all be multilingual and trauma-informed, to identify and address the potentially traumatic events influencing individuals' high mental health burden. As detailed in this study, being trauma-informed also means looking beyond clinical measurements and cut-points that can distort and erase migrant community members' experiences.

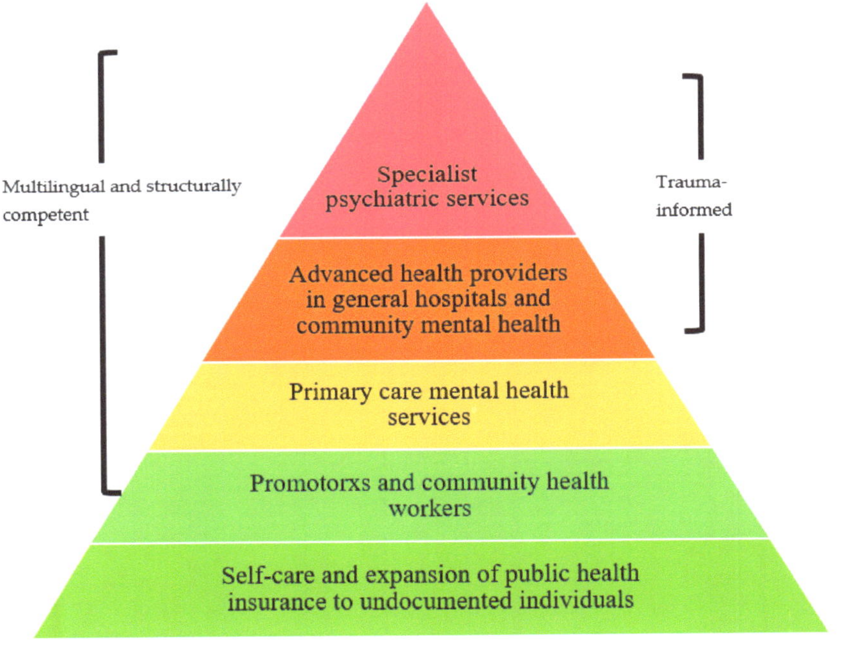

Figure 1. Mental Health Services Pyramid for Latinx (Im)migrant Communities. Note: Adapted from the World Health Organization Optimal Mix of Services Pyramid.

Because many constraints on healthcare capacity derive from funding limitations, comprehensive private and public investment in services and training can improve mental health outcomes for Latinxs. These include expanded insurance coverage for preventative mental health care; increased screening for (im)migrant communities and asylum-seekers; paid, on-site interpreter services including Spanish and Indigenous languages; support for community health workers and promotorxs; and expansion of intensive mental health care services, particularly in rural areas. Further, evaluations of these interventions can inform the implementation of future policymaking and funding strategies.

The findings presented in this paper illuminate multiple directions for future research and evaluation. Researchers should partner with Indigenous language speakers and community leaders to design and implement strategies for decreasing language barriers throughout healthcare systems. Language access is a two-way street. Physicians and other providers need to hear from their patients and understand their perspectives just as much as the other way around. Thus, in addition to assessing factors such as treatment compliance, evaluation of these interventions should also emphasize how providers can improve their efficacy, reach, and impact by working in collaboration with interpreters and community groups. Further, programs for physicians and other healthcare providers to gain structural and cultural competency must be articulated and defined in local contexts. While patterns of exploitation and exclusion create shared patterns of marginalization, lower health access, and worse mental health outcomes, the solutions to these problems must be aligned with local traditions, culture, and leadership.

Author Contributions: Conceptualization, M.A.V.E.-K. and J.P.C.; Data curation, M.A.V.E.-K. and J.P.C.; Formal analysis, M.A.V.E.-K. and J.P.C.; Funding acquisition, M.A.V.E.-K. and J.P.C.; Investigation, M.A.V.E.-K. and J.P.C.; Methodology, M.A.V.E.-K. and J.P.C.; Project administration, M.A.V.E.-K. and J.P.C.; Resources, M.A.V.E.-K. and J.P.C.; Software, M.A.V.E.-K. and J.P.C.; Supervision, M.A.V.E.-K.; Validation, M.A.V.E.-K. and J.P.C.; Visualization, M.A.V.E.-K.; Writing—original draft preparation, M.A.V.E.-K. and J.P.C.; Writing—review and editing, M.A.V.E.-K. and J.P.C. All authors have read and agreed to the published version of the manuscript.

Funding: Authors M.A.V.E.-K. and J.P.C. were supported by the Robert Wood Johnson Foundation through the Health Policy Research Scholars program. M.A.V.E.-K. was also supported by the Health Policy Research Scholars Dissertation Award, Scholars Strategy Network, Community Change Leadership, California Polytechnic State University, San Luis Obispo (Believe, Educate & Empower, Advocate, Collaborate and Nurture (BEACoN) Grant). J.P.C. was also supported by the National Science Foundation Doctoral Dissertation Research Improvement Grant Award 1918769, the Wenner Gren Foundation Dissertation Fieldwork Grant, and the National Institutes of Health Medical Scientist Training Program Grant T32GM136651. The APC was funded by the University of California Santa Barbara Migration Initiative.

Institutional Review Board Statement: This study was conducted in accordance with the Declaration of Helsinki and was approved by the Institutional Review Board (or Ethics Committee) of the University of California, Santa Barbara (Protocol Number: 22-19-0595).

Informed Consent Statement: Informed consent was obtained from all subjects involved in the study.

Acknowledgments: Our thanks go to the participants in both the California and Connecticut studies and to the research assistants at California Polytechnic State University, San Luis Obispo, for the "La Gente Unida" project.

Conflicts of Interest: The authors declare no conflict of interest.

References

1. Pew Research Center. A Brief Statistical Portrait of U.S Hispanics. 2022. Available online: https://www.pewresearch.org/science/2022/06/14/a-brief-statistical-portrait-of-u-s-hispanics/ (accessed on 2 October 2022).
2. Vespa, J.; Medina, L.; Armstrong, D.M. *Demographic Turning Points for the United States: Population Projections for 2020 to 2060*; Current Population Reports; U.S. Census Bureau: Washington, DC, USA, 2020; pp. 25–1144.
3. Noe-Bustamente, L.; Flores, A. Facts on Latinos in America. Pew Research Center's Hispanic Trends Project. 2019. Available online: https://www.pewresearch.org/hispanic/fact-sheet/latinos-in-the-u-s-fact-sheet/ (accessed on 2 October 2022).
4. Ayalew, B.; Dawson-Hahn, E.; Cholera, R.; Falusi, O.; Haro, T.M.; Montoya-Williams, D.; Linton, J.M. The Health of Children in Immigrant Families: Key Drivers and Research Gaps Through an Equity Lens. *Acad. Pediatr.* **2021**, *21*, 777–792. [CrossRef] [PubMed]
5. Berdahl, T.A.; Torres Stone, R.A. Examining Latino Differences in Mental Healthcare Use: The Roles of Acculturation and Attitudes towards Healthcare. *Community Ment. Health J.* **2009**, *45*, 393–403. [CrossRef] [PubMed]
6. Vega, W.A.; Kolody, B.; Aguilar-Gaxiola, S.; Catalano, R. Gaps in Service Utilization by Mexican Americans with Mental Health Problems. *Am. J. Psychiatry* **1999**, *156*, 928–934. [CrossRef]
7. Alegria, M.; Canino, G.; Ríos, R.; Vera, M.; Calderón, J.; Rusch, D.; Ortega, A.N. Mental Health Care for Latinos: Inequalities in Use of Specialty Mental Health Services among Latinos, African Americans, and Non-Latino Whites. *Psychiatr. Serv.* **2002**, *53*, 1547–1555. [CrossRef]
8. Haverluk, T. The Changing Geography of US Hispanics, 1850–1990. *J. Geogr.* **1997**, *96*, 134–145. [CrossRef] [PubMed]
9. Nostrand, R.L. The Hispano Homeland in 1900. *Ann. Assoc. Am. Geogr.* **1980**, *70*, 382–396. [CrossRef]
10. Silva, M.A.; Paris, M.; Añez, L.M. CAMINO: Integrating Context in the Mental Health Assessment of Immigrant Latinos. *Prof. Psychol. Res. Pract.* **2017**, *48*, 453–460. [CrossRef]
11. Substance Abuse and Mental Health Services Administration. *2018 National Survey on Drug Use and Health: Hispanics, Latino or Spanish Origin or Descent*; Substance Abuse and Mental Health Services Association: Rockville, MD, USA, 2020.
12. Lisotto, M.J. *Mental Health Disparities: Hispanics and Latinos*; American Psychiatric Association: Washington, DC, USA, 2017.

13. Alegria, M.; Canino, G.; Shrout, P.E.; Woo, M.; Duan, N.; Vila, D.; Torres, M.; Chen, C.; Meng, X.-L. Prevalence of Mental Illness in Immigrant and Non-Immigrant U.S. Latino Groups. *Am. J. Psychiatry* **2008**, *165*, 359–369. [CrossRef]
14. Acevedo-Garcia, D.; Bates, L.M. Latino Health Paradoxes: Empirical Evidence, Explanations, Future Research, and Implications. In *Latinas/os in the United States: Changing the Face of America*; Springer: Berlin/Heidelberg, Germany, 2008; pp. 101–113.
15. Kann, L.; McManus, T.; Harris, W.A.; Shanklin, S.L.; Flint, K.H.; Queen, B.; Lowry, R.; Chyen, D.; Whittle, L.; Thornton, J.; et al. Youth Risk Behavior Surveillance—United States, 2017. *Surveill. Summ.* **2018**, *67*, 1–114. [CrossRef]
16. Substance Abuse and Mental Health Services Administration. *Behavioral Health Barometer: United States, 2015*; Substance Abuse and Mental Health Services Administration: Rockville, MD, USA, 2015; pp. 1–21.
17. Chu, T.; Keller, A.S.; Rasmussen, A. Effects of Post-Migration Factors on PTSD Outcomes among Immigrant Survivors of Political Violence. *J. Immigr. Minority Health* **2013**, *15*, 890–897.
18. Perreira, K.M.; Ornelas, I. Painful Passages: Traumatic Experiences and Post-Traumatic Stress among US Immigrant Latino Adolescents and Their Primary Caregivers. *Int. Migr. Rev.* **2013**, *47*, 976–1005. [CrossRef] [PubMed]
19. Vogt, W.A. Crossing Mexico: Structural Violence and the Commodification of Undocumented Central American Migrants. *Am. Ethnol.* **2013**, *40*, 764–780. [CrossRef]
20. Vogt, W.A. *Lives in Transit: Violence and Intimacy on the Migrant Journey*; California Series in Public Anthropology; University of California Press: Oakland, CA, USA, 2018; Volume 42.
21. Miller, E.; Decker, M.R.; Silverman, J.G.; Raj, A. Migration, Sexual Exploitation, and Women's Health: A Case Report from a Community Health Center. *Violence Against Women* **2007**, *13*, 486–497. [CrossRef] [PubMed]
22. Watts, C.; Zimmerman, C. Violence against Women: Global Scope and Magnitude. *Lancet* **2002**, *359*, 1232–1237. [CrossRef]
23. Cleaveland, C.; Frankenfeld, C. "They Kill People Over Nothing": An Exploratory Study of Latina Immigrant Trauma. *J. Soc. Serv. Res.* **2020**, *46*, 507–523. [CrossRef]
24. Fortuna, L.R.; Noroña, C.R.; Porche, M.V.; Tillman, C.; Patil, P.A.; Wang, Y.; Markle, S.L.; Alegría, M. Trauma, Immigration, and Sexual Health among Latina Women: Implications for Maternal–Child Well-being and Reproductive Justice. *Infant Ment. Health J.* **2019**, *40*, 640–658. [CrossRef]
25. Kaltman, S.; Hurtado de Mendoza, A.; Serrano, A.; Gonzales, F.A. A Mental Health Intervention Strategy for Low-Income, Trauma-Exposed Latina Immigrants in Primary Care: A Preliminary Study. *Am. J. Orthopsychiatry* **2016**, *86*, 345–354. [CrossRef]
26. Cerdeña, J.P.; Rivera, L.M.; Spak, J.M. Intergenerational Trauma in Latinxs: A Scoping Review. *Soc. Sci. Med.* **2021**, *270*, 113662. [CrossRef]
27. Treisman, R. NPR. Whistleblower Alleges "Medical Neglect", Questionable Hysterectomies of ICE Detainees. 2020. Available online: https://www.npr.org/2020/09/16/913398383/whistleblower-alleges-medical-neglect-questionable-hysterectomies-of-ice-detaine (accessed on 2 October 2022).
28. Cariello, A.N.; Perrin, P.B.; Williams, C.D.; Espinoza, G.A.; Morlett-Paredes, A.; Moreno, O.A.; Trujillo, M.A. Moderating Influence of Enculturation on the Relations between Minority Stressors and Physical Health via Anxiety in Latinx Immigrants. *Cult. Divers. Ethn. Minority Psychol.* **2020**, *26*, 356–366. [CrossRef]
29. Andrews, A.R.I.; Haws, J.K.; Acosta, L.M.; Acosta Canchila, M.N.; Carlo, G.; Grant, K.M.; Ramos, A.K. Combinatorial Effects of Discrimination, Legal Status Fears, Adverse Childhood Experiences, and Harsh Working Conditions among Latino Migrant Farmworkers: Testing Learned Helplessness Hypotheses. *J. Lat. Psychol.* **2020**, *8*, 179–201. [CrossRef]
30. Tran, A.G.T.T.; Lee, R.M.; Burgess, D.J. Perceived Discrimination and Substance Use in Hispanic/Latino, African-Born Black, and Southeast Asian Immigrants. *Cult. Divers. Ethn. Minority Psychol.* **2010**, *16*, 226–236. [CrossRef]
31. Bekteshi, V.; Kang, S. Contextualizing Acculturative Stress among Latino Immigrants in the United States: A Systematic Review. *Ethn. Health* **2020**, *25*, 897–914. [CrossRef] [PubMed]
32. Wang, J.S.-H.; Kaushal, N. Health and Mental Health Effects of Local Immigration Enforcement. *Int. Migr. Rev.* **2019**, *53*, 970–1001. [CrossRef]
33. Martinez, O.; Wu, E.; Sandfort, T.; Dodge, B.; Carballo-Dieguez, A.; Pinto, R.; Rhodes, S.D.; Moya, E.; Chavez-Baray, S. Evaluating the Impact of Immigration Policies on Health Status Among Undocumented Immigrants: A Systematic Review. *J. Immigr. Minor. Health* **2015**, *17*, 947–970. [CrossRef]
34. Becerra, D.; Hernandez, G.; Porchas, F.; Castillo, J.; Nguyen, V.; Perez González, R. Immigration Policies and Mental Health: Examining the Relationship between Immigration Enforcement and Depression, Anxiety, and Stress among Latino Immigrants. *J. Ethn. Cult. Divers. Soc. Work. Innov. Theory Res. Pract.* **2020**, *29*, 43–59. [CrossRef]
35. Garcini, L.M.; Renzaho, A.M.N.; Molina, M.; Ayala, G.X. Health-Related Quality of Life among Mexican-Origin Latinos: The Role of Immigration Legal Status. *Ethn. Health* **2018**, *23*, 566–581. [CrossRef]
36. Vargas, E.D.; Sanchez, G.R.; Juárez, M. Fear by Association: Perceptions of Anti-Immigrant Policy and Health Outcomes. *J. Health Politics Policy Law* **2017**, *42*, 459–483. [CrossRef]
37. Lara-Cinisomo, S.; Fujimoto, E.M.; Oksas, C.; Jian, Y.; Gharheeb, A. Pilot Study Exploring Migration Experiences and Perinatal Depressive and Anxiety Symptoms in Immigrant Latinas. *Matern. Child Health J.* **2019**, *23*, 1627–1647. [CrossRef]
38. Rhodes, S.D.; Mann, L.; Simán, F.M.; Song, E.; Alonzo, J.; Downs, M.; Lawlor, E.; Martinez, O.; Sun, C.J.; O'Brien, M.C. The Impact of Local Immigration Enforcement Policies on the Health of Immigrant Hispanics/Latinos in the United States. *Am. J. Public Health* **2015**, *105*, 329–337. [CrossRef]

39. Bruzelius, E.; Baum, A. The Mental Health of Hispanic/Latino Americans Following National Immigration Policy Changes: United States, 2014–2018. *Am. J. Public Health* **2019**, *109*, 1786–1788. [CrossRef]
40. Hacker, K.; Chu, J.; Leung, C.; Marra, R.; Pirie, A.; Brahimi, M.; English, M.; Beckmann, J.; Acevedo-Garcia, D.; Marlin, R.P. The Impact of Immigration and Customs Enforcement on Immigrant Health: Perceptions of Immigrants in Everett, Massachusetts, USA. *Soc. Sci. Med.* **2011**, *73*, 586–594. [CrossRef] [PubMed]
41. Lopez, W.D.; Kruger, D.J.; Delva, J.; Llanes, M.; Ledón, C.; Waller, A.; Harner, M.; Martinez, R.; Sanders, L.; Harner, M.; et al. Health Implications of an Immigration Raid: Findings from a Latino Community in the Midwestern United States. *J. Immigr. Minority Health* **2017**, *19*, 702–708. [CrossRef] [PubMed]
42. Chishti, M.; Pierce, S.; Bolter, J. The Obama Record on Deportations: Deporter in Chief or Not? Available online: https://www.migrationpolicy.org/article/obama-record-deportations-deporter-chief-or-not (accessed on 17 September 2020).
43. American Immigration Council Summary of Executive Order "Enhancing Public Safety in the Interior of the United States". Available online: https://www.americanimmigrationcouncil.org/immigration-interior-enforcement-executive-order (accessed on 17 September 2020).
44. Ramos-Sánchez, L.; Pietrantonio, K.; Llamas, J. The Psychological Impact of Immigration Status on Undocumented Latinx Women: Recommendations for Mental Health Providers. *Peace Confl.* **2020**, *26*, 149–161. [CrossRef]
45. Trump, D.J. Executive Order: Enhancing Public Safety in the Interior of the United States. Available online: https://www.federalregister.gov/documents/2017/01/30/2017-02102/enhancing-public-safety-in-the-interior-of-the-united-states (accessed on 17 September 2020).
46. Immigrant Legal Resource Center National Map of 287(g) Agreements. Available online: https://datawrapper.dwcdn.net/PKrP1/4/ (accessed on 22 August 2022).
47. U.S. Citizenship and Immigration Services Temporary Protected Status Designated Country: Nicaragua. Available online: https://www.uscis.gov/humanitarian/temporary-protected-status/temporary-protected-status-designated-country-nicaragua (accessed on 17 September 2020).
48. Miller, M.E. Washington Post. 'They Just Took Them?' Frantic Parents Separated from Their Kids Fill Courts on the Border. 2018. Available online: https://www.washingtonpost.com/local/they-just-took-them-frantic-parents-separated-from-their-kids-fill-courts-on-the-border/2018/06/09/e3f5170c-6aa9-11e8-bea7-c8eb28bc52b1_story.html (accessed on 2 October 2022).
49. The Independent "Words Matter": Trump Accused of Fuelling Attacks on Hispanics as Violent Hate Crimes Hit 16-Year High. 2019. Available online: https://www.independent.co.uk/news/world/americas/hate-crimes-racism-violence-us-fbi-hispanic-a9200671.html (accessed on 2 October 2022).
50. Bourgois, P.; Holmes, S.M.; Sue, K.; Quesada, J. Structural Vulnerability: Operationalizing the Concept to Address Health Disparities in Clinical Care. *Acad. Med. J. Assoc. Am. Med. Coll.* **2017**, *92*, 299. [CrossRef] [PubMed]
51. Kasich, J. Personal Responsibility and Work Opportunity Reconciliation Act of 1996. *Contemp. Sociol.* **1997**, *26*, 409–415.
52. Quinn, E.; Kinoshita, S. *An Overview of Public Charge and Benefits*; Immigrant Legal Resource Center: San Francisco, CA, USA, 2020; pp. 1–7.
53. Artiga, S.; Diaz, M. Kaiser Family Foundation. Health Coverage and Care of Undocumented Immigrants. 2019. Available online: https://www.kff.org/racial-equity-and-health-policy/issue-brief/health-coverage-and-care-of-undocumented-immigrants/ (accessed on 2 October 2022).
54. Bucay-Harari, L.; Page, K.R.; Krawczyk, N.; Robles, Y.P.; Castillo-Salgado, C. Mental Health Needs of an Emerging Latino Community. *J. Behav. Health Serv. Res.* **2020**, *47*, 388–398. [CrossRef]
55. Cohen, R.A.; Cha, A.E.; Martinez, M.E.; Terlizzi, E.P. *Health Insurance Coverage: Early Release of Estimates from the National Health Interview Survey, 2019*; National Center for Health Statistics: Atlanta, GA, USA, 2020; pp. 1–18.
56. Office of the Surgeon General; Center for Mental Health Services; National Institute of Mental Health. *Mental Health: Culture, Race, and Ethnicity: A Supplement to Mental Health: A Report of the Surgeon General*; Publications and Reports of the Surgeon General; Substance Abuse and Mental Health Services Administration (US): Rockville, MD, USA, 2001.
57. Hudson, J.L.; Miller, G.E.; Kirby, J.B. Explaining Racial and Ethnic Differences in Children's Use of Stimulant Medications. *Med. Care* **2007**, *45*, 1068–1075. [CrossRef]
58. Kirby, J.B.; Hudson, J.; Miller, G.E. Explaining Racial and Ethnic Differences in Antidepressant Use Among Adolescents. *Med. Care Res. Rev.* **2010**, *67*, 342–363. [CrossRef]
59. Galvan, F.H.; Bogart, L.M.; Klein, D.J.; Wagner, G.J.; Chen, Y.-T. Medical Mistrust as a Key Mediator in the Association between Perceived Discrimination and Adherence to Antiretroviral Therapy among HIV-Positive Latino Men. *J. Behav. Med.* **2017**, *40*, 784–793. [CrossRef]
60. López-Cevallos, D.F.; Harvey, S.M.; Warren, J.T. Medical Mistrust, Perceived Discrimination, and Satisfaction With Health Care Among Young-Adult Rural Latinos. *J. Rural. Health* **2014**, *30*, 344–351. [CrossRef]
61. López-Cevallos, D.F.; Flórez, K.R.; Derose, K.P. Examining the Association between Religiosity and Medical Mistrust among Churchgoing Latinos in Long Beach, CA. *Transl. Behav. Med.* **2019**, *11*, 114–121. [CrossRef] [PubMed]
62. Czeisler, M.É.; Marynak, K.; Klarke, K.E.N.; Salah, Z.; Shakya, I.; Thierry, J.M.; Ali, N.; McMillan, H.; Wiley, J.; Weaver, M.D.; et al. Delay or Avoidance of Medical Care Because of COVID-19–Related Concerns. *MMWR Morb. Mortal. Wkly Rep.* **2020**, *69*, 1250–1257. [CrossRef] [PubMed]

63. Garcini, L.M.; Domenech Rodríguez, M.M.; Mercado, A.; Paris, M. A Tale of Two Crises: The Compounded Effect of COVID-19 and Anti-Immigration Policy in the United States. *Psychol. Trauma Theory Res. Pract. Policy* **2020**, *12*, S230. [CrossRef]
64. Garcini, L.M.; Murray, K.E.; Zhou, A.; Klonoff, E.A.; Myers, M.G.; Elder, J.P. Mental Health of Undocumented Immigrant Adults in the United States: A Systematic Review of Methodology and Findings. *J. Immigr. Refug. Stud.* **2016**, *14*, 1–25. [CrossRef]
65. Caballero, T.M.; Ross DeCamp, L.; Platt, R.E.; Shah, H.; Johnson, S.B.; Sibinga, E.M.S.; Polk, S. Addressing the Mental Health Needs of Latino Children in Immigrant Families. *Clin. Pediatr.* **2017**, *56*, 648–658. [CrossRef]
66. Kim, G.; Loi, C.X.A.; Chiriboga, D.A.; Jang, Y.; Parmelee, P.; Allen, R.S. Limited English Proficiency as a Barrier to Mental Health Service Use: A Study of Latino and Asian Immigrants with Psychiatric Disorders. *J. Psychiatr. Res.* **2011**, *45*, 104–110. [CrossRef] [PubMed]
67. Timmins, C.L. The Impact of Language Barriers on the Health Care of Latinos in the United States: A Review of the Literature and Guidelines for Practice. *J. Midwifery Women's Health* **2002**, *47*, 80–96. [CrossRef]
68. Yun, K.; Jenicek, G.; Gerdes, M. Overcoming Language Barriers in Mental and Behavioral Health Care for Children and Adolescents—Policies and Priorities. *JAMA Pediatr.* **2019**, *173*, 511–512. [CrossRef]
69. Alegría, M.; Álvarez, K.; DiMarzio, K. Immigration and Mental Health. *Curr. Epidemiol. Rep.* **2017**, *4*, 145–155. [CrossRef]
70. Bauer, H.M.; Rodriguez, M.A.; Quiroga, S.S.; Flores-Ortiz, Y.G. Barriers to Health Care for Abused Latina and Asian Immigrant Women. *J. Health Care Poor Underserved* **2000**, *11*, 33–44. [CrossRef]
71. Luque, J.S.; Soulen, G.; Davila, C.B.; Cartmell, K. Access to Health Care for Uninsured Latina Immigrants in South Carolina. *BMC Health Serv. Res.* **2018**, *18*, 310. [CrossRef] [PubMed]
72. Jacob, M.M. *Yakama Rising: Indigenous Cultural Revitalization, Activism, and Healing*; University of Arizona Press: Tucson, AZ, USA, 2013; ISBN 978-0-8165-9921-9.
73. Jolivétte, A.J. *Indian Blood: HIV and Colonial Trauma in San Francisco's Two-Spirit Community*; University of Washington Press: Seattle, WA, USA, 2016; ISBN 978-0-295-99849-7.
74. Rodriguez-Lonebear, D. Building a Data Revolution in Indian Country. In *Indigenous Data Sovereignty: Toward an Agenda*; Kukutai, T., Taylor, J., Eds.; Australian National University Press: Canberra, ACT, Australia, 2016; pp. 253–272.
75. Smith, L.T. *Decolonizing Methodologies: Research and Indigenous Peoples*, 2nd ed.; Zed Books: London, UK, 2012; ISBN 978-1-84813-950-3.
76. Blackwell, M.; Boj Lopez, F.; Urrieta, L. Special Issue: Critical Latinx Indigeneities. *Lat. Stud.* **2017**, *15*, 126–137. [CrossRef]
77. Johnson, H.; Perez, C.A.; Mejia, M.C. *Immigrants in California*; Public Policy Institute of California: San Francisco, CA, USA, 2021.
78. American Immigration Council Immigrants in Connecticut; American Immigration Council: 2015. Available online: https://www.americanimmigrationcouncil.org/research/immigrants-connecticut (accessed on 2 October 2022).
79. Bloss, W. Escalating U.S. Police Surveillance after 9/11: An Examination of Causes and Effects. *Surveill. Soc.* **2007**, *4*. [CrossRef]
80. Hurtado-de-Mendoza, A.; Gonzales, F.A.; Serrano, A.; Kaltman, S. Social Isolation and Perceived Barriers to Establishing Social Networks Among Latina Immigrants. *Am. J. Community Psychol.* **2014**, *53*, 73–82. [CrossRef]
81. Spitzer, R.L.; Kroenke, K.; Williams, J.B.W.; Löwe, B. A Brief Measure for Assessing Generalized Anxiety Disorder: The GAD-7. *Arch. Intern. Med.* **2006**, *166*, 1092–1097. [CrossRef]
82. Villegas, M.; Ebarb, A.; Pytalski, S.; Roubideaux, Y. *Disaggregating American Indian & Alaska Native Data: A Review of Literature*; National Congress of American Indians: Washington, DC, USA, 2016.
83. Potochnick, S.R.; Perreira, K.M. Depression and Anxiety among First-Generation Immigrant Latino Youth: Key Correlates and Implications for Future Research. *J. Nerv. Ment. Dis.* **2010**, *198*, 470–477. [CrossRef]
84. Keller, A.; Joscelyne, A.; Granski, M.; Rosenfeld, B. Pre-Migration Trauma Exposure and Mental Health Functioning among Central American Migrants Arriving at the US Border. *PLoS ONE* **2017**, *12*, e0168692. [CrossRef]
85. National Science Foundation Doctoral Dissertation Research: Biosocial Dynamics of Intergenerational Transmission of Stress. Available online: https://www.nsf.gov/awardsearch/showAward?AWD_ID=1918769&HistoricalAwards=false (accessed on 2 October 2022).
86. Jessica, P. The Wenner-Gren Foundation Cerdena. Available online: https://wennergren.org/grantee/jessica-cerdena/ (accessed on 17 September 2020).
87. Kofman, J. Trint. 2020. Available online: https://trint.com/about-us (accessed on 2 October 2022).
88. Geertz, C. Thick Description: Toward an Interpretive Theory of Culture. In *The Cultural Geography Reader*; Routledge: New York, NY, USA, 2008; pp. 41–51.
89. Jolivétte, A.J. (Ed.) *Research Justice: Methodologies for Social Change*, 1st ed.; Bristol University Press: Bristol, UK, 2015.
90. Collins, P.H. Toward a New Vision: Race, Class, and Gender as Categories of Analysis and Connection. Available online: https://www.taylorfrancis.com/ (accessed on 9 January 2020).
91. Derr, A.S. Mental Health Service Use among Immigrants in the United States: A Systematic Review. *Psychiatr. Serv.* **2016**, *67*, 265–274. [CrossRef]
92. Diaz, Y.; Fenning, P. Toward Understanding Mental Health Concerns for the Latinx Immigrant Student: A Review of the Literature. *Urban Educ.* **2017**, *56*, 959–981. [CrossRef]
93. Gonzales, R.G.; Suárez-Orozco, C.; Dedios-Sanguineti, M.C. No Place to Belong: Contextualizing Concepts of Mental Health among Undocumented Immigrant Youth in the United States. *Am. Behav. Sci.* **2013**, *57*, 1174–1199. [CrossRef]

94. Gorter, J.W.; Stewart, D.; Smith, M.W.; King, G.; Wright, M.; Nguyen, T.; Freeman, M.; Swinton, M. Pathways toward Positive Psychosocial Outcomes and Mental Health for Youth with Disabilities: A Knowledge Synthesis of Developmental Trajectories. *Can. J. Community Ment. Health* **2014**, *33*, 45–61. [CrossRef]
95. Starr, S.; Campbell, L.R.; Herrick, C.A. Factors Affecting Use of the Mental Health System by Rural Children. *Issues Ment. Health Nurs.* **2002**, *23*, 291–304. [CrossRef] [PubMed]
96. Iturralde, E.; Chi, F.W.; Grant, R.W.; Weisner, C.; Van Dyke, L.; Pruzansky, A.; Bui, S.; Madvig, P.; Pearl, R.; Sterling, S.A. Association of Anxiety with High-Cost Health Care Use Among Individuals With Type 2 Diabetes. *Dia Care* **2019**, *42*, 1669–1674. [CrossRef] [PubMed]
97. Arbona, C.; Olvera, N.; Rodriguez, N.; Hagan, J.; Linares, A.; Wiesner, M. Acculturative Stress among Documented and Undocumented Latino Immigrants in the United States. *Hisp. J. Behav. Sci.* **2010**, *32*, 362–384. [CrossRef]
98. Caplan, S. Latinos, Acculturation, and Acculturative Stress: A Dimensional Concept Analysis. *Policy Politics Nurs. Pract.* **2007**, *8*, 93–106. [CrossRef]
99. Hovey, J.D.; King, C.A. Acculturative Stress, Depression, and Suicidal Ideation among Immigrant and Second-Generation Latino Adolescents. *J. Am. Acad. Child Adolesc. Psychiatry* **1996**, *35*, 1183–1192. [CrossRef]
100. Torres, L.; Driscoll, M.W.; Voell, M. Discrimination, Acculturation, Acculturative Stress, and Latino Psychological Distress: A Moderated Mediational Model. *Cult. Divers. Ethn. Minority Psychol.* **2012**, *18*, 17. [CrossRef]
101. Willen, S.S. Do "Illegal" Im/Migrants Have a Right to Health? Engaging Ethical Theory as Social Practice at a Tel Aviv Open Clinic. *Med. Anthropol. Q.* **2011**, *25*, 303–330. [CrossRef]
102. Willen, S.S. How Is Health-Related "Deservingness" Reckoned? Perspectives from Unauthorized Im/Migrants in Tel Aviv. *Soc. Sci. Med.* **2012**, *74*, 812–821. [CrossRef]
103. McGuire, S.S. Agency, Initiative, and Obstacles to Health Among Indigenous Immigrant Women from Oaxaca, Mexico. *Home Health Care Manag. Pract.* **2006**, *18*, 370–377. [CrossRef]
104. Burgess, D.; Lee, R.; Tran, A.; van Ryn, M. Effects of Perceived Discrimination on Mental Health and Mental Health Services Utilization Among Gay, Lesbian, Bisexual and Transgender Persons. *J. LGBT Health Res.* **2007**, *3*, 1–14. [CrossRef] [PubMed]
105. Díaz, R.M.; Ayala, G.; Bein, E.; Henne, J.; Marin, B.V. The Impact of Homophobia, Poverty, and Racism on the Mental Health of Gay and Bisexual Latino Men: Findings from 3 US Cities. *Am. J. Public Health* **2001**, *91*, 927–932. [PubMed]
106. Zea, M.C.; Reisen, C.A.; Poppen, P.J. Psychological Well-Being among Latino Lesbians and Gay Men. *Cult. Divers. Ethn. Minority Psychol.* **1999**, *5*, 371–379. [CrossRef]
107. Mio, J.S.; Iwamasa, G.Y. *Culturally Diverse Mental Health: The Challenges of Research and Resistance*; Routledge: New York, NY, USA, 2013; ISBN 978-1-317-79475-2.
108. World Health Organization. *Improving Health Systems and Services for Mental Health*; World Health Organization: Geneva, Switzerland, 2009.

International Journal of
Environmental Research and Public Health

MDPI

Article

Hoping for a Better Future during COVID-19: How Migration Plans Are Protective of Depressive Symptoms for Haitian Migrants Living in Chile

Yijing Chen [1], Claudia Rafful [2,3], Mercedes Mercado [4], Lindsey Carte [5], Sonia Morales-Miranda [6], Judeline Cheristil [7] and Teresita Rocha-Jiménez [8,9,*]

1 Department of Sociomedical Sciences, Mailman School of Public Health, Columbia University, 722 W 168th St, New York, NY 10032, USA
2 Faculty of Psychology, Universidad Nacional Autonoma de Mexico, Circuito Ciudad Universitaria Avenida, C.U., Mexico City 04510, Mexico
3 Center for Global Mental Health, National Institute of Psychiatry, Calz México-Xochimilco 101, Colonia, Huipulco, Tlalpan, Mexico City 14370, Mexico
4 Faculty of Psychology, Universidad Diego Portales, Santiago 8320000, Chile
5 Núcleo de Ciencias Sociales y Humanidades, Universidad de la Frontera, Francisco Salazar 1450, Temuco 4811230, Chile
6 Consorcio de Investigación sobre VIH SIDA TB CISIDAT, Dwight W. Morrow 8, Apt. 7, Centro, Cuernavaca 62000, Mexico
7 Project "When Reality Overcomes the Intention", Las Condes 7560908, Chile
8 Society and Health Research Center, Facultad de Ciencias Sociales y Artes, Universidad Mayor, Las Condes 4780000, Chile
9 Millennium Nucleus on Sociomedicine (SocioMed), Las Condes 7560908, Chile
* Correspondence: teresita.rocha@umayor.cl

Citation: Chen, Y.; Rafful, C.; Mercado, M.; Carte, L.; Morales-Miranda, S.; Cheristil, J.; Rocha-Jiménez, T. Hoping for a Better Future during COVID-19: How Migration Plans Are Protective of Depressive Symptoms for Haitian Migrants Living in Chile. *Int. J. Environ. Res. Public Health* **2022**, *19*, 9977. https://doi.org/10.3390/ijerph19169977

Academic Editors: Maria De Jesus and Ernesto Castañeda

Received: 14 July 2022
Accepted: 10 August 2022
Published: 12 August 2022

Abstract: This paper explores the migration experiences, perceived COVID-19 impacts, and depression symptoms among Haitian migrants living in Santiago, Chile. Ninety-five participants from eight neighborhoods with a high density of Haitian migrants were recruited. Descriptive statistics, univariate analysis, and logistic regression analysis were conducted. Chi-squared tests were used to confirm univariate results. We found that 22% of participants had major depressive symptoms based on the CESD-R-20 scale, 87% reported major life changes due to COVID-19, and 78% said their migration plans had changed due to the pandemic. Factors associated with more depressive symptoms were being in debt (OR = 3.43) and experiencing discrimination (ORs: 0.60 to 6.19). Factors associated with less odds of depressive symptoms were social support (ORs: 0.06 to 0.25), change in migration plans due to COVID-19 (OR = 0.30), and planning to leave Chile (OR = 0.20). After accounting for relevant factors, planning to leave Chile is significantly predictive of fewer symptoms of depression. Haitian migrants living in Chile had a high prevalence of depression. Planning to leave Chile was a significant protector against depressive symptoms. Future studies should explore how nuanced experiences of uncertainty play out in migrants' lives, mental well-being, and planning for their future.

Keywords: migration; mental and health illness; Chile; COVID-19; social support; racism

1. Introduction

Migration has been linked to multiple risk and stress factors that negatively affect the health of migrants, especially their mental health [1–5]. Research has found various pathways and factors that worsen or ameliorate these negative influences, but most of them do not focus on the complexity of the migration process [2,4,6–10]. As the increase in natural disasters, wars, and internal conflicts have placed a growing population of migrants in cities or countries that they did not intend or plan to move to [4,11–14], few studies have zoomed in on migrants' trajectories and considered the wide range of possible migration patterns within this population [8,10,15–17]. Nevertheless, some studies have found that certain migration trajectories are associated with negative mental health outcomes [2,7,8,10].

During the COVID-19 pandemic, many migrants found themselves in indeterminate circumstances. It is essential to investigate how these migration experiences and patterns impact their mental health status [18,19]. Reports have documented rising levels of anxiety, depression, self-harm, and psychotic symptoms when compared to pre-COVID-19 years [18,20,21]. For some migrant populations, particularly Asians, the limits on movements have posed unique challenges as they could no longer connect with members in their social networks and must cope with rising levels of discrimination [19,20,22]. In general, migrants are often affected by the intersection of class, race, and legal status that hinder their ability to avoid the infection, receive healthcare when needed, and cope with the economic, social, and psychological impacts of the pandemic [23–26]. Furthermore, COVID-19 has increased precariousness and uncertainty for migrant groups that were already in uncertain situations [13,19,20,23,24,26].

Haitian migrants have a history of migrating to countries within Latin America and the Caribbean, such as Colombia and the Dominican Republic, where they have experienced discrimination, xenophobia, and racism. These have issues translated into social and geographical segregation, and issues regularizing their migration status, and thus Haitian migrants eventually decided to migrate to other countries such as Chile and Brazil [27–29]. The first wave of Haitian migrants arrived in Chile in 2015 as this country showed economic and political strength and had relatively welcoming migration policies prior to the 2018 migration reform [30,31]. Furthermore, Chile had an important presence in the United Nations Mission in Haiti (UNMIH) post the 2010 earthquake, which built a relationship between these two countries. In 2015 the Chilean government gave close to 9000 Temporary Resident Visas to Haitians [32]. Nevertheless, the Chilean migration reform in 2018, requiring visa for entry, and other administrative obstacles, countered the ease of entering and staying in Chile for Haitians. Haitians' necessity to find a safe place to migrate makes them susceptible to the effects of new migration and mobility patterns, given their recent migration to non-traditional destination countries such as Chile and more recently Mexico, as well as complicated landscape of migration policies [33].

In addition, while they are staying in places like Chile and Mexico in uncertain times, the exacerbated socioeconomic conditions and the restrictive immigration policies exacerbated by the pandemic may expose them to greater risks of depression and may change their migration plans [18,23,33].

Given the aforementioned context, this paper aimed to analyze the association between specific migration plans such as remaining in the transit country and potential major depressive symptoms among a sample of Haitian migrants living in Chile. Additionally, in the context of the COVID-19 pandemic and the uncertainty with which Haitian migrants live in Chile, and that hopes and plans for the future may be a protective factor for depression [7], we also hypothesized that those who report planning to stay in Chile would have higher odds of having symptoms of depression in comparison who those who are planning to leave.

2. Materials and Methods

2.1. Conceptual Framework

Our analysis was guided by a modified version of Bhugra's Migration Phases and Psychiatric Disorders framework [2]. This framework considers migration experiences or plans while recognizing vulnerabilities (e.g., complex destination migration experiences) and resilience components (e.g., social support) in analyzing the relationship between migration and psychiatric disorders (Figure 1) [2,34–36]. Based on previous studies on transit migrants [7,37], the current global migration context, and the restrictive migration policies in Chile, we hypothesized that those who report planning to stay in Chile would have higher odds of having symptoms of depression in comparison with those who are planning to leave. For this analysis, we focused on the post-migration experiences (i.e., their current life in Chile) and their intended or future migration plans.

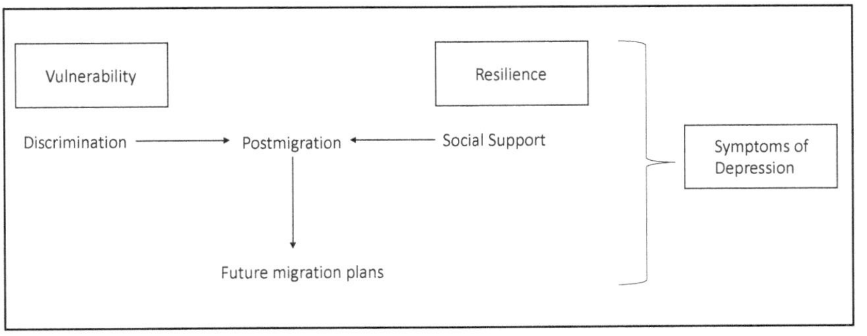

Figure 1. Migration Experiences and Psychiatric Disorders Framework.

2.2. Data Collection

As a part of an ongoing sequential mixed-method project started in February 2021, we recruited 101 Haitian migrants in Santiago de Chile. The qualitative component of this study aimed to understand more in depth the migration trajectories and mental health status of our sample. For the purposes of this article, we report the quantitative results only. Sampling originally started by inviting participants using the respondent-driven sampling (RDS) method to approximate generalizable samples of segregated populations [38–40]. However, as data collection progressed, we observed that the contacts of those who planned to migrate out of Chile were less likely to be invited than the contacts of those planning to stay. Therefore, we decided to switch to a two-stage conglomerate sampling approach. The first stage involved subsampling and stratifying neighborhoods with a higher density of Haitian migrants in the Metropolitan Region of Santiago [41]. The neighborhoods with a higher density of Haitian migrants also have migrant camps inside them where a significant number of Haitian migrants live. We also selected neighborhoods based on the field staff's community presence, and those were also the safest neighborhoods. The neighborhoods selected (e.g., Cerrillos, Estación Central, Santiago Centro) are mainly located in downtown Santiago and in the south of the city and have a historical presence of migrant camps. In the second stage, residents in each selected neighborhood were invited to participate. No one was excluded, and everyone who met the eligibility criteria and gave consent completed the survey.

Eligibility criteria for this study included (a) 18 years old or older; (b) Spanish or Creole speaker; (c) willing and able to provide informed consent; (d) born in Haiti, and (e) living in Chile at the time of the interview. The instruments used for this study were prepared in Spanish and translated to Creole (i.e., written consent forms, informational flyer, survey). Two members of the field staff were bilingual, so the participant could choose to complete the survey in Spanish or Creole. Staff provided a copy of the consent form and explained the study to potential participants, including the purpose, procedures to be followed, and risks and benefits of participation. Along with the consent form, staff provided a flyer with relevant mental health information, resources, and the project psychologist's contact information in case any participant wanted to speak with her in private or schedule an appointment. Upon receipt of written consent, staff conducted face-to-face interviews using Survio, a computer-assisted personal interviewing technology (https://www.survio.com/es/, accessed on 15 February 2021). We conducted all the surveys face-to-face in open spaces (i.e., outside participants' houses, in parks) or, when preferred by the participant, inside their homes or in chapels. The survey took 30–50 min to complete and included questions on sociodemographics, identity, discrimination, social support, migration plans and experiences, perceived consequences of COVID-19, access to health services, geospatial elements (e.g., living and working locations), and a mental health scale to evaluate possible symptoms of depression (i.e., CESD-R-20 items).

2.3. Ethics Procedure

We invited representatives from three key local migrant organizations, one of which was founded by Haitian migrants, to form a Community Advisory Board (CAB). We met with each organization via Zoom to discuss the following items: (a) recruitment and the invitation process, (b) the amount and type of compensation, (c) language, length, and content of the survey, and (d) dissemination strategies. The role of the CAB was essential to recognize the power imbalance between the researchers and participants, and the importance of having the community involved in the decision-making processes of the study [42,43]. After meeting with the CAB, we confirmed the importance of not asking for any private information, including names or personal identification numbers (i.e., RUN, used in official documents and purchases in Chile). Each participant had a code, and we only collected contact information if they wanted to meet with the psychologist or if they wanted to participate in the qualitative component of the study. Participants were compensated with a $6 USD gift card to be used in a grocery store (i.e., Lider) for participating in the interview. The project was approved by the Scientific Ethics Committee of the PI University.

2.4. Dependent Variable

Depressive symptoms were assessed with the self-reported Center for Epidemiologic Studies Depressive Scale—Revised 20-item (CESD-R-20) [44,45]. The CESD-R-20 defines a score equal to or above 16 (out of 60) at risk for clinical depression. An adapted Spanish version of the CESD-R-20 instrument was used in this study [46–49]. Bilingual staff translated the CESD-R-20 scale from Spanish to Creole, then we did a back-translation to ensure that the first translation was accurate. Details of the validation process are explained elsewhere [50]. As the participants had the option to choose their preferred language for the survey, some responded to the original CESD-R-20 in Spanish ($n = 32$) and others in Creole ($n = 63$).

2.5. Independent Variables

Sociodemographic variables included age, gender, marital status (i.e., married or common-law vs. single, divorced, or widowed), self-defined group membership (e.g., migrant and/or Haitian, and/or Chilean), education level, religious affiliation and service attendance, and perceived financial situation (See Table 1).

2.5.1. Migration Experiences

Participants were given a mix of multiple choice and open-ended questions. Participants' history of migration was constructed by asking the age in which they left their country of origin, the length of their stay in Chile, reasons for leaving their country of origin, migration plans (e.g., Did you want to migrate to Chile when you left your country?), reasons for wanting to leave Chile (for those who expressed wanting to depart), and whether their migration plans had changed due to the COVID-19 pandemic (Table 2). We also asked questions about any experiences of discrimination while living in Chile.

Table 1. Sociodemographic characteristics by symptoms of depression among Haitian migrants in Santiago de Chile 2021 (n = 95).

Characteristics	Total Sample (n = 95)	No Symptoms of Depression (n = 74) 78%	Symptoms of Depression (n = 21) 22%
Age [median (IQR)]	33 (28–37)	31 (27–37)	34 (29–39)
Gender			
Male	47 (49%)	39 (53%)	9 (38%)
Female	48 (51%)	35 (47%)	13 (62%)
Self-reported group membership [1]			
Migrant	29 (31%)	18 (24%)	11 (52%)
Haitian	65 (68%)	55 (74%)	10 (48%)
Chilean	4 (4%)	3 (4%)	1 (4%)
Marital status			
Married/with partner	46 (48%)	33 (45%)	13 (62%)
Single/no partner	49 (52%)	41 (55%)	9 (38%)
Level of education			
Less than elementary school	12 (13%)	9 (12%)	3 (14%)
Completed elementary school	42 (44%)	31 (42%)	11 (52%)
Completed secondary school	38 (40%)	32 (43%)	6 (29%)
Completed university	3 (3%)	2 (3%)	1 (4%)
Has children	67 (71%)	50 (68%)	17 (81%)
Religion			
Affiliated with a religion	73 (77%)	67 (91%)	16 (76%)
Planned to move to Chile in the first place	74 (78%)	61 (82%)	13 (62%)
Length of stay in Chile in years [median (IQR)] (n = 86)	4.58 (4–5)	4.59 (4–5)	4.53 (4–5)

[1] These groups are not mutually exclusive.

Table 2. Univariate association with symptoms of depression among Haitian migrants in Santiago de Chile (n = 95).

Predictor	Count [CESD < 16] n = 74	Count [CESD ≥ 16] n = 21	Odds Ratio (95% CI)	p-Value
	Sociodemographic			
Gender (female)	35 (47%)	13 (62%)	1.81 (0.67, 4.88)	0.240
Age	32.51	33.52	-	-
Marital status (married)	33 (45%)	13 (62%)	2.02 (0.75, 5.45)	0.164
Self-reported group membership				
Migrant	18 (24%)	11 (52%)	3.42 (1.25, 9.37)	0.014 *
Haitian	55 (74%)	10 (48%)	0.31 (0.12, 0.86)	0.021 *
Level of education (did not complete primary school)	9 (12%)	3 (14%)	1.20 (0.29, 4.92)	0.797
Have kids	50 (68%)	17 (81%)	2.04 (0.62, 6.73)	0.238
Have children living in Haiti	28 (39%)	5 (24%)	0.51 (0.17, 1.56)	0.236
Language of interview (Creole)	57 (77%)	6 (30%)	0.12 (0.04, 0.36)	<0.001 **
	Financial Situation			
Unemployed	48 (65%)	12 (57%)	0.72 (0.27, 1.94)	0.520

Table 2. *Cont.*

Predictor	Count[CESD < 16] $n = 74$	Count [CESD ≥ 16] $n = 21$	Odds Ratio (95% CI)	p-Value
Self-rated financial situation				
Very good or good	2 (3%)	3 (14%)	8.85 (1.31, 59.80)	0.010 *
More or less	13 (18%)	8 (38%)	3.63 (1.20, 10.98)	0.019 *
Bad or very bad (reference)	59 (79%)	10 (48%)	-	-
In debt ($n = 92$)	8 (11%)	6 (30%)	3.43 (1.03, 11.45)	0.039 *
	Social Support and Discrimination			
Discrimination				
Treated with respect ($n = 93$)	49 (81%)	11 (55%)	0.60 (0.22, 1.64)	0.318
Insulted or offended by people	36 (49%)	11 (52%)	1.16 (0.44, 3.06)	0.764
Treated the same way than others in stores	50 (68%)	15 (71%)	1.20 (0.41, 3.48)	0.738
Unjustly fired from jobs ($n = 94$)	10 (14%)	5 (24%)	1.97 (0.59, 6.57)	0.267
Not able to move to another neighborhood	12 (16%)	9 (43%)	6.19 (1.99, 19.23)	<0.001 ***
Social support: have someone who can ... (nationality of that person)				
Talk about anxieties (82 Haitian, 1 Chilean)	71 (96%)	12 (57%)	0.06 (0.01, 0.24)	<0.001 ***
Help when sick (85 Haitian, 1 Chilean)	71 (96%)	15 (71%)	0.11 (0.02, 0.47)	<0.001 ***
Lend money (69 Haitian, 2 Chilean, 1 Other)	62 (84%)	10 (48%)	0.18 (0.06, 0.51)	<0.001 ***
Show love and affection (88 Haitian, 1 Haitian)	71 (96%)	18 (86%)	0.25 (0.05, 1.36)	0.091
Identify with a religion	67 (91%)	16 (76%)	0.33 (0.09, 1.19)	0.082
Go to services weekly ($n = 83$)	35 (52%)	13 (81%)	3.96 (1.03, 15.19)	0.036 *
	Migration Experiences			
Age at leaving the country of origin (mean)	26.11	26.19	-	-
Reasons for leaving country of origin				
Seek dreams and life changes	49 (66%)	11 (52%)	0.56 (0.21, 1.50)	0.249
My family or partner migrated	6 (8%)	1 (5%)	0.57 (0.06, 4.99)	0.606
No work there	6 (8%)	1 (5%)	0.57 (0.06, 4.99)	0.606
Planned to come to Chile when leaving the country of origin	61 (82%)	13 (62%)	0.35 (0.12, 1.00)	0.047 *
Time in Chile	4.54	4.53	-s	-
Planning to leave Chile	66 (89%)	13 (62%)	0.20 (0.06, 0.62)	0.003 **
Reasons for planning to leave Chile ($n = 79$)				
Work opportunities	1 (2%)	5 (38%)		
Discrimination/racism	36 (55%)	5 (38%)	0.52 (0.15, 1.76)	0.292
Cannot bring family here	5 (6%)	0 (0%)		
	COVID-19-Related			
Had suffered consequences due to the pandemic	64 (86%)	19 (90%)	1.48 (0.30, 7.37)	0.629
Economic issues	57 (77%)	15 (71%)	0.75 (0.25, 2.22)	0.599
Change of living place	7 (9%)	1 (5%)	0.48 (0.06, 4.12)	0.496
Anxiety and worry	12 (16%)	4 (19%)	1.22 (0.35, 4.25)	0.761
Migration plans changed due to COVID-19 ($n = 93$)	61 (84%)	12 (60%)	0.30 (0.10, 0.88)	0.024 *
Move to another country ($n = 70$)	54 (92%)	6 (55%)	0.11 (0.02, 0.50)	0.001 **
Move back to Haiti ($n = 70$)	3 (5%)	1 (9%)	1.87 (0.18, 19.80)	0.602

*: $p < 0.05$, **: $p < 0.01$, ***: $p < 0.001$.

2.5.2. Social Support

We asked four questions of the 19-item Medical Outcome Study Social Support Survey (mMOS-SS) [51]. We included those that the community and CAB recommended (i.e., have someone to talk to about your anxieties, have someone to help you when you get sick, have someone to lend you money when you need it, and have someone to show you love and affection) and we also asked about that person's nationality.

2.6. Statistical Analysis

Descriptive statistics were calculated to provide an overview of recent migrants' demographics by the possible status of clinical major depression. A bivariate analysis was performed on discrete variables to calculate the odds ratio of having a CESD-R-20 score of at least 16 given each predictor (Table 2). We also performed Chi-squared tests as a non-parametric method to confirm our odds ratio results. Since all the *p*-values were very similar, we did not include details about them in the table. Bivariate logistic regression was performed to identify factors associated with possible major depressive symptoms. In the event of two highly correlated covariates, the one with the strongest association with the outcome was retained. To ensure the integrity of the model, interactions between predictors and key independent variables such as gender were calculated, but no significant interaction was found. Only variables significant at $p < 0.05$ were retained in the final multivariate model (Table 3). All regression models are presented with crude and adjusted odds ratios (OR), 95% confidence intervals (95%CI), with $p < 0.05$ considered significant. Analyses were conducted using the readr, dplyr, fmsb, and ltm packages in RStudio Version 1.4.1106 [52–56].

Table 3. Multivariate Logistic Regression of Planning to Stay in Chile and Symptoms of Depression among Haitians in Santiago de Chile ($n = 95$).

Coefficients	Estimate	Std. Error	z Value	*p* Value	OR (95%CI)
(Intercept)	2.3420	1.6937	1.383	0.1667	10.4021 (0.3898, 331.1515)
Planning to leave Chile	−1.7752	0.7154	−2.482	0.0131 *	0.1694 (0.0394, 0.6772)
Have someone to talk about anxieties (social support)	−2.8385	0.8396	−3.381	0.0007 ***	0.0585 (0.0096, 0.2768)
Not able to move to another neighborhood (discrimination)	1.3570	0.7217	1.880	0.0601	3.8844 (0.9388, 16.5659)
Having a religious affiliation	−1.0440	0.8344	−1.251	0.2108	0.3521 (0.0681, 1.8933)
Being female	0.3320	0.6749	0.492	0.6227	1.3938 (0.3643, 5.4273)
Being in a bad financial situation	0.9933	1.1794	0.842	0.3996	2.7003 (0.2607, 31.2644)

*: $p < 0.05$, ***: $p < 0.001$.

3. Results

Among the 101 participants surveyed, only 95 were included in the analyses due to incomplete items on the CESD-20 scale. The sociodemographic characteristics for the overall sample and by presence of clinical major depression are provided in Table 1. With regards to self-reported group membership, we found that even though all of the participants were born in Haiti, only 68% self-identified as belonging to the Haitian group. The remaining viewed themselves as migrants (31%) or Chilean (4%). Those who self-reported as a migrant had more odds of having depressive symptoms. Most of the sample reported some level of formal education (87%), having children (71%), and being affiliated with a religion (77%). About 78% of participants reported planning to move to Chile in the first place (i.e., when they were still in Haiti). On average, our participants had stayed in Chile for 4.58 years. Overall, most of our sample (87%) reported having suffered consequences (mostly economic issues) due to the pandemic. The Cronbach's alpha (α) was calculated to assess the reliability of CESD-R-20 Scale in this study, and values ranged from 0.830–0.927 for the 20 items in the current study sample. The Cronbach's alpha coefficient for the 20-item-scale was 0.895, indicating a high internal consistency and that the removal of any of the items would have reduced the overall alpha marginally [57–59].

Univariate associations between each predictor and symptoms of depression are presented in Table 2. Self-identifying as a migrant (OR = 3.42, 95% CI = 1.25–9.37, $p = 0.014$), having a good self-perceived financial situation (OR = 8.85, 95%CI = 1.31–59.80, $p = 0.010$), and being in debt (OR = 3.43, 95%CI = 1.03–11.45, $p = 0.039$) predicted significantly higher odds of having depressive symptoms, while self-identifying as a Haitian (OR = 0.31, 95% CI = 0.12–0.86, $p = 0.021$) as well as being interviewed in Creole (OR = 0.12, 95% CI = 0.04–0.36, $p < 0.001$) predicted significantly lower odds of scoring as clinically depressed.

Social support and discrimination predictors were significantly associated with odds of having symptoms in the univariate analysis. Participants who were not able to move to another neighborhood had significantly higher odds (OR = 6.19, 95% CI = 1.99–19.23, $p < 0.001$) of having symptoms of depression. All the social support items predicted significantly lower odds of having depression. Identifying with a religion was not a significant predictor (OR = 0.33, 95% CI = 0.09–1.19, $p = 0.082$), but going to services weekly significantly predicted higher odds of presenting clinical depression symptoms (OR = 3.96, 95% CI = 1.03–15.19, $p = 0.036$).

A few predictors examining migration experiences and COVID-19 impacts were found to be significantly associated with lower odds of depressive symptoms: planning to come to Chile when leaving the country of origin (OR = 0.35, 95% CI = 0.12–1.00, $p = 0.047$), planning to leave Chile (OR = 0.20, 95% CI = 0.06–0.62, $p = 0.003$), having migration plans changed due to COVID-19 (OR = 0.30, 95% CI = 0.10–0.88, $p = 0.024$), and deciding to move to a country different than originally planned (OR = 0.11, 95% CI = 0.02–0.50, $p = 0.001$).

The multivariate analysis is presented on Table 3. Although not significant in the bivariate analyses, based on the literature and Bhugra's conceptual framework, we included sex, self-perceived financial situation, and religious affiliation as covariates in the model. After adjusting for the covariates, planning to leave Chile remained a significant protective factor for depressive symptoms (Adjusted odds ratio (AOR) = 0.17, 95% CI = 0.04–0.68, $p = 0.0131$). The social support item of having someone with whom to talk about anxieties had a significant negative association with symptoms of depression (AOR = 0.06, 95% CI = 0.01–0.28, $p = 0.0006$) whereas the discrimination item of not being able to move to another neighborhood was positively associated with having depressive symptoms (AOR = 3.88, 95% CI = 0.94–16.57, $p = 0.06$). Additionally, we report here the nationality results of support persons in their lives.

4. Discussion

The prevalence of symptoms of depression among a sample of Haitian migrants ($n = 95$) living in Chile during COVID-19 was 22%. This is similar to the prevalence of depression in the general Chilean population during the pandemic: 22.6% [60,61]. Although the prevalence is similar to some studies conducted with the general population, such studies were conducted online or by phone which may have influenced the responses and perception of the isolation. Given that previous research found that migrants had a prevalence of depression between 14 and 20%, our sample presented a higher percentage within the migrant population prior to COVID [6,62,63]. As studies found that migrants during COVID had a prevalence of depression between 23 and 28%, our sample of Haitian migrants in Chile had a lower percentage of depression [24,64]. Nevertheless, studies conducted during COVID often used web-based surveys in English, and results could be heavily influenced by migrants' English proficiency and whether they had access to Internet devices. Furthermore, one cross-sectional study in 2001 using structured psychiatric interviews found that about 5.5% of members of private households in Santiago de Chile had depression [65].

As hypothesized, we found that after controlling for relevant covariates, planning to stay in Chile among our respondents was significantly associated with depressive symptoms. The consequences of the COVID-19 pandemic have been especially harsh on populations that work in the informal sector, including migrants [19,20,22], who, given the strict confinement measures implemented in Chile, had very few employment opportunities [66]. An important percentage of this study's participants (77%) reported experiencing economic issues during the COVID-19 pandemic and, when we asked if their migration plans had changed due to the COVID-19 pandemic, 84% of those who were planning to leave responded affirmatively. The changing conditions of migration policies, the pandemic, and US–Mexico border conditions have forced migrants to change their migration trajectories. Deciding on their new migration plans could spark new hopes and make migrants more optimistic about their potential futures, and thus having their plans changed due to COVID and changing their migration destination are both protective of their mental health.

The political climate for migrants in Chile, particularly for Haitian migrants, has been especially difficult as well. The migration reform in 2018 established a consular visa requirement for entry into Chile which had restrictive effects on the arrival of Haitian migrants. In addition, there were administrative obstacles (e.g., the request for a criminal record certificate be sent to Chile from Haiti) which increased monetary costs and waiting times for the completion of regularization procedures and limited the possibilities of regularizing the migratory situation for Haitian migrants already in Chile. These situations had particularly serious effects on the ability of Haitian migrants to obtain and/or maintain a job, increasing the financial difficulties for this group [67]. Simultaneously, the 2020 election of a new president in the United States renewed hopes that Haitian migrants would have the opportunity to enter that country. The hardships faced in Chile coupled with the hope and actual entrance of some migrants from Haiti to the United States drove the Haitian migration flow from Chile to the Mexico–US border [68]. Both the United States and Mexico witnessed an increase in Haitian nationals in case and application numbers [69,70].

In the present study, a high percentage of migrants rated their financial situation as bad or very bad (73%). This is reflective of the tough conditions Haitians are experiencing in Chile as a result of the factors discussed above, many of which were exacerbated by COVID-19. The unemployment rate was high (60%), consistent with reports citing difficulty finding jobs [21,23]. Surprisingly, being in a better self-rated economic situation did not protect individuals from depressive symptoms; rather, it was a risk factor for depression. This might be due to how migrants of poorer financial standings were forced to leave Chile, and planning for a potentially better future gives them hope. On the other hand, those who have better financial standings need to face many obstacles to stay in Chile, putting a heavier mental drain on them. Nevertheless, more research is needed to investigate the interaction effects of economic status and migration plans on mental health [5,25,71,72].

Our results confirmed previous research on the protective effects of social support on mental health. Items from financial to emotional social support were all associated with fewer depressive symptoms, confirming the important role of social support discussed in the literature [4,6,35,73–77]. Our data supported the direct protective effects of social support, measured as the availability of somebody to help, against depressive symptoms. In the multivariate analysis, the social support factor of having someone to talk to about concerns came out as the most influential factor in the social support block. Hence, the present results suggested that having social support for concerns was most impactful against symptoms of depression. However, our sample gave an interesting result on religion. On one hand, identifying with a religion was protective against depression, consistent with previous studies that found religiosity a protective factor of mental health [78,79]. On the other hand, going to services weekly was found to be a risk factor for depression among those who are religious. This might be because migrants who go to services weekly search for help in religion regularly instead of engaging in practical solutions, having a higher odds for depression. Hence, those who identify with a religion but do not go to services weekly enjoy the benefits of religion but do not overly rely on religion for solving their issues. Future studies should examine how various forms of social support may have differential impacts on different aspects of mental health and physical health.

Discrimination is a key risk factor for migrants' mental health, especially during COVID-19. As a moving population, migrants may experience heightened levels of discrimination and stigma and may have worsened mental well-being from these experiences. Racial and ethnic discrimination is significantly associated with worse mental health status [6]. A lower length of residence and higher acculturation level are associated with stronger effects of discrimination [80,81]. According to the WHO Apart Together survey, around 40% of those living on the streets or in insecure accommodation reported discrimination, with the unemployed reporting even higher levels of discrimination [21]. An important part of our sample (68%) identifies themselves as migrants, and such a perception had significantly higher odds of having symptoms of depression, which may be illustrating the perception of not being part of the destination community and self-perceiving the sense of otherness. This has been widely explored and has found to be associated with mental health issues among migrant communities throughout the world [82,83]. We plan to explore the relationship between self-identifying as a migrant and depression in a future paper related to the current project.

Contrary to our expectation that multiple factors of discrimination would be predictive of higher depressive symptoms, only one factor—being unable to move to another place—was significantly associated with depression status. Previous studies on (im)mobility among migrants demonstrated how structural factors such as discrimination and socioeconomic inequality can produce immobility and constitute the sense of insecurity [84,85]. A large portion of our sample also reported coming to Chile as a temporary destination, with the hope of migrating to other countries such as the United States in the future—and the recent situation had pushed some of them to make the decision to leave Chile. Furthermore, given that Chile is not the final destination for a large portion of our sample, it is plausible that the inability to move was especially concerning for this group. This trend is also consistent with studies in other contexts in which migrants who freely chose to move had a lower prevalence of depression [24,62].

Besides the diversity of migrant characteristics, migration encompasses a broad range of experiences and trajectories on spatial and temporal scales that cannot be captured with the migrant versus non-migrant categorization [8,10]. Migration is dynamic and multi-directional: as migrants move from place to place, their plans and resources may change such that they would change the duration of stay, or they would end up in a different place than their original destination [8,13]. These nuances are integral parts of the migration experience and present a multitude of possibilities under the term migration, with risk and protective factors at each step. Bhugra outlined the vulnerability and resilience factors in the process of migration during premigration, selection for migration, the migration experience, and post-migration [2]. At each of the four stages, the migrant might experience a broad range of factors that may either facilitate better mental health or lead to worsened mental health.

The present investigation focused on the condition of transit migration where Haitians came to Chile with the plans of continuing migration in the future. As this migrant collective faced the challenges of policy changes, economic distress, and COVID-19, they could build resilience against mental health issues by having hope for a better future and planning for a journey to achieve that. While conducting this study, we heard from many participants that a family member or friend had been able to cross to the United States, a fact that has been documented in the press [33,68,86]. Thus, this could be another reason for finding a protective effect between the planning to leave Chile and symptoms of depression. Other studies have found a similar effect when plans, resilience, and the future have been analyzed and found to be protective factors for migrants' mental health [7,16,87]. Optimism and a sense of control were protective mediators for migrants' mental health while a lack of hopefulness about the future was associated with worse effects on mental health [5,87].

5. Conclusions

This study surveyed Haitian migrants living in Santiago, Chile about their migration experiences and major depression status. Haitian migrants experienced a myriad of vulnerabilities and uncertainties due to the complex policy environment during the COVID-19 pandemic in Chile. The data revealed that Haitian migrants had a higher level of prevalence of major depression than the general public in Chile, consistent with our hypotheses and previous literature on migrants' mental health during COVID-19. We found that being in debt and discrimination were risk factors associated with the presence of major depression. Protective factors against clinical depression included social support, change in migration plans due to COVID-19, and planning to leave Chile. Multivariate analysis highlighted that planning to leave Chile is significantly predictive of the absence of major depression. These results suggest that Haitian migrants in Chile suffer from a higher prevalence of major depression and present risk and protective factors associated with migrants' experiences in the country.

Although this study showed the important effects of various factors during the migrant's journey on their mental health status and there are no other studies assessing the prevalence of symptoms of depression on Haitian migrants, we cannot generalize the experiences of all Haitians living in Chile as this is a cross-sectional study and includes a small sample. Moreover, our sample size limited the accuracy of our estimates as demonstrated by wide confidence intervals in our analyses. Our study does illustrate an interesting phase of Haitian migrants' journey that may be useful for informing practice of community advocacy groups and health services providers, as well as future studies conducted in Chile but also throughout the Americas as Haitians are migrating northward [86]. Future research should delve into the various parts of the migration process following Bhugra's Migration Phrases and Psychiatric Disorders Framework [2] and investigate how the same factors such as social support and sense of control may have differential impacts on these stages of migration. Longitudinal cohort designs or studies including other destinations of the same migrant group can reveal the nuances of these impacts over time and possibly expose valuable windows for intervention. Studies can also probe the relationship between optimism, sense of control, and other psychiatric disorders.

Author Contributions: Design, conceptualization, and data collection, T.R.-J., J.C. and M.M.; methodology, S.M.-M.; resources, C.R. and L.C.; formal analysis, Y.C.; writing—original draft preparation: Y.C. and T.R.-J.; writing—review and editing, all authors. All authors have read and agreed to the published version of the manuscript.

Funding: This research was funded by the Agencia Nacional de Investigación y Desarrollo, Chile (ANID Fondecyt de Iniciación 11200486 PI: T.R.J.) and by ANID—MILENIO—N° NCS2021_013 (SocioMed). C.R. was funded by Universidad Autónoma de México (IA301320 DGAPA, UNAM).

Institutional Review Board Statement: The study was conducted according to the guidelines of the Declaration of Helsinki, and approved by the Scientific Ethics Committee of the Universidad Mayor, Temuco (project #0169).

Informed Consent Statement: Informed consent was obtained from all subjects involved in the study.

Data Availability Statement: The data presented in this study are available on request from the corresponding author. The data are not publicly available due to ethics and confidentiality concerns for the participants.

Acknowledgments: The authors gratefully acknowledge the participants, community collaborators (Servicio Jesuita a Migrantes, FUPA and Fré), and field study staff in Chile.

Conflicts of Interest: The authors declare no conflict of interest. The funders had no role in the design of the study; in the collection, analyses, or interpretation of data; in the writing of the manuscript, or in the decision to publish the results.

References

1. Beutel, M.E.; Jünger, C.; Klein, E.M.; Wild, P.; Lackner, K.J.; Blettner, M.; Banerjee, M.; Michal, M.; Wiltink, J.; Brähler, E. Depression, Anxiety and Suicidal Ideation among 1st and 2nd Generation Migrants—Results from the Gutenberg Health Study. *BMC Psychiatry* **2016**, *16*, 288. [CrossRef]
2. Bhugra, D. Review Article Migration and Mental Health. *Acta Psychiatr. Scand.* **2004**, *109*, 243–258. [CrossRef]
3. Bourque, F.; van der Ven, E.; Malla, A. A Meta-Analysis of the Risk for Psychotic Disorders among First- and Second-Generation Immigrants. *Psychol. Med.* **2011**, *41*, 897–910. [CrossRef]
4. Collins, C.H.; Zimmerman, C.; Howard, L.M. Refugee, Asylum Seeker, Immigrant Women and Postnatal Depression: Rates and Risk Factors. *Arch. Women's Ment. Health* **2011**, *14*, 3–11. [CrossRef]
5. Hovey, J.D. Psychosocial Predictors of Depression among Central American Immigrants. *Psychol. Rep.* **2000**, *86*, 1237–1240. [CrossRef]
6. Ornelas, I.J.; Perreira, K.M. The Role of Migration in the Development of Depressive Symptoms among Latino Immigrant Parents in the USA. *Soc. Sci. Med.* **2011**, *73*, 1169–1177. [CrossRef]
7. Rocha-Jiménez, T.; Fernández-Casanueva, C.; Suárez-Lopéz, J.R.; Zúñiga, M.L.; Crespo, N.; Morales-Miranda, S.; Goldenberg, S.M.; Silverman, J.G.; Brouwer, K.C. Intercepted Journeys: Associations between Migration and Mobility Experiences and Depressive Symptoms among Substance Using Migrants at the Mexico-Guatemala Border. *Glob. Public Health* **2021**, *17*, 297–312. [CrossRef]
8. Schrooten, M.; Salazar, N.B.; Dias, G. Living in Mobility: Trajectories of Brazilians in Belgium and the UK. *J. Ethn. Migr. Stud.* **2016**, *42*, 1199–1215. [CrossRef]
9. Ward, K.P.; Shaw, S.A.; Chang, M.; El-Bassel, N. Social Support Moderates the Association Between Traumatic Life Events and Depression Among Migrant and Nonmigrant Men in Almaty, Kazakhstan. *J. Trauma Stress* **2018**, *31*, 698–707. [CrossRef]
10. Yang, M.; Dijst, M.; Helbich, M. Migration Trajectories and Their Relationship to Mental Health among Internal Migrants in Urban China: A Sequence Alignment Approach. *Popul. Space Place* **2020**, *26*, e2304. [CrossRef]
11. Caruso, G.; Canon, C.G.; Mueller, V. Spillover Effects of the Venezuelan Crisis: Migration Impacts in Colombia. *Oxf. Econ. Pap.* **2021**, *73*, 771–795. [CrossRef]
12. de la Rizzo Lara, R. La Caminata Del Migrante: A Social Movement. *J. Ethn. Migr. Stud.* **2021**, *47*, 3891–3910. [CrossRef]
13. Sedas, A.C.; Aguerrebere, M.; Juarez, L.A.M.; Zavala-deAlba, L.E.; Itzel Eguiluz, J.B. *Situational Brief: Transit Migration in Mexico during the COVID-19 Pandemic*; Lancet Migration: London, UK, 2020.
14. Cantalapiedraa, E.T.; Navaa, D.M.M. Crossing Borders: Migratory Strategies in Transit of Participants in Migrants Caravans. *Estud. Front.* **2020**, *21*, 1–21. [CrossRef]
15. Collyer, M. In-between Places: Trans-Saharan Transit Migrants in Morocco and the Fragmented Journey to Europe. *Antipode* **2007**, *39*, 668–690. [CrossRef]
16. Gil Everaert, I. Inhabiting the Meanwhile: Rebuilding Home and Restoring Predictability in a Space of Waiting. *J. Ethn. Migr. Stud.* **2021**, *47*, 4327–4343. [CrossRef]
17. Menjívar, C. Liminal Legality: Salvadoran and Guatemalan Immigrants' Lives in the United States. *Am. J. Sociol.* **2006**, *111*, 999–1037. [CrossRef]
18. Programa de Estudios Sociales en Salud (Proessa) Encuesta Sobre COVID-19 a Poblaciones Migrantes. Available online: https://migrantes.mineduc.cl/wp-content/uploads/sites/88/2020/11/Reporte-descriptivo-ENCUESTA-MIGRANTES-Y-COVID19.pdf (accessed on 8 February 2022).
19. Chander, R.; Murugesan, M.; Ritish, D.; Damodharan, D.; Arunachalam, V.; Parthasarathy, R.; Raj, A.; Sharma, M.K.; Manjunatha, N.; Bada Math, S.; et al. Addressing the Mental Health Concerns of Migrant Workers during the COVID-19 Pandemic: An Experiential Account. *Int. J. Soc. Psychiatry* **2021**, *67*, 826–829. [CrossRef]
20. International Rescue Comittee the Cruelty of Containment; 2020. Available online: https://eu.rescue.org/sites/default/files/2020-12/IRC_Cruelty_of_Containment_FINAL.pdf (accessed on 29 March 2022).
21. World Health Organization. *ApartTogether Survey: Preliminary Overview of Refugees and Migrants Self-Reported Imapct of COVID-19*; World Health Organization: Geneva, Switzerland, 2020.
22. Harjana, N.P.A.; Januraga, P.P.; Indrayathi, P.A.; Gesesew, H.A.; Ward, P.R. Prevalence of Depression, Anxiety, and Stress Among Repatriated Indonesian Migrant Workers During the COVID-19 Pandemic. *Front. Public Health* **2021**, *9*, 630295. [CrossRef]
23. Asociación de Municipalidades de Chile. Población Migrante y Sus Problemáticas En El Contexto de La Crisis Sanitaria Derivada del COVID. 2020. Available online: https://amuch.cl/wp-content/uploads/2022/05/Encuesta-Caracterizacion-de-la-poblacion-migrante-y-sus-problematicas.pdf (accessed on 6 January 2022).
24. Attal, J.H.; Lurie, I.; Neumark, Y. A Rapid Assessment of Migrant Careworkers' Psychosocial Status during Israel's COVID-19 Lockdown. *Isr. J. Health Policy Res.* **2020**, *9*, 61. [CrossRef]
25. Brooks, S.K.; Webster, R.K.; Smith, L.E.; Woodland, L.; Wessely, S.; Greenberg, N.; Rubin, G.J. The Psychological Impact of Quarantine and How to Reduce It: Rapid Review of the Evidence. *Lancet* **2020**, *395*, 912–920. [CrossRef]

26. Guadago, L. Migrants and the COVID-19 Pandemic: An Initial Analysis. *Int. Organ. Migr. Migr. Res. Ser.* **2020**, 1–28. Available online: https://publications.iom.int/books/mrs-no-60-migrants-and-covid-19-pandemic-initial-analysis (accessed on 6 January 2022).
27. Paredes, C.L. Catholic Heritage, Ethno-Racial Self-Identification, and Prejudice against Haitians in the Dominican Republic. *Ethn. Racial Stud.* **2019**, *42*, 2143–2166. [CrossRef]
28. Keys, H.M.; Kaiser, B.N.; Foster, J.W.; Burgos Minaya, R.Y.; Kohrt, B.A. Perceived Discrimination, Humiliation, and Mental Health: A Mixed-Methods Study among Haitian Migrants in the Dominican Republic. *Ethn. Health* **2015**, *20*, 219–240. [CrossRef]
29. Keys, H.M.; Noland, G.S.; de Rochars, M.B.; Taylor, T.H.; Blount, S.; Gonzales, M. Perceived Discrimination in Bateyes of the Dominican Republic: Results from the Everyday Discrimination Scale and Implications for Public Health Programs. *BMC Public Health* **2019**, *19*, 1513. [CrossRef]
30. Yaksic Beckdorf, M.S. Introducción. In *Migración y Trabajo. Estudio y Propuestas Para la Inclusión Sociolaoral de Migrantes en Arica*; Rojas Pedemonte, N., Vicuña Undurraga, J.T.S., Eds.; Organización Internacional para las Migraciones: Santiago, Chile, 2014.
31. Texidó, E.; Gurrieri, J.; Artola, J. *Panorama Migratorio de América Del Sur 2012*; Sudamérica: Buenos Aires, Argentina, 2012.
32. Instituto de Políticas Públicas en Derechos Humanos del Mercosur. *Diagnóstico Regional Sobre Migración Haitiana*; OIM: Caba, Argentina, 2017.
33. Ortiz, L.V.; Peña Muñoz, J.J.; Coubès, M.L.; París Pombo, M.D.; de la Barrios, O.M.I.; Mena Iturralde, L.C.; López Reyes, E.A.; Pérez Duperou, G.H. Entre La Espera y El Asentamieto: Lnserción Laboral y Residencial de Inmigrantes y Desplazados En Ciudades Fronterizas Del Norte de México: Los Casos de Tijuana y Ciudad Juárez. Available online: https://www.colef.mx/estudiosdeelcolef/en%20tre-la-espera-y-el-asentamiento-insercion-laboral-y-residencial-de-inmigrantes-y-desplazados-en-ciudades-fronterizas-del-norte-de-mexico/ (accessed on 16 December 2021).
34. Alarcón, R.D.; Parekh, A.; Wainberg, M.L.; Duarte, C.S.; Araya, R.; Oquendo, M.A. Hispanic Immigrants in the USA: Social and Mental Health Perspectives. *Lancet Psychiatry* **2016**, *3*, 860–870. [CrossRef]
35. Mulvaney-Day, N.E.; Alegría, M.; Sribney, W. Social Cohesion, Social Support, and Health among Latinos in the United States. *Soc. Sci. Med.* **2007**, *64*, 477–495. [CrossRef]
36. Cardoso, J.B.; Thompson, S.J. Common Themes of Resilience among Latino Immigrant Families: A Systematic Review of the Literature. *Fam. Soc. J. Contemp. Soc. Serv.* **2010**, *91*, 257–265. [CrossRef]
37. Carroll, H.; Luzes, M.; Freier, L.F.; Bird, M.D. The Migration Journey and Mental Health: Evidence from Venezuelan Forced Migration. *SSM—Popul. Health* **2020**, *10*, 100551. [CrossRef]
38. Heckathorn, D.D. Respondent-Driven Sampling: A New Approach to the Study of Hidden Populations. *Soc. Probl.* **1997**, *44*, 174–199. [CrossRef]
39. Paz-Bailey, G.; Miller, W.; Shiraishi, R.W.; Jacobson, J.O.; Abimbola, T.O.; Chen, S.Y. Reaching Men Who Have Sex with Men: A Comparison of Respondent-Driven Sampling and Time-Location Sampling in Guatemala City. *AIDS Behav.* **2013**, *17*, 3081–3090. [CrossRef]
40. Salganik, M.J.; Heckathorn, D.D. Sampling and Estimation in Hidden Populations Using Respondent-Driven Sampling. *Sociol. Methodol.* **2004**, *34*, 193–239. [CrossRef]
41. Facultad de Arquitectura y Urbanismo Mis Venicas y Venicos Haitianos. Available online: http://www.fau.uchile.cl/noticias/162924/mis-vecinas-y-vecinos-haitianos (accessed on 8 February 2022).
42. Baumann, A.; Domenech Rodríguez, M.; Parra-Cardona, J.R. Community-Based Applied Research With Latino Immigrant Families: Informing Practice and Research According to Ethical and Social Justice Principles. *Fam. Process* **2011**, *50*, 132–148. [CrossRef]
43. Goldenberg, S.M.; Brouwer, K.C.; Jimenez, T.R.; Miranda, S.M.; Mindt, M.R. Enhancing the Ethical Conduct of HIV Research with Migrant Sex Workers: Human Rights, Policy, and Social Contextual Influences. *PLoS ONE* **2016**, *11*, e0155048. [CrossRef]
44. Björgvinsson, T.; Kertz, S.J.; Bigda-Peyton, J.S.; McCoy, K.L.; Aderka, I.M. Psychometric Properties of the CES-D-10 in a Psychiatric Sample. *Assessment* **2013**, *20*, 429–436. [CrossRef]
45. Radloff, L.S. The CES-D Scale. *Appl. Psychol. Meas.* **1977**, *1*, 385–401. [CrossRef]
46. González-Forteza, C.; Jiménez-Tapia, J.A.; Ramos-Lira, L.; Wagner, F.A. Aplicación de La Escala de Depresión Del Center of Epidemiological Studies En Adolescentes de La Ciudad de México. *Salud Pública México* **2008**, *50*, 292–299. [CrossRef]
47. Pinedo, M.; Burgos, J.L.; Zúñiga, M.L.; Perez, R.; Macera, C.A.; Ojeda, V.D. Deportation and Mental Health among Migrants Who Inject Drugs along the US–Mexico Border. *Glob. Public Health* **2018**, *13*, 211–226. [CrossRef]
48. Ros, L.; Latorre, J.M.; Aguilar, M.J.; Serrano, J.P.; Navarro, B.; Ricarte, J.J. Factor Structure and Psychometric Properties of the Center for Epidemiologic Studies Depression Scale (CES-D) in Older Populations with and without Cognitive Impairment. *Int. J. Aging Hum. Dev.* **2011**, *72*, 83–110. [CrossRef]
49. Vilagut, G.; Forero, C.G.; Barbaglia, G.; Alonso, J. Screening for Depression in the General Population with the Center for Epidemiologic Studies Depression (CES-D): A Systematic Review with Meta-Analysis. *PLoS ONE* **2016**, *11*, e0155431. [CrossRef]
50. Marchant, J.P.; Cabezas, J.M.; Rocha-Jiménez, T. *Validación de La Traducción de Español a Creole de La Escala CEDS-R-20*, 2022, *in press*.
51. Moser, A.; Stuck, A.E.; Silliman, R.A.; Ganz, P.A.; Clough-Gorr, K.M. The Eight-Item Modified Medical Outcomes Study Social Support Survey: Psychometric Evaluation Showed Excellent Performance. *J. Clin. Epidemiol.* **2012**, *65*, 1107–1116. [CrossRef]
52. RStudio Team. *R Studio: Integrated Development for R*; RStudio, Inc.: Boston, MA, USA, 2020.

53. Wickham, H.; Hester, J. Readr: Read Rectangular Text Data; 2020. Available online: https://CRAN.R-project.org/package=readr (accessed on 18 July 2022).
54. Wickham, H.; François, R.; Henry, L.; Müller, K. Dplyr: A Grammar of Data Manipulation; 2021. Available online: https://CRAN.R-project.org/package=dplyr (accessed on 18 July 2022).
55. Nakazawa, M. Fmsb: Functions for Medical Statistics Book with Some Demographic Data; 2021. Available online: https://CRAN.R-project.org/package=fmsb (accessed on 18 July 2022).
56. Rizopoulos, D. Ltm: An R Package for Latent Variable Modelling and Item Response Theory Analyses. *J. Stat. Softw.* **2006**, *17*, 1–25. [CrossRef]
57. Haroz, E.E.; Ybarra, M.L.; Eaton, W.W. Psychometric Evaluation of a Self-Report Scale to Measure Adolescent Depression: The CESDR-10 in Two National Adolescent Samples in the United States. *J. Affect. Disord.* **2014**, *158*, 154–160. [CrossRef]
58. Ruiz-Grosso, P.; Bernabe-Ortiz, A.; Diez-Canseco, F.; Gilman, R.H.; Checkley, W.; Bennett, I.M.; Miranda, J.J. Depressive Mood Among Within-Country Migrants in Periurban Shantytowns of Lima, Peru. *J. Immigr. Minority Health* **2015**, *17*, 1635–1642. [CrossRef]
59. Tavakol, M.; Dennick, R. Making Sense of Cronbach's Alpha. *Int. J. Med. Educ.* **2011**, *2*, 53–55. [CrossRef]
60. Duarte, F.; Jiménez-Molina, Á. A Longitudinal Nationwide Study of Psychological Distress During the COVID-19 Pandemic in Chile. *Front. Psychiatry* **2022**, *13*, 204. [CrossRef]
61. Duarte, F.; Jiménez-Molina, Á. Psychological Distress during the COVID-19 Epidemic in Chile: The Role of Economic Uncertainty. *PLoS ONE* **2021**, *16*, e0251683. [CrossRef]
62. Foo, S.Q.; Tam, W.W.; Ho, C.S.; Tran, B.X.; Nguyen, L.H.; McIntyre, R.S.; Ho, R.C. Prevalence of Depression among Migrants: A Systematic Review and Meta-Analysis. *Int. J. Environ. Res. Public Health* **2018**, *15*, 1986. [CrossRef]
63. Lindert, J.; von Ehrenstein, O.S.; Priebe, S.; Mielck, A.; Brähler, E. Depression and Anxiety in Labor Migrants and Refugees—A Systematic Review and Meta-Analysis. *Soc. Sci. Med.* **2009**, *69*, 246–257. [CrossRef]
64. Barbato, M.; Thomas, J. Psychological Wellbeing of Foreign Workers in the United Arab Emirates during the COVID-19 Pandemic. *Int. J. Psychol.* **2021**, *56*, 825–833. [CrossRef]
65. Araya, R.; Rojas, G.; Fritsch, R.; Acuña, J.; Lewis, G. Common Mental Disorders in Santiago, Chile. *Br. J. Psychiatry* **2001**, *178*, 228–233. [CrossRef]
66. Jara-Labarthé, V.; Cisneros Puebla, C.A. Migrants in Chile: Social Crisis and the Pandemic (or Sailing over Troubled Water ...). *Qual. Soc. Work* **2021**, *20*, 284–288. [CrossRef]
67. Mercado, M.; Figueiredo, A. *Construcciones Identitarias de Inmigrantes Haitianos En Santiago de Chile, Desde Una Perspectiva Interseccional*, 2022; *in press*.
68. Gramlich, J. Migrant Encounters at U.S.-Mexico Border Are at a 21-Year High. Available online: https://policycommons.net/artifacts/1804460/migrant-encounters-at-us-mexico-border-are-at-a-21-year-high/2536091/ (accessed on 7 February 2022).
69. Baugh, R. Refugees and Asylums: 2019. 2020. Available online: https://www.dhs.gov/sites/default/files/publications/immigration-statistics/yearbook/2019/refugee_and_asylee_2019.pdf (accessed on 29 March 2022).
70. Comisión Mexicana de Ayuda a Refugiados. Datos de Migrantes al Cierre de Diciembre 2021. 2022. Available online: https://www.gob.mx/cms/uploads/attachment/file/690741/Cierre_Diciembre-2021__1-Enero-2022_pdf (accessed on 29 March 2022).
71. Close, C.; Kouvonen, A.; Bosqui, T.; Patel, K.; O'Reilly, D.; Donnelly, M. The Mental Health and Wellbeing of First Generation Migrants: A Systematic-Narrative Review of Reviews. *Glob. Health* **2016**, *12*, 47. [CrossRef]
72. Qiu, P.; Caine, E.; Yang, Y.; Chen, Q.; Li, J.; Ma, X. Depression and Associated Factors in Internal Migrant Workers in China. *J. Affect. Disord.* **2011**, *134*, 198–207. [CrossRef]
73. Falcon, L.M.; Todorova, I.; Tucker, K. Social Support, Life Events, and Psychological Distress among the Puerto Rican Population in the Boston Area of the United States. *Aging Ment. Health* **2009**, *13*, 863–873. [CrossRef]
74. Gutierrez-Vazquez, E.; Flippen, C.; Parrado, E. Migration and Depression: A Cross-National Comparison of Mexicans in Sending Communities and Durham, NC. *Soc. Sci. Med.* **2018**, *219*, 1–10. [CrossRef]
75. Liu, X.; Lin, X.; Zhou, Q.; Zhou, N.; Li, Y.; Lin, D. Family and Individual Risk and Protective Factors of Depression among Chinese Migrant Children with Oppositional Defiant Disorder Symptoms. *Front. Psychol.* **2017**, *8*, 508. [CrossRef]
76. Meng, X.; Xue, S. Social Networks and Mental Health Outcomes: Chinese Rural–Urban Migrant Experience. *J. Popul. Econ.* **2020**, *33*, 155–195. [CrossRef]
77. Xiao, Y.; Miao, S.; Sarkar, C. Social Ties, Spatial Migration Paradigm, and Mental Health among Two Generations of Migrants in China. *Popul. Space Place* **2021**, *27*, e2389. [CrossRef]
78. Williams, A.; Dixon, J.; Feinn, R.; McCorkle, R. Cancer Family Caregiver Depression: Are Religion-Related Variables Important? *Psycho-Oncology* **2015**, *24*, 825–831. [CrossRef]
79. Braam, A.W.; Koenig, H.G. Religion, Spirituality and Depression in Prospective Studies: A Systematic Review. *J. Affect. Disord.* **2019**, *257*, 428–438. [CrossRef]
80. Finch, B.K.; Kolody, B.; Vega, W.A. Perceived Discrimination and Depression among Mexican-Origin Adults in California. *J. Health Soc. Behav.* **2000**, *41*, 295. [CrossRef]
81. Hatch, S.L.; Gazard, B.; Williams, D.R.; Frissa, S.; Goodwin, L.; SELCoH Study Team; Hotopf, M. Discrimination and Common Mental Disorder among Migrant and Ethnic Groups: Findings from a South East London Community Sample. *Soc. Psychiatry Psychiatr. Epidemiol.* **2016**, *51*, 689–701. [CrossRef]

82. Ata, A.; Morrison, G. Health Care Providers, Bereavement Anxieties and Ethnocentric Pedagogy: Towards a Sense of Otherness. *Aust. e-J. Adv. Ment. Health* **2005**, *4*, 175–178. [CrossRef]
83. Kirmayer, L.J.; Narasiah, L.; Munoz, M.; Rashid, M.; Ryder, A.G.; Guzder, J.; Hassan, G.; Rousseau, C.; Pottie, K. Common Mental Health Problems in Immigrants and Refugees: General Approach in Primary Care. *Can. Med. Assoc. J.* **2011**, *183*, E959–E967. [CrossRef]
84. Iranzo, Á. Sub-Saharan Migrants 'in Transit': Intersections between Mobility and Immobility and the Production of (in) Securities. *Mobilities* **2021**, *16*, 739–757. [CrossRef]
85. Yu, S. "I Am like a Deaf, Dumb and Blind Person": Mobility and Immobility of Chinese (Im)Migrants in Flushing, Queens, New York City. *J. Transp. Geogr.* **2016**, *54*, 10–21. [CrossRef]
86. Alden, E.; Tippet, A. Why Are Haitian Migrants Gathering at the U.S. Border? Available online: https://www.cfr.org/in-brief/why-are-haitian-migrants-gathering-us-border (accessed on 26 July 2022).
87. Chou, K.L. Pre-Migration Planning and Depression among New Migrants to Hong Kong: The Moderating Role of Social Support. *J. Affect. Disord.* **2009**, *114*, 85–93. [CrossRef]

International Journal of
Environmental Research and Public Health

MDPI

Article

"Living in Confinement, Stopped in Time": Migrant Social Vulnerability, Coping and Health during the COVID-19 Pandemic Lockdown in France

Maria De Jesus [1,2,*], Zoubida Moumni [3], Zara Hassan Sougui [4], Neeharika Biswas [1], Raquel Kubicz [1] and Lionel Pourtau [5,6]

1 Center on Health, Risk, and Society, School of International Service, American University, Washington, DC 20016, USA
2 Collegium de Lyon, Université de Lyon, 69002 Lyon, France
3 Psychologie de la Santé, Université Lumière Lyon 2, 69365 Lyon, France
4 Santé Publique, Université Claude Bernard Lyon 1, 69100 Villeurbanne, France
5 Habitat et Humanisme, 69300 Caluire et Cuire, France
6 Pôle Recherche & Innovation, Université Paul Valéry Montpellier 3, 34090 Montpellier, France
* Correspondence: dejesus@american.edu

Abstract: The COVID-19 pandemic has exposed health and social inequities among migrant populations. Less empirical evidence exists about the impact of COVID-19 lockdown measures on migrants. This study aimed to investigate the impact of the first lockdown in France between March and May 2020 on migrants' lives and livelihoods. We adopted a social vulnerability framework to conceptualize how the pandemic and the consequential lockdown in France contributed to a 'compounded crisis' for asylum seekers and undocumented migrants. This crisis encompassed health, protection, and socio-economic challenges for migrants and exposed the shortcomings of existing government policies that exclude migrants and do not address the root causes of health inequities. The study draws on in-depth qualitative interviews conducted with 75 asylum seekers and undocumented migrants during the pandemic lockdown in the French regions of Auvergne-Rhône-Alpes and Île-de-France. The findings of this paper highlight the importance of implementing a cohesive pandemic response approach that views health as a fundamental inclusive right for *all* human beings and *all* policies as health policies to promote well-being for all.

Keywords: COVID-19; lockdown; pandemic; migrants; asylum seekers; crisis; social vulnerability; health inequities; France

Citation: De Jesus, M.; Moumni, Z.; Sougui, Z.H.; Biswas, N.; Kubicz, R.; Pourtau, L. "Living in Confinement, Stopped in Time": Migrant Social Vulnerability, Coping and Health during the COVID-19 Pandemic Lockdown in France. *Int. J. Environ. Res. Public Health* **2022**, *19*, 10084. https://doi.org/10.3390/ijerph191610084

Academic Editors: Paul B. Tchounwou and C. Eduardo Siqueira

Received: 4 June 2022
Accepted: 9 August 2022
Published: 15 August 2022

1. Introduction

The coronavirus disease 2019 (COVID-19) pandemic led to governments in 157 countries introducing lockdowns or re-strictions to people's movement and access to health and welfare support services as well as other rules including social distancing, use of masks, and quarantine. The French government introduced its first mandatory national lockdown on 17 March 2020 due to elevated cases and death rates of COVID-19 in the country [1]. This public health measure required the general population to stay at home except those carrying out an essential job (referred to as a 'key worker' in the domains of transportation, education, food, and health), to buy necessary items, or to engage in physical activity.

Evidence demonstrates that the pandemic disproportionately affected socially vulnerable populations, including migrants [2–5]. The pandemic exposed and exacerbated health and social inequities among migrant and ethnic/racial groups [6]. Less is known about the firsthand impact of the COVID-19 lockdowns, specifically on migrant populations in France. One recent French qualitative study in Lyon and Paris on homeless individuals and migrants (undocumented, asylum seekers, or refugees) in shelters revealed the negative impact of the first lockdown on these populations [2]. Similarly, another qualitative article on migrants in France described the negative effects of confinement related to the COVID-19 pandemic on French-speaking Sub-Saharan undocumented migrants [3]. Similarly, our study contributes to this understudied area of research by exploring the impact of the first lockdown in France on migrants' lives and livelihoods from their perspectives. This information is critical to inform future preparedness response plans that include migrants so as not to further exacerbate vulnerabilities among these populations.

1.1. Defining Migrant Terminology Used in the Study

While the term refugee is precisely defined in the 1951 Convention relating to the Status of Refugees and the 1967 Protocol 3, migrants are a heterogeneous group with no international consensus [7]. The umbrella term 'migrant' is defined as a person who moves away from his or her place of usual residence, whether within a country or across an international border, temporarily or permanently, and for a variety of reasons [8]. Table 1 describes a common typology of migrants. For the purposes of this study, we adopt the term "migrant" which includes the labels in Table 1.

Table 1. Defining common migrant terminology, adapted from International Organization for Migration (Reprinted/adapted with permission from ref. [8]. Copyright 2021, J. Redpath-Cross & R. Perruchoud).

Asylum Seeker	A person who seeks safety from persecution or serious harm in a country other than his or her own and awaits a decision on the application for refugee status under relevant international and national instruments.
Economic Migrant	A person leaving his or her habitual place of residence to settle outside his or her country of origin in order to improve his or her quality of life. This term is often loosely used to distinguish from refugees fleeing persecution and is also similarly used to refer to persons attempting to enter a country without legal permission and/or using asylum procedures without bona fide cause. It may equally be applied to persons leaving their country of origin for the purpose of employment.
Irregular Migrant	A person who, owing to unauthorized entry, breach of a condition of entry or the expiration of his or her visa, lacks legal status in a transit or host country. The definition covers, inter alia, those persons who have entered a transit or host country lawfully but have stayed for a longer period than authorized or subsequently taken up unauthorized employment (also called clandestine/undocumented migrant or migrant in an irregular situation). The term 'irregular' is preferable to 'illegal' because the latter carries a criminal connotation and is seen as denying migrants' humanity.

This is a condensed list and is not exhaustive.

Their asylum case at the host country with the aim of obtaining refugee status, they may also be documented or 'undocumented' ("*sans papiers*" in French). There is also no universally accepted definition of 'irregular' migration. The International Organization for Migration (IOM) defines it as "movement that takes place outside the regulatory norms of the sending, transit, and receiving country" [8]. From the perspective of destination countries, it refers to entry, stay, or work in a country without the necessary authorization or documents required under immigration regulations. Migrants escaping conflict and persecution in their countries and seeking protection in another country may be counted as undocumented migrants at the moment of crossing the border, but their status may change once they apply for asylum [9,10] or are regularized.

1.2. Social Vulnerability: A Conceptual Lens to Understand the Experiences of Migrants

The concept of social vulnerability is used across a variety of fields and disciplines, including global health, development, disaster management, economics, sociology, anthropology, geography, and environmental studies. The concept emerged within the natural hazards and disaster management literature, emphasizing the exposure risk and the amount of damage caused by a particular hazard from a technical or engineering sciences perspective [11,12]. Rather than simply examining risk exposures, social scientists transformed the concept to consider the vulnerability that pre-exists in a system before it encounters a hazard.

The negative impact of a pandemic on migrant health and well-being are exacerbated by antecedent social determinants, including poverty, discrimination, social exclusion, low levels of education, poor public infrastructure, and uneven distribution of resources that amplify social vulnerability [5,11,13]. From this perspective, the COVID-19 pandemic is conceptualized as a crisis or disruptive event that occurs at a rate and magnitude that exceeds normal capacity (e.g., increasing cases, hospitalization, and death rates of COVID-19).

In this article, we adopt the lens of social vulnerability as a conceptual framework to help interpret the impact of the pandemic and consequential lockdown. The notion in this framework is that a 'compounded crisis', which encompasses a health crisis, a protection crisis, and a socio-economic crisis [14], arises from existing vulnerabilities reinforcing each other and is amplified during a pandemic and subsequent lockdown, creating a detrimental cycle (Figure 1).

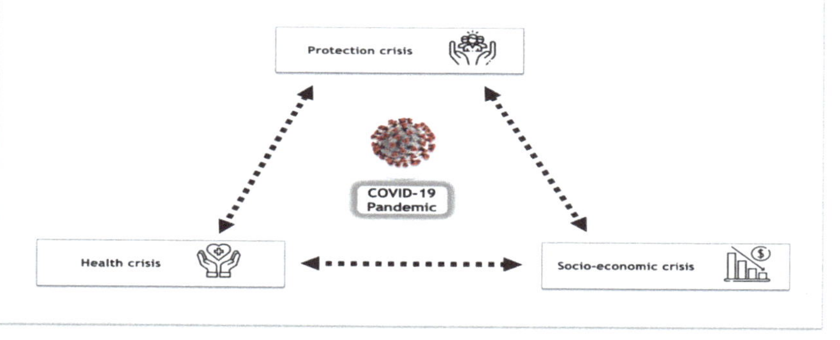

Figure 1. Social vulnerability: a conceptual framework to interpret the impact of the COVID-19 pandemic and subsequent lockdown on migrants (adapted from UN Sustainable Development Group) (Reprinted/adapted with permission from ref. [15]. Copyright 2021, UN Sustainable Development Group).

1.3. A Health Crisis

Data from the World Health Organization (2020) demonstrated that 93% of countries experienced disruption in one or more of their services for mental, neurological, and substance use disorders [16]. Mental health services were cut during the pandemic, given the insufficient number of health workers, the lack of personal protective equipment (PPE), and the conversion of mental health facilities to quarantine/treatment facilities [17]. The pandemic, therefore, led to worsened pre-existing mental health outcomes or to new con-ditions among migrants [17–21].

Apart from the U.K, Norway, Sweden, Denmark, Finland, and Iceland, European countries did not report COVID-19 statistics according to migrant status or ethnicity [22]. Scandinavian countries reported higher rates of COVID-19 cases, mortality, and morbidity among migrant populations [23]. For example, in Sweden, in comparison to Swedish-born individuals, migrants from Somalia faced a ninefold excess risk in mortality, sixfold for migrants from Lebanon, fivefold for migrants from Syria, and a two-to-threefold for migrants from Turkey, Iran, and Iraq [23]. In Denmark, migrants of non-Western origins comprised 15% of COVID-19 hospital admissions despite constituting 9% of the total population [23]. In France, population-wide data on morbidity and healthcare are not col-lected according to ethnic and migrant status [24]. However, data on all-cause mortality rates revealed that persons who are foreign-born had, on average, double the rates of all-cause mortality (some of which were due to COVID-19) compared with the native-French population between March and April 2020, when the virus was surging [25]. Excess COVID-19-related mortality (i.e., a 118% increase compared with the preceding year) was also observed in Seine-Saint-Denis (located in the North of Paris), the poorest district in France with the highest immigrant population (30% in comparison to France's at 10%) [26,27].

Furthermore, the stringent measures towards migrants regarding healthcare provision in France have made it more difficult for migrants to seek healthcare. The 2019 *L'aide médicale de l'État* (AME), or Federal Medical Assistance reform, meant that asylum seekers must complete a 3-month "délai de carence" (waiting period) in France prior to accessing basic healthcare coverage. New restrictions on the type of care available were also introduced, for example, excluding psychiatric support [28].

1.4. A Protection Crisis

Most governments instituted measures such as social distancing, lockdown procedures, and mask mandates in response to COVID-19 case and death rates at the time [29–31]. Implementing government-mandated COVID-19 precaution measures proved particularly challenging for migrants residing in precarious living conditions, which con-tributed to increased vulnerabilities and a protection crisis, and in turn, elevated risk for COVID-19 infection and death among this population, as described above.

Unsanitary and overcrowded living conditions were already an existing issue prior to the COVID-19 pandemic and were exacerbated during the lockdown and the pandemic. For example, the Moria camp in Lesbos, Greece dubbed as "Moria jungle," housed 17,000 migrants above capacity and eventually burnt down in September 2020, leaving over 20,000 residents without shelter [32]. Perilous conditions were not restricted to migrant camps in the Mediterranean; many urban and perceived 'progressive' states have fostered the same adverse living conditions. In November 2020, the French police destroyed a mi-grant camp at the Place de la République in central Paris [33]. The substandard living conditions in the French capital saw migrants with little to no access to sanitation facili-ties and reliant on food donation points by local organizations and civil society [33]. Over 85% of respondents slept in tents, under bridges, or on damp mattresses on the floor [33]. Between 2015 and 2017, the unhygienic and overcrowded conditions combined with a lack of essential resources (e.g., hygiene products) led to recurring outbreaks of scabies [34]. Overall, these adverse physical environmental conditions further augment the popu-lation's vulnerability to disease outbreaks. These living conditions were worsened during the COVID-19 lockdown and the pandemic.

1.5. A Socioeconomic Crisis

Migrants face major hurdles in economic integration in France, given that they have little to no access to the labor market [35]. Undocumented migrants face *de jure* work restrictions (i.e., not legally permitted to work given that they are not afforded the same labor rights in law as citizens) and de facto struggles when working illegally [35]. Most migrants who work are limited to the informal sector with no protections and, thus, higher vulnerabilities.

Evidence highlights the economic and labor challenges faced by migrants due to the COVID-19 pandemic, including increased difficulty in accessing informal labor market participation [29]. The International Labour Organization (ILO) found that these informal sectors were highly impacted by the pandemic, leading to the widespread loss of livelihood and the resultant poverty increase among migrants in Europe [36]. The loss of jobs and informal income-generating opportunities, therefore, led to even deeper financial and food insecurity for migrants than before the pandemic [33].

2. Methods

This study was part of a larger mixed methods research project in collaboration with a community partner, *Habitat et Humanisme*. In 2016, *Habitat et Humanisme* expanded its mission to aid asylum seekers and refugees in France. Its three main aims are (1) to provide accommodation centers for asylum seekers and refugees where they can obtain social, administrative, legal, and integration support; (2) to develop integration programs through training, employment, housing, and culture for refugees; and (3) to conduct research on migrants and their experiences in the host country. Approval for this study was obtained from the Institutional Review Board of the Université de Lyon.

Between September 2019 and February 2020, we began our field research with asylum seekers and refugees. We contacted 16 centers that served migrants in the southeast-central region of Auvergne-Rhône-Alpes and in the north-central region of Île-de-France. Twelve of the centers were affiliated with *Habitat et Humanisme*. Our partnership facilitated our entry into the centers. The first three authors went to each of the centers and held study information sessions to describe the study and the eligibility criteria (at least 18 years of age; migrant status; and currently residing in France) and answer any questions from potential participants. We also emphasized that participation was voluntary. Following the information session, interested participants enrolled in the study. Data collection for the larger research project consisted of ethnographic observations, in-depth, semi-structured interviews, and a survey.

Our field data collection was halted abruptly due to the COVID-19 pandemic. On 16 March 2020, President Macron announced a mandatory home lockdown for 15 days starting at noon on 17 March 2020. This was extended twice and ended on 11 May 2020. Given the pandemic and lockdown situation, we decided to expand our research and developed a semi-structured qualitative interview with the aim of gaining an in-depth understanding of the real-time impact of the pandemic and lockdown from the perspectives of migrants who were either asylum seekers or undocumented. Six months of fieldwork on the larger research project with migrants allowed for much more rapid access to conduct this follow-up research than would normally be the case for community-based qualitative research.

We employed a qualitative, inductive research design, which is concerned with an emic, idiographic approach to research [37]. This approach is focused on the experiences of specific participants (i.e., migrants) and the unique richness of a phenomenon (i.e., their perspectives and experiences living through a pandemic and lockdown). This was the design of choice given the lack of information about this research topic. A semi-structured interview guide was developed to ensure consistency across interviews. Participants were asked open-ended questions with probing questions.

This article presents data from the hour-long phone interviews we conducted with 75 migrants during the pandemic lockdown between March and May 2020. Approximately 120 asylum seekers were contacted, and the purpose of the study were clarified; we were not able to reach about one-third, and several refused to participate in the study. We first collected demographic information from those participants who agreed to participate in the study and then scheduled the interviews. Due to sensitivity regarding obtaining written consent from a migrant population who was seeking asylum and/or undocumented, we obtained informed oral consent instead from each participant prior to the interview. The interviews were conducted in English or French, and an interpreter was used for the participants who stated that they preferred to do the interview in their native language. Each interview was recorded and transcribed into English. Data saturation, that is, when more interviews were not adding any new themes or concepts to what was already known, was achieved [38].

Data Analysis

Qualitative thematic analysis was used to analyze the interview data [39]. Based on Corbin and Strauss' qualitative analytic methods, this analytic technique is grounded in the process of coding similar responses from the sample and using those codes to discern important themes and patterns across participants [39]. The first three authors followed an iterative process of independently reading the interview transcripts, developing a codebook, applying a priori codes, and comparing and revising codes using ATLAS.ti (version 8.0, Berlin, Germany). Using a line-by-line coding method, we each added emergent codes from the data and modified the codebook as needed during the analytic process. Subsequently, we located patterns in the codes and collapsed codes into themes. This was an interpretive process where we searched for meanings at the level of coding as well as contextualized understandings within the data at the level of interpreting findings [39].

During weekly online debrief meetings, we discussed points of disagreement. Stability and agreement are the most relevant types of reliability for textual data. After revisions, we achieved an interrater reliability of 95 percent. To see if this agreement was due to chance, the intercoder reliability was tested using Cohen's Kappa [40]. The overall Kappa coefficient was 0.96. To further ensure data validity, the lead author conducted a member check with a smaller subgroup of migrants (n = 5) who did not participate in the study but possessed similar sociodemographic characteristics as the study participants. Consensus was reached on key themes related to the perceived impact of the lockdown.

3. Results

Table 2 summarizes the sociodemographic characteristics of the study sample. Most participants were male (85%), and the median age for the sample was 26 years old. Approximately 75% of the sample had a primary or secondary level education. While almost 62% of participants had an intermediate level of French language comprehension, more than half (56%) had only a beginner level of oral expression in French. Slightly more than half of the participants were from an African country (55%), while 45% were from Afghanistan. The sociodemographic data for this study is comparable to similar studies with migrants in France [2,3].

Table 2. Sociodemographic characteristics of study sample (n = 75).

Gender, *n* (%)	
Male	64 (85.33)
Female	11 (14.67)
Age (years), median	26
Education, *n* (%)	
Primary	22 (29.33)
Secondary	34 (45.33)
Post-secondary	17 (22.67)
Little or no schooling	2 (2.67)
Level of Comprehension in French, *n* (%)	
Beginner	19 (25.33)
Intermediate	46 (61.33)
Advanced	10 (13.34)
Level of Oral Expression in French, *n* (%)	
Beginner	42 (56.00)
Intermediate	28 (37.33)
Advanced	5 (6.67)
Country of Origin, *n* (%)	
Afghanistan	34 (45.33)
Guinea	7 (9.33)
Mali	6 (8.00)
Ivory Coast	5 (6.67)
Nigeria	4 (5.33)
Senegal	4 (5.33)
Sudan	3 (4.00)
Somalia	3 (4.00)
Eritrea	2 (2.67)

Table 2. *Cont.*

Gender, n (%)	
Congo	2 (2.67)
Chad	2 (2.67)
Madagascar	2 (2.67)
Pakistan	1 (1.33)

The salient themes reflecting the impact of the pandemic and lockdown from the perspectives of the migrants themselves are reported below. Pseudonyms are used for all the participants. The findings below depict how the pandemic and subsequent lockdown contributed to a 'compounded crisis' (i.e., a health, a protection, and a socioeconomic crisis). A social vulnerability lens elucidates how the vulnerabilities experienced by the migrants during the lockdown reinforce and amplify each other.

3.1. Challenges in Following the Public Health Guidelines for Stopping the COVID-19 Spread

Although most of the migrants stated their desire to follow public health guidelines, they recounted not being able to easily follow the guidelines of social distancing and handwashing. Moussa, a 23-year-old male migrant from Guinea, expressed the challenges posed by his living conditions: *"It is practically impossible to follow the social distancing rule. We live in a small physical space and it is overcrowded"*. Another migrant from Nigeria, 25 years of age, spoke about informational and resource barriers to implementing the COVID-19 public health measures: *"Some of the guys are not wearing masks. There is a lack of resources and information. Some are not wearing it correctly. They are placing it underneath their nose or letting it hang by one ear. We also do not always follow the hand sanitization rule. Sometimes we are missing hand soap or hand sanitizer here"*. In addition to a protection crisis, the migrants also experienced challenges related to food and financial insecurity.

3.2. Food and Financial Insecurity

Approximately three-quarters of the migrants spoke of a disruption in their food intake during the lockdown because of lack of money and other resources, which was ex-acerbated due to the lockdown and the pandemic. Mariame, a 28-year-old female from Guinea, recounted her experience: *"During the lockdown, I do not have enough money to buy enough food for the week. To get to those stores that sell food more cheaply, I need a tram ticket, and I do not have money for that. There are days when I go hungry". Other migrants expressed feeling stressed and worried due to their financial situation during the lockdown.* Abdul, a 27-year-old male from Afghanistan stated: *"With the lockdown I am very stressed thinking that I do not have enough money for myself nor to send to my wife and kids back home"*. The pandemic and lockdown also negatively affected migrants' social environment, and, in turn, took a toll on their physical and mental health, as described below.

3.3. Formal Social Networks Disrupted

During the lockdown, most expressed that they felt cut off from their more formal social networks comprised of center staff, social workers, and volunteers. These formal networks were disrupted during the lockdown because there were fewer staff members at the migrant reception centers during that period. Without direct support from staff, the migrants also experienced barriers to scheduling needed administrative, medical, and social service appointments. For many of the migrants, the staff members were their main source of connection to a French person. The disruption of these relationships contributed to feelings of loneliness and social isolation among many of the migrants. Oumou, a 22-year-old male migrant from Mali recounted his experience during the lockdown period:

> *I am completely lost. The people I depend on at the center are not here. Days pass, and I cannot get anything done. I can't schedule my asylum application appointment. Everything is shut down. I need a signature from the center staff on one of the forms and*

> *they are not here. There is nothing to do but wait. I am getting more anxious as the days go on. It seems like it is never-ending, and I feel very alone and desperate without the staff here.*

A few migrants described how they were able to obtain some staff phone support, but it was very limited, which made it difficult for them to adapt to this unprecedented situation.

Most of the asylum seekers also described not having all the necessary information related to COVID-19 and the lockdown and described feeling abandoned by the staff members. Abdul-Ali, a 26-year-old male Afghan migrant reported: "*It is like they (staff at center) left us all alone to fend for ourselves with minimal resources. We need the support from staff in such a difficult situation. There is a lot of confusion and a lack of information during the lockdown. I am not sure what to do or where to go. There is no one here. I do not speak French and do not have any papers or other resources …* " In addition to disrupted formal social networks, all the participants mentioned how the pandemic and lockdown negatively affected their daily and weekly routines.

3.4. Daily and Weekly Routines Disrupted

The lockdown affected the migrants' routines. All the asylum seekers would typically attend French as a second language courses twice a week with an instructor who was a native speaker. For these asylum seekers, the instructor was a consistent source of contact with the French language and culture, and therefore, no longer having this connection made them feel even more disconnected from French society. Some participants shared that their instructor had tried to continue the course via WhatsApp, but this proved to be too challenging and was discontinued. Volunteers were also not able to come to the centers where migrants resided during the lockdown. A 26-year-old male Afghan asylum seeker stated:

> *I look forward to seeing the college students who come every week to the center. We play games, exchange, and have tea together. I learn more about French culture and the language by talking with the volunteers. I miss doing things with them. I spend my time doing nothing all day. The volunteers are all gone. When will I get to see and talk with them again?*

A few migrants who were more proficient in French also volunteered in different organizations. These opportunities had ceased abruptly and indefinitely due to the pandemic. These disruptions meant less interaction and support from their social networks. As a 23-year-old female migrant from Mali stated: "*Volunteering gave me a good excuse to get out and make myself useful. I also made new friends*". Being cut off from their social networks and breaking with their everyday routines and activities contributed to a health crisis, including experiences of social isolation and loneliness.

3.5. Social Isolation and Loneliness

All the participants stated that their social isolation intensified during the lockdown. During this period, the French government had decreed that people should only leave their homes for essential activities, for example, to shop for food or other necessities or to exercise, and that they should limit their distance to one kilometer (0.62 miles) from their home. A Somalian 20-year-old male, Abdirahim, stated, "*I feel confined in my room. There is no one around me. I feel very lonely. Without papers, I feel even more confined as I am not a full member of this society*".

Similarly, another 20-year-old male asylum seeker from the Ivory Coast, Kouakou, described his experience this way: "I am living in confinement, stopped in time. I could not really go anywhere or see anyone other than the people who live with me in the container. I feel isolated from the rest of the world". Although they could physically go outside during the lockdown period, slightly more than half of the participants had no interest in doing so, stating that they felt "depressed," "stressed", or "bored".

Most of the migrants also shared that they had lost interest in eating, personal hygiene, or keeping their living space tidy. All the participants also shared that during the lockdown they experienced poor sleep quality, either "*not sleeping well at all*" or "*too little*" or the other extreme of "*sleeping all day*" or "*most of the day*". In addition to feeling socially isolated and lonely, all the participants reported that they felt an added layer of worry and stress with being away from their families during the pandemic.

3.6. Intense Worry for Themselves and Their Distant Family Members

During the lockdown, most of the participants expressed that they felt even more vulnerable given that they were worried and stressed about the pandemic for themselves and their distant family members. As Seydou, a Malian 26-year-old male asylum seeker, relayed: "*If one of us gets sick, what will happen to us? Where will we go? Where will they put us? Who will help us? Many of us are here alone with no one to help us if we get sick. We do not have legal papers, which will make it more difficult*".

All the migrants also shared concerns about the health and well-being of their distant family members. These family members were in countries with less resources, an inadequate health infrastructure, and where there was a lack of information or misinformation about COVID-19. As Djoëlle, a 24-year-old female asylum seeker from the Democratic Republic of the Congo explained: "*I miss my kids and family back home and I am very worried for their well-being. COVID-19 is scary and there is nothing and nobody there to help them. They do not even have access to the right information. The healthcare system is bad there. What will they do if they get sick?*" Most of the migrants also felt excluded from mainstream society during the lockdown.

3.7. Social Exclusion, Marginalization, and Fear of Deportation

During the lockdown, migrants experienced intensified social exclusion, marginalization, and fear of deportation. Nawaskhan, a 25-year-old male migrant from Afghanistan stated, "*We are not French. We do not speak the language well. As migrants, what rights do we have to complain? We are here, yet we are excluded. During this stay-at-home time, we cannot do anything. Where do we go for help if we need it? We have not been granted refugee status, so we are marginalized*".

Many asylum seekers shared that they felt "*uncomfortable*" or "*fearful*" leaving their room, apartment, center, or container where they lived. Given their undocumented status, many of them did not feel comfortable completing a paper copy or online version of the "Attestation de déplacement" (i.e., government-issued travel certificate), which was required every time one left one's home during the lockdown period to "prove" their purpose for leaving home. Genet, a 28-year-old female migrant from Eritrea, stated, "*I do not have my French papers, so I do not feel at ease filling out an 'Attestation' (travel certificate)*". Similarly, Mohamed, a 27-year-old male Congolese asylum seeker's narrative revealed his fear of being deported:

> *It is too risky to go outside, especially because I do not have my resident permit or any papers. Without my papers, I am excluded. Now they are stopping people and asking them for their attestation de déplacement (travel document). I also do not want to be stopped by the police and risk paying a fine of 135 euros for not having my attestation. I am afraid of going outside. I could get stopped and deported.*

The asylum seekers were already in a "limbo" situation having to wait a longtime (in some cases, several years) to hear news about the outcome of their asylum case and whether they could remain in France with legal status. Along with the lockdown in place, this produced even stronger feelings of uncertainty among migrants regarding their future.

3.8. Uncertain Futures

Due to the lockdown, the asylum administrative processes had all been halted given that government offices had been temporarily closed until further government notice. As a result, all the participants expressed feeling greater uncertainty about their future and the outcome of their asylum case. In the words of Bahiri, a 24-year-old male Afghan asylum seeker: "*It is even harder now during the lockdown to work towards future goals. I am just waiting*". Tabish, also a 24-year-old male migrant from Afghanistan, explained: "*When will my asylum application be processed? I have been waiting for 13 months already and now with the lockdown, it will take even longer. I feel even less confident about my future*". Four participants who already had court appointments for their asylum proceedings received news of their appointments being postponed indefinitely.

Not being able to plan for their futures took a heavy toll on the migrants' mental and physical health and well-being. Many of them stated that they were experiencing headaches, backaches, anxiety, depression, and suicidal thoughts. Nine participants also mentioned that they could not go to the doctor due to structural barriers. Abdo, a 23-year-old male Sudanese migrant, explained: "*I was waiting and waiting for my French healthcare insurance card. Before the pandemic, there was a delay already; you had to wait at least three months. But with the pandemic and the lockdown now, I do not know when I will get it. If I get sick, I do not know what will happen to me*". Despite all the challenges they were facing during the lockdown, the migrants demonstrated different forms of coping too. They turned to each other for different types of support when they needed it most.

3.9. Migrant Solidarity and Reliance on Informal Support Networks

About a third of the asylum seekers mentioned that there was a strong sense of solidarity and social support among fellow asylum seekers during the lockdown. Aboubacar, a 29-year-old male migrant from Guinea stated: "*We decided to form an informal sport group during the lockdown. We use the space outside the container to work out together. It is a great way to feel less lonely and get energy for ourselves and from each other*".

Kamal, a 20-year-old male Sudanese asylum seeker, expressed relying on these informal networks for tangible support during the lockdown: "*We depend on one another right now. When I need money, my friends at the center help me out and give me some money. They know I am more desperate, and they help me out during this hard time during the lockdown*". Most of the participants also recounted being able to depend on fellow asylum seekers for emotional support. Babacar, a 26-year-old male migrant from Senegal, explains: "*This is tough right now with the confinement. I am down. I have not been out of my room in three weeks. This is the first time today that I went to the salon to talk to the other guys there. When I am down, I isolate myself in my room. They help me feel better. We listen to music and watch some YouTube videos together. They help me feel a little better*". There were many other examples of solidarity among migrants during the lockdown period. They also revealed different forms of coping.

3.10. Forms of Coping

Besides mutual social support, most migrants found other ways to cope with the negative consequences of the lockdown. Many of them spoke about needing to stay strong for themselves and their families, including those relatives with whom they stayed in touch via social apps on their phones, such as WhatsApp. Seydou, a 24-year-old male migrant from the Ivory Coast, expressed: "*What choice do I have? I need to be there for my wife and three children in the country. I need to put a smile on their faces. I talk to them three times a week. I do not burden them with my worries. I tell them everything is ok, even though we are having a lockdown here*".

Omran, a 28-yer-old male asylum seeker from Afghanistan, shared how the lockdown situation was beyond his control and how he used his spiritual faith as a coping mechanism: "The confinement is not something I can control. We must make the best out of this situation. *In sha'Allah!* I leave it in Allah's hands. He will help me, and all of us make it through this difficult time. I pray and ask Allah for strength". Many of the Arabic-speaking migrants verbalized the common Arabic term "*In sha'Allah*", an equivalent to the English expression "God willing" or "if God wills" when they were referring to "*getting through*" the lockdown. The term expresses the belief that nothing happens unless God wills it, and that God's will supersedes all human will. Most of the participants demonstrated different forms of coping as they faced multiple challenges during the mandatory lockdown.

4. Discussion

The findings reveal that migrants experienced increased food and financial insecurity as well as disruptions of formal social networks and routines. These vulnerabilities led to more social isolation and loneliness, as well as more worry for themselves and for their relatives who were left behind in their countries of origin. During the lockdown, feelings of social exclusion, marginalization, and fear of deportation among migrants escalated. In addition, they worried about the consequences of the pandemic on both their immediate and future lives.

Analysis of the migrants' narratives showed how these negative effects on their social, physical, and psychological well-being converged during the lockdown. Our study findings are consistent with similar studies conducted in France [2,3,41]. First, the gap in mental and physical healthcare for migrants only worsened during the lockdown as migrants were cut off from their regular social networks of volunteers and aid workers. The unmet needs of migrants piled onto the already large burden of being a migrant without documentation in France.

Second, the financial challenges that migrants were experiencing during the pandemic added another layer of vulnerability to their lives as stipends that they typically received from the government were either unreliable or stopped completely, especially as funds were being diverted to pandemic healthcare efforts [33,36]. Moreover, informal income-generating opportunities were now unavailable, contributing to the financial insecurity experienced by many migrants. This also led to food insecurity as many migrants who relied on aid organizations for food were left with little to no resources.

Third, there was a lack of security and protection for migrants, many of whom were living in precarious living conditions, making it nearly impossible to follow public health measures and putting them at an increased risk for contracting COVID-19. The health, socio-economic, and protection crises exacerbated by the COVID-19 pandemic and lockdown disproportionately affected migrants, given their severely limited ability to access health-care, education, work, social protections, and other fundamental human rights even prior to the pandemic. Furthermore, the pandemic exposed the negative health and social outcomes among migrant groups that have resulted from long-standing structural inequities.

On a larger scale, the gaps left for migrants call into question policies for the general population. The global pandemic was a test for our policies and social protection measures, and we failed. The difficulties the migrants were experiencing during the pandemic served as a litmus test that exposes failures in policies and practices that do not address the social determinants of health, as evidenced by the negative outcomes for migrants, who are among the most vulnerable populations on the front line.

Specifically, in France we observe that a major barrier to address migrant health and well-being is the lack of data on migrants and their social conditions [24]. These practices and norms stem, in part, from an assimilationist view and practice of foreign-born individuals and 'color-blindness' ideology. The lack of data, including epidemiological data about migrants, poses multiple challenges for researchers and policymakers, such as the underestimation of the number of '*sans papiers*' (i.e., undocumented) and the inability of researchers to document the full extent of the problem.

The COVID-19 response plan in place during the onset of the pandemic and lockdown was a policy that excluded migrants and therefore worsened their health and well-being. Migrant aid organizations have filled the gaps left by the state by providing migrants with as much care as they were able to provide. The vaccine rollout added another layer of complexity as the French government was hesitant to offer vaccinations to undocumented migrants [42]. Aid organizations once again stepped in to fill the gaps in healthcare left by the state, and in July 2021, *Médecins Sans Frontières* (Doctors Without Borders) began offering vaccines to migrants [41,42].

4.1. Study Limitations and Strengths

Limitations of this study include a small sample, which makes it difficult to know whether the findings are valid for the overall migrant population in France. This was the design of choice given the lack of information about this research topic and the difficulty in reaching this marginalized population. Despite the limitation, this study was innovative, and the use of a rigorous, qualitative methodology allowed us to generate in-depth knowledge from the perspectives of migrants living through the first pandemic lockdown in France. We were also able to achieve data saturation with the sample. Other study strengths include adopting a community-academic research partnership model, using multiple coders to check reliability, and conducting member-checks to ensure data validity.

4.2. Policy and Practice Implications

Study findings highlight the importance of understanding the negative effects of the COVID-19 pandemic and lockdown measures on migrants' lives and livelihoods to develop effective policies and measures that can either prevent or mitigate these effects in a future pandemic. First and foremost, vulnerable populations such as migrants require special attention from policymakers in their response to a pandemic, given the migrants' adverse living situations. Safe living conditions that ensure appropriate personal protective equipment and non-crowded living quarters are essential to prevent the exposure and spread of a virus among migrants and spread to others outside their living spaces. Moreover, inclusive policies that ensure equitable access to healthcare, including prevention and treatment, testing, and new therapeutics, are critical to protecting the whole population.

Second, the collection and dissemination of surveillance data and sociodemographic data including age, country of birth, migration status, and self-reported race/ethnicity will help determine the relative contribution of each of these driving factors for the observed health disparities and identify areas of unmet need. We must also advocate for the strengthening of public health datasets so that data can be collated and shared more effectively, as this is an essential step to guide policy, healthcare provision, prevention, and intervention efforts. These data systems will be important in both supporting the response to a future pandemic as well as new surges and in ensuring a long-term response to better tackle health inequities.

Third, public health efforts that provide messaging and interventions adapted to the linguistic, cultural, and social circumstances of migrants will be crucial to effectively prevent transmission within and beyond these communities.

Fourth, it is important to recognize the vital role that civil society organizations and other non-governmental actors play in providing different types of much-needed support to migrants during a pandemic. Their efforts highlight how the French government needs to adopt an intersectoral approach to mitigating the effects of a pandemic.

Fifth, the COVID-19 pandemic has shone a spotlight on health inequities and has created an opportunity to address the social determinants of health underlying these inequities. To date, policymakers have yet to adopt an approach that views *all* policies (including immigration policy) as health policies. This approach, referred to as the *Health in All Policies* approach, highlights how all sectors in the government, such as transportation, education, housing, and employment, have healthcare implications [43–45]. For example, during the COVID-19 pandemic, transportation policy is important because an individual who has COVID-19 who relies on public transportation for work can be exposed to the virus easily and then spread the virus to many people through close contact, which makes wearing masks, regular cleaning, and more frequent buses and trains a necessity to cut down on crowds and curb the spread of the virus.

In addition, implementing a *Health in All Policies* approach through the lens of migration during a global pandemic underscores the importance of achieving regional and global policy coherence. As we observed with the case of COVID-19, response policies varied by country, which made it difficult to curb the spread of COVID-19. The statement that "no one is safe until everyone is safe" highlights the need for a united global response to a pandemic [46]. Having regional and global coordination of response policies headed by health ministers across countries would ensure policy coherence across the board and a universal standard of practices that could potentially curb the global spread of a contagious disease like COVID-19.

Lastly, creating these coherent pandemic policies would also potentially help to depoliticize COVID-19 and healthcare for migrants. A case in point is Portugal. At the beginning of the pandemic, the Portuguese government implemented a policy that treated migrants within its borders as if they were residents, giving them full access to public services, including healthcare [47]. Portugal's policy serves as an example of incorporating a multisectoral approach and depoliticizes the care of migrants under the state system. Future studies examining how policy changes that promote equity and inclusion influence health outcomes among migrants are recommended.

5. Conclusions

Health is a fundamental human right for *all* human beings despite income, ethnicity/race, gender, age, country of origin, and other factors, and is indispensable for the exercise of other human rights. Thus, the right to health is an inclusive right that extends not only to healthcare but also to the underlying determinants of health, such as adequate sanitation, sufficient and nutritious food, and safe living and working conditions. Inclusive, responsive, and coherent policies and practices that apply health and healthcare to *all* sectors and regardless of migration status, are essential. Ultimately, this is the way forward to minimizing the burden and transmission of infectious diseases and promoting health equity for all.

Author Contributions: Conceptualization, M.D.J.; Formal analysis, M.D.J.; Funding acquisition, L.P.; Investigation, M.D.J., Z.M. and Z.H.S.; Methodology, M.D.J.; Resources, M.D.J. and L.P.; Supervision, M.D.J.; Visualization, M.D.J. and Z.M.; Writing—original draft, M.D.J.; Writing—review & editing, M.D.J., N.B. and R.K. All authors have read and agreed to the published version of the manuscript.

Funding: This research was funded by the Institute for Advanced Studies, Collegium de Lyon within the Université de Lyon and Habitat et Humanisme.

Institutional Review Board Statement: The study was conducted in accordance with the Declaration of Helsinki and approved by the Institutional Review Board of Université de Lyon.

Informed Consent Statement: Informed consent was obtained from all subjects involved in the study.

Data Availability Statement: Data can be made available upon reasonable request.

Acknowledgments: The authors would like to thank the study participants who shared their perspectives.

Conflicts of Interest: The authors declare no conflict of interest. The funders had no role in the design of the study; in the collection, analyses, or interpretation of data; in the writing of the manuscript, or in the decision to publish the results.

References

1. French Public Health Agency. COVID-19: Point Épidémiologique du 10 mars 2020. 2020. Available online: https://www.santepubliquefrance.fr/maladies-et-traumatismes/maladies-et-infections-respiratoires/infection-a-coronavirus/documents/bulletin-national/covid-19-point-epidemiologique-du-10-mars-2020 (accessed on 21 January 2021).
2. Crouzet, L.; Scarlett, H.; Colleville, A.-C.; Pourtau, L.; Melchior, M.; Ducarroz, S. Impact of the COVID-19 pandemic on vulnerable groups, including homeless persons and migrants, in France: A qualitative study. *Prev. Med. Rep.* **2022**, *26*, 101727. [CrossRef] [PubMed]
3. Carillon, S.; Gosselin, A.; Coulibaly, K.; Ridde, V.; Desgrées du Loû, A.; The MAKASI Study Group. Immigrants facing COVID-19 containment in France: An ordinary hardship of disaffiliation. *J. Migr. Health* **2020**, *1–2*, 100032. [CrossRef]
4. Greenaway, C.; Hargreaves, S.; Barkati, S.; Coyle, C.M.; Gobbi, F.; Veizis, A.; Douglas, P. COVID-19: Exposing and addressing health disparities among ethnic minorities and migrants. *J. Travel Med.* **2020**, *27*, taaa113. [CrossRef]
5. Page, K.R.; Venkataramani, M.; Beyrer, C.; Polk, S. Undocumented U.S. immigrants and COVID-19. *N. Engl. J. Med.* **2020**, *382*, e62. [CrossRef] [PubMed]
6. Marmot, M.; Allen, J. COVID-19: Exposing and amplifying inequalities. *J. Epidemiol. Commun. Health* **2020**, *74*, 681–682. [CrossRef] [PubMed]
7. UN General Assembly. *Convention Relating to the Status of Refugees*; United Nations, Treaty Series, 189, 137; Institute of Jewish Affairs: London, UK, 1951; Available online: https://www.refworld.org/docid/3be01b964.html (accessed on 24 January 2021).

8. Redpath-Cross, J.; Perruchoud, R. *Glossary on Migration*; IOM: Geneva, Switzerland, 2019; Available online: https://www.iom.int/glossary-migration (accessed on 24 January 2021).
9. Vespe, M.; Natale, F.; Pappalardo, L. Datasets on Irregular Migration and Irregular Migrants in the EU. IOM, 2017; pp. 26–33. Available online: https://publications.jrc.ec.europa.eu/repository/handle/JRC107749 (accessed on 22 January 2021).
10. International Organization for Migration. IOM World Migration Report. International Organization for Migration, 2018; pp. 1–359. Available online: https://www.iom.int/sites/g/files/tmzbdl486/files/country/docs/china/r5_world_migration_report_2018_en.pdf (accessed on 24 January 2021).
11. Ge, Y.; Dou, W.; Zhang, H. A new framework for understanding urban social vulnerability from a network perspective. *Sustainability* **2017**, *9*, 1723. [CrossRef]
12. Burton, C.; Rufat, S.; Tate, E. Social Vulnerability: Conceptual Foundations and Geospatial Modeling. In *Vulnerability and Resilience to Natural Hazards*; Cambridge University Press: Cambridge, UK, 2018. [CrossRef]
13. Kim, S.J.; Bostwick, W. Social vulnerability and racial inequality in COVID-19 deaths in Chicago. *Health Educ. Behav.* **2020**, *47*, 509–513. [CrossRef] [PubMed]
14. Kruczkiewicz, A.; Klopp, J.; Fisher, J.; Mason, S.; McClain, S.; Sheekh, N.M.; Moss, R.; Parks, R.M.; Braneon, C. Compound risks and complex emergencies require new approaches to preparedness. *PNAS* **2021**, *118*, e2106795118. [CrossRef] [PubMed]
15. UN Sustainable Development Group. Policy Brief: COVID-19 and People on the Move. 2020. Available online: https://unsdg.un.org/resources/policy-brief-covid-19-and-people-move (accessed on 24 January 2021).
16. World Health Organization. COVID-19 Disrupting Mental Health Services in Most Countries, WHO Survey. 2020. Available online: https://www.who.int/news/item/05-10-2020-covid-19-disrupting-mental-health-services-in-most-countries-who-survey (accessed on 22 January 2021).
17. Pinzón-Espinosa, J.; Valdés-Florido, M.J.; Riboldi, I.; Baysak, E.; Vieta, E. The COVID-19 pandemic and mental health of refugees, asylum seekers, and migrants. *J. Affect. Disord.* **2021**, *280*, 407–408. [CrossRef] [PubMed]
18. Júnior, J.G.; de Sales, J.P.; Moreira, M.M.; Pinheiro, W.R.; Lima, C.K.T.; Neto, M.L.R. A crisis within the crisis: The mental health situation of refugees in the world during the 2019 coronavirus (2019-nCoV) outbreak. *Psychiatry Res.* **2020**, *280*, 407–408. [CrossRef]
19. Dalexis, R.D.; Cénat, J.M. Asylum seekers working in Quebec (Canada) during the COVID-19 pandemic: Risk of deportation, and threats to physical and mental health. *Psychiatry Res.* **2020**, *292*, 113299. [CrossRef] [PubMed]
20. Kenny, M.A.; Grech, C.; Procter, N. A trauma informed response to COVID 19 and the deteriorating mental health of refugees and asylum seekers with insecure status in Australia. *Int. J. Ment. Health Nurs.* **2022**, *31*, 62–69. [CrossRef]
21. Mukumbang, F.C.; Ambe, A.N.; Adebiyi, B.O. Unspoken inequality: How COVID-19 has exacerbated existing vulnerabilities of asylum-seekers, refugees, and undocumented migrants in South Africa. *Int. J. Equity Health* **2020**, *19*, 141. [CrossRef] [PubMed]
22. Simon, P. The failure of the importation of ethno-racial statistics in Europe: Debates and controversies. *Ethn. Racial Stud.* **2017**, *40*, 2326–2332. [CrossRef]
23. Vist Gunn, E.; Arentz-Hansen, E.H.; Vedoy, T.F.; Spilker, R.S.; Hafstad, E.V.; Giske, L. Incidence and Severe Outcomes from COVID-19 among Immigrant and Minority Ethnic Groups and among Groups of Different Socio-Economic Status: A Systematic Review. Available online: https://www.fhi.no/globalassets/dokumenterfiler/rapporter/2021/incidence-and-severe-outcomes-from-covid-19-among-immigrant-and-minority-ethnic-groups-and-among-groups-of-different-socio-economic-status-report-2021.pdf (accessed on 21 January 2021).
24. Melchior, M.; Desgrées du Loû, A.; Gosselin, A.; Datta, G.D.; Carabali, M.; Merckx, J.; Kaufman, J.S. Migrant status, ethnicity and COVID-19: More accurate European data are greatly needed. *Clin. Microbiol. Infect.* **2021**, *27*, 160–162. [CrossRef] [PubMed]
25. Papon, S.; Robert-Bobée, I. Une hausse des décès deux fois plus forte pour les personnes nées à l'étranger que pour celles nées en France en mars-avril 2020. *INSEE Focus* **2020**, *198*, 160–162. Available online: https://www.insee.fr/fr/statistiques/4627049 (accessed on 21 January 2021).
26. L'Institut Paris Region. La Surmortalité Durant L'épidémie de COVID-19 Dans les Départements Franciliens. 2020. Available online: https://www.ors-idf.org/nos-travaux/publications/la-surmortalite-durant-lepidemie-de-covid-19-dans-les-departements-franciliens.html (accessed on 24 January 2021).
27. Fouillet, A.; Pontais, I.; Caserio-Schönemann, C. Excess all-cause mortality during the first wave of the COVID-19 epidemic in France. *Eur. Commun. Dis. Bull.* **2020**, *25*, 34. [CrossRef]
28. Stone, J. Macron Plans to Bar Refugees from Accessing Medical Care. The Independent, 2019. Available online: https://www.independent.co.uk/news/world/europe/emmanuel-macron-migrants-refugee-access-medical-care-immigration-latest-a9188166.html (accessed on 24 January 2021).
29. Organisation for Economic Co-Operation and Development (OECD). The Territorial Impact of COVID-19: Managing the Crisis across Levels of Government. 2020. Available online: https://www.oecd.org/coronavirus/policy-responses/the-territorial-impact-of-covid-19-managing-the-crisis-across-levels-of-government-d3e314e1 (accessed on 22 January 2021).
30. Financial Times Visual & Data Journalism Team. Lockdowns Compared: Tracking Governments' Coronavirus Responses. 2021. Available online: https://ig.ft.com/coronavirus-lockdowns (accessed on 27 January 2021).
31. Haug, N.; Geyrhofer, L.; Londei, A.; Dervic, E.; Desvars-Larrive, A.; Loreto, V.; Pinior, B.; Thurner, S.; Klimek, P. Ranking the effectiveness of worldwide COVID-19 government interventions. *Nat. Hum. Behav.* **2020**, *4*, 1303–1312. [CrossRef] [PubMed]

32. BBC. Lesbos: Greek Police Move Migrants to New Camp after Moira Fire. Available online: https://www.bbc.com/news/world-europe-54189073 (accessed on 21 January 2021).
33. Byrne, M. On the streets of Paris: The experience of displaced migrants and refugees. *Soc. Sci.* **2021**, *10*, 130. [CrossRef]
34. Par, C.B. Paris: Retour de la Gale Parmi les Réfugiés. LeParisien, 2017. Available online: https://www.leparisien.fr/paris-75/paris-75018/paris-retour-de-la-gale-parmi-les-refugies-15-06-2017-7055208.php (accessed on 21 January 2021).
35. Louarn, A.-D. The Risks of Working Illegally in France. 2018. Available online: https://www.infomigrants.net/en/post/7067/the-risks-of-working-illegally-in-france (accessed on 24 January 2021).
36. International Labour Organization (ILO). Impact of Lockdown Measures on the Informal Economy. 2020. Available online: https://www.ilo.org/wcmsp5/groups/public/---ed_protect/---protrav/---travail/documents/briefingnote/wcms_743534.pdf (accessed on 24 January 2021).
37. Watson, L.C.; Watson-Franke, M.-B. *Interpreting Life Histories: An Anthropological Inquiry*; Rutgers University Press: New Brunswick, NJ, USA, 1985.
38. Morse, J.M. The Significance of Saturation. *Qual. Health Res.* **1995**, *5*, 147–149. [CrossRef]
39. Corbin, J.; Strauss, A. *Basics of Qualitative Research (3rd ed.): Techniques and Procedures for Developing Grounded Theory*; Sage: Thousand Oaks, CA, USA, 2008.
40. Bernard, H.R. *Social Research Methods: Qualitative and Quantitative Approaches*; Sage: Los Angeles, CA, USA, 2013.
41. Gautier, L.; Nguengang Wakap, S.; Verrier, F.; Miranda, E.; Négré, V.; Hamza, J.; Poveda, J.-D.; Bouchon, M. Responding to increasing health and social needs of unprotected unaccompanied minors in Paris in the context of COVID-19: A mixed methods case study. *J. Immigr. Refug. Stud.* 2022; 1–20, *ahead-of-print*. [CrossRef]
42. Pedram, A. Aid Group Vaccinates Migrants as France Expands Virus Pass. ABC News, 2021. Available online: https://abcnews.go.com/Health/wireStory/aid-group-vaccinates-migrants-france-expands-virus-pass-79141632 (accessed on 22 January 2021).
43. De Jesus, M.; Williams, D.R. The Care and Prevention in the United States Demonstration Project: A call for more focus on the social determinants of HIV/AIDS. *Public Health Rep.* **2018**, *133*, 28S–33S. [CrossRef] [PubMed]
44. Rudolph, L.; Caplan, J.; Ben-Moshe, K.; Dillon, L. *Health in All Policies: A Guide for State and Local Governments*; American Public Health Association and Public Health Institute: Washington, DC, USA; Oakland, CA, USA, 2013.
45. Clavier, C. Implementing health in all policies—Time and ideas matter too! Comment on Understanding the role of public administration in implementing action on the social determinants of health and health inequities. *Int. J. Health Policy Manag.* **2016**, *5*, 609–610. [CrossRef] [PubMed]
46. UNICEF. No-One Is Safe until Everyone Is Safe—Why We Need a Global Response to COVID-19. UNICEF, 2021. Available online: https://www.unicef.org/press-releases/no-one-safe-until-everyone-safe-why-we-need-global-response-covid-19 (accessed on 24 January 2021).
47. Reuters Staff. Portugal to Treat Migrants as Residents during Coronavirus Crisis. Reuters, 2020. Available online: https://www.reuters.com/article/us-health-coronavirus-portugal/portugal-to-treat-migrants-as-residents-during-coronavirus-crisis-idUSKBN21F0N7 (accessed on 24 January 2021).

International Journal of
Environmental Research and Public Health

MDPI

Article

Reskilled and Integrated, but How? Navigating Trauma and Temporary Hardships

Cihan Aydiner [1,*] and Erin L. Rider [2]

[1] Homeland Security Program, Department of Security and Emergency Services, College of Arts & Sciences, Worldwide Campus, Embry-Riddle Aeronautical University, Daytona Beach, FL 32114, USA
[2] Department of Sociology and Political Science, College of Social and Behavioral Sciences, Jacksonville State University, Jacksonville, AL 36265, USA
* Correspondence: aydinerc@erau.edu

Abstract: Immigrants are often pressed to show how they will contribute to a host country, thus proving through their conditions of entry and human capital whether they will be perceived as an asset or burden, and this is juxtaposed with the host country's institutions offering an improved quality of life, mainly through employment. Seeking employment is often a key factor to be economically assimilated, and in the case of highly educated Turkish migrants, the opportunity to reclaim their previous professional and quality of life statuses. Based on qualitative research, we have examined the experiences of highly educated Turkish people (n = 42) in the recently forced migrant population. Following events including terrorism and the coup on 15 July 2016, Türkiye experienced the highest forced migration in her history. With exiled Turkish migrants, the forced aspect of their migration prompts them to seek a host country that provides safety, and they are also driven to transfer their educational degrees and professional credentials. However, changing careers to become educated and certified in new fields takes time and resources, contributing to a fluctuating economic status and loss of well-being. Once this is regained, their economic situation is improved, but there is still the lost time from the immigration and transfer period. Thus, the process has positive and negative components, but understanding this nuanced process provides opportunities for policy reform that can shorten the time of re-education, increase employability, and support well-being.

Keywords: forced migration; exile; well-being; highly educated migrants

Citation: Aydiner, C.; Rider, E.L. Reskilled and Integrated, but How? Navigating Trauma and Temporary Hardships. *Int. J. Environ. Res. Public Health* **2022**, *19*, 13675. https://doi.org/10.3390/ijerph192013675

Academic Editors: Ernesto Castañeda and Maria De Jesus

Received: 5 October 2022
Accepted: 19 October 2022
Published: 21 October 2022

1. Introduction

1.1. Migration of Large Turkish Population to the USA

Immigrants, especially forced ones, generally prefer neighboring countries to migrate to due to main reasons such as affordability, proximity, and similarity to their origin states. Moving too far away from the origin country requires more economic, social, and cultural capital. In the case of modern Türkiye, large groups of Turkish migrants have taken residence within Europe mainly for economic reasons and family reunification in the 1960s. Turks contribute to the highest immigrant population, with more than five million in Europe now [1].

Due to immigration laws, Turkish immigrants to the USA were a smaller migration population, but were more educated, with around 23,000 in the same period [2]. Following World War II, the U.S. attracted many professionals with its rise in science and technology. Highly skilled and educated Turks, including doctors, engineers, and academics, also took their place in this brain drain in the USA until the 1980s and increased the population up to 50,000 [3,4]. Between the 1980s and 2010, the Turkish population reached close to 200,000 based on US census data (2010). During this period, Türkiye faced a military coup and the Kurdish conflict. As a result, Kurdish-origin Turks and other less educated and semi-skilled Turks migrated to the U.S. due to political unrest and economic reasons [2].

The Turkish migration to the U.S. following the coup in Türkiye on 15 July 2016 was dramatically different from previously forced migrations. The foundation of democracy has been undergoing recent threats, and authoritarianism is rising in many countries. Some semi-democratic regimes are using staged events such as coups or terrorism for the sake of their survival, transition to autocracy, and empowerment. Türkiye is an explicit example of this transition process under Erdogan's rule. On 15 July 2016, staged events such as the coups were organized and directed by Erdogan's government and its partners to oppress opposing groups and people on the side of democracy, freedom of speech, and rule of law. Erdogan described the events of 15 July as a "gift from God". Regarding the critical events and indications of democratic erosion in Türkiye before and after 15 July 2016, coup-like events provide a larger picture of the causes of targeting some people in the country. Those opposing groups on the side of democracy have been silenced, isolated, jailed, exiled, and/or forced to migrate systematically to accomplish the transition process to the anti-democratic regime by Erdogan's government. Specifically, the ruling AKP (Adalet ve Kalkinma Partisi—Justice and Development Party) declared a state of emergency, imprisoned or fired hundreds of thousands of high-profile civil servants, and closed thousands of schools and hundreds of news outlets. During the crackdown, many officials in Western countries, including diplomats, foreign ministry officials, and academics, refused to return home following government orders due to a lack of evidence and the risk of imprisonment. Some of them returned and experienced imprisonment or mobbing, abuse, and eventual dismissal from their posts. This political climate has prompted former state officials to consider the option of permanent residence in the host country. As a result of these political conditions, Türkiye experienced the third highest immigration pattern in her modern history. Over 250,000 Turks emigrated in 2017 after the events, which was a 42% increase from 2016. Asylum applications worldwide increased by 10,000 to over 33,000 in 2017 [5]. The number of Turkish immigrants obtaining lawful permanent resident status in the USA was approximately 5000 yearly from 2017 to 2021. However, the number of individuals granted asylum affirmatively was only 15 in 2017. Asylum rates increased to 475 in 2018, 1714 in 2019, and 1568 in 2020 [6]. The Turkish population is estimated to be around 350,000 in the U.S. currently, including increased unauthorized arrivals, especially through the El Paso/Texas entryway, reaching more than 10,000 Turkish nationals in 2022 [7].

The main reason for professionals' migration was opposition to the ruling party. Almost all of them were highly educated, skilled, and legal migrants. Professionals included judges, teachers, doctors, journalists, police officers, ministry officials, and military career officers, including cadets and retired officers. If they were not arrested, most of them were denied passports, disqualified, humiliated, and stamped in the country. This atmosphere has forced many to leave the country through legal or illegal means to Europe and North America. Many of them were fluent in English and familiar with life in the U.S. due to having educational and occupational experience prior to the 2016 events. However, despite some familiarity with the U.S., most of them had never envisioned living in another country because their identity and loyalty were centered on serving their homeland (Aydiner and Rider 2021). Many of these displaced professionals have been granted special visas, green cards, asylum, or refugee status. Managing the migration process and providing suitable jobs for this talented immigrant group is, therefore, a challenge [8].

1.2. Purpose of the Research

The recently immigrated Turkish migrant population creates a compelling case for researching higher education connections and the administration of justice in migration policies/practices related to highly educated individuals' integration into the U.S. as well as supporting their well-being. Understanding this nuanced process provides opportunities for policy reforms that can reduce re-education and recredential time, increase employability, and promote well-being. We anticipate there are benefits to the U.S. in employing this professional labor group and inclusion strategies for new immigration populations from different countries following global crises and events similar to those experienced by exiled Turkish professionals. Uniquely, this professional labor group occupies a higher economic status as a group of professional, skilled workers with presumably greater economic options in the U.S. and a strong likelihood of permanent integration.

The most important research questions guiding this study were: What are the long-term effects of immigrants' new career paths, their strategies/solutions to cope with policy issues, and the psychological issues that follow them? and What are the outcomes for the temporary deskilling of highly educated immigrants? The current study focuses on Turkish emigration following the 2016 coup-like event. This migrant population is unique, given that they were forced to flee their relatively stable lives built around their family, education, and profession in order to seek safety. Their forced migration was unplanned and required significant maneuvering to re-establish their lives in a foreign country. In acknowledgment of the dire factors of the immigration process, many Turkish immigrants had high human capital with regard to education and their profession. Higher human capital tends to indicate the self-selection of a host country that can offer adequate labor opportunities. However, for Turkish immigrants, despite their high levels of education and professional status, the forced aspect of their migration and the level of urgency complicated their immigration experience and ability to secure stability, maintain their high human capital, and regain their former professional status. This study examines the economic assimilation experiences of forced yet highly educated Turkish immigrants to better understand complex factors that either aid or hinder economic integration in a destination society. This project suggests direct benefits for the management of highly educated migrants by learning the characteristics of the migrant population and proposing solutions/innovative alternatives for inclusion and integration. The study helps to understand the development of a policy reform by showing the nuanced differences of the population. This may support the creation of a fast-tracked integration model by collaborating with employers and organizations to strategize efforts for streamlined accreditation and training processes.

2. Literature Review

Immigration studies have largely focused on the dichotomy between push and pull factors that impact immigrants in different ways based on their immigration type—voluntary and involuntary [9,10]. It has long been supported that economic migrants (voluntary) have greater decision-making ability and financial capital planning for migration [10,11]. For political refugees, their migration journey is determined often immediately with little opportunity to plan [12–14]. The unique circumstances of Turkish migrants can be predicted based on push and pull factors. Push factors are related to their country's political and economic instability and lack of safety, while pull factors are associated with safety and economic opportunity in the host society. Regarding social capital, previous experience in the U.S. and other Western countries, educational and professional skill sets, degree of English fluency, and social networking with other Turks, these factors can afford Turkish immigrants a smoother integration transition [8,15]. However, some factors could be barriers; these include challenges associated with forced migration and trauma, foreign credentials, lack of work experience in a host country, and less direct professional and social networks with native workers.

The literature has characterized the challenges of immigrant assimilation in a variety of contexts, such as social, professional, and civic, and the nature of the immigration process initially, either forced or voluntary. In the literature, it is often presumed that forced or voluntary migrants with little human capital will face greater barriers to improving their quality of life and social and economic integration [16]. On the other hand, destination countries tend to advertise for a need to accept highly educated professionals to fill gaps in work industries [17–19]. Sapeha [20] finds "during the application process, the Canadian immigration system allocates more points to immigrants with higher levels of education. This assumes that those with higher human capital would have a smoother process of integration into the receiving society. However, findings from the present study do not support this assertion". This study finds levels of satisfaction to be lower [20]. In the case of highly educated Turkish immigrants, the assumption of being sought after for their educational background, skill sets, and professional experience underscores another factor that their economic integration is not always easy nor streamlined. Specifically, Western developed countries' demand for professional skilled immigrants assumes there will be less barriers and public welfare concerns [21], enabling immigrants to efficiently integrate into the skilled labor market, which is an ultimate mutual benefit to destination countries' skilled employment and immigrants' quality of life. However, several studies have come to find that foreign credentials hold lower value and are not comparable to native citizens' credentials [22–24]. Significantly, Sweetman, McDonald, and Hawthorne find that this leads to consequences for immigrants, specifically "lower earnings and job dissatisfaction" and "to the host country in terms of lost productivity" [25].

There are several factors unique to highly educated/skilled migrants that pose barriers to economic integration and workplace participation: the foreign credential recognition process [25,26], occupational mismatches [27,28], hiring chances [26], and long-term earnings gaps [25,29]. These barriers have been generally attributed to or categorized as ethnic penalties [30,31] and are noticeable in comparison to native citizens. The foreign credential recognition process is complex as it is not standardized across professions. In general, foreign degrees are often more challenging to verify regarding equivalency and quality in comparison to the ease of determination for native citizen degrees. Research on STEM-educated immigrants by Boyd and Tian finds that in comparison to Canadian-educated citizens, immigrants educated in "Canada, the U.S., the U.K., and France, do earn less, but the earnings gap are lower than for immigrants educated elsewhere" [32]. As Boyd and Tian assert, "degrees from Eastern Europe and Asia are not as portable" [32]. These findings reveal both ethnic penalties and assumptions about which countries' degrees are viewed as equivalent. Here, Western countries standardize foreign degrees from other Western-identified countries. Michalikova, in her research on Eastern European immigrants, finds that they are hindered by socioeconomic differences based on their educational systems, pre-emigration labor market experiences, and the language barrier [31].

Certain professions, such as those in the medical field, encounter a more arduous process that may require education and training to be done in the destination society rather than be transferred in, while other professions that do not have licensure may find an easier transfer process. Occupations with associated credentialing tend to be more difficult for immigrants to access, and immigrants are less likely to gain employment in these professions [33]. Despite these access barriers, these jobs tend to be coveted because they are associated with "higher wages and their wage disadvantage is lower" [33]. This leads to the previously mentioned notion that host countries can attract highly educated immigrants with the promise of skilled professions, but in reality, the access to these jobs and transferability are low. The time and money invested in an occupation, thus, may not be matched with opportunities to continue in that occupation in the destination society. Notably, in a study examining the outcomes of occupational licensure, Redbird and Escamilla-Garcia found a positive linkage in the ability for licensure to "increase inclusion and transferability of educational credentials" [34]. Other research has shown similar findings that licensure can enable immigrants to access professions based on verification (see Fu and Hickey [35]). Similarly, Haberfield et al., in their research on highly skilled German immigrants, found that factors such as highly skilled, transferability of human capital, self-selection of the host country, and reception in the host country all added to their ability to reach "full earnings parity with natives of similar attributes" [36]. Other research has added that immigrants with "standardized and occupation-specific profiles" can access greater advantages [26].

Immigrants may also find themselves unable to continue in their profession due to barriers in the credential recognition process, lack of available jobs in the destination society, and time spent waiting for re-education/certification. Some immigrants may choose to seek out a new occupation, thus embarking on new educational and skill development. These circumstances demonstrate problems associated with an occupational mismatch [28,37]. In this sense, immigrants' education, skills, and professional experience are unused and potentially wasted. Guo observes a glass gate effect in which "professional communities" restrict qualified immigrants because of the perception that their education and skill credentials are deemed lower [23]. This is further compounded by the glass door and glass ceiling effects; former education is not perceived as transferrable [23]. In a study by Dahlstedt, they found differences in the mismatch between vocationally educated and generally educated populations. Specifically, "the vocationally-educated population are more likely to be occupationally matched, but also that they are unlikely to advance past their educational level", while the reverse is true for the generally educated population who experience "occupational mismatch and advance to employment exceeding their educational level" [27]. Some of these initial barriers can be improved with recertification or by seeking new education or credentials and with built-up experience in the workforce based on settlement length [38,39]. Further, there may be other emerging barriers related to soft skills, such as degree of cultural awareness, language barriers [40], and cultural factors.

The inability to have foreign credentials transferred, thus leading to short-term or long-term differences in jobs or careers, can lead to lower levels of occupational commitment. Changing career pathways may indicate that the second career choice is less complementary to an immigrant's preferred career and professional identity and instrumental to their need to seek a career for economic capital. Referring back to occupational mismatch, the reason for changing careers is for economic opportunity, not one's connection to a particular field. For example, in our previous research [8] on a separate sample of Turkish immigrants, individuals made new career selections based on the current demands of employers, thus seeking out industries in higher demand, careers that would have a shortened timeframe between training to job placement, and jobs that pay well. The instrumental reason to seek a career that brings about economic stability contradicts one's passion for the field. It may be that the original career was closer to one's interest and the secondary career was instrumentally based. Although, it could very well be that the first career was also instrumentally based. Research has shown that, over time, lower levels of occupational commitment led individuals to end career positions prior to retirement [41].

In recognizing that highly educated immigrants seek out new career pathways in order to speed up their economic integration into a destination society, we can compare the amount of time invested in pursuing two or more career fields. Previously, Turkish migrants were educated and had professional employment in Türkiye, but following their forced immigration experience, for some, they sought new careers with re-education or training that could take one or more years to complete. During this time, they were typically employed in the secondary sector until establishing their new career. Although they found temporary employment, wages were low, work conditions were likely to be more exploitative and demoralizing, and difficulties emerged with balancing work–education–family. Over time, this temporary hiatus from their career demonstrates an overall earnings gap impacting both earned income and retirement benefits.

This study extends the literature on economic integration by examining the U.S. context specifically and migrants from different career types. It also broadens the focus to include the pre-conditions for migration, and a career focus related to the initial adjustment to the U.S. and the degree of success in regaining professional status. Similar to other studies, the barriers, challenges, and any negative outcomes are understood through a focus on immigrants' agency.

3. Materials and Methods

Much of the literature tends to focus on the forced aspect of migration experienced by undocumented migrants or refugees with lower social capital levels; however, this study will examine the unique conditions of highly educated, forced migrants that offer the U.S. a professional labor stock, and how they navigate the immigration process to regain status and reach economic integration. Instead of focusing on the time of immigration to the destination country, we have broadened our focus to the holistic migration journey of the immigrants, starting with the details of societal and individual events forcing them to move to the decision-making process and, finally, to the economic and psychological process of regaining their status. Based on recent qualitative data, including tracking some interviewees from our previous study in 2019, we have interviewed 42 (12 of them tracked from our first study) highly educated Turkish people in the U.S. In our first comparative study, we interviewed 30 forced or exiled Turkish people in eight different countries, including six European countries, Canada, and the U.S. Half of the respondents were from the U.S. [8]. They were living in historically highly Turkish-populated areas (more than 10,000) in the U.S. in the order of: New Jersey/NY, Dallas/TX, Houston/TX, California, and Virginia. The Turkish population increased between 15% to 50% from 2015 to 2020 in these selected cities [6]. These longitudinal data efforts have increased our ability to both generalize findings and garner rich information. The focus of our study is specifically on highly educated Turkish people who moved or were exiled to the U.S. due to increasing oppression, economic instability, unhappiness, and polarized relations after the 15 July 2016 events in Türkiye. Since we worked in-depth with vulnerable individuals who were targeted in their homeland, our methodology was shaped by the sensitive political and psychological circumstances of the forced and/or exiled community. The study is qualitative.

3.1. Recruitment Procedures

The first author is a Türkiye-born researcher who came to the USA one year before the coup-like staged events and has a good network with the recent Turkish exiled community. The study and its procedures have been approved by the Institutional Review Board (IRB). The collected data are from four main areas in the U.S., consistent with the most Turkish-populated regions. These cities are New Jersey, Houston, Dallas, and Virginia Beach. The researchers created a flyer, an informed consent form, and a detailed call about the study to recruit interviewees and provided Amazon gift cards as incentives. The requirements to participate in the study are stated as follows: being a highly educated Turkish person who has a college/university degree from a 4-year university/college or attends a college/university currently and who moved, decided to stay, or is planning to stay in the U.S. within the last six years. The researchers disseminated flyers to Turkish network groups and organizations. Some organizations, including the Blue Tulip Human Rights Center, based in Virginia and founded by Turkish veterans and American professionals, featured the study and shared it with their networks. This organization describes its mission as "increasing local and global awareness of sufferings of isolated and silenced women and children" on its webpage [42]. They have scholarships, psychological support, and empowering women and human rights awareness programs, especially for Turkish migrants who moved to the U.S. following the 15 July events. As a result, many of the volunteers in their network decided to support the study. The lead researcher also has a connection with Turkish Professionals US, which is very active in social media and has almost 9000 members. They support each other in information sharing, job searches, and integration into the U.S. Some of the interviewees were affiliated with this group. Lastly, the researcher also has connections with former state officials (i.e., bureaucrats and senior NATO officers). In accordance with our snowball sampling techniques, they also supported the study, and some shared their experiences during exile and the forced migration process.

Interviewees signed their informed consent forms before the face-to-face interviews. Participants were assured of the confidentiality of the procedure, including the fact that no personal identifiers were included in the transcripts, each interviewee was assigned a pseudonym, and results were reported as grouped data. Additionally, participants were informed they would have access to the study results, and Amazon gift cards were shared after the interviews. All interested participants gave informed consent and completed their interviews.

3.2. Interviews

Semi-structured interviews were conducted between May and September 2022. Forty-two people agreed to and finished an interview. Twelve of the interviewees were tracked among fifteen individuals in the U.S. from our previous comparative study conducted in 2019. Three of them were not available in our travels to target regions [8].

We conducted audio interviews in places based on participants' requests (i.e., participants' offices and library rooms) to protect their privacy. Furthermore, we conducted video interviews with the eleven volunteered participants to better observe their body language and facial expressions in places based on participants' requests. The risks of participating in this study were no more than what was experienced in daily life. The participants of the interviews did not have to answer any questions they were uncomfortable answering. Interview sessions, on average, took approximately one hour. However, some of the interview sessions lasted up to two hours due to the speaking pace of the participant, some emergency calls during the recording, or individuals having a hard time responding to emotional/sensitive questions. Although all interviewees were fluent in English, the interview language was Turkish to completely reflect the psychological and emotional circumstances of the participants.

The semi-structured interview guide enabled the interview to flow in a conversational way, and interviewees were asked to share their stories and experiences about the process. However, if the interviewees did not elaborate or had a limited response, we provided follow-up prompts such as, "How did you earn money until getting your work permit?" or "Have you ever had PTSD in your migration process?"

We observed body and facial expressions during the sessions and analyzed them along with the transcripts. Qualitative data were transcribed, coded, and analyzed using Atlas Ti 8 following the grounded theoretical design of Charmaz [43]. The coding procedure involved highlighting phrases, terms, and topics within the transcribed text that were repeated during unstructured conversation and grouping them under themes.

3.3. Demographics

Forty-two highly educated people participated in the study. They live in New Jersey (11), Dallas (9), Houston (8), Virginia (7), and 7 of them live in other places, namely California, Pennsylvania, Chicago, and Florida. Some of them, including tracked individuals from the previous study, had moved to new places different than their first location in the U.S. due to better jobs or living opportunities. They were all legally in the U.S.

The participants' ages were in the thirties to mid-fifties. Ten of them were 30–35 years old, seven of them 35–40 years old, thirteen of them 40–45 years old, five of them 45–50 years old, and seven of them 50–55 years old. Most participants were male (37), and five of them were female. All of them were married with Turkish spouses because having a good marriage was one of the social criteria selected for representing roles abroad for highly educated Turkish exiles. Thus, we also asked questions about their spouses' experiences. During the July 15 events, 22 of the participants were in Western countries due to professional roles representing Türkiye, pursuing a graduate degree, or on short-term vacation following job-related meetings/courses. All of them were called back within one year following the events in Türkiye with state orders to return immediately. Three of them returned and worked under pressure and in extraordinary situations for a while. Then, they understood that they did not have any alternatives to being imprisoned and, thus, decided to return to the U.S. Other participants had enough time to evaluate what could happen to themselves if they returned. Because those who return immediately have faced jail, probation, torture, mobbing, or abuse for flimsy reasons, they decided to stay in their locations until they saw a clear picture of the events. However, the state of emergency was extended seven times for three months and ended after two years. During this period, the government started to dismiss (including our interviewees) hundreds of thousands of state officials in critical positions (e.g., president and members of the supreme court, high-level judges, lawyers, opposition politicians/leaders, military generals, heads of police departments, human rights defenders, and journalists). Following these events, Türkiye transitioned from a parliamentary system to a Turkish-type presidency system, and Erdogan became the first president. The highly educated participants who were abroad understood that they were in exile until democracy came back to their homeland. Four out of twenty-two participants who were abroad moved from European countries to the U.S. due to their positive feelings during their previous experiences in the U.S., specifically including the language barrier in Europe, job opportunities, and a better future for their children. Twenty participants were in Türkiye during the events. Most of them have experienced difficult times, including imprisonment, abuse, mobbing, and social death, and experienced many challenges during their journey to the U.S. The jobs of the interviewees were high-level military officers, physicians, engineers, academics, and college students in closed institutions during the 15 July events.

4. Results and Discussion

4.1. Perspectives and Experiences of Highly Educated Exiled Turks in Their Journey to the USA

We examined the journey of Turkish professionals under three themes that emerged from the interviews: issues migrating with them, short-term poverty, and filling the gap.

4.2. Issues Migrate with Them

This section focuses on Turkish migrants' previous trauma and its barrier to the potential success of their migration. The interviewees were directly affected by the post-July 15 events in Türkiye. They (39 out of 42) were dismissed from their prestigious positions in governmental jobs in waves of purges after their long service without a logical reason. The rest of the interviewees (3 out of 42) were cadets in closed/transformed schools at that time. Those professionals have been blamed and labeled as "terrorists or sympathizers" by Erdogan's government. Some of them were detained or jailed following state of emergency decrees, while some others were exiled to hot zones including the Syrian border for unrelated missions with regard to their background and experience. They could not find new jobs after losing their jobs in the country because they were registered in state records. It was a highly difficult decision to migrate from the country, but they understood that it was not possible to have a normal life for themselves or their families in the country. So, even though they faced the risk of death in the migration journey, some of them decided to try. For example,

> *I've been purged from my job with Erdogan's law decrees. I stayed two years in jail and was released. After 1-year effort to be able to make work in the homeland, I understood that it was impossible. I got judiciary calls every three months, and the police knocked on my door at inappropriate times. I could not focus on or be motivated to do anything. Employers were reluctant to hire me though I was the best candidate for the positions they were looking for (Male, 40–45, Senior Data Scientist, New York).*

The interviewee has experienced each stage of the difficulties starting with dismissal. He tried to adapt to changes, but it was not possible. In another example, a participant had not experienced detention or jail, but it was still hard to adapt to dramatic changes. He recalled:

> *It is like you are a leper. If someone greets you, they can be taken to prison as a "terrorist" [Erdogan's government labeled them] sympathizer. A few years later, it was the anniversary of 15 July. I didn't want to go out that day. Lynching culture was very widespread in the country. There were vandals everywhere. But my kid wanted ice cream, so we went out. If they knew that I was a discharged soldier and someone said that they knew me in that crowd and slandered me, they would have killed me next to my wife and child (Male, 30–35, IT professional, Chicago).*

This quote shows the participant's emotional distress after the events. He was not content with the increasing radicalization and lynching culture at all. He shows the bravery and risk involved in engaging in a simple activity due to his discredited status. Another immigrant was in a professional position to observe the emotional trauma of other fellow citizens. She stated,

> *I've had my bachelor's and doctorate degrees at the top two universities in Türkiye. My husband was like me. He was a faculty at a prestigious college. Since we know we are innocent [it was a bad assumption, though], we continued to work at our colleges after 15 July. One week later, my husband was detained for a week [normally, it should be 24 h] in very bad conditions. He doesn't want to talk about those days. Then, he was discharged from his job, although he was released and acquitted. We opened our own psychology clinic and served people, including those people/families affected by Erdogan's law decrees. We know they were innocent like us. So, while every other government and private institution rejects serving them, we tried to help them by hiding their identities. I've listened to people's stories, my lips chapped, and I couldn't get rid of the effects of the people's stories for days.*
>
> *... after 3 years of judicial control, even though there is nothing new in my husband's file, the judge decided that he was involved in the incidents [15 July] and gave an arrest warrant for imprisonment. He had to leave without saying goodbye. ... I thought if we had a child, he would have a memory left. I thought I couldn't see him again (Female, 30–35, Psychologist, New York).*

Although professionals, including the participant, are aware of the experiences of other similarly situated individuals, they did not expect the same situations to find them later. Their agency was based on attempting to adapt to the current atmosphere hoping that, in a rational sense, they would be able to be found innocent and continue their careers and way of life. Other interviewees described victimization of psychological and physical torture.

> *After 15 July, I worked for a week. Everything was okay. I had a holiday ticket to ... [European country] with my wife on 21 July. I asked my supervisor what to do if I should cancel, and he said yes, cancel, wait for the mess. On 22 July, the prosecutor came and took all of us, 400 people got off the buses, and we opened our eyes to Sincan [known jail in Ankara]. There was a right-left police raid like the football players went down to the stadium. I can't tell you how they cursed, kicked, and slapped. We waited 4 h in the very cold at the tent gym saloon of Sincan. I have seen the tortured state of the friends they took before us ... I was sleeping next to the toilet. They gave us a small piece of bread, 1 L of water, and a small, spoiled cheese. So, people needed to go to the bathroom. But they closed most of the restrooms. There were 4 open restrooms for 500–1000 people. We waited in line for 4–5 h. Sometimes the police come and beat someone they choose decently. I didn't eat for 1.5 days ... someone older than me said you couldn't get anything. We got used to it for 10 days, he said, come and eat mine.*
>
> *... I translated a book [Military Psychology, Second Edition: Clinical and Operational Applications by Carrie H. Kennedy and Eric A. Zillmer] from English into Turkish with my colleagues about the stages of psychological torture when I was working on psychology. They [police] practiced all steps of it. The sub-master relationship has been eroded. They [police] made the soldiers beat the generals. The windows are closed. You don't know if it's 8 a.m. or 1 a.m. The time perception has been lost. The spotlights were on, there was a strong sound of air conditioning. Where am I, what am I doing?*
>
> *... They woke me up at night and testify. I said, what expression of what did I do? The lawyers were like prosecutors ... The expression has begun. ... destroying the constitutional order, bombing the parliament, assassinating the president, deliberately killing people ... I said hold on; I was a teacher. Where am I on this story? (Male, 35–40, IT Analyst, New Jersey).*

This statement shows how highly educated professionals were unaware of the events. They were not even aware of their so-called crimes, but they knew what the government was trying to do to professionals. Another participant supports this argument:

. . . since we are public lawyers, we are people who have read the history of the coups. How does a coup happen, why does it happen, who does it, and against whom? At that time, there were no conditions for a coup in Turkey. This is exactly what I said to my wife; I said that day [15 July 2016], "If someone is going to stage a coup right now, it will be none other than the President."

. . . They [police] detained us at the university. They illegally locked us in a room at the university for two days. They mistreated us there. Two days later, at midnight, they took us to a place we did not know before. I can say that it was the day I feared the most in my life. It was a sports hall. The first sight, there was very frightening. Six hundred or seven hundred people. Blood everywhere, blood on the walls, blood on the floors, blood on people's heads. All dressed in orange. At the bottom, some have black, some brown trousers. Many of them had blood on them. Their jaws, their heads, their eyes . . . They were all wrapped in bandages. Everyone was still tortured when we left. Screams, crying . . .

. . . there were two people who were severely tortured in my ward. One of them was the rector [president] of our university. For three months, he could not recover, for three months, he cried. I mean, a sixty years old man, a rector, a professor of medicine was severely tortured . . . he cried for three months. . . . he wanted to die. He didn't think he would ever get out of the prison alive (Male, 45–50, Educator, Florida).

The experiences they suffered left them little agency except to try to survive. Some focused their worries on the impact on their children, which prompted them to migrate. For example,

The psychological operation applied to me does not give any results. It can't make me a terrorist, it can't radicalize me, but in this environment and this psychology, a child who grows up could be abused by any radical organization in the future. I turned to my wife and said, let's get out of here. And she said okay (Male 35–40, Security Analyst, Virginia).

Another statement of an interviewee supports the quote above:

I was on a short vacation after a work trip in Europe when 15 July happened. My boss called me to return as soon as possible, and I did. However, since I had many courses and missions in the USA and was at the top of my cadre, they've looked at me as a potential criminal. The purged officers were, in my profile, successful and hard-working people. Colleagues and superior officers did continuous mobbing on me. The commander of the unit threatened me. Then, the forces command exiled me to a terror region though I completed my mandatory duty in that region. When I went there and see a big poster of Erdogan's regime related to 15 July, which depicts an unlisted soldier beaten by the so-called public on the Bosphorus Bridge, I asked myself, whom am I working for? For those [public] slaughtering his own Mehmetcik [soldier]. I thought that my children should not grow up in this society (Male, 45–50, Senior Cybersecurity Analyst, Virginia).

The events following 15 July have changed the feeling of professionals against the government and its supporters. In one case, the interviewee reflected on his extreme situation,

. . . one feels trapped. I remember looking at my gun at one point. I wonder if the way to get rid of this pressure is inside the barrel of the gun (Male, 35–40, Data Scientist, Texas).

In these extreme cases, interviewees could not feel safe. They felt even their human rights are not under protection. For example, one participant was worried about her passport,

After my husband had to leave home, hide from the police, and prepare to move abroad, police from TEM [anti-terror branch] came to my house at 2 am midnight. We were living in . . . [high-status people living area]. They [police] went on a terrorist hunt in the middle of the metropolis. It was ridiculous. They wanted to search my home, and I allowed them. I remembered my passport. . . . how much a passport can be a burden to a person. I wanted to hide it ten floors below the ground. It's a document that I have a right to take, but, in this atmosphere, they can take it. . . . and losing it is like losing your future, means losing your spouse, means breaking away from life (Female, 30–35, Psychologist, New York).

Some interviewees could not easily decide to leave their homeland and thought it might work if they did not see people. They tried to accomplish it by isolating themselves. One recalled,

... Finally, my friend (ex-helicopter pilot) and I decided to escape from society and raise chickens on a farm far away from the city (Male, 40–45, Senior Data Scientist, Virginia).

Running away from society did not work for the participants. Most (16 out of 20) exiled immigrants experienced similar cases to those mentioned above statements and decided to risk their lives for the sake of freedom. However, psychological problems and PTSD migrated with some of them, too:

I see nightmares frequently. Felt like someone would hold my shoulder from the back, and I would experience the same things (Male, 40–45, Pilot, Texas).

Another participant has seen nightmares, too:

For a long time, I have seen nightmares. I was in Turkiye in my nightmares. I was angry with myself about why I left my family in the USA and came here [Turkiye] (Male, 45–50, Professor, Texas).

Since most of the participants had to deal with new problems of the transition to new life, they could not have had a chance to consider the events they experienced until our interview. One reported,

I spent all my life on duty, honor, and country until my dismissal from service. In order to protect the prestige and interest of the country, we flew many hours over the Aegean Sea to show the Turkish flag and presence, deployed many times to other bases for scramble duties.. During the Syrian crisis, I flew at least 300 hours of air patrolling missions along the border to defend our airspace.. I had to neglect my family and made many sacrifices. We are [crying ...] how they can dare to judge our patriotism? How can they dare to label us as "ter ... " [terrorists—could not complete the word for 50 s and forced himself not to cry] (Male, 40–45, Business Owner, Texas).

In another experience, the participant recalled how he tried to deal with his psychological issues by thinking of others who were not as lucky as himself.

After me, 19 people who tried to cross to Greece from where I passed lost their lives by drowning by boat. Because I had my wife and children with me, I considered myself the happiest and luckiest person in the world. The psychological trauma was a luxury for me, and I needed to relax to live it (Male, 30–35, Senior Cyber Security Analyst, Pennsylvania).

These psychological traumas migrated with exiled Turkish professionals. They have felt, and some still feel, trauma and developed different strategies to deal with them. As shown in the interviewees' described experiences, they encountered risk in identification, detention, and other forms of penalties. Many of them discussed either directly facing torture and abuse or the threat of abuse. Their sense of normalcy, safety, and understanding of their human and citizenship rights were drastically taken away. In response, their agency was then refocused on survival. Although migration afforded many a chance at renewed safety, despite the many risks of being detected or the migration journey failing, the trauma was pervasive and impacted their way of life. It also shows that their old way of life and what they were accustomed to culturally, professionally, and socially changed and likely would never be re-experienced. Thus, by examining how trauma impacts the lived realities of migrants, we find that migration may not bring about a full sense of normalcy and sense of satisfaction. Migration may be a new set of insecurities added to the previous insecurities and distress.

4.3. Short-Term Poverty

Thus, previous experiences of trauma undermine Turkish migrants' ability to adjust to a new country and maintain their status. All interviewees experienced financial loss after their dismissal from their previous jobs. However, some experienced short-term poverty fiercely, especially those having an exhausting journey from jail to release and illegal migration to neighboring countries. Some interviewees experienced major financial issues to have this journey. One recalled,

> *I had to spend all my money on smugglers and other expenditures to be able to come here (Male, 30–35, Data Scientist, Virginia).*

Another participant had a similar experience to this:

> *We were thinking a lot about how to do it [migration] financially. I had a ban on leaving Turkey abroad, and I didn't have a passport. Even just buying a plane ticket was very expensive. We disposed of our savings, sold the immovables, turned them into cash, and borrowed money from family. I asked for help from friends who went out before me. Someone gave me a phone number [smuggler]. I came to the USA through six countries. When I arrived eight weeks later, all the savings were over, I had $500 in my pocket. I spent $30,000 on flight tickets and smugglers' money for a passport. We stayed with 6 people in the 1 + 1 house of a friend I know. . . . after 1 week, I found an hourly job (Male, 30–35, Senior Cyber Security Analyst, Pennsylvania).*

Another participant from a different location experienced similar short-term poverty, though he was on an abroad mission during the events. He recalled,

> *Our income sources were completely cut off in an instant. In that context, I started as a taxi driver, a . . . [one of the top American colleges] graduate taxi driver. I was, at that time, forty-odd years old. But let me say that being able to bring money back to my family, I was lucky enough to experience that after two or three months of interruption (Male 45–50, Professor, Virginia).*

Some other participants experienced short-term poverty and could not buy their essential needs for a while. One stated,

> *I had no money to buy furniture for my rented apartment. I was looking for free items on the Facebook marketplace to use or resale (Male, 40–45, Pilot, Texas).*

These four quotes show the general experiences of people who have an exhausting journey from their homeland to the USA. As their experiences show, their financial capital was quickly depleted by the forced migration process. Based on an urgency to flee, less planning could occur, and more risk mounted as they had to find quick ways to escape. A total of 22 out of 42 participants who were abroad during the events still had financial hardships until receiving their work permits and using their savings. Poverty was a completely new phenomenon for all of them, and their once-held high human capital diminished quickly. One stated,

> *I came from an upper-middle-class family. I never experienced poverty in my life until my dismissal from the job and losing Türkiye's sponsorship during my post-doc in the USA (Male, 45–50, Professor, Texas).*

One important reason to overcome short-term poverty as soon as possible was related to the interviewees' sense of responsibility for their families. Although they had significant enthusiasm and interest to continue their previous careers, they had to be more realistic and make fast economic integration decisions while searching for jobs in the destination areas. One interviewee said,

> *If I were alone, I would stay in the park [decrease expenditures to a minimum] and try. However, it was not possible to continue my previous job with my family responsibility and spend more time and money on accreditation (Male, 40–45, Data Scientist, Virginia).*

Another respondent stated,

If I wanted to continue with piloting, I should freeze the life for 8 months [not earning money in odd jobs], give money on it [credentials in pilot courses], take my time, and make it happen. So, it was a very difficult road for a married man with two children. So, I preferred a cybersecurity job (Male, 30–35, Cybersecurity Analyst, Virginia).

Here, the desire to pursue his professional work was disrupted by the need to make money and support his family. With depleted resources and an inability to make adequate money, life choices were based on how quickly money could be earned comparable to the previous livelihood. Other interviewees in the data science field have reported reasons similar to the above statement. They could not continue their previous professions while managing the living and household expenditures of their families.

Although they experienced financial issues at this level for the first time in their lives, they were aware that this situation was temporary because their ultimate plan was to rebuild their lives in the U.S. and regain their economic stability and professional status [44]. Additionally, they motivated themselves by thinking about people in their homeland in worse conditions.

4.4. Fill the Gap (Overload)

This portion allows us to examine the struggles of the interviewed professionals in regaining their former status and the hardships of finding a professional job. Exiled professionals felt the stress of regaining their previous status and providing ideal living standards for their families. They were overwhelmed and took significant risks for the sake of reaching their goals soon. They understood that they could not do their previous jobs without making many sacrifices and losing time [45,46]. However, some of them (two doctors, two pilots, and six academics) insisted on pursuing their previous jobs by accepting junior-level positions. The rest of them preferred to regain new skills in completely new fields for them, including data science and trade [47]. This process brought extraordinary overload to both groups. One stated,

I have taught 13 courses at 4 different universities at the same time. I was thinking I needed to earn money; I shouldn't make my children feel the difficulty of staying here (Male, 45–50, Professor, Texas).

Another person experienced this overload by doing many jobs. However, this overload also included gaining new skills as fast as possible to reach their former statuses [8,46].

I did 7–8 different jobs: heavy work in the warehouse, container loading, waiter and cooker in a restaurant, electricity handyman, entertaining children, and delivery. The side works continued for 13 months until November 2020. If there was a scholarship opportunity, it would pay my kitchen expenses and rent for a while, and I could get my license for commercial piloting in 6 months and do my old job. But . . . it was unrealistic. When I got my work permit, I started working as an Uber driver. It was like a promotion for me. I started a fast boot camp in the cyber security field. I've been working hard for 6 months. I was able to provide for my family's livelihood by doing Uber for 4–5 h a day. I attended most of the classes with my headset while driving an Uber. 2 weeks after the course ended, I found a six-figure work (Male 35–40, IT Security Specialist, Virginia).

Our participants shared similar experiences about doing daily jobs to make money as much as they could and making sacrifices to learn new jobs [22,45]. The following statement shows the general behaviors of the interviewees:

While driving and waiting for my working permit, I was taking data science camp courses at night and watching as many tutorials and courses as I could to learn more about the field. I did not know even basic terms in the field like "terminal" I googled everything I heard new. Listened to very short free learning videos at first and watched longer ones when I found a chance. After a year-long effort, I was familiar with almost everything, and people were asking me about any issues they faced (Male, 40–45, Senior Data Scientist, New York).

Although it was hard to transition their previous skills into new jobs directly, their backgrounds, hardworking skills, and other soft skills were rewarded in their new jobs. For example, the following statements support this transition process:

> *Because my previous experiences [20 years of engineering in government] are different from the field I applied for, I started in a junior position. However, I moved to senior positions faster than the others. You can reflect on your experience after entering the first job (Male, 40–45, Senior Software Engineer & Team Leader, Virginia).*

> *I made the delivery half day to make money and followed Udemy, Coursera courses, and YouTube videos in data science for a year. Applied for any job post for three months and took an offer from three different companies and started to one of them and changed it with a better job option in another company. Since I've felt myself behind in the new field, I forced myself to learn all new terms I've heard daily. When our leading senior data scientist with ten-plus years of experience left for another job, the manager asked me to take over his role (Male, 40–45, Senior Data Scientist, New York).*

The participants were rewarded for their hard work after finding their first job or starting a new position in a new field in a short amount of time. Some interviewees even took significant financial risks to regain their former statuses in a short amount of time. For instance,

> *I took over a store with a debt of $250 k. I did two-man jobs for three years; I had to learn design, sales and how to run a business; we closed the debts, and we made a profit. We are doing kitchen and bathroom design very well (Male, 40–45, Business Owner, Texas).*

His previous experiences were completely different from the requirements of the new job. However, he was aware of his soft skills to learn new things quickly. Therefore, this risk was reasonable for the participant. However, some interviewees could not accept this career change easily:

> *When I came here, I thought that burning the diplomas they were useless. . . . whomever I talk to says the same thing. My left brain is convinced to pursue the IT course, but my right brain says no, you have worked so much for psychology, you have spent years, and you should continue working on it. (Female, 30–35, Psychologist, New York).*

The participants and other highly educated immigrants know the market needs in IT fields in the USA. Their background, math skills, and education are advantages in finding a job in these fields. However, it is not an easy decision, especially for academics. On the other side of the same coin, we have found the negative consequences of this filling-the-gap process. This kind of overloading and risk taking caused a loss of well-being for exiled immigrants. Some reported,

> *I gained a lot of weight in these two years. I have been working hard with an ambition to close the gap. This process left permanent effects on my health.*

> *COVID-19 made this process harder for professionals.*

> *In times of lockdown due to COVID, I was going for handyman jobs like the assembly of trampolines or basketball hoops and risking my life and health to make money for my family (Male, 40–45, Senior Data Scientist, New York).*

Another statement from a different location reflects a similar feeling:

> *While everyone sitting in their homes and trying to avoid COVID, I was making food delivery in Instacart (Male 35–40, IT Security Specialist, Virginia).*

Moreover, after finding an ideal full-time job, interviewees (33 out of 42) encouraged their spouses to find a full-time job, especially in the data science field (e.g., cybersecurity, QA, Salesforce), by taking more responsibility at home. Then, many spouses (21 out of 33) found full-time jobs in these fields. Some spouses preferred to pursue their education in new or previous fields, especially in the fields of law and education, while some of them transitioned their hobbies to online store jobs. One interviewee observed this change in spouses,

> *90% of my [exiled] friends' spouses found full-time jobs in our region [New York] (Male, 40–45, Senior Data Scientist, New York).*

Most of the interviewees reported that they continued their side jobs and extra work even after getting very good jobs. The motivation that lies behind this may be related to their connection with people in their home country. Interviewees' motivation to help others and support professionals in similar situations encouraged them to take more risks and start new initiatives. These initiatives supported silenced and isolated people emotionally and financially in their homeland and abroad [48]. For example, the following statement shows the psychological support they provide for others:

> *We've founded a psychological institute with volunteer psychologists and doctors to help forced migrants and people who experienced trauma. We've provided free service to 1400 people so far. After two years, we also started to help people who were forced to migrate all around the world (Female, 30–35, Psychologist, New York).*

Another statement shows the support for gaining new skills and financial well-being. The participant recalled,

> *You know professionals like us [discharged with Erdogan's law decrees] cannot do any work in Turkiye. So, while gaining new skills in a new country, I've also thought of giving away to people in Turkiye and here [USA]. I founded an IT school with my friends, we worked very hard and slept less, and within four years, we were selected as one of the top IT schools in the U.S. and Europe (Male, 40–45, Founder of an IT school, Virginia).*

The experiences of the participants were similar to each other in terms of regaining their statuses. They worked hard and used every opportunity to accomplish their goals as soon as possible. Although they encountered challenges finding temporary income and regaining their professional credentials or seeking new education and credentials altogether [44], one aspect that does stand out is their agency evident in their ability to take on innovative strategies, commit to initiative and motivation, and find success. This ability is linked to their professional credentials and experiences, and the ability for them to build on previous social and cultural capital to be successful. However, despite their success, there is concern that their profession and educational skills were not automatically deemed verifiable and usable, and the time lost either regaining credentials or seeking new careers reveals a loss of earning potential, lower job and life satisfaction, a poorer quality of life generally, and a drop in occupational commitment [45,46].

5. Conclusions

The findings of this study highlight that Turkish migrants experience challenging conditions throughout the migration period, beginning with the violence that prompts them to migrate quickly out of safety concerns, the short-term poverty they experience in the migration journey itself and in settling into the host country, and the temporary loss of professional jobs and status as they engage in the credentialing process. We anticipated both the challenges that come with urgent forced migration, as has been well-documented in the literature regarding the dire plights immigrants face when forced to flee, and the economic assimilation liminality that comes with finding new jobs and adjusting to a new society [8,16]. However, the findings give us a more nuanced understanding of the insecurities and barriers within the migration process. First, higher forms of human capital are not as stable; however, high human capital can increase agency. Despite having economic security, specifically financial capital, namely income, savings, and resources, Turkish immigrants found that this was depleted quickly at the start of the migration process. Their ability to receive income to support their entry and settlement experiences in the U.S. was not a stable resource. However, due to high human capital, they could rely on professional skills, experience, and networks to regain their economic security and career, leading to an opportunity to regain their quality of life economically [8,44]. Second, the insecurities in each stage of the migration process (deciding to migrate, migration journey, and assimilation/settlement) are compounded because they build on each other. Thus, the process is not made of discrete issues that can be resolved before addressing any new insecurities. In the case of many Turkish migrants in this study, trauma was an ongoing component in their life, and the economic and professional loss that occurred, although mostly temporary, ended up having long-term consequences: the stress of rebuilding, the loss of their professional status, and the lack of presence with their family, all of which impacted their quality of life. Economically, it meant the loss of earnings, and emotionally, the inability to engage in mental health intervention to improve emotional well-being. One last conclusion we found relates to their new way of life in relation to their previous sense of identity. In addition to many Turkish migrants seeking new fields for their careers, all experienced a change in their way of life. Their upbringing, connection to their homeland, friends, family, acquaintances still residing in Türkiye, their cultural customs, and way of life can never be returned to in the same way they had once experienced them. The harmful and lasting effect of events, such as the coup, has reshaped their cultural connection, pride, and well-being associated with their homeland. Even though we could generally imply that the U.S. and other European countries promise safety from the regime in Türkiye, their trauma and insecurities are replaced with new insecurities as they adjust to a different culture.

This study provides a greater understanding of immigrants' agency to regain professional status, mostly using their own professional skill sets, experiences, and social networks. This study provided a broader context to exploring the trajectory of the migration process as immigrants sought to regain their professional livelihoods in the U.S. The study also is comparable to other studies that focus on specific Western countries, particularly Canada and Western Europe, by showing both the challenges in transferring skills and education and the short-term disruption to regaining their professional careers.

In addition to the important contributions of the paper, it has some limitations in the generalizability of the results. The snowball sample includes many professional participants representing Türkiye in Western countries. Therefore, they may have better language, education, and professional skills than other highly educated people in the general migration population after the 15 July events. Interested researchers can test our findings that migration can bring new insecurities to previous issues starting with pre-migration decisions of highly educated immigrants. Quantitative and qualitative inquiries on the integration process and degree of agency can help provide an understanding of the short- and long-term impacts of deskilling, seeking new education and credentials or transferability of credentials, and the earnings gap. Further, highly educated immigrants from economically disadvantaged countries may deplete their financial capital to reach the U.S. through illegal ways, but they may depend on their high human capital and network for economic integration since the U.S. provides many opportunities to use them accordingly. Both comparative studies across countries and country-specific economic integration can be further extended to build on findings in the literature that suggest integration is underdetermined by a multitude of economic and social factors, policies, immigrant reception, and types of professions. Future research may test these findings in other highly educated migrant groups such as the recent highly educated Ukrainian population who were forced to migrate to the U.S. and other European countries. To further understand the process of exiled professionals, future research could study their legal status experiences as well as the comparison between their assumptions and facts since their migration decisions were unprepared and quick. The nuanced understanding of the experiences of selected exiled professionals provided us the opportunity to view the policy issues they faced. These professionals offer the U.S. a unique labor stock in less-found expertise areas. However, policy reform is needed to facilitate the immigration status of migrants and create a smooth integration process by lessening the time taken to verify foreign credentials and enabling professionals to continue in their line of training and career.

Author Contributions: Conceptualization, C.A. and E.L.R.; methodology, C.A.; software, C.A.; validation, C.A. and E.L.R.; formal analysis, C.A.; investigation, C.A.; resources, C.A. and E.L.R.; data curation, C.A. and E.L.R.; writing—original draft preparation, C.A. and E.L.R.; writing—review and editing, C.A. and E.L.R.; visualization, C.A. and E.L.R.; supervision, C.A. and E.L.R.; project administration, C.A.; funding acquisition, C.A. All authors have read and agreed to the published version of the manuscript.

Funding: This research was funded by Embry-Riddle Aeronautical University, grant number GC87022.

Institutional Review Board Statement: The study was conducted in accordance with the Declaration of Helsinki and approved by the Institutional Review Board of Embry-Riddle Aeronautical University (22-095 and 25 February 2022).

Informed Consent Statement: Informed consent was obtained from all subjects involved in the study.

Data Availability Statement: Not applicable.

Acknowledgments: This research was partially supported through Embry-Riddle Aeronautical University's Faculty Innovative Research in Science and Technology (FIRST) Program.

Conflicts of Interest: The authors declare no conflict of interest.

References

1. Güveli, A. 2000 Families Research: Some Findings and Potential for Future Research. *J. Econ. Cult. Soc.* **2019**, *60*, 87–104. [CrossRef]
2. Akcapar, S.K. Turkish Associations in the United States: Towards Building a Transnational Identity. *Turk. Stud.* **2009**, *10*, 165–193. [CrossRef]
3. Karpat, K. Turks in America. In *Les Annales de L'Autre Islam*; Stephane, T.D., Ed.; Erism: Paris, France, 1995; Volume 3, pp. 231–252.
4. Micallef, R. Turkish Americans: Performing Identities in a Transnational Setting. *J. Muslim Minor. Aff.* **2004**, *24*, 233–241. [CrossRef]
5. Gall, C. Spurning Erdogan's Vision, Turks Leave in Droves, Draining Money and Talent. 2019. Available online: https://www.nytimes.com/2019/01/02/world/europe/turkey-emigration-erdogan.html (accessed on 1 September 2022).
6. United States Department of Homeland Security. *2020 Yearbook of Immigration Statistics*; U.S. Department of Homeland Security, Office of Immigration Statistics: Washington, DC, USA, 2022.
7. Border Report. *El Paso Becoming Favored U.S. Entryway for Turkish Nationals*. 2022. Available online: https://www.borderreport.com/immigration/el-paso-becoming-favored-u-s-entryway-for-turkish-nationals/ (accessed on 10 August 2022).
8. Aydiner, C.; Rider, E. Migration Policies and Practices at Job Market Participation: Perspectives of Highly Educated Turks in the US, Canada and Europe. *Int. J. Sociol.* **2021**, *42*, 399–415. [CrossRef]
9. Lee, E. A Theory of Migration. *Demography* **1966**, *3*, 47–57. [CrossRef]
10. Massey, D.; Arango, J.; Hugo, G.; Kouaouci, A.; Pellegrina, A.; Taylor, J.E. Theories of International Migration: A Review and Appraisal. *Popul. Dev. Rev.* **1993**, *19*, 431–466. [CrossRef]
11. Castles, S. Towards a sociology of forced migration and social transformation. *Sociology* **2003**, *37*, 13–34. [CrossRef]
12. Conte, A.; Migali, S. The Role of Conflict and Organized Violence in International Forced Migration. *Demogr. Res.* **2019**, *41*, 93–424. [CrossRef]
13. Davenport, C.; Moore, W.H.; Poe, S. Sometimes You Just Have to Leave: Domestic Threats and Forced Migration, 1964–1989. *Int. Interact.* **2003**, *29*, 27–55. [CrossRef]
14. Moore, W.; Shellman, S. Whither Will They Go? A Global Study of Refugees' Destinations, 1965–1995. *Int. Stud. Q.* **2007**, *51*, 811–834. [CrossRef]
15. Andrejuk, K. Strategizing Integration in the Labor Market. Turkish Immigrants in Poland and the New Dimensions of South-to-North Migration. *Pol. Sociol. Rev.* **2019**, *206*, 157–176.
16. Disbudak, C.; Purkis, S. Forced Migrants or Voluntary Exiles: Ethnic Turks of Bulgaria in Turkey. *J. Int. Migr. Integr.* **2016**, *17*, 371–388. [CrossRef]
17. Koikkalainen, S.; Linnakangas, R.; Suikkanen, A. Does International Migration Pay Off?: The Labor Market Situation of Finnish Return Migrants Based on Longitudinal Register Data. *Nord. J. Work. Life Stud.* **2016**, *6*, 49–66. [CrossRef]
18. Kulu-Glasgow, I.; Schans, D.; Smit, M. The Dutch Battle for Highly Skilled Migrants: Policy, Implementation and the Role of Social Networks. *Migr. Lett.* **2018**, *15*, 517–532. [CrossRef]
19. Spadavecchia, C. Migration of Women from Sub-Saharan Africa to Europe: The Role of Highly Skilled Women. *Sociol. Y Tecnociencia* **2013**, *3*, 96–116.
20. Sapeha, H. Explaining Variations in Immigrants' Satisfaction with Their Settlement Experience. *Int. Migr. Integr.* **2015**, *16*, 891–910. [CrossRef]

21. Tzeng, R.; Tsai, M.-C. Good for the Common Good: Sociotropic Concern and Double Standards toward High- and Low-Skilled Immigrants in Six Wealthy Countries. *Soc. Indic. Res.* **2020**, *152*, 473–493. [CrossRef]
22. Akkaymak, G. A Bourdieuian Analysis of Job Search Experiences of Immigrants in Canada. *Int. Migr. Integr.* **2016**, *18*, 657–674. [CrossRef]
23. Guo, S. Economic Integration of Recent Chinese Immigrants in Canada' Second-Tier Cities: The Triple Glass Effect and Immigrants' Downward Social Mobility. *Can. Ethn. Stud.* **2013**, *43*, 95–115. [CrossRef]
24. Somerville, K.; Walsworth, S. Admission and Employment Criteria Discrepancies: Experiences of Skilled Immigrants in Toronto. *Int. Migr. Integr.* **2010**, *11*, 341–352. [CrossRef]
25. Sweetman, A.; McDonald, T.; Hawthorne, L. Regulated Occupations and Foreign Qualification Recognition: An Overview. *Can. Public Policy* **2015**, *41*, 1–13. [CrossRef]
26. Stumpf, F.; Damelang, A.; Abraham, M.; Ebensperger, S. How National Institutions Shape Skilled Immigrants' Chances of Getting Hired: Evidence from Harmonised Factorial Surveys with Employers in Germany and England. *KZfSS Kölner Z. Für Soziologie Und Soz.* **2020**, *72*, 351–373. [CrossRef]
27. Dahlstedt, I. Occupational Match: Over- and Undereducation Among Immigrants in the Swedish Labor Market. *Int. Migr. Integr.* **2011**, *12*, 349–367. [CrossRef]
28. Pecoraro, M.; Wanner, P. Does the Recognition of Foreign Credentials Decrease the Risk for Immigrants of Being Mismatched in Education or Skills? In *Migrants and Expats: The Swiss Migration and Mobility Nexus*; Steiner, I., Wanner, P., Eds.; Springer: Cham, Switzerland, 2019; pp. 161–180.
29. Zorlu, A. Occupational Adjustment of Immigrants in The Netherlands. *Int. Migr. Integr.* **2013**, *14*, 1711–1731. [CrossRef]
30. Brinbaum, Y. Incorporation of Immigrants and Second Generations into the French Labour Market: Changes between Generations and the Role of Human Capital and Origins. *Soc. Incl.* **2018**, *6*, 104–118. [CrossRef]
31. Michalikova, N. Segmented Socioeconomic Adaptation of New Eastern European Professionals in the United States. *Comp. Migr. Stud.* **2018**, *6*, 8. [CrossRef] [PubMed]
32. Boyd, M.; Tian, S. Is STEM Education Portable? Country of Education and the Economic Integration of STEM Immigrants. *Int. Migr. Integr.* **2018**, *19*, 965–1003. [CrossRef]
33. Rohrbach-Schmidt, D. Licensing, Educational Credentialing, and Wages Among Foreign Skilled Workers in Germany. *Kölner Z. Für Soziologie Und Soz.* **2020**, *72*, 375–400. [CrossRef]
34. Redbird, B.; Escamilla-García, A. Borders within Borders: The Impact of Occupational Licensing on Immigrant Incorporation. *Immigr. Occup.* **2020**, *6*, 22–45. [CrossRef]
35. Fu, C.; Hickey, R. The Costs of Regulatory Federalism: Does Provincial Labor Market Regulation Impede the Integration of Canadian Immigrants? *Int. Migr. Integr.* **2014**, *16*, 987–1002. [CrossRef]
36. Haberfield, Y.; Birgier, D.; Lundh, C.; Elldér, E. Migration Across Developed Countries: German Immigrants in Sweden and the U.S. *Int. Migr.* **2020**, *58*, 171–194. [CrossRef]
37. De Alwis, S.; Parr, N.; Guo, F. The Education–Occupation (Mis)Match of Asia-Born Immigrants in Australia. *Popul. Res. Policy Rev.* **2018**, *39*, 519–548. [CrossRef]
38. Adamuti-Trache, M. First 4 Years in Canada: Post-Secondary Education Pathways of Highly Educated Immigrants. *Int. Migr. Integr.* **2011**, *12*, 61–83. [CrossRef]
39. Amit, K.; Bar-Lev, S. Immigrants' Sense of Belonging to the Host Country: The Role of Life Satisfaction, Language Proficiency, and Religious Motives. *Soc. Indic. Res.* **2015**, *124*, 947–961. [CrossRef]
40. Étémé, G.; Girard, A.; Massé, J.-C.; Sercia, P. Do acculturation Strategies Have Impacts on the Self-Declared Health, Well-Being and Lifestyle of First-Generation Allophone Immigrants in Montreal, Canada? *Int. J. Migr. Health Soc. Care* **2016**, *12*, 66–82. [CrossRef]
41. Riegle-Crumb, C.; Peng, M.; Russo-Tait, T. Committed to STEM? Examining Factors that Predict Occupational Commitment among Asian and White Female Students Completing STEM U.S. Postsecondary Programs. *Sex Roles* **2020**, *82*, 102–116. [CrossRef]
42. Blue Tulip Human Rights Center. How We Help. 2022. Available online: https://www.blue-tulip.org/how (accessed on 5 August 2022).
43. Charmaz, K. *Constructing Grounded Theory*; Sage: Thousand Oaks, CA, USA, 2014.
44. Kelly, M.; Hedman, L. Between Opportunity and Constraint: Understanding the Onward Migration of Highly Educated Iranian Refugees from Sweden. *J. Int. Migr. Integr.* **2016**, *17*, 649–667. [CrossRef]
45. Creese, G.; Wiebe, B. Survival Employment: Gender and Deskilling among African Immigrants in Canada. *Int. Migr.* **2012**, *50*, 56–76. [CrossRef]
46. Nowicka, M. Migrating Skills, Skilled Migrants and Migration Skills: The Influence of Contexts on the Validation of Migrants' Skills. *Migr. Lett.* **2014**, *11*, 171–186. [CrossRef]
47. Yanasmayan, Z. *The Migration of Highly Educated Turkish Citizens to Europe: From Guestworkers to Global Talent*; Routledge: London, UK, 2020.
48. Yildiz, A.; Verkuyten, M. Inclusive Victimhood: Social Identity and the Politicization of Collective Trauma Among Turkey's Alevis in Western Europe. *Peace Confl.* **2011**, *17*, 243–269. [CrossRef]

International Journal of
Environmental Research and Public Health

MDPI

Article

"Step by Step We Were Okay Now": An Exploration of the Impact of Social Connectedness on the Well-Being of Congolese and Iraqi Refugee Women Resettled in the United States

Caitlin Bletscher * **and Sara Spiers**

Department of Human Development, Washington State University, Vancouver, WA 98686, USA
* Correspondence: caitlin.bletscher@wsu.edu

Abstract: Little is known about the gendered impacts of the displacement and resettlement process. Women are known to struggle more with feelings of belonging and the creation of social networks to access essential information, resources, and social and emotional support to enhance their overall health and well-being. The purpose of the present study was to qualitatively explore female refugee perceptions of belongingness and social connectedness post-resettlement into their U.S. host community. Conducted between January and June of 2016, through the partnership of multiple governmental, nonprofit, and community-based organizations, two female focus groups were conducted among Congolese (n = 6) and Iraqi (n = 6) U.S. resettled refugees. Descriptive surveys were distributed to participants, providing valuable insights into participant demographics and indicators that could impact the integration process (i.e., age, language, country of origin, ethnicity, education, length of time spent in the U.S., housing). Participants discussed the social connections (individuals, communities, organizations) that acted as facilitators or inhibitors of developing social capital. The importance of building strong transformational bonding (family members, other refugees) and bridging (host community) relationships, alongside transactional ties with linking agencies (resettlement social services), was critical for a positive resettlement experience. The strength of their network ties among these social connections contributed to their perceptions of belongingness and well-being post-resettlement into their host community.

Keywords: gender; refugee; resettlement; social capital; belonging; isolation

Citation: Bletscher, C.; Spiers, S. "Step by Step We Were Okay Now": An Exploration of the Impact of Social Connectedness on the Well-Being of Congolese and Iraqi Refugee Women Resettled in the United States. *Int. J. Environ. Res. Public Health* **2023**, *20*, 5324. https://doi.org/10.3390/ijerph20075324

Academic Editors: Maria De Jesus and Ernesto Castañeda

Received: 24 December 2022
Revised: 9 March 2023
Accepted: 27 March 2023
Published: 30 March 2023

1. Introduction

The well-being of an increasing number of displaced people has become a global public health concern [1,2]. According to the Guiding Principles on Internal Displacement [3], displaced people include:

> "Persons or groups of persons who have been forced or obliged to flee or to leave their homes or places of habitual residence, in particular as a result of or in order to avoid the effects of armed conflict, situations of generalized violence, violations of human rights or natural or human-made disasters, and who have not crossed an internationally recognized border."

Such populations experience loss of family, social support, and identity. Most displaced people are resettled to a secondary country, while about 1% of the migrant population is resettled into a third host country such as the United States (U.S.). This compounding displacement creates additional complications and barriers to the resettlement process and integration post-resettlement.

Gender has been identified as one such barrier to successful resettlement [4]. Even though gender has been consistently identified as an individual indicator to successful integration among migrant populations [5,6], most research and discourse on migration instead tells a homogenous gendered story [7,8]. This narrative shows refugees as unitary, non-gendered entities, assuming a 'gender blind' stance that ignores the ways that gender shapes the experiences and risks in migration [9].

Thus, a shift of attention or a 'womanist framework' [10] is needed to understand the experiences of migrant women [9], due to the millions of women experiencing forced displacement worldwide [4]. Historically, about 50% of the world refugee population are women [11], and numbers continue to increase. Female refugees face significant obstacles to coping with the many challenges of migration in comparison to their male counterparts. Obstacles include fear and persecution [4], gender-based discrimination and physical and/or sexual violence [5,11–16], cultural displacement, inequitable gender norms or confluence of cultural gender role expectations, language barriers, lack of resources and education, and an increase of structural and situational stressors [1,5,7,16,17]. Women's social identities also reside in disadvantaged locations in the hierarchical social sphere [18,19], creating significant social tensions [17].

Upon resettling to their third host communities, refugee women face a wide array of challenges and obstacles, especially for refugees from non-western and non–white countries [20]. After female refugees migrate, they experience conflict within their personal identify development. On one hand, they have their perceptions of their ethnic, religious, and linguistic identities; on the other hand, they are embedded within their new host community [4], which has different expectations, which can significantly impact their sense of well-being [20].

Because women often migrate as dependents of their male partner or family members, the focus tends to fall on the male migrants' needs, dismissing women's unique health concerns and well-being [21], not to mention the significant challenges facing resettled women with navigating the U.S. healthcare system [22,23]. Thus, during resettlement, female refugees face significant barriers to appropriate healthcare, due to a lack of health literacy, cultural differences, communication issues, and challenges with access [24]. This highlights why gender (females) has been significantly positively associated with symptoms of depression, anxiety, Post-Traumatic Stress Disorder, and risky behavioral problems such as Alcohol Use Disorder [25,26].

Many times, refugee women are caught in a 'cycle of isolation' upon resettlement, stemming from religious and ethnic backgrounds, alongside the host country's social, political, and institutional processes [27]. This cycle is continuously reinforced throughout the integration process, through ongoing internal ethnic factors and external marginalizing factors [27] such as discrimination, racism, and prejudice from their host community.

While the research on what drives public perceptions and attitudes toward refugee populations (versus immigrants at large) is limited [28], findings have showcased negative perceptions such as discrimination and profiling towards resettled refugees in the U.S. [29,30], mainly as potential security threats to U.S. safety and well-being [28]. Results of a 2016 study of American adults showed preferences towards Syrian refugees who are female, highly skilled, English speaking, and Christian [28]. Religious and gender identities were significant variables among American preferences of their newcomers. Religious bias towards Christianity was especially significant [28], in agreement with previous research on American anti-Muslim bias and discrimination [31], especially towards women [4,32,33]. These findings build on previous literature that found that Muslim women experience more discrimination against their religious group than their Muslim male counterparts [34].

As the research suggests, the refugee migration experience significantly differs by gender, where each gender responds differently and their corresponding realities impact all stages of migration (pre-, during, and post-resettlement) [9]. Not only do refugee women face significant obstacles to successful resettlement, but the isolation and marginalization that female refugees experience as the 'outsider' among their new host community can further harm or inhibit access to resources to support their well-being. In order to better understand their integration process into their new community, the following migration literature review provides insights into gender inequities throughout the resettlement process (focusing on post-resettlement), with intentional focus on refugee social connectedness and perceptions of belongingness.

1.1. Social Connectedness and Belongingness among Refugee Populations

Kohut's [35] self-psychology theory defined social connectedness as a construct which allows people to feel they are "being human among humans" (p. 200) in order to identify with others who may be dissimilar. A decrease in connectedness leads to isolation, where the individual finds it hard to accept his or her social role [36]. Therefore, if refugees have limited social connectedness and limited feelings of belonging among their new communities, the more isolated they may become.

An individual's formation of social networks significantly benefits their overall well-being. Individuals with a high sense of connectedness can develop relationships easily, while others without social connectedness may experience low self-esteem, anxiety, and depression [36]. With these benefits in mind, Ager & Strang's [6] Indicators of Integration framework demonstrated that the values of social connections shared among refugees are vital to positive integration experiences post-resettlement.

Similarly, a significant amount of research has been dedicated to exploring the impact of belongingness or '(non)belonging' on overall refugee well-being (i.e., [37,38]). Belongingness is not only linked to community acceptance [6], but it is also one of the most important components of resettlement [37]. Considering the transitory nature of refugee populations, where connections are lost as individuals are displaced from their homes, they often form relations of (non)belonging [37] with new places and communities that are not always receptive to their arrival [38].

Carey-Wood et al. [39] conducted a survey among refugees resettled in the United Kingdom exploring their perceptions and attitudes of integration, concluding that seeing Britain as their permanent home was a significant contributing factor to their sense of belonging. Similarly, Spoonely et al. [40] suggested that the acceptance of identity and individuality is a dimension of feeling part of one's host community. They illustrated the critical need for refugees to first feel a sense of connectedness with their host community before they can start developing social connections elsewhere. Without this initial sense of belongingness, refugees are more susceptible to vulnerability, unable to access essential support, resources, or information obtained from their social networks.

Yuval-Davis et al. [41] suggested that there is a complex relationship between belongingness and social cohesion among British migrants and their host community. Their research concluded that belongingness is context-specific, including demographic information like one's country of origin, host country, religion, ethnicity, and culture. Therefore, migrants have the potential to achieve social cohesion among their new community by socially excluding migrants who do not entirely 'integrate' (i.e., adopt the language and culture) into the host community.

1.2. Female Refugees and Social Capital

Research has shown that refugee women hold successful resilient strategies to overcome the disproportionate number of obstacles they face [1,7]. Most importantly, the makeup of their social networks [11,19,42], as well as their social positioning [12] and social experiences [5], have been shown to influence coping ability and can significantly impact (support or inhibit) social, emotional [5,42], mental [5,24,43], and physical [5,11] health and well-being. Social connections have been shown to not only reduce isolation, but also increase access to healthcare [24].

Previous research has showcased the impacts of gender on bonding, bridging, and linking social capital. Zetter et al. [44] concluded that refugee women are more likely to generate *bonding social capital*, or social connections with similar populations (i.e., same resettled ethnic groups, family members). In their longitudinal photo voice study among U.S.-resettled Congolese refugee women, Saksena and McMorrow [5] revealed that social bonding within their own ethnic community (especially those living in close proximity) combatted some of the challenges with integration experienced by participants. Congolese women would turn to each not only for social support, but also for economic and physical support (i.e., meals).

The findings from Saksena and McMorrow [5] suggest that members of multi-cultural communities should also engage in social interactions among differing ethnic groups (*bridging social capital*) in order to expand their social capital; in turn, generating greater reciprocity and increased levels of trust within their host community [45]. Without these opportunities to develop social networks among differing ethnic groups, refugees may develop strong bonds of solidarity and segregation with similar groups, impeding access to resources, limiting social mobility, reducing social trust, and possibly perpetuating social exclusion [46]. Bridging social capital, through community-based interactions like religious activities or even friendly neighborhood conversations [6], provide important opportunities for belongingness, security [6], and essential emotional, social [47], mental [48], and health-related [24] support.

Female refugees have also disproportionally lacked *linking social capital*, such as career readiness or education courses [49], which provides social connectedness with hierarchical institutions of power and access to support [50]. For example, female refugees tend to have less access to social services that provide English language classes compared to their male counterparts [51] and hold a more silenced voice among service providers and governmental agencies [47], missing out on important connections that could possibly increase belongingness, overall well-being, or even opportunities for an increase in power and participation in their host community.

Kingsbury et al. [12] conducted personal social network analysis among U.S.-resettled Bhutanese recent mothers. They explored social network ties, demographic characteristics of ties, frequency of communication, length of relationships, and the strength of social networks among mothers prior to being resettled and upon giving birth in the U.S. Researchers found that three close personal connections were essential during their pregnancy, including family members that participants knew prior to resettlement. Considering public health strategies, results suggest that family is an important social connection for refugees that could be leveraged to improve the flow of information and resources, supporting female refugee well-being during and after the resettlement process. The authors' findings support other migration research (i.e., [51]) that suggests that social connections in general are not only useful in ensuring refugees' health and well-being, but can also be useful in developing effective programming, services, and policy surrounding migration and resettlement.

While the establishment and development of social ties after resettlement has been shown to positively impact female refugee experiences and remains critical to the integration experience [52], there is limited research addressing the social networks themselves, including their reliance on those social connections and who is and is not part of those connections [53]. While social connectedness is not the only source of support for female refugees (i.e., religion and spiritually [4,42,54]), it is clearly essential in their overall health and well-being.

1.3. Critical Feminist Approach

Acknowledging global and local systems (political, economic, social structures) of gender inequities and oppression, Critical Feminist Perspective (CFP) centralizes women's unique lived experiences through an intersectional approach to gender identity [8,55–57]. In alignment with this approach, the exploration of immigrant and refugee women's health and well-being requires:

> "... new ways of inquiry, ones that move beyond the traditional ways of conceptualizing and operationalizing research... creat[ing] space for the exploration of how various dimensions of social identity, such as race, gender, and class, as well as education, citizenship, and geographical locations, intersect to influence the health of immigrant and refugee women" (p. 33) [13].

Intersectionality has been useful in analyzing power among relationships developed while in migration, which are the source of much social inequality and discrimination, especially for women fleeing persecution [58]. The authors therefore utilized this CFP lens to frame the present study, combatting the sentiment that genders form homogenous experiences by examining shifts in identity, power, social positions, and oppression [57,59] post-resettlement.

Intersectionality acknowledges that gender, race, class, ethnicity, sexuality, and nationality form interdependent systems of power that continuously shape individuals' lives [55,60,61]. Theorists within this field have rejected the separation of these categories and have instead vocalized the need to both engage with and analyze how these groups intersect among one another symbolically and in practice [61–63]. Therefore, social service providers and policymakers alike should not only become familiar with intersectionality but must also become aware of its significance and familiar with its practicality when developing policy and implementing programming among vulnerable populations. Without looking through an intersectional lens, governmental institutions and social service agencies run the risk of further discrimination, possibly creating or enhancing inequitable and oppressive power relations among its communities (whether intentional or not).

A vast amount of research (especially among governmental frameworks) has been conducted to provide an operational standardization for 'successful' (positive outcomes) integration post-resettlement, where refugees progress towards fully engaged participation in their host country [64]. Although the framework for refugee integration by Ager and Strang [6] commissioned by the United Kingdom provided foundational scholarship on integration, ultimately, there is no all-encompassing meaning or definition of the term, which varies among host countries [65]. Without being clearly defined, intersectionality has been used to combat the complexity of integration within migration literature. A need has risen to look beyond simplistic language in order to more fully capture the complexity of the integration and resettlement process; "this level of complexity regarding the understanding of integration is reinforced by a lack of understanding in common discussion as to what exactly refugees are expected to integrate into and how" (p. 5) [6]. Without looking beyond some of these static categories, practitioners and policymakers run the risk of ignoring the complex histories and multitude of identities that go into community formation among female refugees [66].

The impact of complex intersections of social identities on the health of immigrant and refugee women has grown in recognition in recent decades [18]. Researchers have suggested that indicators and definitions of integration vary across historical contexts, regional locations [40], and cultural dimensions [67]. Social service providers, healthcare professionals, and policymakers must consider the cultural dimensions of social injustice and the many systemic and individual barriers to integration that migrant populations face, including forms of indifference, discrimination, and social exclusion from their host community [40].

Previous migration research has highlighted these many factors that impact the migration and integration process and overall well-being of refugee populations; addressed in this present study were categories of city or residence, language, age, English comprehension, marital status, employment, education, length of time living in the U.S., and housing. Intersectionality was specifically addressed through the analysis of both systemic (qualitatively, focus groups) and individual (demographic survey) indicators that lead to refugee integration experiences post-resettlement. This research provides an important contribution to the existing literature (i.e., [11,19,47]) that acknowledges the significance of social connectedness as a determinant of refugee health and well-being for women, contributing to their resettlement outcomes.

1.4. Congolese and Iraqi Female Refugees

A refugee's ethnicity and cultural context impacts their integration outcomes post-resettlement [5,45,68]. Critically understanding the cultural and historical components of a population is the first step to facilitating more positive integration outcomes [69]. This study specifically explored Congolese and Iraqi female U.S.-resettled refugees. Around the time of this study (2014–2015), the largest groups of refugees admitted into the U.S. were from Iraq, Burma, Somalia, and Bhutan [70,71]. Acknowledging the differences in culture among the study's participants is an essential component for understanding the meaning that is given to gender, their migration experience, and their social networks—all of which impact social inequities. Therefore, the following brief cultural background provides a foundation for this study's specific population of Congolese and Iraqi refugees resettled in the U.S.

Congolese Refugees. During the time of this study, one of the United Nations' (U.N.) largest foci in Africa was the Democratic Republic of the Congo (D.R.C.), as they tried desperately to find homes for more than 50,000 Congolese refugees over the upcoming years [72]. Despite the fact that over 470,000 Congolese people took refuge in the D.R.C.'s nine neighboring countries [73], due to the heightened unrest, many needed to be resettled outside of the continent of Africa into a third host country. Over the span of five years during the time of this study (2013–2018), the U.S. Bureau of Population, Refugees, and Migration announced that tens of thousands of displaced Congolese refugees would be resettled in the U.S. [71–73], joining the 10,000+ that were already resettled in the U.S. since 2001 [73].

Two (+) decades of armed conflict and unrest in the D.R.C has recently contributed factor to the increasing numbers of Congolese refugees. A majority of displaced Congolese people are ethnic minorities from the Eastern D.R.C [72]. The conflict stemmed from the 1996 Rwandan invasion in pursuit of those who had taken refuge from the genocide in the Eastern D.R.C., followed by the first and second Congolese wars in 1996 and 1998 [73]. The heightened brutality and mass numbers of various countries involved in conflict during this time procured the name 'Africa's World War' [73], the deadliest conflict since World War II [73]. Despite the official end of the second Congo War in 2003, the Congolese continued to suffer the aftermath of decades of conflict and violence [74]; by 2013, more than 2.4 million Congolese were displaced [73]. Gender is essential when considering displacement and conflict in the D.R.C. due to gender-based violence; sexual violence has been and is still currently so commonly used as a weapon of war in the country that "human rights groups have called the area 'the most dangerous place in the world to be a woman'" (p. 2) [73].

A majority of Congolese refugees come to the U.S. with work experience as farmers and herders from rural areas, unskilled workers and professionals from urban areas, and small traders [73]. Similar to other refugee ethnic groups, the Congolese have arrived in the U.S. with high expectations, without preparation for the difficulties that await them in the U.S. [73]. Compounding these difficulties is ethnicity; research has shown social and cultural discrimination is especially heightened for Black female refugees in the United States [5] and is a central component of their integration experience [20].

During the time of this study, almost all (96%) Congolese refugees were pronounced Christians, finding churches to be a tremendous resource for both fiscal and emotional support upon their arrival, similar to the function of churches in the D.R.C. [73]. Due to past history of personal violence and trauma in their country, many Congolese have shown high rates of Post-Traumatic Stress Disorder, which is often masked due to cultural values and attitudes [73]. Therefore, many U.S.-resettled Congolese turn to religious faith for healing and support as an important role in personal and community life [73].

Iraqi Refugees. Just prior to the time of this study, "the U.N. High Commissioner for Refugees (UNHCR) estimated that more than four million Iraqis [were] displaced by the war in Iraq and its aftermath" (p. 5) [75]. During this time, about half (two million) of these Iraqi refugees fled nearby to secondary host countries of Syria, Jordan, Egypt, Iran, Lebanon, and Turkey. However, it's important to note that Iraqi refugees were resettled to the U.S. even prior to the Iraq war, with an estimated 12,000 admitted during the 1991 Gulf War [75].

Refugees have fled from Iraq for various reasons, including ethnic, religious, and political persecution. Ethnic targeting has included Sunni-Shi'I violence against Muslims, religious targeting of non-Muslim minorities (Baha'is, Christians, Jews, Sabean-Mandaeans, and Yazidis), and political targeting of supporters of the former regime, the insurgency, the current Iraqi government, or multinational forces [74]. Since most Iraqi communities are targets for other groups, the country has experienced numerous breaches to human rights and is not always able to protect its citizens; hence, resettlement back to Iraq or in a neighboring country is not available to most refugees. Therefore, Iraqi people must flee to a third host country resettlement, such as the U.S. [75]. Since large-scale Iraqi refugee processing for admission into the U.S. was initiated in February of 2007, the U.S. committed to increasing Iraqi acceptance numbers into the U.S. as a worldwide commitment during the time of this study [76].

2. Materials and Methods

2.1. Purpose

The purpose of the present study was to qualitatively explore female refugee perceptions of belongingness and social connectedness post-resettlement into their U.S. host community.

2.2. Study Design

This study was conducted between January and June of 2016, with the partnership of the U.S. Department of Children and Family Service's Refugee Services Program, three Voluntary Agencies, one governmental agency, three community-based organizations, two nonprofit organizations, and two churches. These partnering organizations were essential due to their established trust, credibility, and ongoing contact with the study's hard to reach population.

Research was conducted in two metropolitan cities that resettle some of the largest number of refugees in the state of Florida. Two female focus groups were conducted in this study, consisting of Iraqi (n = 6) and Congolese (n = 6) refugee participants. Depending on the participants' English language fluency, the guidance of the focus group was either conducted partially in English or entirely translated between English and participant native language with use of community representatives. Representative leaders within the local community were identified by a governmental liaison and confirmed by local service provider partners in the study. The representatives were heavily involved in participant recruitment, translating back-and-forth during focus groups, and data analysis through member checking, ensuring the retention of the original meaning of the researcher questions and participant responses, and further explaining concepts that participants used that were unfamiliar to the researcher [77]. After concluding each workshop, the researcher debriefed with the representative to determine the accuracy of their summary. Although beneficial to have a translator as a member of the participants' own ethnic community (i.e., trust, *bonding social capital*), the authors note the significant challenges that exist with interpreters in terms of bias, power dynamics, language diversity, and cultural approaches traditional to Western research practices [78].

Prior to the focus groups, each participant received two printed copies of the informed consent document (in their native language) and questionnaire (in their native language). These surveys provided valuable insights into participant demographics, as well as additional indicators that could impact the integration process (i.e., age, language, country of origin, ethnicity, education, length of time spent in the U.S., housing). This descriptive survey was essential in understanding how women experience multiple domains [3]. Quantitative data from the descriptive survey were analyzed with frequencies and mean scores.

Using a postpositivist perspective, the questions for the open-ended, semi-structured focus group were determined utilizing an expert-oriented approach [79]; questions were designed based on the professional expertise of the panel of experts and previous literature (i.e., [38]). The guide for the focus group instrument and procedure can be found in the entire report [80]. Each focus group consisted of 6 participants each and lasted approximately 1.5 h.

When considering the environment of working with refugee populations, the most culturally appropriate means of collecting data has been shown to be conducted through focus groups, storytelling, or outreach conversations, versus solely surveys or scalar types of evaluation [81]. By utilizing focus groups, this study allowed space for "participant ideas to build from one interviewee to another" (p. 445) [82] and allowed for the researchers to explore how people, organizations, and structures impact the refugee resettlement process [83]. Furthermore, due to the complex nature of the relationships formed throughout the integration process, qualitative data best suited the nature of this study, providing the richest contextual data necessary to understand the social connections that impact refugee well-being. This methodology allowed for 'interpreting interpretations' of the understanding of the relation of migration, rather than solely explaining it [83]. Qualitative methodologies allowed the researchers to obtain a "fuller expression of refugee experiences in their own terms" and were "essential in revealing subjective aspects of integration ... [which was significant because] how refugees feel about their experiences was as important an indicator as are objective indicators of adaption such as employment, income, and socio-economic mobility" (p. 53) [81].

The focus groups were audio recorded and then transcribed into English utilizing an online translation service. The analysis was completed on the translated transcripts. The authors note the limitations of this process due to the many challenges facing translators and interpreters with possible misunderstandings or differences in semantics [78], with the potential of even contributing to further participant marginalization [84]. With this consideration, the authors note that migrant researchers using both qualitative and quantitative data must acknowledge that both language and culture play a significant role in successfully addressing the needs of U.S.-resettled refugees [85].

The authors applied Braun and Clarke's [86,87] six-phase thematic analysis approach to gain familiarity with the data, code the data, and interpret the data. In order to become familiar with all data sources (phase 1 [86,87]), the authors independently read and re-read the focus group transcripts thoroughly and reread the focus group guides before beginning the qualitative analysis [86,87]. This step enhances the study's validity, ensuring that the findings of the study accurately reflect the data [86–88]. The authors then followed phase 2 and independently identified codes within the focus group data [86,87]. Throughout the interpretation process, the researchers sought to be empathetic in order to consider how the world looks to refugee populations [89], as well as reflexivity, considering the power of the research findings on the population and limitations of the authors' perspectives [90]. To ensure rigor in the analysis process, the authors met to discuss their codes through an iterative comparison process, which allowed them to find themes (phase 3) that were specific to each focus group, as well as emerging themes that cut across all focus groups [86,87]. Themes were revisited and refined once all codes were identified.

2.3. Sample

Refugee participants included Congolese and Iraqi refugees currently residing in the state of Florida in the U.S. (n = 12), who were recruited from local partnering organizations. Informed consent was obtained from all subjects involved in the study. Demographics among Congolese and Iraqi participants varied, especially among self-reported city of residence, age, employment status, education, and number of individuals living in their household. For more detailed information regarding a comparison of participant demographics among the two focus groups, please see Table 1.

It is important to note that a majority of women in this study were unemployed and lived in semi-permanent housing (rented). In addition to housing concerns, their lived experiences have the potential to place them in economic dependence and restrict mobility with members of their family or community, increasing their overall vulnerability [4]. Additionally, considering the higher amount of educational experience among Congolese women in the present study, previous research has found that, despite arriving with higher education and professional credentials, some refugee women may not get such credentials recognized in the U.S. [31]. Similarly, Stempel and Alemi [31] found that less educated women, as well as women whose received education outside of the U.S., were most targeted or harmed by discrimination among multiple refugee groups.

Table 1. Female-only focus group demographics comparison.

Demographics	Congolese	Iraqi
City of Residence	Orlando (n = 6)	Jacksonville (n = 6)
Primary Language	French (n = 5) Swahili (n = 1)	Kurdish (n = 5) Arabic (n = 1)
Secondary Language	English (n = 2) Lingala (n = 1) Kikongo (n = 1) None (n = 2)	English (n = 3) None (n = 3)
Average age	M = 45.5 (SD = 14.511)	M = 32 (SD = 7.16)
Average English comprehension (read and understand)	M = 2.5 (Slightly well–Well) SD = 1.00	M = 2.17 (Slightly well) SD = 1.34
Marital status	Married (n = 0) Separated (n = 1) Widowed (n = 1) Never Married (n = 4)	Married (n = 3) Separated (n = 1) Widowed (n = 1) Never Married (n = 1)
Employment	Not employed (n = 4) Employed (n = 2)	Not employed (n = 3) Employed (n = 3)
Education	M = 8.8 years (SD = 3.56)	M = 3.4 years (SD = 6.29)
Length (range) of time living in City	2 months–8 years	6 months–6 years
Rent vs. Own housing	Rent (n = 6) Own (n = 0)	Rent (n = 4) Own (n = 2)
Number of individuals in household (average)	M = 2.83 (SD = 0.90)	M = 4.17 (SD = 0.90)
Total number of children (under 18 years old) in household	2 children (n = 0) 1 child (n = 2) 0 children (n = 4)	2 children (n = 1) 1 child (n = 0) 0 children (n = 5)

2.4. United States Political Climate

It is important to note that the present study was conducted during a very polarizing time in public discourse on migration, with the 2016 U.S. presidential election. However, considering the years that have passed since the time of this study, ongoing shifts in the U.S. political climate surrounding migration continue to exist. Thus, the results of this study provide service providers and policymakers with a necessary foundation for existing (and in many cases, *growing*) vulnerabilities among U.S.-resettled refugees. For example, the drastic decrease in U.S. refugee resettlement (and migration at large) during the global pandemic, as well as the harsh cuts to the refugee resettlement program (including significant resettlement agency downsizing and closures) by the Trump administration developed further vulnerabilities for the U.S. Refugee Program, undermining the U.S. placement as the world's top country for third-country refugee admissions [91].

Lastly, considering the ongoing (if not heightened) opposing discourse on immigration across partisan lines, this study holds significant weight into the perceived experiences of female refugees. Even as of recent, there continues to be an increase in stigmatized targeting of Muslim religious identities as migration becomes more politicized [31]. Considering current U.S. President Biden's hope to expand the domestic resettlement program [91], the results of this study provide insights into successful strategies and policies that could combat current inequities among female refugees resettled or in the process of resettling in the U.S.

3. Results

Despite the plethora of evidence outlining the adversities faced by female refugees post-resettlement, both focus groups mentioned the welcoming nature they experienced in their community (especially Iraqi participants). Although this connectedness started initially upon resettlement, developing a sense of belongingness required a significant amount of time and trust, especially among their host community and service providers. Established and reciprocal trust was essential for the development of bonding, bridging, and linking social capital.

The development of *bonding* social capital varied among focus groups. Although both focus groups found essential social connections through church and spiritual outlets, important bonding networks for Congolese participants were established at work and developed among fellow female refugees, while Iraqi networks were strong among family members and other refugee groups (without gender specificity). Differences in language and culture made it challenging for both focus groups to develop strong (*bridging*) ties with their host community. Despite these barriers, Iraqi women still vocalized important social connections among American community members to provide them with practical support and assistance.

Lastly, while Iraqi participants gleaned essential information and resources through their *linking* networks, Congolese participants emphasized their insufficiencies in cultural awareness, communication, and genuine care/concern; similar to *bridging* social capital, lack of English language fluency was also a barrier to support from social connections. Both focus groups emphasized the lack of quality resources provided by social service agencies, resulting in increased isolation. This lack of *linking* social capital created self-dependency and further perpetuated their isolation, creating additional stressors for participants (i.e., employment, housing, physical healthy) that negatively impacted their well-being post-resettlement, especially among Congolese participants.

In the discussion that follows, the authors further elaborate on these emerging themes, drawing from participant voices to highlight perceptions of belongingness and reciprocal trust among their social connections. Table 2 summarizes the themes and codes that emerged from both focus groups.

Table 2. Themes and codes.

Belongingness and Trust					
Bonding Capital		**Bridging Capital**		**Linking Capital**	
Congolese and Iraqi		**Congolese and Iraqi**		**Congolese and Iraqi**	
• Church and religious social connections		• Language and culture		• Lack of quality social services • Isolation	
Congolese	**Iraqi**	**Congolese**	**Iraqi**	**Congolese**	**Iraqi**
• Work social connections • Supportive female social connections	• Fellow refugee social connections • Family		• American Social Connections	• Lack of cultural competence • Perceived apathy • Poor communication • Language	• Essential information and resources

3.1. Belongingness and Trust

Despite the many adversities faced by female refugee participants, both Congolese and Iraqi participants mentioned the welcoming nature and sense of belonging they experienced in their community. This sense of belongingness was established upon their initial resettlement; *"it feels like it's your home the first part that you arrived in"* (IJF2). In fact, when asked if they felt welcomed, all Iraqi refugee focus group participants indicated that they felt welcomed by their host community upon arrival to the United States, as if *"you're part of America"* (IJF1).

When asked about the possibility or desire for future migration in the U.S., as they began to build their social network outside of their immediate city of residence, participants mentioned the ease to move to a place where they felt more belongingness and connected:

> *"People in New York. People in Indiana* [have moved elsewhere outside of [City] and they feel more welcomed]. *Like some friends will meet them, but in Indiana they enjoy. If we tell them what we are facing, they are like just move"* (COF3).

Participants indicated that both *bridging* (host community) and *linking* (social service agencies) ties contributed to their sense of belongingness. Participants acknowledged the kindness (social and emotional support) they received from their local neighbors and community: *"For now we have to stay over here because people to be honest with you from here they're really kind and nice"* (IJF4).

One Congolese participant tied their sense of 'welcoming' to the direct support (healthcare, employment) they were receiving:

> *"You have come here, but you have not yet get any card. You only benefits is in Orlando. Its all America. They're the same, but you be welcome in America. You have to wait until you get all those benefit. You've got the hospital. You work, and at least you have something for you to move"* (COF3).

Although the sense of belongingness was more clearly articulated among Iraqi participants than Congolese participants (who expressed mixed feelings of belongingness), both focus groups acknowledged that welcoming took time. Successful outcomes and integration take time to adjust and develop social connections. Starting out, refugee women felt *"alone"* (IJF4) until relationships started to develop (*"they were talking and making jokes"* (IJF4); "[we started to] *talk and* [then I] *trust them"* (COF)) and feelings of belongingness within their host community began to shift (*"and we're happy now"* (IJF4); *"step by step we were okay now"* (IJF4)).

Iraqi participants expressed an essential shift of feelings of belongingness when trust was developed. Towards the initial stages of resettlement, most Iraqi participants highlighted that trust was only found through religion (*"First she trusts God and then she trusts the government, then* [resettlement agency]*"* (IJF4)) and family (*Interviewer: "How much do you trust your husband to do their best? "* ... *"Alot."* (IJF3); *"Because he's* [husband] *the only one in here that I need to talk and trust him"* (IJF4)). After some time has been allotted to develop social connections, Iraqi participants were then able to develop mutual trust among *bridging* and *linking* networks, such as friends (*"Friend that you really trust"* (IJF4)), host community members, and resettlement agencies (*Interviewer: "Pick the person you trust the most."* ... *"Case worker"* (IJF2)).

3.2. Bonding Capital

Church and religious social connections. Research has shown that relationships established between refugees and the wider community differ by gender; for example, women may be more likely to make friends with other parent(s) at school, while men tend to develop their social network through work [45]. Despite the aforementioned isolation in the present study, several women have found social connectedness and support through church and religion. Church, one of the most frequently discussed social connection, provided both Congolese and Iraqi participants with social (*"She will pray to God. Talk to her kids"* (IJF4)) and emotional support, as well as a heightened sense of trust (*"If we didn't trust the people from here or trusted God, we wouldn't be here* (IJF4)) above most other social connections (*Interviewer: "Who do you trust the most?"* ... *"Family first. Church is second"* (COF)). Even in an emergency, one participant said, *"Call 911 and pray to God"* (IJF3).

Work social connections (*Congolese*). Congolese participants developed bonding social capital not only through religious outlets, but also through work and among their female colleagues. Unlike previous gender research [45], and in alignment with others (i.e., [90]), work was also an important place to build and develop social connections for female refugees. However, despite work being a source for relationship building, the development of strong social connections still remained fairly slow: *"Most of us they will say that we have friends from work. That is where you meet new people, because they are working with them. I get to know you slowly by slowly making friends"* (COF).

Work provided women with an outlet to leave the physical space of their home and focus on non-household responsibilities, and an opportunity to cultivate friendships: *"It's difficult* [to make friends] *because you don't work. You are just staying at home"* (COF).

Supportive female social connections (*Congolese*). Fellow female refugee relationships provided an essential support for a variety of problems that Congolese participants faced. Such social connections provided unique assistance to problems; they provided *"hope"* (COF) and guidance (*"show me"* (COF)) in moving forward with the issues they were facing. This aligns with previous migration research [91] that showcased that refugee women tend to establish higher levels of *bonding* (i.e., homogenous genders) versus *bridging* social capital.

Fellow refugee social connections (*Iraqi*). Iraqi refugees expressed a shared understanding of the difficulty of the resettlement process. Especially after resettlement, Iraqi refugees had limited interactions with networks outside of their immediate family or ethnicity (*"Everyone is Kurdish"* (IJF3)). They also missed many aspects of their homeland that they had to leave behind, as well as parts of their home culture that was starkly different from their new host community's culture. When they find others from their same culture or experience, this commonality provides an instant bond and underlying desire to support one another in the same or similar challenges. One way an Iraqi woman developed connection with her fellow refugee neighbor was by bringing him food: *"Because there is a neighbor right here and he's a old guy but when he cook something we always give it to him, because he's a refugee too, so we helped him"* (IJF4).

Family (*Iraqi*). In contrast to Congolese participants, Iraqi participants would often turn to their only social connections, which was often their family members (*"mom," "father," "husband," "boyfriend," "sister," "brother," or "child"* (IJF2, IJF3, IJF4)), or in some cases, close friendships. Family members became available and were immediately accessible for support because they were some of the only social connections that participants interacted with regularly, even if they were not physically nearby; *"when I talk to them* [my sister on FaceTime], *I feel better"* (IJF4). When asked about various characteristics of their social connections, including qualities of importance, power, and safety, participants generally prioritized family due to their reciprocal trust (*"close in trust"* (IJF3)) developed among these relationships.

> *"Does she have any close relationship here with people that are not Kurdish? "No. Just only she has... She just comes to our home and goes to my sister's home, that's it. Her mother-in-law and sister-in-law and that's it. She doesn't have anybody just only us"* (IJF4).

3.3. Bridging Capital

Language and culture. Participants in both focus groups acknowledged that making friends is *"not really easy"* (COF), *"very difficult"* (COF), and *"hard"* (IJF2). For several women, developing bridging connections is a slow and burdensome process, due to differences in language and culture with their local host community. Language proved to be a significant barrier to developing *bridging* social capital, making connections with differing ethnicities or American host community members challenging. Integrating into their host community was *"harder... because another language"* (IJF3, IJF4).

> *"One thing which I would say is making friends depends on someone. It depends on someone, how that person is, their personality, how they talk. Then what could be also to be challenge on the refugee women, most of them they don't speak their language. How can you make a friend with someone? You can meet me but I want to become your friend. We don't have the collaboration in language"* (COF).

> *"Let me say it in general. Whites are not like us Africans. For us African we are kind of friendly. I hope you understand that, but Whites they have that kind of something which is kind of privacy but for us as we grow, as our culture, I can come to your house. I go there waiting for the food. I eat. Something like that but that is not of the Whites. I have to come at the right time, if I was invited"* (COF).

American social connections (*Iraqi*). In some instances, Iraqi participants suggested that the connections made with their American host community were just as essential as relationships developed among fellow refugees. These social connections provided essential trusting (*"Yes, I have a friend, she's American and then I also have another friend he was an army that I trust him a lot"* (IJF4)) support for refugees post-resettlement. However, the nature of these ties varied in strength; while fellow Kurdish refugees provided emotional and social support, American connections were more transactional with direct, tangible assistance. Two participants described the transactional relationship through their encounter with their American friends at the airport. The interviewer asked, "Do you have any close relationships with people here that are not Kurdish?" The participants responded: *"They're Americans. One man and woman... they came to pick us up from the airport"* (IJF3) and *"Some American... by the airport when they come and pick us [up]"* (IJF4). Host community members often helped refugee participants with navigating complex U.S. systems and helped them feel welcomed when they first arrived by picking them up at the airport. One participant acknowledged the limited strength of such ties with their host community, where support was provided under the conditions and convenience of the community member: *"A couple of friends if we need anything call them and when they're not busy, they come here and help us. Yeah, the Americans"* (IJF4).

3.4. Linking Capital

Linking social capital [50] proved to be the most challenging for participants to establish and further build upon. Participants mentioned this difficulty, starting with the first day they resettled to the U.S. Access to resources or additional social connections for support was very challenging, due to a lack of cultural competence, as well as perceived apathy and lack of emotional connection among resettlement service providers. Congolese participants also expressed the obvious deficiency of social service resources, poor communication, and language barriers that further inhibited their development of *linking* social capital. Due to these obstacles, building and developing social capital is very challenging. Refugees are left to advocate for their needs, find their own solutions to everyday stressors (i.e., broken phone, internet issues), or navigate complex U.S. systems by themselves, due to the limited support from social service agencies or other community resources.

Essential information and resources (*Iraqi*). Similar to their *bridging* connections, Iraqi participants also established weak ties among their *linking* connections to gain essential information and resources. Although somewhat transactional, these networks (resettlement agencies) were critical for providing them with 'the most information since coming to the U.S.' (Interviewer question); *"...if I need to go somewhere they [resettlement agency] can come pick me and take me and find me some ways to do good things"* (IJF2). Although weak, these institutions also provided a direct link to essential resources to support refugee health and well-being, extending beyond the initial point of resettlement: *"Whenever I need them [resettlement agency], twice a month maybe... they gave us social security, DCF, Medicaids"* (IJF3).

Lack of cultural competence (*Congolese*). Starting with their first day of resettlement in their new host community, Congolese participants mentioned difficulty with building strong connections with *linking* institutions due to the organization's lack of cultural competency and sensitivity.

Upon arrival into the U.S., refugees are required to repay (reimburse) their travel expenses on the interest-free loan that was used to cover the cost of their airline ticket provided for refugee resettlement to the U.S. [92]. Refugees are then allegedly supported by agencies that specialize in resettlement services. The U.S. State Department provides refugee furnishing, rent, food, and clothing for three months; nonprofit, charity, or faith-based community members provide all remaining support during this time.

Following this brief period of governmental support, assistance shifts to the Department of Health and Human Services and other nonprofit organizations that provide additional supportive services (i.e., medical assistance, language classes, employment preparedness) [91] through a public-private partnership model that draws from (generally faith-based) local community networks [93]. Although well-intentioned, one Congolese woman specifically remarked on the contractual feeling of this weak social tie, providing resources (i.e., food, furniture) with limited knowledge of cultural differences:

"They take money. We are from Africa. We don't know. We don't eat food. Then, they come. What do we eat? If they... a bigger thing for the [church support] and then they cannot put in the house. On the first day you come, and you don't know anything. They will start counting even those thing food. We got this. We bought this. Only your money. We don't even wait for you to come because they don't know the food you eat" (COF3).

Perceived apathy (*Congolese*). The common sentiment of caseworkers and social service providers *"not even caring"* (COF) was mentioned several times by Congolese women. Participants acknowledged that this perceived lack of genuine care and *"emotional connection"* (COF) stemmed from the service provider being overworked (*"She* [service provider] *was like, 'Oh that day I will be so busy. I have two jobs'"* (COF)), as well as having a lack of language commonality (*"If I can easily communicate with you, most likely I'm going to look after you. If I cannot, emotionally I'm not connecting, language is a barrier, you are a gone case"* (COF5)) and lack of desire to support or connect refugees with additional resources (*"it's there, but they don't want to give it to you"* (COF)).

Poor communication (*Congolese*). According to Congolese participants, alongside (and perhaps hand in hand with) culturally insensitive and deficient resources resides poor communication between social service providers and their refugee clients. Participants remarked that the most frequent point of contention, in terms of ineffective communication, was the lack of availability over the telephone. Many participants emphasized the lack of answering phone calls and responding to voicemails in a perceived timely manner. Through their elaborations and narratives, participants provided further elaboration as to the frustrations and expectations of what constitutes 'timely' and 'effective' communication.

According to participant experiences, social service provider or caseworker responses to client phone calls included: *"she was like, 'I'm busy"* (COF3), *"sometimes they don't answer the phone"* (COF3), or "[they] *take time to... answer"* (COF3). This 'time' to call back was quantified by two participants as *"after two or three days"* (COF6) and *"hours and hours... maybe after two days"* (COF1). Considering the lack of power and social connections held by refugee women, especially after she *"keep[s] on calling"* (COF3), or in urgent or emergency situations, these unmet expectations for timely communication may cause further vulnerability, feelings of distrust, or isolation.

"One thing so far, why do they put their numbers in voicemail every time? Someone can have an emergency. You call them, maybe you have an emergency. I'm new here. I don't want a policy like that" (COF1).

Several participants acknowledged that the wait time for support and communication response is lengthy, even when meeting for in-person care as well:

"If you go there ["charities"], they will make you sitting there. You wait for long time then they attend you. They say go back. I already made a client in the internet so if they answer I will call you. It's just like that. Then you come, you sit, wait for even one month" (COF).

Despite their deficient allocation of services and poor communication tendencies, participants still mentioned that these entities were (at some point in their resettlement process, to varying degrees) a resource where *"you have to go"* (COF). A sense of familiarity and necessity, despite its frustrations and weakness, was paired with this social *linking* tie.

Language (*Congolese*). Similar to *bridging* social capital, language proved to be a significant barrier among Congolese participants in developing *linking social* capital as well. Language was a barrier to accessing appropriate help or resources from authoritative institutions of power, such as resettlement agencies, emergency services, healthcare facilities, and the police. One participant felt, *"If I can easily communicate with you, most likely I'm going to look after you. If I cannot, emotionally I'm not connecting, language is a barrier, you are a gone case"* (COF5). In another instance the misunderstanding from the language barrier involved a moment of emotional distress and further vulnerability by bringing in law enforcement:

> *"The person who knocked called the police. They had a misunderstanding of the language. The police was asking, "What can I do?" Committed the kid to the hospital. The kid was hurt, the mother was crying, shaking. After a minute, and then someone came, "Those people they're speaking like African language"* (COF1).

Lack of quality social service resources. One of the most prevalent themes among all participants that emerged as a barrier for support and well-being was the deficient lack of quality social service resources. Congolese participants specifically raised several issues of retention and high turnover (*"they just sent me to another person"* (COF)), increased caseloads, and shortened times for availability (*"I'm calling because I know if I call her after 3:00 PM, she will be off"* (COF1)) for support. *"There are some agencies are overwhelmed. Case specialists or case managers are being given a lot of cases that, I would say, legally it should not be allowed"* (COF5).

> *"We're running through that a lot, but the biggest concern I am having is the case specialists having too many cases to handle and they are dropping the ball on someone. All the agencies in town, yes"* (COF).

> *"They have also called the food stamps. Then they know that she's not working. The income of the two, its very low. In her age, she doesn't know how to read. She doesn't go to school. really the government, by the time they knew about her, about all the clothing she have. really is the government want just to leave her like that. Even the food stamp, it's cut. Everything is cut"* (COF3).

Both Congolese and Iraqi participants addressed the overall lack of quality (*"waste money for nothing which would help me"* (COF3), *"they are diving into mediocrity"* (COF5)) or insufficient services among agencies. When addressing daily issues or problems long term, both Congolese and Iraqi participants overall preferred *bonding* (family, other refugees) or *bridging* (friends, host community) social connections—or even no one at all (they would take care of the matter themselves)—in comparison to social service agencies. When asked what social connections were most helpful when they first arrived in the U.S., Iraqi focus group members mentioned: *"Yeah, but they* [friends] *help us more than* [refugee resettlement agency] *to be honest with you, yes"* (IJF4).

> *"They* [friends] *help us more than* [refugee resettlement agency]. *They take us to interview like Walmart, when we need something we told them, but* [refugee resettlement agency] *just bring us over here and take care of the people that's it, but they* [friends] *help us a lot"* (IJF4).

The lack of quality and quantity of social services resulted in refugee self-dependency and further perpetuated their isolation, creating additional stressors for participants that negatively impacted their well-being post-resettlement.

Self-agency. Building social connections to access support, information, and resources is very challenging, and participants (especially Congolese women) conveyed the lack of facilitation or support from caseworkers and social service providers in this networking process. Therefore, many participants were forced to take matters into their own hands by advocating for and solving problems by themselves. Participants seemed to express a sense of feeling defeated by the lack of support, so they decided to move forward independently (*"I went there and I applied by myself"* (COF)). Such strategies have the potential to be problematic, considering the lack of social connections (and therefore limited access to resources, information, and support) and ongoing feelings of isolation that many had already previously expressed.

> *"You have to face that by yourself. Then once those people [social service providers] start to return to you, they will just tell you they have no solution. Your benefit got finished. They will just give you number to try to call the government and claim the government's got to help. That's what they do"* (COF3).

Many times, when Congolese participants reflected on which social connections they would reach out to for support when facing an issue, they instead discussed that they would solve the problem themselves. In response to whom they would speak or talk with about their problem, many responses resounded with a similar comment: *"Nobody because I don't know any"* (COF).

To counter this barrier to *linking* social capital, refugee participants began self-advocating for their own needs, problem-solving the issues themselves, or sought out alternative networks for support. Some sentiment suggested that women already knew that the development of social networks would be a slow process; instead, they are self-advocating on behalf of future generations of female refugees:

> *"It's also better you talk, and sometime when you feel like you want to cry, you cry. We hope one day a chance. Others which are coming behind will get a chance. Only because we are thirsty. We won't get a chance. No, that's... for us. We are fighting for those ones who are behind. Maybe the children of the children only... those"* (COF3).

Isolation. Overall, both Congolese and Iraqi participants discussed the challenges with developing and maintaining social connections post-resettlement. The challenges of not feeling connected with their host community and a lack of linking support aided in negative outcomes. A lack of social connections caused *"suffering"* (COF)), loneliness, and social/emotional distress among participants; *"miss home, so we were coming from Arab to here, we don't see anybody"* (IJF4). Isolation was also expressed through feelings of not receiving adequate support from social service agencies, resulting in further loneliness and negative health outcomes, especially among Congolese participants.

Lack of support in resources and information regarding housing, employment, transportation, childcare, food, and healthcare proved to be significant barriers to well-being. Additionally, considering the unique finances associated with refugee populations, such as the repayment to the federal government of the original resettlement flight to the U.S. (*"still we have to pay the ticket which brought us here"* (COF3)), these populations are starting with an unimaginable task with limited resources and support.

Many refugees emphasized the impact of employment–especially unemployment—on successful integration. Such *"low"* (COF1) or non-existent wages have significant impact on other factors, such as affordable housing.

> *"You start working on the 17th. Then they tell we have let you go. You have to pay the rent. How can I pay rent when I start working on 17th? I have to wait that because when I'm working, they pay two weeks. I have to wait for those two week"* (COF3).

The makeup of the participant's family unit also played a significant role in how much employment (or lack thereof) became a significant stressor:

> *"They give them the food stamps of the kid only thirty days for the whole month. They she's working. They have to pay for housing. They have to pay for electricity.* ***They have to pay everything****"* (COF3, emphasis added).

For women with children or without a husband, financial challenges became a significant inhibitor to well-being. Low income became a stark and difficult realization, considering the additional financial burden that is placed on mothers.

> *"The challenge which I know that they are facing is her with a daughter and a son, the income is very low"* (COF).

> *"At least you know, "My child she's on day care. It has worked peacefully. Let me go to work." Other they're failing to go to work because of the kids and then at the same time, if it does not work they cannot afford a house"* (COF1).

For single refugee women, the lack of a dual-household income and domestic support also places additional compounding pressure to pay for all the household expenses:

> *"The good thing, it would be better if the husband is around because the husband could be also working. At least that's more income they could be sharing and they share the bills. Now only two people in the house are working and then the income is very low"* (COF).

Several participants highlighted the high expense and burden of rent. Affordable housing cannot be obtained; what minimal affordable housing is available is not large enough or adequate/appropriate housing for a family unit.

> *"One month you are telling the landlord to wait at least, to hold on. You don't have the money, but once you get your payment you pay that, but in America, it's all like that. Once you given your purse on day, they challenge you for that. That one day. You have to pay a hundred and something"* (COF3).

Considering that a majority of the study's participants are renting their housing, this leaves a heightened possibility for continual migration and a lack of permanency in their dwelling space, which further perpetuates risks of vulnerability.

> *"They have an issue with like whether they're working. Now where they are staying, the owner of the house want to sell the house"* (COF3).

For several refugee participants, due to unattainable housing costs, alongside compounding taxes and credit interest, the security of housing was prioritized over food for the family. However, one participant mentioned that, with the limited financial security of employment (despite the low income mentioned previously), there is an opportunity to pay for *"at least my housing and get my food"* (COF3).

> *"When she failed to pay the rent, she has to go and take a credit. Then you have to take 500. You have to return that 555 dollar. Then after paying that... when you are getting 1200. Thats not just that passed into that check. Then you pay the tax. You are paying the house maybe 800 or 900. You have nothing put on food"* (COF3).

Such stressors not only have serious implications for mental and emotional well-being, but also physical well-being. It was aforementioned that the prioritization of food (nutritious or otherwise) was low, in comparison to other living essentials (such as housing). Additionally, medical bills and affordable healthcare were also indicated as financial challenges and stressors, which proved to be a significant burden. With a lack of employment, many participants lacked any healthcare benefits; *"She doesn't work. On the top of that she doesn't have Medicaid"* (COF).

> *"If she throws sick or go to the hospital, the bills do come very much. She doesn't work. How is she going to pay them?"* (COF3).

4. Discussion and Conclusions

Drawing from the results of this study, the researchers conclude with a discussion on future research directions and tangible recommendations for policy considerations, integration process revision, and infrastructure development for resettlement advocates and practitioners.

4.1. Moving beyond Homogenous Identities

In alignment with previous research [26], the diverse, complex history, and unique concerns [24] of a female refugee's ethnicity must be taken into account in relation to health outcomes and well-being. Considering the differences observed between the focus groups, refugee programming and policy must take refugee ethnicity (as well as other intersecting identities) into account. Conjoining 'all refugee women' into one distinct category or group is a disservice to the oppressed identities and advantageous strengths that each individual holds. For example, in the present study, Iraqi participants highlighted that extended family, friends, and *bridging* social ties were essential to support their well-being significantly more than their fellow Congolese women. Researchers, policymakers and social service providers must consider the intersections of gender and race, ethnicity, and national origin [66]. An integrated, multi-system approach is needed to improve female refugee well-being and health outcomes [24]. For policymakers specifically, this includes combatting gender neutral terms in migration policy, which ignores power dynamics and socio-economic and -cultural systems that create a differentiated gendered experience [9].

Echoing previous calls for social service reforms to build knowledge and skillsets for navigating U.S. society [5], the authors also encourage resettlement agencies to include the historical contexts of race, ethnicity, national origins, and gender as they relate to the United States as part of the cultural orientation training for refugees post-resettlement.

4.2. Belongingness and Trust

While Iraqi women still experienced loneliness and isolation post-resettlement, results suggest that they emphasized their level of connection and sense of welcome with their host community more than the Congolese women. Due to this increase in vocalized social connectedness, the researchers consider the following questions: Are Iraqi women better connected in terms of *bridging* social capital? Do they experience a greater sense of belongingness accordingly?

Results also suggest that this heightened level of belongingness stems from a shift (*"it's just different"* (IJF)) in trust among their social connections. Previous trust literature among migrant populations defines 'trust' as a community's capacity to generate reciprocity among residents [94]; this reciprocity suggests that there is an expectation that relationships developed within the community will be available when needed [48]. The results of this study align with previous scholarship, which concludes that, in order for social networks to develop into social capital for the individual, the relationship must be built on reciprocal trust [95]. When considering the complex nature of refugee resettlement, trust becomes more of an abstract concept. Refugees need to place trust not only in their social connections, but also in the larger "humanitarian commitment" (p. 338) of social services and aid within their host country [96].

Iraqi participants in the present study highlighted that trust was found first through religion (*"God"* (IJF)), then family, and later (after some time was allotted to develop social connections) among *bridging* and *linking* social ties. Trust is a significant factor especially when developing *bridging* social capital; this capital stimulates cooperation and familiarity, leading to knowledge-based, interpersonal trust and an increased generalizable trust [50].

The authors found it interesting that, although religion provided a foundation for the development of trust, there was a lack of discussion among participants regarding religion as a facilitator of distrust among non-Muslim community members or possible discrimination, as discussed in previous research highlighting gender-based, anti-Muslim bias and prejudice in the U.S. (i.e., [3,30,33–36,97]). Future research on how this spiritual connection impacts other social networks or contributes to other aspects of refugee well-being or belonging should be explored. For example, although not well studied, how might anti-Muslim discrimination influence economic outcomes [30] or financial stressors discussed in this study?

Stolle et al. [98] explored the impact of ethnic diversity in Canada on social unity, specifically considering its relationship with trust. They found that individuals who consistently engage with their neighbors are less influenced by the ethnic characteristics of their surroundings than people who lack consistent social interactions. Therefore, social networks could mediate negative effects of diverse populations on trust; ongoing social interactions among "diverse others" [98] make ethnic differences less threatening. Drawing from these findings, in the present study, results suggest that ongoing social connections with 'diverse others' (refugees of other ethnicities, American host community members, resettlement agency personnel) could have shifted perceptions of Iraqi female refugees to become more trusting, despite their differences.

Conversely, several consequences arise from distrust of social connections. Due to their limited contact or exposure, the distrust that many refugees hold towards both service providers and their host communities [99] further perpetuates a state of vulnerability and isolation. The absence of trust as an emerging theme among Congolese participants in the present study is concerning, possibly contributing to or even bolstering negative outcomes yet to be explored.

4.3. Social Capital

Building on previous research [47], the results of this study also confirm that refugee social connectedness has a gendered dimension regarding social capital resources. Bonding, bridging, and linking social capital proved to be essential to refugee well-being, providing various degrees, ways of developing, and types of support.

Social bonding. To support women's successful integration, trusting their social connection of kinship was more important for Iraqi than Congolese participants. The present study contributes to previous research [47,92] that suggests that higher levels of *bonding* social capital (i.e., family, close friendships) exist among female refugee networks than *bridging* social capital. Such strong kinship ties have previously been shown to improve the quality of life for refugees, ironically for men more so than women [100]. However, research has also suggested that an increase in *bonding* social capital has the potential to make it harder for individuals to trust their surrounding diverse community [101]. Did Congolese participants experience heightened levels of distrust towards their host community? Although not directly seen in the present study's findings, the authors suggest that further migrant research considers the gendered nature of trust among highly bonded refugee communities.

Despite the isolation many participants experienced, the results of the present study concluded that the church was an important network in the development of social *bonding*, contributing to social and emotional support, while spirituality (*"God"*) was rooted in significant trust. Findings support previous research [30,42,47,54], affirming the contribution of religious institutions to essential socioemotional support for female refugees. Similarly, the trust of spirituality vocalized among participants in the present study could also contribute to female refugee resilience and coping, as shown in previous research [4].

The authors note the lack of religious dependency as expected in the Congolese female focus group. During the time of this study, as previously mentioned, almost all (96%) Congolese refugees were pronounced Christians, finding churches to be a tremendous resource for both fiscal and emotional support upon their arrival, similar to their lives in turmoil back in the D.R.C. [73]. Many U.S.-resettled Congolese turn to religious faith for healing and support as an important role in personal and community life [83]. Perhaps these results point to a possible shift in spiritual dependency as a significant source of *bonding* capital or coping mechanism among female Congolese refugees.

Social bridging. In alignment with previous research [102], the workplace proved to be a source for Congolese participants to build and develop social connections. These results contradict previous gender research that has suggested that men (more so than women) tend to develop networks through work, while women may be more likely to build relationships with other parents at school [47]. These differing results could be due to the demographic make-up of Congolese women in the present study, considering that most participants were never married and had little to no children living in their homes, encouraging them to spend more time at work (to address their single household income) and limited interactions with parents at school.

Regardless, considering the importance of the workplace as a platform for social connectedness, the authors suggest that future research should consider the importance of employment not only to combat financial stressors emphasized in this present study, but also as an opportunity to further develop *bridging* social capital. Economic integration research among U.S.-resettled refugees tends to focus on how fast refugee groups can find employment [5], as well as how much they rely on support services beyond the initial 90-day federal resettlement support [103], versus the opportunity to develop social connections through the workplace.

Previous studies have highlighted the low levels of employment among highly educated refugee women and the lack of economic niches for those less educated, which significantly impacts their lower earnings [33]. Employment has also been shown to vary depending on gender (women experience lower employment rates than their male counterparts [16]), as well as the length of time an individual has resided in the U.S. [104] and citizenship status [105]. While female refugees have lower levels of employment within their first year post-resettlement (especially women who have had children more frequently and earlier [105]), male and females experience have shown to hold similar employment effects in later years [106]. However, it is important to note that other research has yielded mixed results and employment differences among gender; for example, one study concluded that U.S.-resettled refugee women are actually employed at a higher rate than their male equivalent [107].

Despite these mixed results, an overwhelming about of literature points to the significant benefits of employment for refugee women, not only for themselves (i.e., greater autonomy, opportunities, social support, and combatting isolation) [108], but also for the economic vitality of their host country [105] and community. There are many challenges that face employment research among migrant populations, such as the limited refugee labor market data and scarce disaggregated refugee data by gender [109]. Additionally, challenges arise with data collection and analysis, considering the interdependent barriers and political and social issues that vary across contexts and impact employment data [109]. Although the authors acknowledge these many obstacles, they still promote the importance of future research on exploring the gendered differences of employment as forms of both *bridging* and *linking* social capital.

While the multiple identities of female refugees must be considered to better analyze the development of *bridging* social capital (not only among work colleagues), the results of the study also suggest that relationships established between refugees and the wider community are gendered and take time to develop. The lengthy and difficult process of making friends is due to differences in language and culture with their fellow refugees of different ethnicities and languages, as well as their local host community. Female refugees disproportionally lack *linking* social capital such as career readiness or education courses [49] and are less likely to have access to social services that provide English language classes [51] in comparison to their male counterparts. This directly impacts their ability (or inability) to make social connections with individuals in their host community.

The difficulty expressed by participants in developing *bridging* networks could also be due to tensions in identity development. For example, a case study approach was used to identify how female refugees construct social networks and how these networks aid or restrict identity development in a new place [19]. Similar to the results of the present study, many of the women held weak (or non-existent) ties with members of their host community. Missing that strong *bridging* social connection restricts network connectivity [19]; *bridging* social capital is fairly limited with many refugees. Relationship ties formed during the rebuilding process impact identity redevelopment, as female refugees attempt to balance the past self with the future self and mourn the loss of their old self. The authors suggest that future research explores how the rebuilding of female identities is shaped by the resettlement process among varying demographics. For example, in the present study, Iraqi participants suggested that the connections made with their American host community were just as essential as relationships developed among fellow refugees, although the nature of these ties varied in strength. Did the strength and quantity of *bridging* ties among Iraqi women alter their rebuilding of identity post-resettlement? Was this process different for Congolese women, who possibly had less *bridging* social capital? Future migration research should attempt to address these questions through an intersectional lens.

Social linking. Congolese and Iraqi participants held varying perspectives on how social service institutions provide support. While Iraqi participants capitalized on these transactional weak ties to gain essential information and resources to support their well-being, Congolese participants are caught in the tension of acknowledging their necessity for support and the frustration of the lack of cultural competence, perceived apathy, lack of emotional connection, and poor communication among these institutions. This discontented feeling is concerning, when considering the significant stressors emphasized by Congolese participants; increased distrust and discouragement surrounding a lack of support leads to further distress. The authors consider the unique dynamics of these findings, when considering other previous research, such as the Refugee Well-being Project [99]. Data from a large, randomized control study called the Refugee Well-Being Project used a mixed methodology to answer how social ties impact the refugee resettlement process in the U.S. among refugees from Afghanistan, Iraq, Syria, and the Great Lakes region of Africa. Both strands showed that stronger ties with service providers generally created greater distress [99]. A reason for this dynamic comes from the transactional relationship that service providers tend to have with refugees, where they are called in a time of crisis or great need; this contrasts to the transformative relationships established with non-service provider support found in bonding and bridging ties.

Both focus groups agreed that *linking* social capital was the most challenging to establish, where a deficient allocation of quality social service resources left refugees to advocate for their own needs, find their own solutions to everyday stressors (i.e., broken phone, internet issues), or navigate complex U.S. systems by themselves due to the limited support from social service agencies or other community resources. Resources obtained through *linking* social capital have significant implications not only for the development of *bonding* and *bridging* social capital, but are also essential for them to thrive in their integration process [47].

As aforementioned, the lack of quality and quantity of social services resulted in refugee self-dependency and further perpetuated their isolation, creating additional stressors for participants that negatively impacted their well-being post-resettlement. Considering that many obstacles that contributed to refugee isolation and loneliness were caused by financial stressors, the authors suggest that refugee advocates and policymakers shift an intentional focus on cultural orientation courses specifically aimed at financial literacy with an understanding of the U.S. credit system.

Additionally, prevention strategies for social service providers are essential in addressing the mental health symptoms resulting from the entire resettlement process, including pre-migration trauma, the difficulties and challenges with initial integration [42,43,110], and significant hardships and trauma that post-resettlement [11]. Such prevention strategies have the potential to impact other areas of refugee well-being, beyond the direct mental health benefits. For example, the mental and physical health among refugee populations has been associated with their educational attainment and English language ability [31], which were both found to be potential obstacles to further social capital development in the present study. One way to address these mental health issues (especially heightened levels of loneliness and isolation) is by partnering with ethnic-based community organizations (who have established trust) to deliver psychoeducational materials and workshops [26]. Drawing from previous suggestions (i.e., [24]), social service providers can work with community leaders to foster dialogue, education, and collaborations among local organizations to bolster community social networks. Such community engagement strategies have been shown to improve mental health symptoms among new arrivals to their host community [111]. Despite the increase of community social support, it's important to note the aforementioned challenges female refugees face when navigating the U.S. healthcare system [22,23]. Therefore, there is a further need to address language barriers and improve overall provider-patient communication [24]. Considering the variations in strength among female refugee social network ties, and their corresponding impacts on refugee access to support, information, and resources, future research should be conducted to better understand the types of networks and their degrees of support. Future questions include: If participants had more social connections, would their health and (in turn) well-being be positively impacted? How does the strength of their social connectedness influence everyday stressors? What about in emergency or crisis situations? How do social connections influence levels of loneliness and isolation? In alignment with previous research, the findings of the present study suggest that an increase in social capital could provide opportunities to enhance refugee health and well-being; however, refugees listed a multitude of barriers to forming social connections that ultimately increased their loneliness and isolation, contributing to further vulnerabilities and lack of resources. While each person will experience barriers differently based on various cultural and demographic identities (including gender), each focus group did face a multitude of barriers. What barriers could be combatted with strengthened bonding, bridging, and/or linking ties? Further research is needed to identify, address, and increase policy interventions to curb such barriers.

4.4. The Role of the Researcher

Considering the CFP lens used to explore refugee social connectedness in the present study, the authors note the unequal distribution of power held by the researcher. As aforementioned, the researchers acknowledged reflexivity, considering the power of the research findings on the population and the limitations of the authors' perspectives [78]. However, it is critical to note that both focus groups were initially somewhat distrustful towards the research process, suggesting that the researcher had affiliations with governmental entities, even questioning the altruism of her intentions. The researcher clarified her role as a representative of a university and provided culturally appropriate compensation to show appreciation for their time and investment in the study. A commonality between the researcher and participants is their identification as cis-gender women. While we all experience gender differently, some subliminal shared identities could create trust or credibility. Regardless, the role of the researcher as a position of power among female migrants (among all vulnerable populations) must be considered in the entire research process: its design, implementation (data collection and analysis), and distribution of the results.

4.5. Limitations

The small sample of the present study limited our analysis capabilities; due to the sampling approach, results cannot be generalized to other refugee populations with similar identities. Considering that both focus groups were female only, there was also a lack of a comparison group of male refugees; therefore, the authors were unable to compare the unique experiences of resettlement to that of their male counterparts [4]. Additionally, since the focus group process and guide were translated from English to the participant's native language, then back once again for the researcher, there is the potential that the questions were not fully understood or culturally resonated with participants, leading to further misunderstandings, o even possibly a loss of nuance to the posed questions. However, the results of this exploratory study can still lend powerful insights to the impact of female refugee social connectedness and levels of belongingness and well-being.

Lastly, the authors only explored cis-gendered, heterosexual refugee women. Among migration research, there is a significant lack of attention paid to the health (including sexual/reproductive rights, risks, and needs) and well-being of queer immigrant women [9,19]. Therefore, the authors call for future migration research that takes an intersectional approach to highlight diverse gender identities that might otherwise be overlooked.

5. Conclusions

U.S.-resettled female refugees face unique challenges and barriers compared to their male counterparts. Previous literature has primarily focused on the obstacles facing refugees during the resettlement process without discussing the differing gendered experiences. This paper adds to the recent emerging research and conversation revolving around how different genders experience the resettlement process; this includes all levels of engagement with federal, state, and local systems, as well as informal systems such as neighbors, friends, work colleagues, and communities. While support is generally needed by both formal and informal systems, each one plays a distinct role in the refugee's unique resettlement experience, with social service providers providing more transactional interactions. The informal networks of neighbors, friends, and community members provided critical social and emotional support. These transformational relationships strengthened *bonding* and *bridging* social capital, improving overall well-being. The strong isolation experienced among refugee women highlights the need for changes in resettlement policy and supportive programs to enhance gender equity among U.S.-resettled refugees.

Author Contributions: Conceptualization, C.B.; methodology, C.B. and S.S.; software, C.B. and S.S.; validation, C.B. and S.S.; formal analysis, C.B. and S.S.; investigation, C.B.; resources, C.B.; data curation, C.B..; writing—original draft preparation, C.B.; writing—review and editing, C.B. and S.S.; visualization, C.B.; supervision, C.B.; project administration, C.B.; funding acquisition, C.B.. All authors have read and agreed to the published version of the manuscript.

Funding: This research was funded by the Association of Academic Women (University of Florida).

Institutional Review Board Statement: The study was conducted according to the guidelines of the Declaration of Helsinki and approved by the Institutional Review Board of the University of Florida (2015).

Informed Consent Statement: Informed consent was obtained from all subjects involved in the study.

Data Availability Statement: The data presented in this study are available on request from the corresponding author. The data are not publicly available due to IRB restrictions of confidentiality.

Conflicts of Interest: The authors declare no conflict of interest.

References

1. Denzongpa, K.; Nichols, T. We can't step back: Women specifically...: A narrative case study on resilience, independence, and leadership of a Bhutanese refugee woman. *J. Women Soc. Work* **2020**, *35*, 129–145. [CrossRef]
2. Reebs, A.; Yuval, K.; Bernstein, A. Remembering and responding to distressing autobiographical memories: Exploring risk and intervention targets for posttraumatic stress in traumatized refugees. *Clin. Psychol. Sci.* **2017**, *5*, 789–797. [CrossRef]
3. United Nations Human Rights [UNHCR]. International Standards: Special Rapporteur on the Human Rights of Internally Displaced Persons. 2022. Available online: https://www.ohchr.org/en/special-procedures/sr-internally-displaced-persons/international-standards (accessed on 20 December 2022).
4. Shaw, S.A.; Peacock, L.; Ali, L.M.; Pillai, V.; Hussain, A. Religious coping and challenges among displaced Muslim female refugees. *Affilia* **2019**, *34*, 518–534. [CrossRef]
5. Saksena, J.; McMorrow, S. At the intersection of gender and discrimination: Experiences of Congolese refugee women with social and cultural integration in the United States. *Women's Stud. Int. Forum* **2021**, *88*, 102517. [CrossRef]
6. Ager, A.; Strang, A. Understanding integration: A conceptual framework. *J. Refug. Stud.* **2008**, *21*, 166–191. [CrossRef]
7. Shishehgar, S.; Gholizadeh, L.; DiGiacomo, M.; Green, A.; Davidson, P.M. Health and socio-cultural experiences of refugee women: An integrative review. *J. Immigr. Minor. Health* **2017**, *19*, 959–973. [CrossRef] [PubMed]
8. Winkler, K. Reflecting on European migration and refugees: From a feminist perspective. *J. Mass Commun.* **2017**, *7*, 90–96. [CrossRef]
9. Hennebry, J.L.; Petrozziello, A.J. Closing the gap? Gender and the global compacts for migration and refugees. *Int. Migr.* **2019**, *57*, 115–138. [CrossRef]
10. Haffejj, B.; East, J. African women refugee resettlement: A womanist analysis. *Affilia* **2016**, *31*, 232–242. [CrossRef]
11. Kingsbury, D.M.; Bhatta, M.P.; Castellani, B.; Khanal, A.; Jefferis, E.; Hallam, J.S. The personal social networks of resettled Bhutanese refugees during pregnancy in the United States: A social network analysis. *J. Community Health* **2018**, *43*, 1028–1036. [CrossRef]
12. Falb, K.L.; McCormick, M.C.; Hemenway, D.; Anfinson, K.; Silverman, J.G. Violence against refugee women along the Thai–Burma border. *Int. J. Gynecol. Obstet.* **2013**, *120*, 279–283. [CrossRef] [PubMed]
13. Guruge, S. Gender Roles, Power Relations, and Social Supports in the Context of Post-Migration Domestic Violence in the Sri Lankan Tamil Community of Toronto. Doctoral Dissertation, University of Toronto, Toronto, ON, Canada, 2004. Available online: https://www.collectionscanada.gc.ca/obj/thesescanada/vol2/002/NR28053.PDF?is_thesis=1&oclc_number=461541088 (accessed on 20 December 2022).
14. Hyndman, J. Introduction: The feminist politics of refugee migration. *Gend. Place Cult.* **2010**, *17*, 453–459. [CrossRef]
15. Walgenbach, K.; Dietze, G.; Hornscheidt, L.; Palm, K. *Gender as an Interdependent Category: New Perspectives on Intersectionality, Diversity, and Heterogeneity*; Opladen: Leverkusen, Germany, 2012; ISBN 978-3-86649-131-1.
16. Cheung, S.Y.; Phillimore, J. Gender and refugee integration: A quantitative analysis of integration and social policy outcomes. *J. Soc. Policy* **2017**, *46*, 211–230. [CrossRef]
17. Dadush, U.; Neibuhr, M. *The Economic Impact of Forced Migration*; OCP Policy Center: Rabat, Morocco, 2016. Available online: https://carnegieendowment.org/files/RP-_16-03_Final.pdf (accessed on 20 December 2022).
18. Guruge, S.; Khanlou, N. Intersectionalities of influence: Researching the health of immigrant and refugee women. *Can. J. Nurs. Res.* **2004**, *36*, 32–47. [PubMed]
19. Smith, L.R. Female refugee networks: Rebuilding post-conflict identity. *Int. J. Intercult. Relat.* **2013**, *37*, 11–27. [CrossRef]
20. Magan, I.M. On being Black, Mulsim, and a refugee: Stories of Somalis in Chicago. *J. Immigratn Refug. Stud.* **2020**, *18*, 172–188. [CrossRef]

21. Guruge, S.; Collins, E. Emerging trends in Canadian immigration challenges for newcomers. In *Working with Immigrant Women: Issues and Strategies for Mental Health Professionals*; Guruge, S., Collins, E., Eds.; Centre for Addictions and Mental Health: Toronto, ON, Canada, 2008; pp. 3–15.
22. Qutranji, L.; Silahli, N.Y.; Baris, H.E.; Boran, P. Refugee women's well-being, needs, and challenges: Implications for health policymakers. *J. Public Health* **2020**, *42*, 506–512. [CrossRef]
23. Siddiq, H.; Alemi, Q.; Mentes, J.; Pavlish, C.; Lee, E. Preventative cancer screening among resettled refugee women from Muslim-majority countries: A systematic review. *J. Immigr. Minor. Health* **2020**, *22*, 1067–1093. [CrossRef] [PubMed]
24. Hawkins, M.M.; Schmitt, M.E.; Abedbayo, C.T.; Weitzel, J.; Olukotun, O.; Christensen, A.M.; Ruiz, A.M.; Gilman, K.; Quigley, K.; Dressel, A.; et al. Promoting the health of refugee women: A scoping literatura review incorportating the social ecological model. *Int. J. Equity Health* **2021**, *20*, 45. [CrossRef] [PubMed]
25. Horyniak, D.; Melo, J.S.; Farrell, R.M.; Ojeda, V.D.; Strathdee, S.A. Epidemiology of substance use among forced migrants: A global systematic review. *Political Sci. One* **2016**, *11*, e0159134. [CrossRef]
26. Kim, I. Behavioral health symptoms among refugees from Burma: Examination of sociodemographic and migration-related factors. *Asian Am. J. Psychol.* **2018**, *9*, 179–189. [CrossRef]
27. Northcote, J.; Hancock, P.; Casimiro, S. Breaking the isolation cycle: The experience of Muslim refugee women in Australia. *Asian Pac. Migr. J.* **2006**, *15*, 177–199. [CrossRef]
28. Adida, C.L.; Lo, A.; Platas, M.R. Americans preferred Syrian refugees who are female, English-speaking, and Christian on the eve of Donald Trump's election. *PLoS ONE* **2019**, *14*, e0222504. [CrossRef]
29. Lajevardi, N.; Oskooi, K. Old-fashioned racism, contemporary islamophobia and the isolation of Muslim Americans in the age of Trump. *J. RaceEthn. Politics* **2018**, *3*, 112–152. [CrossRef]
30. Hainmueller, J.; Hopkins, D.J. The hidden American immigration consensus: A conjoint analysis of attitudes toward immigrants. *Am. J. Political Sci.* **2015**, *59*, 529–548. [CrossRef]
31. Stempel, C.; Alemi, Q. Challenges to the economic integration of Afghan refugees in the U.S. *J. Ethn. Migr. Stud.* **2021**, *47*, 4872–4892. [CrossRef]
32. Connor, P.; Krogstad, J.M. *The Number of Refugees Admitted to the U.S. Has Fallen, Especially among Muslims*; Pew Research Center: Washington, DC, USA, 2018. Available online: https://www.pewresearch.org/fact-tank/2018/05/03/the-number-of-refugees-admitted-to-the-u-s-has-fallen-especially-among-muslims (accessed on 20 December 2022).
33. Perry, B. "All of a sudden, there are Muslims": Visibilities and Islamophobic violence in Canada. *Int. J. Crime Justice Soc. Democr.* **2015**, *4*, 4–15. [CrossRef]
34. Litchmore, R.V.H.; Safdar, S. Perceptions of discrimination as a marker of integration among Muslim-Canadians: The role of religiosity, ethnic identity, and gender. *J. Int. Migr. Integr.* **2015**, *16*, 187–204. [CrossRef]
35. Kohut, H. *How Does Analysis Cure?* International Universities Press: New York, NY, USA, 1984.
36. Lee, R.M.; Robbins, S.B. Measuring belongingness: The social connectedness and the social assurance scales. *J. Couns. Psychol.* **1995**, *42*, 232–241. [CrossRef]
37. Nunn, C.; Spaaij, R.; Luguetti, C. Beyond integration: Football as a mobile, transnational sphere of belonging for refugee-background young people. *Leis. Stud.* **2022**, *41*, 42–55. [CrossRef]
38. Chopra, V.; Dryden-Peterson, S. Borders and belonging: Displaced Syrian youth navigating symbolic boundaries in Lebanon. *Glob. Soc. Educ.* **2020**, *18*, 449–463. [CrossRef]
39. Carey-Wood, J.; Duke, K.L.; Karn, V.; Marhsall, T. *The Settlement of Refugees in Britain. Home Office Research Studies (141)*; His Majesty's Stationery Office (HMSO): London, UK, 1995. Available online: https://eprints.mdx.ac.uk/id/eprint/13854 (accessed on 20 December 2022).
40. Spoonley, P.; Peace, R.; Butcher, A.; O'Neil, D. Social cohesion: A policy and indicator framework for assessing immigrant and host outcomes. *Soc. Policy J. N. Z.* **2005**, *24*, 85–110.
41. Yuval-Davis, N.; Anthias, F.; Kofman, E. Secure borders and safe haven and the gendered politics of belonging: Beyond social cohesion. *Ethn. Racial Stud.* **2005**, *28*, 513–535. [CrossRef]
42. Khanlou, N. Migrant mental health in Canada. *Can. Issues: Immigr. Ment. Health* **2010**, 9–16. Available online: https://multiculturalmentalhealth.ca/wp-content/uploads/2019/07/Immigrant_mental_health_10aug10.pdf (accessed on 20 December 2022).
43. Schlaudt, V.A.; Bosson, R.; Williams, M.T.; German, B.; Hooper, L.M.; Frazier, V.; Carrico, R.; Ramirez, J. Traumatic experiences and mental health risk for refugees. *Int. J. Environ. Res. Public Health* **2020**, *17*, 1943. [CrossRef]
44. Zetter, R.; Griffiths, A.; Sigona, N.; Flynn, D.; Pasha, T.; Beynon, R. *Immigration, Social Cohesion and Social Capital: What Are the Links?* Joseph Rowntree Foundation: North Yorkshire, UK, 2006. Available online: https://www.jrf.org.uk/sites/default/files/jrf/migrated/files/9781899354440.pdf (accessed on 20 December 2022).
45. Strang, A.; Ager, A. Refugee integration: Emerging trends and remaining agendas. *J. Refug. Stud.* **2010**, *23*, 589–607. [CrossRef]
46. Villalonga-Olives, E.; Kawachi, I. The dark side of social capital: A systematic review of the negative health effects of social capital. *Soc. Sci. Med.* **2017**, *194*, 105–127. [CrossRef]
47. Elliot, S.; Yusuf, I. 'Yes we can: But together': Social capital and refugee resettlement. *Kotuitui N. Z. J. Soc. Sci. Online* **2014**, *9*, 101–110. [CrossRef]
48. Bagci, S.C.; Turnuklu, A.; Bekmezci, E. Cross-group friendships and psychological well-being: A dual pathway through social integration and empowerment. *Br. J. Soc. Psychol.* **2018**, *57*, 773–792. [CrossRef]

49. Harris, M.; Young, P. Building bridges: The third sector responding locally to diversity. *Volunt. Sect. Rev.* **2010**, *1*, 17. Available online: https://publications.aston.ac.uk/id/eprint/26687/1/Third_sector_responding_locally_to_diversity.pdf (accessed on 20 December 2022). [CrossRef]
50. Putnam, R.D. *Bowling Alone: The Collapse and Revival of American Community*; Simon and Schuster: New York, NY, USA, 2000. [CrossRef]
51. Ibrahim, Y. Sounds of the jungle: Rehumanizing the migrant. *JOMEC J. J. Media Cult. Stud.* **2012**, 1–18. Available online: https://core.ac.uk/download/pdf/77039509.pdf (accessed on 20 December 2022). [CrossRef]
52. Cheung, S.Y.; Phillimore, J. Refugees, social capital, and labour market integration in the UK. *Sociology* **2014**, *48*, 518–536. [CrossRef]
53. Ryan, L.; D'Angelo, A. Changing times: Migrants' social network analysis and the challenges of longitudinal research. *Soc. Netw.* **2018**, *53*, 148–158. [CrossRef]
54. Liev, M.H. Adaptation of Cambodians in New Zealand: Achievement, Cultural Identity, and Community Development. Doctoral Dissertation, University of Auckland, Auckland, New Zealand, 2008. Available online: https://researchspace.auckland.ac.nz/handle/2292/3362 (accessed on 20 December 2022).
55. Berry, A.G. Survival at Risk: Evaluating Refugee Policy towards Survivors of Sexual and Gender-Based Violence (Student Publication No. 8536293). Master of Arts Thesis, University of Ottawa, Ottawa, ON, Canada, 2022. Available online: http://hdl.handle.net/10393/43910 (accessed on 20 December 2022).
56. Collins, P.H. Intersectionality's definitional dilemmas. *Annu. Rev. Sociol.* **2015**, *41*, 1–20. [CrossRef]
57. Tastsoglou, E. Transnational, feminist and intersectional perspectives on immigrants and refugees in Canada: An introduction. *Can. Ethn. Stud. J.* **2019**, *51*, 1–17. [CrossRef]
58. Spies, T. Violence gender ethnicity: Intersectionality in the discursive context. In *Migration and Gender: Theoretical Approaches and Empirical Results*; Mechthild, B., Ricker, P., Schnitzer, A., Eds.; Juventa: Tokyo, Japan, 2012; pp. 105–125.
59. Mehrotra, G. Toward a continuum of intersectionality theorizing for feminist social work scholarship. *J. Women Soc. Work* **2010**, *25*, 417–430. [CrossRef]
60. Collins, J. "You don't know what they translate": Language contact, institutional procedure, and literary practice in neighborhood health clinics in urban Flanders. *Linguist. Anthropol.* **2006**, *16*, 249–268. [CrossRef]
61. McCall, L. The complexity of intersectionality. *Signs J. Women Cult. Soc.* **2005**, *30*, 1771–1800. Available online: http://www.jstor.org/stable/10.1086/426800 (accessed on 20 December 2022). [CrossRef]
62. Aguayo-Romero, R.A. (Re)centering black feminism into intersectionality research. *Am. J. Public Health* **2021**, *111*, 101–103. [CrossRef]
63. Hovorka, A.J. Women/chickens vs. men/cattle: Insights on gender-species intersectionality. *Geoforum* **2012**, *43*, 875–884. [CrossRef]
64. Nunn, C.; Gifford, S.; McMichael, C.; Correa-Velez, I. Navigating precarious terrains: Reconceptualizing refugee-youth settlement. *Refuge* **2017**, *33*, 45–55. [CrossRef]
65. Donato, K.M.; Ferris, E. Refugee integration in Canada, Europe, and the United States: Perspectives from research. *Am. Acad. Political Soc. Sci.* **2020**, *690*, 7–35. [CrossRef]
66. Aberman, T. Gendered perspectives on refugee determination in Canada. *Refuge* **2014**, *30*, 57–66. [CrossRef]
67. Humpage, L.; Marston, G. Cultural justice, community development and onshore refugees in Australia. *Community Dev. J.* **2005**, *40*, 137–146. [CrossRef]
68. Clinton-Davis, L.; Fassil, Y. Health and social problems of refugees. *Soc. Sci. Med.* **1992**, *35*, 507–513. [CrossRef] [PubMed]
69. Asian & Pacific Islander American Scholarship Fund. *Invisible Newcomers: Refugees from Burma/Myanmar and Bhutan in the United States*; Asian & Pacific Islander American Scholarship Fund: Washington, DC, USA, 2014. Available online: http://apiasf.org/research/APIASF_Burma_Bhutan_Report.pdf (accessed on 20 December 2022).
70. Gordon, M.R.; Smale, A.; Lyman, R.U.S. Will Accept More Refugees as Crisis Grows. *N. Y. Times* **2015**. Available online: http://www.nytimes.com/2015/09/21/world/europe/us-to-increase-admission-of-refugees-to-100000-in-2017-kerry-says.html?_r=0 (accessed on 20 December 2022).
71. Zong, J.; Batalova, J. *Refugees and Asylees in the United States*; The Migration Policy Institute: Washington, DC, USA, 2015. Available online: http://www.migrationpolicy.org/article/refugees-and-asylees-united-states (accessed on 20 December 2022).
72. Here & Now. U.N., U.S. Resettling 50,000 Congolese Refugees. 2015. Available online: http://hereandnow.wbur.org/2015/05/14/refugees-congo-uwiringiyimana (accessed on 20 December 2022).
73. Cultural Orientation Resource Center. Congolese Refugees. 2014. Available online: http://www.culturalorientation.net/learning/populations/congolese-refugees (accessed on 20 December 2022).
74. Refugee Council USA. Displaced Persons from the Democratic Republic of the Congo. 2016. Available online: http://www.rcusa.org/displaced-persons-from-the-drc (accessed on 20 December 2022).
75. Cultural Orientation Resource Center. Refugees from Iraq: Their History, Cultures, Background and Experiences. 2008. Available online: http://www.culturalorientation.net/learning/populations/iraq (accessed on 20 December 2022).
76. United States Citizenship and Immigration Services. Iraqi Refugee Processing Fact Sheet. 2013. Available online: http://www.uscis.gov/humanMitarian/refugees-asylum/refugees/iraqi-refugee-processing-fact-sheet (accessed on 20 December 2022).
77. Bazeley, P. *Qualitative Data Analysis: Practical Strategies*; Sage Publications: Thousand Oaks, CA, USA, 2013; ISBN 978-1-84920-303-6.

78. Bletscher, C.G.; Galindo, S. Challenges with Using Transformative Mixed Methodologies among Vulnerable Populations: Reflections from a Study among US-Resettled Refugees. *J. Mix. Methods Res.* 2023, *in press*.
79. Worthen, B.R.; Sanders, J.R.; Fitzpatrick, J.L. *Program Evaluation: Alternative Approaches and Practical Guidelines*, 2nd ed.; Addison Wesley Longman: Boston, MA, USA, 1997.
80. Bletscher, C.G. Community Connectedness: An Examination of the Social Dynamics of Resettled Refugees in the State of Florida. (Publication No. 10646316). Doctoral Dissertation, University of Florida, Gainesville, FL, USA; p. 2016.
81. Korac, M. Creating solutions: The role of social networks and transnational links in shaping migration choices of forced migrants from the former Yugoslavia. In Proceedings of the 9th International Conference of the International Association for the Study of Forced Migration (IASFM), Sao Paulo, Brazil, 9–13 January 2005.
82. Sweetman, D.; Badiee, M.; Creswell, J.W. Use of the transformative framework in mixed methods studies. *Qual. Inq.* **2010**, *16*, 441–454. [CrossRef]
83. Zapata-Barrero, R.; Yalaz, E. Qualitative methods in migration research. In *Introduction to Migration Studies: An Interactive Guide to the Literatures on Migration and Diversity*; Scholton, P., Ed.; Springer: Berlin/Heidelberg, Germany, 2021; pp. 424–441.
84. Kercood, S.; Morita-Mullaney, T. Health Perceptions and Practices of Burmese Refugee Families: A Participatory Mixed Method Study. *J. Southeast Asian Am. Educ. Adv.* **2015**, *10*, 1–30. Available online: https://docs.lib.purdue.edu/cgi/viewcontent.cgi?article=1124&context=jsaaea (accessed on 20 December 2022). [CrossRef]
85. Mertens, D.M.; Olavarria, C.; Peroni, A. Transformative mixed methods training for the next generation of researchers and evaluations in southern countries. *Int. J. Mult. Res. Approaches* **2018**, *10*, 390–402. [CrossRef]
86. Braun, V.; Clarke, V. *Thematic Analysis*; American Psychological Association: Washington, DC, USA, 2012.
87. Braun, V.; Clarke, V. Using thematic analysis in psychology. *Qual. Res. Psychol.* **2006**, *3*, 77–101. [CrossRef]
88. Harding, J. *Qualitative Data Analysis from Start to Finish*; Sage Publishing, Inc.: Thousand Oaks, CA, USA, 2013.
89. Hennink, M.; Hutter, I.; Bailey, A. *Qualitative Research Methods*; Sage Publishing, Inc.: Thousand Oaks, CA, USA, 2011.
90. Creswell, J.W. *Qualitative Inquiry & Research Design: Choosing among Five Approaches*; Sage Publishing, Inc.: Thousand Oaks, CA, USA, 2007.
91. Klobucista, C.; McBride, J.; Roy, D. *How Does the U.S. Refugee System Work?* Council on Foreign Relations: New York, NY, USA, 2022. Available online: https://www.cfr.org/backgrounder/how-does-us-refugee-system-work-trump-biden-afghanistan?gclid=CjwKCAiAv9ucBhBXEiwA6N8nYB_z2tZkoeiloVMOHflp2bW9lAtju9l_ZvejBvWOhIiqwH2irgaMwBoCT1sQAvD_BwE (accessed on 20 December 2022).
92. United States [US] Committee for Refugees and Immigrants (n.d.). Travel Loan Services. Available online: https://uscripayments.org/#:~:text=When%20refugees%20are%20admitted%20to,over%20a%20pre%2Ddetermined%20period (accessed on 20 December 2022).
93. Eby, J.; Iverson, E.; Smyers, J.; Kekic, E. The faith community's role in refugee resettlement in the United States. *J. Refug. Stud.* **2011**, *24*, 586–605. [CrossRef]
94. Green, G.P.; Haines, A. *Asset Building and Community Development*, 3rd ed.; Sage Publishing, Inc.: Thousand Oaks, CA, USA, 2012. [CrossRef]
95. Paxton, P. Is Social Capital Declining in the United States? A Multiple Indicator Assessment. *Am. J. Sociol.* **1999**, *105*, 88–127. Available online: https://www.jstor.org/stable/10.1086/210268?origin=JSTOR-pdf (accessed on 20 December 2022). [CrossRef]
96. Lamba, N.K.; Krahn, H. Social capital and refugee resettlement: The social networks of refugees in Canada. *J. Int. Migr. Integr.* **2003**, *4*, 335–360. [CrossRef]
97. Pew Research Center. Muslims Concerned about Their Place in Society, but Continue to Believe in the American Dream. 2017. Available online: https://www.pewforum.org/wp-content/uploads/sites/7/2017/07/U.S.-MUSLIMS-FULL-REPORT-with-population-update-v2.pdf (accessed on 20 December 2022).
98. Stolle, D.; Soroka, S.; Johnston, R. When does diversity erode trust?: Neighborhood diversity, interpersonal trust, and the mediating effect of social interactions. *Political Stud.* **2008**, *56*, 57–75. [CrossRef]
99. Im, H. Falling through the cracks: Stress and coping in migration and resettlement among marginalized Hmong refugee families in the United States. *Fam. Soc. J. Contemp. Soc. Serv.* **2021**, *102*, 50–66. [CrossRef]
100. Greene, R.N. Kinship, friendship, and service provider social ties and how they influence well-being among newly resettled refugees. *Socius* **2019**, *5*, 1–11. [CrossRef]
101. Putnam, R.D. E Pluribus Unum: Diversity and community in the twenty-first century: The John Skytte Prize Lecture. *Scand. Political Stud.* **2007**, *30*, 134–167. [CrossRef]
102. Kenny, S.; Mansouri, F.; Smiley, D.; Spratt, P. *Arabic Communities and Well-Being: Supports and Barriers to Social Connectedness*; The Centre for Citizenship and Human Rights, Deakin University: Melbourne, Australia, 2005. Available online: https://static1.squarespace.com/static/5b0fd5e6710699c630b269b1/t/5b41fc77f950b7059f903ab2/1531051135874/Arabic+Communities+and+Wellbeing.pdf (accessed on 20 December 2022).
103. Kallick, D.D.; Mathema, S. *Refugee Integration in the United States*; Center for American Progress: Washington, DC, USA, 2016. Available online: https://www.americanprogress.org/article/refugee-integration-in-the-united-states/ (accessed on 20 December 2022).
104. Brell, C.; Dustmann, C.; Preston, I. The labor market integration of refugee migrants in high-income countries. *J. Econ. Perspect.* **2020**, *34*, 94–121. Available online: https://www.jstor.org/stable/26873531 (accessed on 20 December 2022). [CrossRef]
105. Abdelhadi, E. The hijab and Muslim women's employment in the United States. *Res. Soc. Stratif. Mobil.* **2019**, *61*, 26–37. [CrossRef]

106. Mask, J. Consequences of immigrating during a recession: Evidence from the U.S. Refugee Resettlement Program. *IZA J. Dev. Migr.* **2020**, *11*, 1–21. [CrossRef]
107. Capps, R.; Newland, K. *The Integration Outcomes of US Refugees: Successes and Challenges;* Migration Policy Institute: Washington, DC, USA, 2015. Available online: https://www.migrationpolicy.org/research/integration-outcomes-us-refugees-successes-and-challenges (accessed on 20 December 2022).
108. Var, S.; Pyrazli, S.; Grahame, K.M. Personal well-being and overall satisfaction of life of Asian and African immigrant and refugee women. *J. Asia Pac. Couns.* **2013**, *3*, 77–90. [CrossRef]
109. Kabir, R.; Klugman, J. Georgetown Closing Economic Gaps to Benefit All. Georgetown Institute for Women, Peace, and Security. 2019. Available online: https://gbvaor.net/sites/default/files/2019-08/Unlocking-Refugee-Womens-Potential.pdf (accessed on 20 December 2022).
110. Berzengi, A.; Berzenji, L.; Kadim, A.; Mustafa, F.; Jobson, L. Role of Islamic appraisals, trauma-related appraisals, and religious coping in the posttraumatic adjustment of Muslim trauma survivors. *Psychol. Trauma Theory Res. Pract. Policy* **2017**, *9*, 189–197. [CrossRef] [PubMed]
111. Small, E.; Kim, Y.K.; Praetorius, R.T.; Mitschke, D.B. Mental health treatment for resettled refugees: A comparison of three approaches. *Soc. Work Ment. Health* **2016**, *14*, 342–359. [CrossRef]

International Journal of
Environmental Research and Public Health

MDPI

Article

A Qualitative Study of Adolescents from Refugee Backgrounds Living in Australia: Identity and Resettlement

Nigar G. Khawaja * and Robert D. Schweitzer

School of Psychology and Counselling, Queensland University of Technology, Victoria Park Road, Kelvin Grove, QLD 4059, Australia; r.schweitzer@qut.edu.au
* Correspondence: n.khawaja@qut.edu.au

Abstract: Identity formation among young people from refugee backgrounds is complex, as it occurs while they are both integrating into a novel cultural landscape and navigating the intricacies of adolescence. The present study explored sense of identity and experiences among refugee youth in the context of resettlement. Nineteen young people (15–18 years) from refugee backgrounds, settled in Brisbane, Australia, took part in the study. An individual semi-structured interview, drawing upon the Tree of Life method, was used. The thematic analysis (TA) methodology was adopted, and several themes emerged: experiencing changes in family roles; experience of belonging; experience of bonds with lost loved ones; dealing with emotions in a new context; experience of self in the context of change. There was one emergent overarching theme of meaning-making in the context of change. These themes were explicated within the framework of social identity and sociocultural theories, which emphasises the dynamic co-construction of identity through the interplay of belonging and meaning-making within specific contextual settings. This study highlights the fundamental role of social context, particularly the fostering of school belonging, in the multifaceted process of identity construction. The findings identify the importance of integrating multiple identities and experiences to develop a comprehensive and resilient sense of personal cohesion and selfhood.

Keywords: acculturation; adolescent; Australian; identity; meaning-making; refugee; resettlement

Citation: Khawaja, N.G.; Schweitzer, R.D. A Qualitative Study of Adolescents from Refugee Backgrounds Living in Australia: Identity and Resettlement. *Int. J. Environ. Res. Public Health* **2024**, *21*, 281. https://doi.org/10.3390/ijerph21030281

Academic Editor: Alberto Borraccino

Received: 20 December 2023
Revised: 13 February 2024
Accepted: 21 February 2024
Published: 28 February 2024

1. Introduction

Identity formation is an intricate process for all adolescents [1]. In the context of young people from refugee backgrounds, an additional layer of complexity emerges, given the interplay of various psychological, social, cultural, ethnic, religious, and personal factors which contribute to identity [2]. While the field of identity research is heterogenous, there is a consensus that life experience plays a central role in the formation of identity [1,3]. For adolescents from refugee backgrounds, rupturing life experiences are recurrent and profound. Trauma, loss, displacement, and resettlement all have the potential to cause immense disruption to young people's sense of personal coherence, bringing identity issues to the fore [2]. In addition, the increased salience of cultural context and unfamiliar group membership in the position of other [4], as well as pre-migration experiences, acculturation processes, and post-settlement challenges exert significant influences on the complicated tapestry of identity development [2].

This paper seeks to explore and articulate the experiences of identity and resettlement among refugee youth. It achieves this by identifying and interpreting qualitative data obtained from recently resettled young individuals from refugee backgrounds in Brisbane, Australia. The data analysis has been informed by social identity and sociocultural theories that amalgamate insights from anthropology, sociology, and psychology to the understanding of the construction of self and identity. Such theories emphasise the notion of co-construction in identity formation, that is, the importance of the dynamic relationship between an individual and their environment in shaping their sense of self [5]. In essence, co-construction of identity is not an individual effort but involves the reciprocal influence of collective and personal narratives, values, beliefs, and experiences which are internalised and adapted [6]. Hence, identity formation for multicultural individuals is influenced by both the persons' new cultural context and their "home" culture. Social identity theory (SIT), a widely known theoretical framework, lends itself to an understanding of how individuals from refugee backgrounds may renegotiate their social identities within their host countries. Further, identity is understood as being constructed in sociocultural settings.

1.1. Theoretical Perspectives

1.1.1. Social Identity Theory

Social identity theory (SIT) is a widely acclaimed theory; according to SIT, individuals ascertain part of their identity from their perceived affiliation with relevant social groups [7]. As a part of growing up, young persons are part of family, school, and several interest, leisure, religious, ethnic, and community groups. They interact with these groups and belong to these groups at various points in their lives [8]. These social interactions can be positive or negative. The positive interactions can lead to a tendency for people to express a preference for in-group members compared to out-group members [9]. Along with personal identity and achievements, the group affiliation and the achievements of the group reinforce a positive social identity and foster self-esteem [10]. Group memberships are associated with a sense of belonging and connectedness [3]. Conversely, if a negative social identity is maintained through experience, people may disassociate from their group. Thus, social identity is subject to fluctuations based on experience and meaning-making. It is further elaborated upon from the sociocultural perspective.

1.1.2. The Sociocultural Perspective

Within this model, the sense of self and environment are intrinsically linked and interdependent, with human action shaped by sociocultural context and vice versa [11]. Individuals exist in "figured worlds", that is, the socially and culturally constructed lenses through which we see and engage with the world [12]. In this framework, particular aspects of experience are assigned significance and value [12]. By thinking, feeling, and behaving in line with a particular template or set of rules, the figured world is preserved and further developed [13]. When individual and collective interpretations within our figured world conflict with one another, we develop new ways of thinking, feeling, and behaving, which in turn, constitute identity [14]. Consequently, we are constantly renegotiating our identity to accommodate new experiences and the meanings we derive from these experiences [15].

Identity formation is the never-ending process of integration and reconstruction of our own unique life experiences [15]. When we engage in this process, our own subjective meaning of the experience is removed from the context in which it emerged and "placed in meaningful relation ... to the existing semiotic architecture of the self in generalized form" [16]. Thus, we are constantly engaging with the world, in a perpetual state of flux, and reconstructing our self-structure to accommodate the subjective meanings derived from each new experience [17,18]. Generally, this process is not conscious. However, under certain circumstances, this process becomes overt and more deliberate, as we try to derive meaning from experiences that do not fit neatly into our carefully constructed mosaic, comprising a number of self-states.

1.1.3. Identity of Young People from Refugee Backgrounds

Young people from refugee backgrounds are members of multiple groups. They have families, which could be atypical because of the traumatic loss of family members [19]. Despite varying life circumstances, they are all part of educational institutions. Further, they tend to have affiliations with ethnic and cultural groups [20]. Their identity is considered to develop through their participation with their cultural traditions, norms, roles, and contexts [21]. Further, this social participation exposes them to cultural values and beliefs which influence the way they give meaning to their own self and construct their identities.

Identity is shaped by historical circumstances [22]. Young people with refugee backgrounds may be directly or indirectly impacted by war, trauma, and other atrocities. These young people were originally members of collectivistic, authoritarian, and hierarchical societies [6]. Therefore, they may see themselves as a part of their heritage group. They may look up to authority figures for support and direction, and may accept specific roles in hierarchical setups that are geared towards caring for their families and communities [23].

As the social environment changes in one's life, one's identity is also subject to change [1,6]. As young people from refugee backgrounds enter a highly developed and individualistic Australian society, their identity may undergo a shift. As they interact with a different language, culture, religious beliefs, and norms, they have to navigate their new environment by constructing a hybrid identity [10]. The identification of their personal, ethnic, religious, and national context may have to be negotiated [2,15]. This shift in socio-cultural context and group loyalties is further impacted by potential trauma and adverse experiences, influencing social networks and interactions within communities [21]. Under these circumstances, young people from refugee background may encounter "rupturing otherness" [24]. However, these rupturing experiences are managed to regain a sense of coherence. For young people who are refugees in particular, these repeated adversities are likely to profoundly disrupt their self-structure. Consequently, it is assumed that the process of identity construction will frequently enter their conscious awareness [4,25]. Refugees who successfully integrate their experiences and context tend to cultivate a more cohesive self-concept. This process has been described by Papadopoulos as adversity-activated development [26].

1.2. The Current Study

Presently, there is a paucity of research looking specifically at young people from refugee backgrounds, particularly in Australia. The current study was designed to be exploratory in nature, adopting an inductive approach, placing the voices of the participants at the forefront. The study involved guided discussion around how young people from refugee backgrounds see themselves and perceive the world around them, thus reflecting their sense of self or identity in the context of resettlement. By explicating themes related to identity and resettlement, the current study contributes to the existing body of literature on identity among refugee youth and identifies issues that may be unique to participants in an Australian context.

2. Method

2.1. Design

The current study utilised a qualitative approach with a semi-structured interview based on the narrative Tree of Life tool [27,28]. This qualitative research methodology was selected for the following reasons: (1) to enhance participant control over the research process, reducing the likelihood of a power imbalance occurring between participant and researcher [29]; (2) to allow for new information to be introduced by the young people [30].

2.2. Participants

Nineteen young people (13 females and 6 males) from refugee backgrounds, aged 15–18, participated in the study. The participants had migrated from 12 different countries across South Asia, Africa, and the Middle East. They had entered on humanitarian visas, with the majority of participants being granted a permanent visa. Table 1 provides an overview of participant demographic information. Pseudonyms are used to preserve their anonymity.

Table 1. Participant gender, age, ethnicity, visa status, and length of time in Australia.

Participants [a]		Gender	Age	Ethnicity	Visa Status	Time in Australia
1	Salim	Male	18	Iraqi	Bridging	11 months
2	Khin	Male	18	Burmese	Bridging	15 months
3	Mairi	Female	17	Iranian	Permanent	11 months
4	Lucy	Female	17	Sierra Leonean	Provisional	6 months
5	Juliet	Female	15	Liberian	Provisional	11 months
6	Farhia	Female	16	Somali	Permanent	15 months
7	Ariana	Female	16	Northern African	Permanent	11 months
8	Matida	Female	16	South Sudanese	Permanent	1 month
9	Matthew	Male	18	South Sudanese	Permanent	1 month
10	Sana	Female	15	Pakistani	Permanent	15 months
11	Mirembe	Female	16	Ugandan	Permanent	4 months
12	Rima	Female	18	Syrian	Permanent	7 months
13	Ajmal	Male	18	Afghan	Bridging	24 months
14	Hani	Female	17	Somali	Permanent	20 months
15	Kalan	Male	15	Afghan	Permanent	13 months
16	Estelle	Female	16	Ivory Coast	Permanent	7 months
17	Alima	Female	17	South Sudanese	Permanent	8 months
18	Mariam	Female	16	Afghan	Permanent	19 months
19	Nazir	Male	15	Afghan	Permanent	15 months

[a] Pseudonyms issued to each participant to preserve anonymity. A Bridging Visa is a temporary visa granted to individuals who are in Australia and have lodged an application for a substantive visa (such as a protection visa or partner visa) but have not yet received a decision on that application. A Permanent Visa is a visa that allows an individual to live and work in Australia indefinitely. The most common permanent visa is the Protection Visa (subclass 866). The Provisional Visa category is for individuals who are in a genuine and ongoing relationship with an Australian citizen, permanent resident, or eligible New Zealand citizen. It allows the visa holder to enter and stay in Australia temporarily while their permanent partner's visa application (subclass 100) is being processed.

2.3. Materials

Tree of Life (ToL)

The interviews with the participating young people were structured around the Tree of Life tool (ToL) [27,28]. The template is based on guidelines provided by Ncube [28]. These guidelines were condensed into a template. Initially developed to assist children affected by HIV/AIDS in Southern Africa, the ToL is a narrative tool designed to facilitate self-awareness and create a more positive and coherent self-narrative [27,28,31].

The ToL uses the metaphor of a tree to map aspects of a young person's life. In the ToL, the roots signify a person's family, community, and/or place of origin, while the ground is representative of their current day-to-day routine (e.g., school, work, living arrangements). At the trunk of the ToL, individuals are invited to reflect on their strengths, which may include characteristics or personality traits that are seen as positive by the person (e.g., nurturing) or a particular skill (e.g., cooking). At the branches of the ToL, individuals are encouraged to reflect on their hopes and dreams for the future, while the leaves are reserved for people with whom the individual shares a significant relationship. Gifts received by others are represented in the fruit of the ToL. These include tangible gifts, as well as the fulfilment of emotional and interpersonal needs (e.g., love, support) and the modelling or transmission of certain values within a family or community. The ToL process provided the basis for the qualitative data underpinning the study.

Art Supplies: To complete the drawing component of the Tree of Life interview, all young people were provided with paper, pencils, an eraser, a pencil sharpener, and connector pens.

2.4. Procedure

2.4.1. Ethics

Ethical approval was gained by the university's research committee prior to the commencement of the study. Permission was also granted by the school at which the research was conducted.

2.4.2. Recruitment

Participants were recruited from a transitional school for newly arrived refugee and migrant young people aged 11–18 years. The school was established to teach young people English, and to provide information and support to prepare them for life and study in Australia. Young people typically attend the school for a period of 6–18 months. Initial contact was made with teachers via email, with the facilitation of the school guidance officer. Relevant teachers and the school guidance officer were provided with information about what participation would involve and were given the opportunity to provide feedback on the research methodology to ensure that data collection methods were appropriate for the target population. Recruitment was undertaken over an extended period with sensitivity to the need to build rapport with potential participants prior to the commencement of research. That is, members of the research team had ongoing contact with the school for about five years and attended school functions and developed familiarity with members of the school community. This process was deemed essential in developing trust within the school community.

2.4.3. Inclusion Criteria

Students were informed that they could participate in the study if they met the following criteria: (1) they were from a refugee background; (2) they were aged 15–18 years inclusive; (3) they were confident in their English language ability; (4) they had arrived in Australia on one of the humanitarian visas. Young people on work, migration, research, and training visas were excluded from the study. English language ability was desired to limit the dependence on the interpreter, as changes to language inevitably occur through the process of translation [32,33], which can alter the meaning of words or sentences [26]. All participants were recruited from advanced classes, which are reserved for students who have achieved the competencies required for the entry classes, ensuring intermediate or advanced English language ability. Participation was voluntary and no compensation was offered.

2.4.4. Data Collection

Informed consent was obtained from the young people and their parents or guardians if necessary. The interviews were conducted by a postgraduate student completing her Professional Doctorate in Clinical Psychology. She had extensive experience working with vulnerable people with mental health issues and was supervised by the authors. She met with the participants individually and provided a summary of the study and information about confidentiality. The interviewer then met with the young people at the designated times and conducted semi-structured interviews and the drawing activity based on the ToL tool. The participants received instructions to draw a tree; it was explained that different parts of the tree tell us about different parts of ourselves. They were informed that the roots of the tree were about where they came from. The ground was explained as where they were lived currently, with whom they lived and what they did every day. As they moved up the tree, they had different parts to fill in. They were asked to draw and comment on what they were good at, different people in their lives, and the things these people have given them. It was explained that these things could be real things, like a bicycle, or it could be about something they have inherited, like their parents' sense of humour, love, or support. The participants were informed that they could do the activity any way they wanted as there was no right or wrong way. The participants had the option of drawing or writing, and they were assured that the drawing or writing did not have to be perfect. The interviewer emphasised that it was important to learn about where the participant came from and what life was like for them at that point in time.

The interviewer asked the participant to elaborate on their drawing throughout the process (e.g., "Can you tell me more about where you come from?") to promote and enhance discussion around identity and resettlement. Drawings were used to enhance the comfort of the participants and to use them as anchor points to have a conversation with the participant. Drawings and the associated verbal or written comments were interpreted along with the interview data. To facilitate communication, all participants were offered the option of using a phone interpreter; however, only one participant took up this option.

Interviews ranged from 16 to 82 min, with 18 of the 19 interviews conducted in English. One interview was conducted in Farsi and translated by a telephone interpreter service following a request by the participant. All interviews were audio-recorded and transcribed verbatim. The number of interviews completed was determined by the point at which data saturation occurred. To identify the saturation point, the researchers analysed and interpreted interview content throughout the data collection process, coding themes as they emerged. Once the researchers were satisfied that no new themes were emerging from the dataset (i.e., when content had reached the point of saturation), data collection was concluded.

2.5. Data Explication

The postgraduate student analysed the data in collaboration with the authors. Common themes related to identity and resettlement were explicated through a five-stage process of thematic analysis based on Braun and Clarke's [34] method. Thematic analysis was selected as it is theoretically flexible and allows the researcher to code broadly and diversely using an inductive approach emerging from the data [34]. The process involved coding and collapsing the data before examining the more prominent themes in the context of the aims of the study, that is, to explicate themes related to identity and resettlement. This process was completed with the aid of a qualitative software analysis program, NVivo 12. In Stage 1, the student and the authors familiarised themselves with the data, listening to the recorded interviews and reading through interview transcripts whilst noting pertinent observations. In Stage 2, the student and the authors generated codes for the data, focusing primarily on features related to identity and resettlement, noting those that occurred repeatedly across the dataset. In Stage 3, themes were explicated, with existing codes collated to correspond with each theme. These themes were reviewed in Stage 4, with the authors examining each theme to determine whether they told a coherent story both independently and together. In Stage 5, the student and the authors defined and named each theme, focusing on the 'essence' of each theme and how they fit into the overall 'story' of the wider dataset. Due to the subjective nature of thematic analysis, it was anticipated that the personal biases, values, and judgments of the authors may significantly impact the coding and interpretation of data. To acknowledge these biases and how they shaped the data, analyses were documented in a reflexivity journal. The postgraduate student, who led this stage of the explication of the data, consulted regularly with the other authors to examine the data and discuss the themes, to further enhance the trustworthiness of the findings.

Reflexive Comment: The authors are academic researchers with a long-standing relationship with the school involved in the research. The first named author is female and was born in Pakistan and completed her post graduate training in clinical psychology in Australia, where she holds a senior position as an academic and research supervisor. She has lived experience of conflict and resettlement. The second author is a male academic, with a long history of researching refugee-related issues. The authors conceptualised the study and supervised the data collection and analyses. Both authors shared a commitment to undertaking research informed by principles of social justice and leading to practical outcomes.

3. Findings

3.1. Overview of Themes

Five prominent themes related to identity and resettlement were explicated: experiencing changes in family roles; experience of belonging; experience of bonds with lost loved ones; dealing with emotions in a new context; and experience of self in the context of change. These all fell within an overarching theme of meaning-making in the context of change. These themes are described below.

3.2. Experiencing Changes in Family Roles

Young people often spoke of role changes and shifts in the formation of their families. Due to the death or disappearance of the parents, half of the participants reported having an aunt or an uncle or an older sibling as a carer and guardian. This was a shift from the previous family structure and involved accepting a new person as a head of the family. For the majority of the participants, schooling had been disrupted in their home countries or previous countries of asylum. They reported not attending school at all or attending for some short periods of time. Subsequently, they were engaged in caring roles or domestic chores. Other members of their family had become accustomed to seeing them contributing to everyday responsibilities. According to one participant, "Back in Liberia... from school, I come home, go to market, buy food, cook, finish, that's it" (Julliet). After settling in Australia, all the participants had to re-adjust to the role of being a full-time student. For some participants, the commitment to education made it impossible to fulfil roles they held previously in their country of origin, which they experienced as causing disruption to the family system. There was an expectation form the relatives that they would still complete their other duties. Juliet perceived her role in the family as disrupted by her return to full-time study, while Juliet's uncle and aunt (carers) reportedly struggling to adjust to the loss of Juliet as caretaker. She reported:

Sometimes [my uncle] gets upset with me and then not talk to me ... Like, when we were in Africa, [I was] working, washing ... doing the housework ... Not like that anymore ... [Now] I have to go to school (Juliet).

Similarly, nearly half of the participants found that language barriers often precipitated a shift in family roles, with younger family members needing to interpret for the rest of the family:

Because [my elder sister/guardian] can't speak English ... when she has a problem, she talks to me and if there is no solution, I have to talk to another people, then they give me some idea, then I would just come and talk to her like my own idea ... like when I first came to this school for interview and then they tried to ask her and she can't speak the language and I talked to the teachers so they could understand (Lucy).

In some cases, the demand of language brokering kept them away from their education. According to Kalan, "I have to leave school for my father, for my mother, because they do not know the language".

3.3. Experience of Belonging

A lived sense of belonging and being part of a group were common threads woven throughout participants' narratives. Many of the young people described being displaced more than once and were often subjected to discrimination and racial abuse in previous countries of asylum. These experiences of displacement and discrimination often triggered a feeling of otherness, with the young people becoming acutely aware of issues surrounding their sense of difference and cultural identity.

When the participants arrived in Australia, the majority of the young people alluded to a strong sense of belonging within their school context, which was a transitional language school (whose population comprises refugees and migrants from different backgrounds). At school, the young people revealed a sense of unity in relation to shared identities of (a) migrant and (b) student.

Hani spoke very positively about her experiences of resettling in Australia ('Everything is great ... in Australia') and did not share any difficulties associated with the transition. Another participant saw school as a place of support and comfort. According to her, "When I come to school, having my friends, laughing, and then I talk to the teachers sometimes and my teacher will have fun, laugh together" (Julliet).

3.4. Experience of Bonds with Lost Loved Ones

All participants reported having lost a significant relative or community member to war, disease, or physical separation. The lost family members were parents, grandparents or siblings ("Taliban killed my brother"—Kalan). For many of the young people, it felt important to sustain a bond with those who had passed away or been left behind. For some young people, the experience of bonds (or attachment) was about pursuing a dream shared with their lost loved one: "My elder brother ... he liked [dentistry]. And he says for me, I have to become a dentist" (Nazir). For others, emotional bonds were experienced by internalising the traits or beliefs of the lost loved one. For example, many reported having adopted values of compassion and kindness, which they attributed to the influence of a lost parent, sibling, or other relative.

The loss of significant others was often associated with valuing a sense of responsibility, ambition, and diligence. The young people described feeling close to their lost loved one by acting in accordance with these values, thereby keeping the memory of the loved one alive in a country far from home. For many participants, carrying a loved one with them appeared to add value and meaning to their existence. Very often, the young people were able to intentionally integrate an aspect of their lost loved one into their identity without subjugating their own emerging values and beliefs. This was revealed by Kalan's comment, who said "My brother said never go with the bad boys., You have to be a good man".

3.5. Dealing with Emotions in a New Context

All the young people interviewed reported experiencing separation from friends and family in their home country or first country of asylum. A number of them talked about experiences of separation and how they considered themselves to be the lucky few who were able to relocate to a safer country. This 'lucky one' identity was linked with participants downplaying and potentially disavowing distressing emotional experiences and difficulties associated with resettlement. This phenomenon was particularly striking in young people whose futures appeared uncertain (e.g., those on temporary visas). Khin, for example, stated, "I am so happy in Australia", followed by:

I'm so lucky to get here. Because you are now Australian, you're freedom now, they tell me. They told me that. I can look my family. Because they are still in situation they are in now. They are still in refugee camp. How can we live? ... Our people [are still in the] refugee camp ... They tell me, you apply for us. I say I don't have any visa now—you must wait 6 years ... until I get citizenship ... It's good [to have that responsibility], it's really good. Because I want that. My family is great (Khin).

During this conversation, Khin was noticeably distressed. However, he attributed his emotional ambivalence solely to the plight of the Rohingyan people and his family's suffering in the refugee camp. Absent from Khin's discussion were any distressing feelings attributable to resettlement in Australia, including the uncertainty associated with a bridging visa and the possibility of returning to the country of origin. This showed his capacity to disengage from potentially distressing experiences.

Further, Salim was on a Bridging Visa and his future was uncertain. His drawing (Figure 1) with black, white with grey shades, sharp lines and a stump near the tree, indicated underlying anxiety. Despite this uncertainty, he showed resilience by keeping himself in the present moment and focussing on his experiences in Australia. He reported, "I don't think about the future. I just think about today and tomorrow. Nothing more than that".

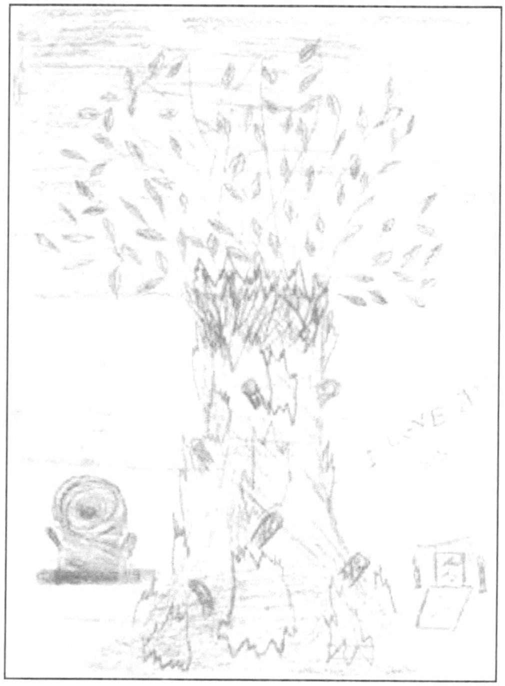

Figure 1. Salim's drawing of the tree.

3.6. Experience of Self in the Context of Change

The process of meaning-making was implicit in the narratives of all participants. All participants shared a number of significant life events, including recurrent trauma, loss, displacement, and resettlement in Australia. In the context of identity, these events all have the potential to profoundly disrupt the person's sense of personal coherence. So, what determines the likelihood of a rupture occurring? In the current study, the degree of disruption depended on the subjective meaning derived from the event. For example, Mairi, who had been in Australia for less than 12 months, stated:

In Iran, in the school, I'm best in class . . . but in Australia . . . I'm last one . . . so I'm very sad for this. Sometimes [I] cry, I can't do it, anything in class and [my teacher] say [to] me, I'm listening . . . but . . . I can't understand. I don't like. I'm very sad . . . [I say to myself] why you can't understand? . . . I don't know why I [cannot understand] (Mairi).

In this excerpt, Mairi is struggling in an area of her identity, her capacity to learn, that had previously been very easy for her and evidently a great source of pride. The disparity between past self and current self can be seen as causing a rupture in Mairi's self-structure, with Mairi unable to make sense of the disparity. This discontinuity in her sense of personal coherence leads her to feel emotionally distressed. Her drawing of the tree (Figure 2) also shows her frustration with acquiring English language and the impact it had on her sense of self.

Mairi's experience stands in contrast to that of 15-year-old Kalan, who lost his elder brother in Afghanistan. Ordinarily, we would expect this loss to cause a rupture in personal coherence of some degree. However, Kalan recognised that his brother died because they lived in dangerous country:

My big mistake of my father is when he leave Pakistan [to go to Afghanistan] with . . . my big brother. Our life is good in [Pakistan] but . . . my father love his country [Afghanistan] too much (Kalan).

Kalan had already experienced significant trauma in Afghanistan ("They put bombs in our home") and wanted to move abroad to safety. The meaning Kalan derived from his brother's death aligned with his preexisting experience of Afghanistan, which prevented him from experiencing a profound rupture to his own sense of personal coherence. After fleeing Afghanistan, Kalan sustained a continuing bond with his deceased brother by striving for a more meaningful and successful life in a new country. Kalan made sense of his experience by continuing to carry his brother with him, which also assisted in the maintenance of a more cohesive identity, often referred to as a cohesive sense of self.

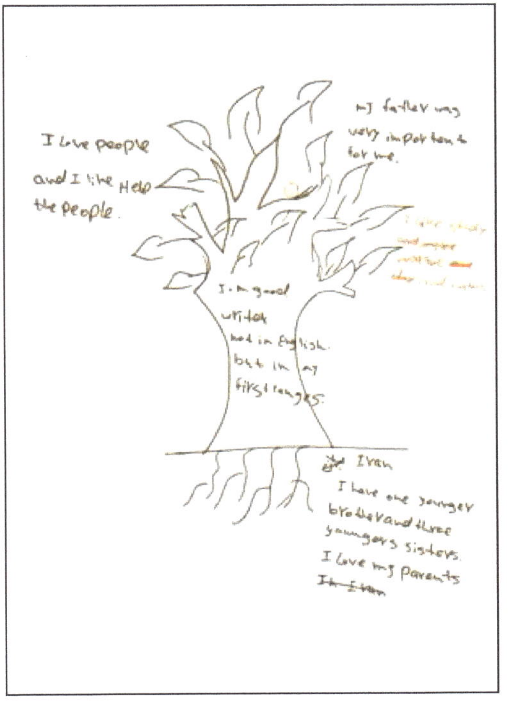
I Love people
and I like Help
the people.
my father was
very important
for me.
Iran
I have one younger
brother and three
youngers sisters.
I love my parents

Figure 2. Mairi's drawing of the tree.

4. Discussion

While identity has been studied in several papers, the topic of identity in young people from refugee backgrounds has received less scrutiny. The current findings, drawing upon the explication of interview data, provide a novel exploration of the complex interplay between identity formation, meaning-making, and the resettlement experiences of young people from refugee backgrounds newly settled in Australia. The data highlight issues faced by young people during the early stages of relocating to a new country and the ways in which people construct meaning in the context of their reconstructed lives.

From a theoretical lens, the themes elucidated in the paper—addressing encompassing experiences of changes in family roles, experiences of belonging, experiences of bonds with lost loved ones, the process of dealing with emotions in a new context, and experience of self in the context of change—all contribute to the formation of a person's identity, in terms of their membership of social groups [1,2,35]. Aligned with social identity theory, the interview data revealed that the participants adopted one or more social identities, mirroring their experience of repeated displacement and resettlement in different countries. Many of the young people also described their sense of self in dynamic terms, that is, as a process of change. This process is conceptualised within an overarching theme of ongoing meaning-making, as per social identity theory and sociocultural perspectives [15].

In Australia, young people from refugee backgrounds continue to occupy a position of marginalisation and difference; however, most participants in the current study did not refer to experiences of exclusion. In the current study, a sense of belonging strongly supported by the school appeared to buffer against feelings of otherness in the wider social context, with young people sharing at least two social identities of (a) student and (b) migrant. For young people from refugee backgrounds, school is one of the most important social contexts for promoting wellbeing and resettlement in a new country [36], with higher levels of connection and commitment to school reportedly being associated with lower levels of depression and higher levels of self-efficacy in young people with refugee backgrounds [37]. Unsurprisingly, school belonging has been found to weaken when transitioning from a specialist English Language School (ELS) to a mainstream school, with refugee young people in Australia reporting lower levels of support and higher levels of discrimination at mainstream schools compared to ELS schools [36]. Current findings lend support to the idea that feelings of marginalisation and difference might be attenuated by a strong sense of belonging within school and peer groups. However, more research into school belonging and sense of otherness is needed before firm conclusions can be drawn.

In the current study, meaning-making was implicit in all the young people's narratives [17,18]. Across the dataset, participants shared several significant life events (e.g., loss, displacement, and resettlement). All these events had the potential to create a rupture in the person's sense of coherence and sense of belonging. The extent of this rupture—if any—depended on the meaning derived from the experience. Consistent with the sociocultural context of identity theory and research, the young people in this study negotiated the restructure in the family and accepted people other than their parents as their carers and guardians. They were also motivated to make sense of their experiences, drawing on previously internalised voices and dialogues to determine how their experiences fit with their bricolage of self [15,38]. Young people may construct their sense of self by assembling different elements of their experience from their environment, sociocultural context, relationships, and personal factors, thereby creating a unique and multifaceted sense of identity [14,15].

With reported experiences of loss, continuing bonds with the loss of a loved one was a way of making sense of what had happened, with many young people internalising the beliefs and values held by lost loved ones. This finding is consistent with the contemporary bereavement literature [39], which suggests continuing bonds assist individuals to integrate and accept the loss of loved ones, so long as they accept that they cannot regain physical proximity with the person who is deceased.

Overall, participants shared experiences of emotional distress associated with rupturing life experiences that could not be placed meaningfully into the self-structure (e.g., the case of Mairi and Salim) [24]. For some young people, there was a tendency to engage in behaviour which may be understood in terms of disavowal [40], that is, to separate themselves from distressing emotions and/or difficulties associated with resettlement, as these did not fit with their self-identity of the 'lucky ones' who escaped war and persecution in their countries of origin.

The current findings inform our understanding of identity in a group of young people from refugee backgrounds. They support the idea that identity is constructed through a continuous process of configuration and re-configuration of self, usually in interaction with others, including their sociocultural context and where the person "fits" in relation to others. Additionally, the narratives of the participants illustrate a continual process of identity development, commencing in early childhood and supported by their social context (i.e., a specialist school dedicated to supporting youth with refugee backgrounds, newly arrived in Australia). The ultimate attainment of a fixed sense of identity endpoint remains uncertain; for these individuals, the evolution of their self-structure occurred in response to new experiences, alongside the development of collective memories. The group's shared narrative implies an indefinite continuation of self-reconfiguration [41], supporting the idea that identity formation is an ongoing process and not a fixed entity [1–3,35].

From a clinical standpoint, these observations underscore the integral role of meaning-making in the resettlement and acculturation process. The findings highlight the need for clinical interventions that prioritise the exploration and interpretation of life experiences, supporting the construction a unified self-narrative. Moreover, providing education that underscores the intricate and multifaceted nature of identity and emotions could prove beneficial. This is particularly the case as the refugee young people in this study experienced distress, often associated with a sense of guilt, as they grappled with thoughts of those left behind in their countries of origin.

There were several challenges associated with research involving refugee young people. The current study took great care to manage these challenges throughout the research process, to improve the overall trustworthiness of the data and reduce the risk of research-related harm. To enhance the credibility of the data, the interviewer kept a reflexive journal and met regularly with the authors to discuss the interviews and the data [42]. To increase data integrity, the young people were reminded that participation was voluntary, and data would be de-identified. Participants were offered a range of response options (i.e., interview, drawing, writing) to enhance research control and autonomy, increasing the likelihood of participants feeling comfortable enough to provide rich and truthful information [36]. The semi-structured interview approach and ToL were both designed to be participant-centred, enhancing young people's control over research participation, thereby shifting the balance of power between researcher and participant [29]. The inclusion of the ToL metaphor and the provision of the opportunity to draw or write allowed some emotional distance from more challenging topics [27,43], again increasing the likelihood of young people feeling safe enough to provide a rich and accurate picture.

4.1. Implications

The findings of this study have theoretical and practical implications. Firstly, the study highlights the importance of understanding changes in family roles. It is crucial to recognise the substantial role transitions that young people experience within their families, including the restructuring of the family as well as the shift from acting as caretakers and helpers in the household to becoming full-time students. The potential impact of these changes contributes not only to the individual's social identities, but also the broader sociocultural construction of identity within the family unit. This is a valuable insight into the acculturation process and identity formation for youth with refugee backgrounds. Thus, it is important to provide support and resources to help young people navigate their new roles and responsibilities, balancing their familial and educational obligations within their cultural context.

The study endorses the significance of a sense of belongingness and connection for young people from refugee backgrounds. This is particularly relevant when considering their experiences of displacement and discrimination, and the subsequent possibility of a negative social identity. Experiences of belonging positively contribute to the health and wellbeing of refugee youth and facilitate the cultivation of a cohesive identity [3,22]. The availability of specialised schools in Australia plays a crucial role in this process. Hence, it is fundamental to create inclusive environments where young people feel welcomed, valued, and supported in exploring their cultural identities. Relatedly, the data promoted school connectedness. The school environment is seen as important in providing a supportive and inclusive environment for young people, where they can both transition into their new cultural milieu and develop social connections, academic skills, and a sense of purpose. A number of strategies may be implemented at a local level to enhance school belongingness and peer support, such as peer mentoring programs and cultural exchange activities within the school setting.

Lastly, the findings recognised the significance of the emotional bonds of young people from refugee backgrounds with lost loved ones. Importantly, they highlighted the deliberate integration of an aspect of the departed loved one into their identity. This result provides valuable insights into identity reconstruction in the context of loss. It is essential to provide opportunities for young people to respect and/or preserve the memories of their lost loved ones through activities such as storytelling, creative expression, or commemorative activities.

4.2. Limitations and Future Directions

The study was not free from limitations. The sample was small and not reflective of all refugee groups in Australia. Further, there were very small numbers for various visa categories, and it was not possible to compare the subgroups. A larger sample with participants from a range of communities with varying demographics and visa statuses should be recruited in the future to build a better understanding of the roles that different contexts play in the identity development among the youth from a refugee background. Further, a larger group would allow the researchers to draw conclusions surrounding the similarities and differences among former refugee youth living in different circumstances.

Further, data were collected in a single session. Despite efforts to enhance rapport, it is possible that some participants may have been inhibited from sharing their experiences. Future studies may use multiple meetings with the young people to understand the role of their social environment in the development of their identity. Further, the present study did not provide the participants with an opportunity to check their responses. Future studies could engage in member checking [42] (p. 277), which would provide the young people with an opportunity to provide feedback on how well they felt the interpretations captured their experience [44]. This exploration holds the potential to provide deeper insights into the nuanced nature of identity formation within this population.

4.3. Conclusions

This study highlights the salient identity challenges faced by young people from refugee backgrounds residing in Australia. Intricately woven throughout the dataset is the persistent endeavour of these young people to derive meaning from their past and present life events within the context of their family, school, and community setting, striving to reconstruct a coherent sense of self. These observations align with a conceptualisation of identity that emphasises ongoing processes, demanding the meaningful integration of each new experience and relationship into an individual's evolving self-structure.

Overall, the study highlights the imperative for interventions aimed at supporting young people from refugee backgrounds that foster the exploration and interpretation of life experiences and facilitate the development of a more cohesive sense of identity. This approach is particularly salient in working with young individuals who have encountered significant adversity, displacement, and relocation. The significance of school connectedness is notably emphasised, with a sense of belonging serving as a crucial buffer against further ruptures in personal coherence. This finding is congruent with prior research that has alluded to the pivotal role of peers in the identity construction process for refugee youth [45–47].

Author Contributions: Conceptualization, N.G.K. and R.D.S.; Methodology, N.G.K.; Data collection, N.G.K.; Data analysis, N.G.K. and R.D.S.; Writing, N.G.K. and R.D.S.; funding acquisition, R.D.S. All authors have read and agreed to the published version of the manuscript.

Funding: This research received seed funding from Milpera State High School.

Institutional Review Board Statement: The authors assert that all procedures contributing to this work comply with the ethical standards of the relevant national and institutional committees on human experimentation and with the Helsinki Declaration of 1975, as revised in 2008.

Informed Consent Statement: Informed consents were obtained from the participants.

Data Availability Statement: Data will be made available on request.

Acknowledgments: We wish to express our thanks the previous principal of Milpera State High School, Thomas Beck, and to the students and staff involved in the project. We are also grateful to Jessica Halloran for her assistance with the data collection and analysis and to Rohani Mitchell and Yi Wang for their contribution to the editing and preparation of the manuscript for publication.

Conflicts of Interest: The authors declare no conflicts of interest.

References

1. Hayes, S.W.; Endale, E. "Sometimes my mind, it has to analyze two things": Identity development and adaptation for refugee and newcomer adolescents. *Peace Confl. J. Peace Psychol.* **2018**, *24*, 283–290. [CrossRef]
2. Wehrle, K.; Klehe, U.-C.; Kira, M.; Zikic, J. Can I come as I am? Refugees' vocational identity threats, coping, and growth. *J. Vocat. Behav.* **2018**, *105*, 83–101. [CrossRef]
3. Chen, S.; Schweitzer, R.D. The experience of belonging in youth from refugee backgrounds: A narrative perspective. *J. Child Fam. Stud.* **2019**, *28*, 1977–1990. [CrossRef]
4. Ziaian, T.; Puvimanasinghe, T.; Miller, E.; De Anstiss, H.; Esterman, A.; Dollard, M. Identity and belonging: Refugee youth and their parents' perception of being Australian. *Aust. Psychol.* **2021**, *56*, 123–136. [CrossRef]
5. Hermans, H.J.M. Conceptions of self and identity towards Dialogical view. *Int. J. Educ. Relig.* **2001**, *2*, 43–62. [CrossRef]
6. Shahimi, F.; Block, K.; Alisic, E. Sense of identity among young people with refugee backgrounds: A scoping review. *Child. Youth Serv. Rev.* **2024**, *157*, 107378. [CrossRef]
7. Tajfel, H.; Turner, J.C.; Austin, W.G.; Worchel, S. An integrative theory of intergroup conflict. In *Organizational Identity: A Reader*; Oxford University Press: Oxford, UK, 1979; Volume 56, p. 9780203505984-16.
8. Stets, J.E.; Burke, P.J. Identity Theory and Social Identity Theory. *Soc. Psychol. Q.* **2000**, *63*, 224–237. [CrossRef]
9. Jackson, J.W. Intergroup Attitudes as a Function of Different Dimensions of Group Identification and Perceived Intergroup Conflict. *Self Identity* **2002**, *1*, 11–33. [CrossRef]
10. Guzder, J. Second skins: Family therapy agendas of migration, identity and cultural change. *Fokus Fam.* **2011**, *39*, 160–179. [CrossRef]
11. Hughes, G. Finding a voice through 'The Tree of Life': A strength-based approach to mental health for refugee children and families in schools. *Clin. Child Psychol. Psychiatry* **2014**, *19*, 139–153. [CrossRef]
12. Oikonomidoy, E.; Karam, F. 'Flatbread and lollipops': Social funds of identity in the trilingual journey of a refugee-background student. *Innov. Lang. Learn. Teach.* **2023**, 1–14. [CrossRef]
13. Urrieta, L. Identity Production in Figured Worlds: How Some Mexican Americans Become Chicana/o Activist Educators. *Urban Rev.* **2007**, *39*, 117–144. [CrossRef]
14. Caraballo, L. Being "loud": Identities-in-practice in a figured world of achievement. *Am. Educ. Res. J.* **2019**, *56*, 1281–1317. [CrossRef]
15. Grignolio, A.; Mishto, M.; Faria, A.M.C.; Garagnani, P.; Franceschi, C.; Tieri, P. Towards a liquid self: How time, geography, and life experiences reshape the biological identity. *Front. Immunol.* **2014**, *5*, 153. [CrossRef] [PubMed]
16. Bergquist, G.; Soliz, J.; Everhart, K.; Braithwaite, D.O.; Kreimer, L. Investigating layers of identity and identity gaps in refugee resettlement experiences in the Midwestern United States. *West. J. Commun.* **2019**, *83*, 383–402. [CrossRef]
17. Kinefuchi, E. Finding home in migration: Montagnard refugees and post-migration identity. *J. Int. Intercult. Commun.* **2010**, *3*, 228–248. [CrossRef]
18. Vahali, H.O. *Lives in Exile: Exploring the Inner World of Tibetan Refugees*; Taylor & Francis: Abingdon, UK, 2020.
19. Betancourt, T.S.; Newnham, E.A.; Layne, C.M.; Kim, S.; Steinberg, A.M.; Ellis, H.; Birman, D. Trauma history and psychopathology in war-affected refugee children referred for trauma related mental health services in the United States. *J. Trauma. Stress* **2012**, *25*, 682–690. [CrossRef]
20. Karam, F.J.; Kibler, A.K.; Johnson, H.E.; Molloy Elreda, L. Identity, positionality, and peer social networks: A case study of an adolescent refugee background student. *J. Lang. Identity Educ.* **2020**, *19*, 208–223. [CrossRef]
21. Hassan, G.; Kirmayer, L.J.; Mekki-Berrada, A.; Quosh, C.; El Chammay, R.; Deville-Stoetzel, J.-B.; Youssef, A.; Jefee-Bahloul, H.; Barkeel-Oteo, A.; Coutts, A. *Culture, Context and the Mental Health and Psychosocial Wellbeing of Syrians: A Review for Mental Health and Psychosocial Support Staff Working with Syrians Affected by Armed Conflict*; UNHCR: Geneva, Switzerland, 2015.
22. Edge, S.; Newbold, K.B.; McKeary, M. Exploring socio-cultural factors that mediate, facilitate, & constrain the health and empowerment of refugee youth. *Soc. Sci. Med.* **2014**, *117*, 34–41. [CrossRef]
23. Rabiau, M.A. Culture, migration, and identity formation in adolescent refugees: A family perspective. *J. Fam. Soc. Work* **2019**, *22*, 83–100. [CrossRef]
24. Märtsin, M. Rupturing otherness: Becoming Estonian in the context of contemporary Britain. *J. Integr. Physiol. Behav. Sci.* **2010**, *44*, 65–81. [CrossRef]
25. Van Blerk, L.; Shand, W.; Prazeres, L.; Bukenya, B.; Essaid, A.A.; Hunter, J.; Kasirye, R. Youth transitions in protracted crises: Conceptualising the 'rupture' of refugees' pathways to adulthood in Uganda and Jordan. *Trans. Inst. Br. Geogr.* **2022**, *47*, 315–330. [CrossRef]

26. Papadopoulos, D. In the ruins of representation: Identity, individuality, subjectification. *Br. J. Soc. Psychol.* **2008**, *47*, 139–165. [CrossRef] [PubMed]
27. Denborough, D. *Collective Narrative Practice: Responding to Individuals, Groups, and Communities Who Have Experienced Trauma*; Dulwich Centre: Adelaide, Australia, 2008.
28. Ncube, N. The Tree of Life Project: Using narrative ideas in work with vulnerable children in Southern Africa. *Int. J. Narrat. Ther. Community Work* **2006**, *1*, 3–16.
29. Barker, J.; Weller, D. "Is it fun?": Developing children centred research methods. *Int. J. Sociol. Soc. Policy* **2003**, *23*, 33–58. [CrossRef]
30. Block, K.; Warr, D.; Gibbs, L.; Riggs, E. Addressing ethical and methodological challenges in research with refugee-background young people: Reflections from the field. *J. Refug. Stud.* **2013**, *26*, 69–87. [CrossRef]
31. Schweitzer, R.D.; Vromans, L.; Ranke, G.; Griffin, J. Narratives of healing: A case study of a young Liberian refugee settled in Australia. *Arts Psychother.* **2014**, *41*, 98–106. [CrossRef]
32. Squires, A. Methodological challenges in cross-language qualitative research: A research review. *Int. J. Nurs. Stud.* **2009**, *46*, 277–287. [CrossRef]
33. Gee, J.P. *Social Linguistics and Literacies: Ideology in Discourse*; Falmer Press: London, UK, 1990.
34. Braun, V.; Clarke, V. *Thematic Analysis: A Practical Guide*; Sage: Thousand Oaks, CA, USA, 2021.
35. Michalovich, A.; Kendrick, M.; Early, M. Youth from refugee backgrounds positioning their Identities through reaction videos. *J. Lang. Identity Educ.* **2022**, 1–16. [CrossRef]
36. Gifford, S.M.; Correa-Velez, I.; Sampson, R. *Good Starts for Recently Arrived Youth with Refugee Backgrounds: Promoting Wellbeing in the First Three Years of Settlement in Melbourne, Australia*; La Trobe Refugee Research Centre: Mildura, Australia, 2009.
37. Kia-Keating, M.; Ellis, B.H. Belonging and connection to school in resettlement: Young refugees, school belonging, and psychosocial adjustment. *Clin. Child Psychol. Psychiatry* **2007**, *12*, 29–43. [CrossRef]
38. Märtsin, M. Self-regulation by signs: A social semiotic approach to identity. In *Multicentric Identities in the Globalizing World*; Salvatore, S., Gennaro, A., Valsiner, J., Eds.; Information Age Publishing: Charlotte, NC, USA, 2014; pp. ix–xx.
39. Im, H.; Neff, J. Spiral loss of culture: Cultural trauma and bereavement of Bhutanese refugee elders. *J. Immigr. Refug. Stud.* **2021**, *19*, 99–113. [CrossRef]
40. Wolf, E.S. *Treating the Self: Elements of Clinical Self Psychology*; Guilford Press: New York, NY, USA, 1988.
41. Wertsch, J.V.; Jäggi, O.L. Habits of collective memory. *Prog. Brain Res.* **2022**, *274*, 149–166. [CrossRef]
42. Anney, V.N. Ensuring the quality of the findings of qualitative research: Looking at trustworthiness criteria. *J. Emerg. Trends Educ. Res. Policy Stud.* **2014**, *5*, 272–281.
43. Handler, L.; Thomas, A.D. *Drawings in Assessment and Psychotherapy: Research and Application*; Routledge: Oxfordshire, UK, 2014.
44. Onwuegbuzie, A.J.; Leech, N.L. A call for qualitative power analyses. *Qual. Quant.* **2007**, *41*, 105–121. [CrossRef]
45. Lewis, L.D. Social Networking and the School Adjustment of Karen Refugee Youth from Burma: Determining the Effects of Ethnic Identity, Bonding Social Capital, and Facebook Use. Ph.D. Thesis, University of North Carolina, Chapel Hill, NC, USA, 2013. Available online: https://libres.uncg.edu/ir/uncg/listing.aspx?id=10060 (accessed on 20 February 2024).
46. Moran, L. Constructions of race: Symbolic ethnic capital and the performance of youth identity in multicultural Australia. *Ethn. Racial Stud.* **2016**, *39*, 708–726. [CrossRef]
47. Ndengeyingoma, A.; de Montigny, F.; Miron, J. Development of personal identity among refugee adolescents: Facilitating elements and obstacles. *J. Child Health Care* **2014**, *18*, 369–377. [CrossRef] [PubMed]

International Journal of
Environmental Research and Public Health

MDPI

Article

Do Resettled People Adapt to Their Current Geographical Environment? Evidence from Poverty-Stricken Areas of Northwest Yunnan Province, China

Liquan Qu, Weidong Xiao * and Weidong Gao

School of Geography, Geomatics and Planning, Jiangsu Normal University, Xuzhou 221116, China
* Correspondence: xiaowd@jsnu.edu.cn; Tel.: +86-150-5082-4860

Abstract: The geographical environment adaptation of the resettled population is a deep-seated problem that determines whether the goal of the poverty alleviation resettlement (PAR) policy can be achieved. Scientific assessment of adaptive capacity (AC) and adaptation level (AL) provides a basis for subsequent policy formulation, which is of practical significance. This study took the poverty-stricken areas of northwest Yunnan as the study area and calculated the adaptive capacity index (ACI) and adaptation level index (ALI) based on survey data of 1002 resettled households and regional socioeconomic statistics by constructing the vulnerability as expected poverty (VEP) model and multi-factor analysis model. The results showed that (1) The ACI and ALI were 0.660 and 61.2 respectively, indicating that the resettled population has obvious environment adaptation barriers and a relatively high risk of returning to poverty. (2) The AC and AL of the resettled population had significant geographical differentiation. In general, Diqing Prefecture was significantly better than Nujiang Prefecture and the problems in Gongshan County, Fugong County and Lanping County were more prominent. (3) AC is a determinant of AL. However, these two indices in Gongshan and Lanping counties deviated from the general trend due to different policy effects. Based on the evaluation results and differentiation mechanism analysis, the study finally emphasized the importance of formulating and implementing the follow-up development plan of the resettled population and put forward measures to promote the resettled population to adapt to the geographical environment around the three core tasks of employment income increase, public service and bottom guarantee.

Keywords: poverty alleviation resettlement (PAR); adaptive capacity (AC); adaptation level (AL); differentiation mechanism; poverty-stricken areas of northwest Yunnan

Citation: Qu, L.; Xiao, W.; Gao, W. Do Resettled People Adapt to Their Current Geographical Environment? Evidence from Poverty-Stricken Areas of Northwest Yunnan Province, China. *Int. J. Environ. Res. Public Health* **2023**, *20*, 193. https://doi.org/10.3390/ijerph20010193

Academic Editors: Ernesto Castañeda and Maria De Jesus

Received: 16 November 2022
Revised: 15 December 2022
Accepted: 19 December 2022
Published: 23 December 2022

1. Introduction

Poverty remains an existential challenge shared by all humanity. Eradicating poverty is the primary goal of the UN sustainable development goals (SDGs) [1]. Over time, countries such as China, Brazil and Vietnam have contributed significantly to poverty alleviation around the world [2,3]. Among them, the implementation of China's series of poverty reduction policies has lifted millions of rural poor out of poverty. Due to the complex causes of poverty [4], some areas of China were still trapped in "spatial poverty" [5]. In response, China launched a targeted poverty alleviation strategy (TPA) in 2013, which has ultimately been a great success in poverty alleviation [6]. By the end of 2020, China has eliminated the absolute poverty problem been under the current standard [7–9]. The central government demands that poverty alleviation areas sort out shortfalls to prevent a widespread return to poverty and view the consolidation and expansion of poverty alleviation achievements as a crucial task in the coming years.

Poverty alleviation resettlement (PAR) is an important measure of TPA [10]. PAR aims to relocate 10 million poor people living in poor conditions to suitable areas and fundamentally change their living conditions [11]. Nevertheless, resettlement under administrative intervention has not only broken the original low-level human–land symbiosis but also brought about a series of socio-economic problems such as the lack of fundamental production means, social network disruption and multi-ethnic cultural conflicts [12]. The resettled population has reached the poverty alleviation goal according to the current evaluation standard. However, they historically resided in relatively segregated areas. They are inherently sensitive and vulnerable to changes in the living environment. Therefore, we must pay attention to the resettled population. Do they adapt to the current geographical environment? What mechanisms influence their adaptation to the current geographical environment? These problems determine whether the resettled population can develop sustainably and eliminate poverty stably, which has practical significance for consolidate the successes of poverty alleviation.

This study aimed to reflect the current pattern of resettled population's adaptation to the new environment and explain its formation mechanism by evaluating adaptive capacity (AC) and adaptation level (AL) based on a random survey of 45 relocation sites and 1002 resettled households in poverty-stricken areas of northwest Yunnan. In this way, it could provide a basis for the local formulation of measures to consolidate poverty alleviation work and reduce the risk of returning to poverty. Considering the reproducibility of China's poverty reduction experience in developing countries, this study can also serve as a reference for relevant studies conducted in other areas of the world where carry out PAR.

2. Literature Review and Conceptual Framework

2.1. The Theory of Man–Land Areal System

The theory of man–land areal system is the cornerstone of studying the geographical environment adaptation of relocated population. According to the system theory and the theory of man–land areal system, the elements of "man" and "land" are interwoven with each other according to certain rules to form a complex and open giant system, which has a certain structure and functional mechanism inside and a certain geographical scope in space [13]. Under the interaction and mutual feedback between man and land and the external force of the system, the man–land areal system always evolves in the manner of "balance–unbalance–rebalance", exhibiting vulnerability, risk, resilience and adaptation characteristics [14,15]. The geographical environment adaptation obstacle is the external manifestation of the mutual influence and feedback between man and nature after the sudden change of the relationship between man and land and the breaking of the system balance before and after the relocation. The core goal of man–land areal system research is to coordinate the man–land relationship [16], which is consistent with the SDGs and provides a perspective and theoretical basis for studying the geographical environment adaptation of resettled population. The basic research methods of the man–land system mainly include classification, zoning, quantitative analysis, model building and evaluation [17]. For instance, some researchers utilize the coupling degree to reflect an objective representation of the interaction stress and interaction dependence relationship between various systems or various system components and to characterize the evolution trend of the regional system at a certain moment [18,19].

2.2. Geographical Environment Adaptive Capacity of Migrant Population

The concept of adaptive capacity (AC) originates from natural science [20]. Steward first applied AC to human systems, studying how people adjust their behavior to the natural environment [21]. The research on the natural environment AC of population mainly involves the fields of climate change [22–24], disaster risk [25,26]. Due to the vulnerability of humans and the complex relationship between humans and land, there is still a lack of research on how to link daily life with adapting to environmental changes. Meanwhile, research on meso–micro scales such as cities and communities has not received much attention [27]. We retrieved all periodical literature with the keywords of "resettlement" and "adaptation" on China's CNKI (http://www.cnki.net/, accessed on 4 May 2022) and found that the majority focuses on sociology and ethnology. It covers social adaptation [28], administrative ethical care [29], multiple spatial remodeling of migrants [30], community governance of relocated migrants [31], citizenship of relocated population [32] and social integration of relocated populations [33]. As can be observed, there is still a dearth of geographic study on the AC of the relocated population.

2.3. Follow-Up Development of Resettled Population

PAR aims to create conditions for subsequent poverty alleviation and development by relocating the rural poor. In developed countries, similar concepts to PAR are environmental migration [34,35] and ecological migration [36]. The research mainly involves six aspects: biodiversity conservation, poverty and pro-poor environment, climate change and regional conflicts, resettlement areas, emigration areas and sociological issues of environmental refugees. It has macro, policy, comprehensive and cross-regional characteristics [37].

Although relocation directly improves the living conditions of the resettled, the poverty problem is not resolved naturally. The poverty incidence rate of many resettlement sites is still high, so the follow-up development of the resettled population is a crucial issue. The relevant research results can be classified into two categories: one is a comprehensive study of the poverty alleviation effect and subsequent development of the resettled population [38,39]. For example, using panel data and fixed effects models, Leng et al. explored the impact of PAR on household income. They found that relocation reduces the transaction costs of poor households in accessing technology, markets and other information, improves agricultural production efficiency and the quality of agricultural products and thus leads to an increase in household farm business income [11]. Wang et al. measured the vulnerability of relocated farming households and make recommendations to increase the precision and sustainability of anti-poverty policies [40,41]. Hu et al. explored the changes in the scope of social interaction and social support under the PAR policy [42]. The second is the study of specific ways to increase income, such as the rational use of rural homesteads, employment transfer and eco-compensation [43–45]. These studies discuss how to improve the well-being of resettled people from different perspectives and have important reference value for relevant local governments to formulate measures to consolidate the achievements of poverty alleviation.

To sum up, the existing studies provide references for our study. However, there are still some deficiencies: first, although many scholars emphasize the importance of the follow-up development of the relocated people and put forward many measures to increase their income, few mention that the mutation of the man–land areal system and the resulting difficulty in adapting to the geographical environment are the root causes of the difficulty in the follow-up development of the resettled population and the risk of returning to poverty. Second, the current research mostly qualitatively discusses the adaptation of the resettled population to the social and cultural environment from the perspective of sociology and ethnology and the studies of quantitative evaluation of the resettled population's geographical environment adaptation from the perspective of man–land relationship are rare. Third, China's relocation policy applies to areas with fragile ecological environments, a lack of productive resources and difficulties in improving the living conditions of farm households, mainly in mountainous areas. Located in the Hengduan Mountains on the eastern edge of the Tibetan Plateau, Northwest Yunnan has significant geographical characteristics. First, it has a relocation population share of 14.5%, the highest in the country. Second, it has a remote national border with weak non-agricultural industries and a lack of infrastructure and public services. Third, there is a population of Tibetan, Lisu and other major ethnic minorities with low cultural quality and a tradition of living by the mountains. These factors add to the difficulties of population relocation and subsequent poverty eradication. This region has the characteristics of large-scale relocation and a high risk of returning to poverty, which should have been paid particular attention to.

Therefore, based on existing research, we took the theory of the man–land areal system as the theoretical basis and emphasized the adaptation of the population participating in PAR to the geographical environment. This study first constructed an evaluation model to quantify the AC and AL of the relocated population to the geographical environment.

Secondly, using the field survey data in Northwest Yunnan, it was judged and analyzed the spatial differentiation of the AC and AL of the geographical environment of the relocated population on the county level. Through the analysis of the formation mechanism of spatial differentiation, policy recommendations to improve the AC and AL of the relocated population were finally put forward (Figure 1).

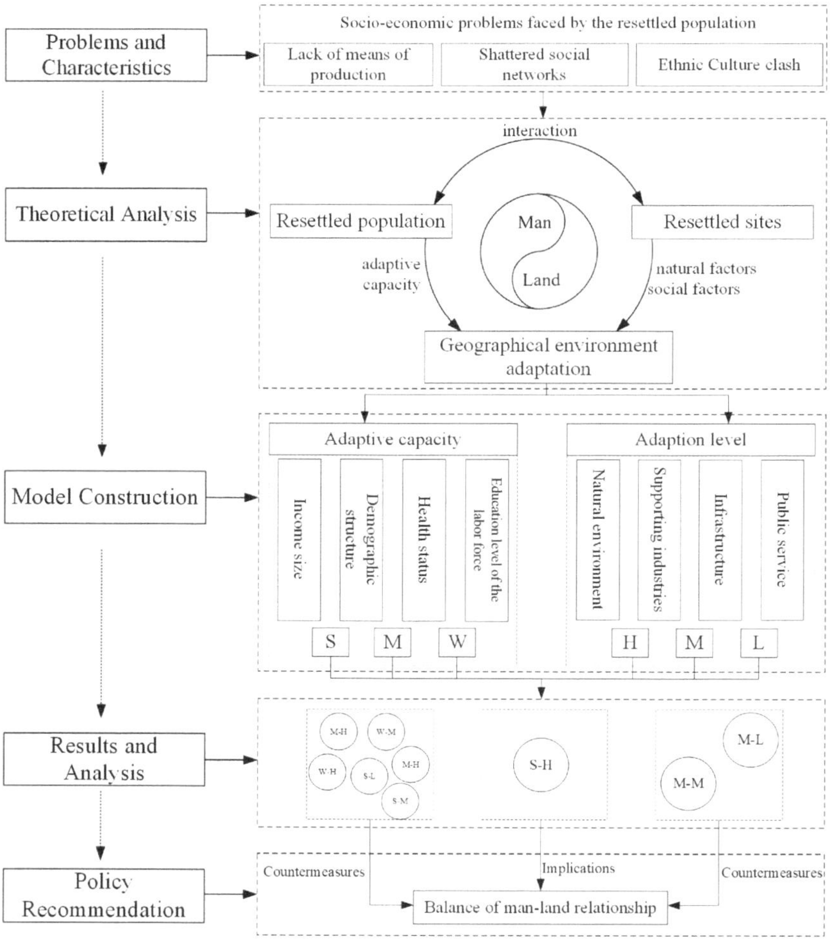

Figure 1. Conceptual framework. Note: In the conceptual framework, "S", "M" and "W" represent that AC is strong, medium and weak, respectively; "H", "M" and "L" represent that AL is high, medium and low, respectively.

3. Materials and Methods

3.1. Study Area

The poverty-stricken areas of northwest Yunnan refer to the two ethnic minority autonomous prefectures of Diqing and Nujiang, with five counties and two cities. Nujiang Prefecture is located in the mountainous area on the border of western Yunnan, with a total population of 553,000. Ethnic minorities account for 93.9% of the population, of which the three "directly-entering-socialism ethnic groups", Lisu, Dulong and Nu, account for 58.8%. Diqing Prefecture is located in the transition zone between Yunnan-Guizhou Plateau and

Qinghai-Tibet Plateau at the junction of Yunnan, Tibet and Sichuan provinces and is adjacent to Nujiang Prefecture in the south. Of the 387,000 people in Diqing Prefecture, Tibetans, Lisu, Naxi and and other ethnic minorities account for 89.1% of the total population. Nujiang and Diqing Prefecture have similar natural environments, with mountains and rivers distributed vertically. Their reclamation coefficient is less than 4% and farmland resources are scarce. Due to the long-term constraints of unfavorable factors, this region's socioeconomic development is relatively lagging and it is one of the poorest areas in Yunnan Province and even the whole country. Therefore, the poverty-stricken areas of northwest Yunnan have dual attributes of typicality and importance.

3.2. Evaluation Indicator

(1) Adaptive capacity (AC) and adaptive capacity index (ACI). AC refers to the capacity of the resettled population to cope with potential external risks and the ability to adjust themselves to deal with negative impacts [46]. It is determined by a series of household characteristic variables such as income size, demographic structure, education level of the labor force and health status of the relocating household. A relative index to it is poverty vulnerability, which expresses the likelihood that the basic living conditions of the poor will fall below the socially accepted level of the region due to household exposure to risk [47]. The number of risks that the resettled population may face and their ability to resolve risks are negatively correlated with their ability to adapt to the geographical environment. Conceptually, poverty vulnerability is an important indicator to test the adaptation of the resettled population. Therefore, we applied poverty vulnerability to measure the ACI.

Poverty vulnerability is usually defined by some relative benchmarks, such as Vulnerability as Expected Poverty (VEP) [48], Vulnerability as Low Expected Utility (VEU) [49] and Vulnerability as Uninsured Exposure to Risk (VER) [50]. Compared with VEU and VER, VEP has advantages in practical applications [51]. First, its data requirements are relatively low. Second, VEP is an ex-ante measure, which fully considers the future welfare of farmers or risks related to the future welfare and is more instructive for policy optimization [52].

VEP refers to the probability that the farmers' expected future income is below the poverty line. Its value is subject to the distribution characteristics of the family's future welfare level and is ultimately determined by the characteristic variables of the resettled family and the local poverty line [53]. The VEP value is between 0–1. The smaller the VEP is, the smaller the probability of future poverty, which also shows that the AC to the new environment is stronger. 1-VEP indicates the probability that the future income of farmers is higher than the poverty line, reflecting the resettled population's environmental AC and poverty elimination ability. Therefore, this study defines 1-VEP as the environmental adaptive capacity index (ACI). ACI is also between 0 and 1. The larger the value, the stronger the AC to the new environment and vice versa.

(2) Adaptation level (AL) and adaptation level index (ALI). AL refers to the adaptation of the resettled population to the new geographical environment. It is affected by many factors such as the ability to adapt to the geographical environment, the implementation of the PAR policy and the regional natural and social environment. As PAR has a policy objective of "immigrant out of the bad environment, obtaining stability, achieving prosperity", therefore, we measured AL by establishing an evaluation index system from these three aspects in this study.

We divided the ACI and ALI values into three intervals and then through the combination of the two, there will be nine possibilities. In addition to the "strong-high" combination, the remaining eight combinations will reflect different adaptation problems. Studying these problems and their formation mechanism is of great significance and is the basis for solving the problem.

3.3. Evaluation Method

3.3.1. Calculation Method of ACI

(1) VEP

According to the definition of Chaudhuri et al. [53], the VEP formula is:

$$VEP_{i,t} = P(y_{i,t+1} < pl) \tag{1}$$

where $VEP_{i,t}$ represents the vulnerability of the resettled household i in the current period; $y_{i,t+1}$ represents the per capita income of the household in period $t + 1$, that is, the expected income; and pl represents the poverty line in the corresponding period; $P(y_{i,t+1} < pl)$ indicates the probability that the expected income is less than the poverty line.

It is generally believed that the income characteristics of high-income groups conform to the Pareto distribution, while the log-normal distribution is more suitable for describing the status of low-income groups [54]. For a specific period, the poverty line pl is the minimum annual per capita income needed to sustain a normal livelihood as measured by the level of local socioeconomic development. Therefore, let $p = lnpl$, Equation (1) can also be expressed as follows:

$$VEP_{i,t} = P(\ln y_{i,t+1} < p) \tag{2}$$

As mentioned above, the expected future income of the resettled farmers is mainly subject to the characteristic variables of the family, such as the education level of the main labor force, the proportion of the elderly and the health status of family members. Therefore, $\ln y_{i,t+1}$ can be expressed as a function of a set of family characteristic variables X_i:

$$\ln y_{i,t+1} = X_i\beta + e_i \tag{3}$$

where X_i represents the observable family characteristics of household i; β is the variable coefficient of family characteristics; e_i is the fluctuation term of expected income. Among them, e_i comes from the risk shock and is subject to the variable of family characteristics and obeys the following equation:

$$e_i^2 = X_i\theta + \varepsilon \tag{4}$$

where θ is the parameter vector to be estimated; ε is the error term.

To convert the above model into an econometric model, we need to estimate the income function. This study uses the feasible generalized least square (FLGS) to estimate β and θ to reduce the estimation error caused by heteroscedasticity. The process is as follows:

First, the ordinary least squares (OLS) method is used to estimate Equation (3) and the estimated error term is used in Equation (4) to obtain the following:

$$\hat{e}_i^2 = X_i\hat{\theta}_{OLS} + \hat{\varepsilon} \tag{5}$$

where $\hat{\varepsilon}$ is the random error term. By dividing the both sides of Equation (4) by $X_i\hat{\theta}_{OLS}$, we can obtain the following equation:

$$\frac{e_i^2}{X_i\hat{\theta}_{OLS}} = \left\{\frac{X_i}{X_i\hat{\theta}_{OLS}}\right\}\theta + \frac{\varepsilon}{X_i\hat{\theta}_{OLS}} \tag{6}$$

Next, we perform OLS regression on Equation (6) to obtain the asymptotically effective estimate of θ, as follows.

$$\hat{e}_{i,FGLS}^2 = X_i\hat{\theta}_{FGLS} \text{ or } \hat{e}_{i,FGLS} = \sqrt{X_i\hat{\theta}_{FGLS}} \tag{7}$$

Removing both sides of Equation (3) with in Equation (7), we obtain the following:

$$\frac{lny_{i,t+1}}{\hat{e}_{i,FGLS}} = \frac{X_i}{\hat{e}_{i,FGLS}}\beta + \frac{e_i}{\hat{e}_{i,FGLS}} \tag{8}$$

By estimating Equation (8), the asymptotic effective estimation value $\hat{\beta}_{FLGS}$ of the coefficient β of the family characteristic variable is obtained. According to the estimation results $\hat{\beta}_{FLGS}$ and $\hat{\theta}_{FGLS}$, we can obtain the expectation and variance of the expected logarithm of income:

$$\hat{E}(lny_i|X_i) = X_i\hat{\beta}_{FGLS} \tag{9}$$

$$\hat{V}(lny_i|X_i) = X_i\hat{\theta}_{FGLS} \tag{10}$$

Finally, we can obtain the econometric model of VEP of resettled households:

$$\widetilde{VEP}_{i,t} = \widetilde{P}(lny_{i,t+1} < p|X_i) = \varnothing\left(\frac{p - X_i\hat{\beta}_{FGLS}}{\sqrt{X_i\hat{\theta}_{FGLS}}}\right) \tag{11}$$

(2) ACI

According to the previous analysis of the relationship between the ACI and the VEP, the measurement model of the ACI can be expressed as follows:

$$\text{ACI} = 1 - \varnothing\left(\frac{p - X_i\hat{\beta}_{FGLS}}{\sqrt{X_i\hat{\theta}_{FGLS}}}\right) \tag{12}$$

ACI is the probability that a relocated household's per capita expected annual income (net of necessary expenditures) is above the poverty line. Since household characteristics variables determine expected income, constructing a regression model of the two makes it possible to quantify AC based on household characteristics variables.

(3) Family characteristic variables of resettled farmers

The expected per capita net income of the resettled households is affected by various factors such as the size of the family population, the number of laborers, the education level of the labor force, the situation of out-migrant work, the situation of receiving skill training and the situation of enjoying public welfare jobs. Since some assistance policies will be gradually canceled after the completion of poverty elimination, this study deducts rigid expenditures such as education, medical care and debt interest from the net income of households. Therefore, the family characteristic variables that affect the future expected income and rigid expenditure of the resettled households are the focus of the field survey, as detailed in Table 1.

Table 1. Household characteristic variables of resettled farmers (2020).

Variable Symbol	Variable	Description
sal	Proportion of salary income	Proportion of salary income in total household income
sca	Family scale	The total population of household registration
pla	Proportion of labor force	Labor force/total household population
non	Proportion of migrant workers population	Number of workers outside their county/total household population
chr	Serious or long-term chronic patients	Do they have serious or long-term chronic patients (the population with major diseases or long-term chronic diseases designated by rural medical insurance) at home? Yes = 1, No = 0
def	Proportion of disabled people	Number of disabled people/total family population
ced	Proportion of population in compulsory education stage	Number of people attending compulsory education/total family population
hig	Proportion of population with high school and above	Number of people attending high school, junior college, university, postgraduate/total family population

Table 1. *Cont.*

Variable Symbol	Variable	Description
tra	Income of land transfer	Income from land transfer in the form of leases, shares, etc.
wel	Public welfare positions	Have they enjoyed the public welfare positions (including forest rangers, river managers, border guards, road guards, cleaners and so on arranged by local governments)? Yes = 1, No = 0
mla	Situation of enjoying the minimum living allowance (MLA)	Enjoy class A of MLA = 3, class B of MLA = 2, class C of MLA = 1, not = 0
edu	Education level of householder	0 for elementary school and below, 1 for middle school, 2 for high school and above

3.3.2. Calculation Method of ALI

(1) Conceptual model of AL

As mentioned above, the AL of resettled households to the geographical environment is affected by AC, degree of relocation policy implementation and other subjective and objective factors. Therefore, AL is a function of many influencing factors and the conceptual model of AL can be expressed as:

$$\mathrm{AL} = \mathrm{f}\ (E_1, E_2, E_3 \ldots\ldots E_n\ ) \tag{13}$$

where E_i represents the influencing factor; n represents the number of influencing factors.

(2) Index system and index weight

With the principles of comprehensiveness, weak mutual correlation, accessibility and quantification, we selected indicators of the AL to the geographic environment of the relocated population. Dimensional layer index weights were determined by the Delphi method. Indexes layer weights were determined by the hierarchical analysis method. The index weights were calculated by two comparisons using Matlab platform programming and the judgment matrix passes the consistency test and the indexes and their weights are detailed in Table 2. Finally, the weights of each index were obtained by multiplying the dimensional layer weights and the category layer weights by the multiplication method.

As seen from the table, the weights of indexes such as X_{17}, X_{10}, X_3, X_{19}, X_{11}, X_{18}, and X_5 are relatively large. In the future, measures to improve the AL should be developed with a focus on these aspects.

Table 2. Evaluation indexes and their weights of geographical environment adaptation level.

Dimensional Layer	Category Layer	Indexes Layer		Weight
		Indexes	Explanation	
Immigrant out of the bad environment 0.20	Physical	Degree of relocation plan (X_1)	Actual number of resettled households/planned number of resettled households	0.254
		Proportion of resettled households breaking the contract (X_2)	Number of households refusing to relocate in breach of contract/planned number relocation households	0.170
	Psychology	Degree of relocation regret (X_3)	Number of households that expressed regret after relocation/number of households resettled under field survey	0.407
		Proportion of households returning to farming (X_4)	Number of households returning to farming after relocation/number of resettled households under field survey	0.169

Table 2. *Cont.*

Dimensional Layer	Category Layer	Indexes Layer		Weight
		Indexes	Explanation	
Obtaining stability 0.45	Life and culture	Adaptation of basic living (X_5)	Number of households with clean household environment and correct use of household appliances and sanitary facilities/number of resettled households	0.111
		Inheritance of ethnic culture (X_6)	Good cultural heritage = 1, general = 0.5, poor = 0 (by interviewing community administrator)	0.080
		Multi-ethnic cultural integration (X_7)	Good participation in cultural activities = 1, general = 0.5, poor = 0 (by interviewing community administrator)	0.096
	Social relations	Maintenance of original social relations (X_8)	Number of households contacting relatives and friends "increased" and "unchanged" after relocation/number of surveyed resettled households	0.079
		Establishment of new social relations (X_9)	Number of households that "communicate more and become more familiar with the resettled population that they did not know before" after relocation/number of households surveyed	0.092
	Income	Annual per capital income (X_{10})	Per capita net income in 2018 (unit: CNY)	0.136
		Non-agricultural income share (X_{11})	Household non-agricultural income/total household income	0.119
	Social security	Distance to the nearest primary school (X_{12})	Distance from placement to nearest primary school (unit: km)	0.052
		Distance to the nearest clinic (X_{13})	Distance from the resettlement site to the nearest clinic (unit: km)	0.052
		Proportion of households enjoying public welfare posts (X_{14})	Number of households enjoying public welfare positions/number of households resettled under investigation	0.074
		Proportion of households enjoying low insurance (X_{15})	Number of households enjoying low insurance/number of resettled households under investigation	0.070
		Coverage rate of bottom protection (X_{16})	Number of households with a bottom protection/number of households that should enjoy the bottom line	0.039
Achieving prosperity 0.35	Industry support	Per capita non-agricultural economic output value (X_{17})	Total output value of secondary and tertiary industries/total regional population in 2018	0.224
	Flexible employment	Proportion of local workers (X_{18})	Number of workers in their counties/number of labor force of resettled households under investigation	0.176
		Proportion of migrant workers (X_{19})	Number of migrant workers outside the county/number of labor force of resettled households under investigation	0.200
	Asset income	Per capita eco- compensation income (X_{20})	Eco-compensation income/household population	0.086
		Per capita land transfer income (X_{21})	Land transfer income/household population	0.133
		Per capita village reclamation income (X_{22})	Village reclamation income/household population	0.067
		Per capita collective economic benefits (X_{23})	The collective economic benefits/household population	0.114

(3) Index normalization processing

The index was dimensionless processing by the assignment method. First, we assigned a score of 100 to the best of the j-item indexes (j = 1, 2... 23) in all county-level regions. Then, according to the difference between the worst index value and the best index value, the corresponding score of the worst index value was determined, denoted as A_{jmin} ($A_{jmin} \geq 0$).

Finally, we used the range standardization Equations (14) and (15) to convert the positive and negative indicators into corresponding scores and eliminated the index units.

$$A_{ij} = A_{jmin} + \frac{(100 - A_{jmin})(X_{ij} - X_{jmin})}{X_{jmax} - X_{jmin}} \tag{14}$$

$$A_{ij} = A_{jmin} + \frac{(100 - A_{jmin})(X_{jmax} - X_{ij})}{X_{jmax} - X_{jmin}} \tag{15}$$

where A_{ij} is the score corresponding to j indicators in i region, X_{ij} is the index value of j indexes in i region, X_{jmax} and X_{jmin} are the best index value and the worst value of j indexes in the study area.

(4) The econometric model of ALI

According to the general method of multivariate analysis, the measurement model of ALI can be listed:

$$\mathrm{ALI} = \sum_{1}^{j} A_j W_j \tag{16}$$

where A_j and W_j are the scores and weights corresponding to the index X_j. Because A_j is a constant between 0–100 and $\sum_{1}^{j} W_j = 1$, it can be seen that the ALI is between 0–100. The larger the ALI value, the higher the AL and vice versa. ALI is a relative number that reflects the relative size of the degree of adaptation to the geographical environment of the relocated population in different regions. Unlike ACI, ALI combines various factors such as household characteristics, social security and policy support and is an objective reflection of relocated households' adaptation status to the new environment. A comparative study of ACI and ALI using counties as a unit makes it easier to identify problems in the implementation of relocation policies.

3.4. Data Sources

(1) Field Investigation

From August to September 2019, our research team carried out fieldwork on the geographical environment adaptation of the resettled population in the study area. In selecting the sample for the survey, we used a stratified sampling method. Firstly, relocation sites were classified according to scale, with those with more than 100 households being medium and large settlements and those with less than 100 households being small settlements. Secondly, to ensure the sample size of the survey, we randomly selected the interviewed households mainly in the medium and large resettlement sites.

The survey objects were resettlement site administrators and resettled households. The survey for resettlement site administrators is to obtain the primary conditions of the emigration and settlement areas, including the relocation distance, ethnic customs, occupancy, the resources and environment of the out-migration area and the farming methods of farmers, the industrial support of the settlement area and the construction of basic public service facilities. The survey of resettled households is mainly to grasp the family population, income source, relocation willingness, cultural inheritance, concept change, employment situation, life security and dependence on agricultural production in the place of relocation. Finally, this study investigated administrators of 45 resettlement sites and 1008 resettled households. After excluding six invalid questionnaires, we obtained 1002 valid questionnaires. The spatial distribution of the valid survey sample is shown in Figure 2.

(2) Nujiang and Diqing Prefectures Poverty Alleviation and Development Management System

The poverty alleviation and development management system registers the primary household information of all local resettled poor households and other poor households registered from the previous year of registration. It covers geographic location, family population, income breakdown, causes of poverty, poverty alleviation status, assistance policies enjoyed and effectiveness, etc. The data update every October and the results are under check and clean of the national and Yunnan provincial data, so the relevant data are more accurate and have sound currency.

(3) Statistical Bulletin of National Economic and Social Development of Diqing Prefecture and Nujiang Prefecture in 2019.

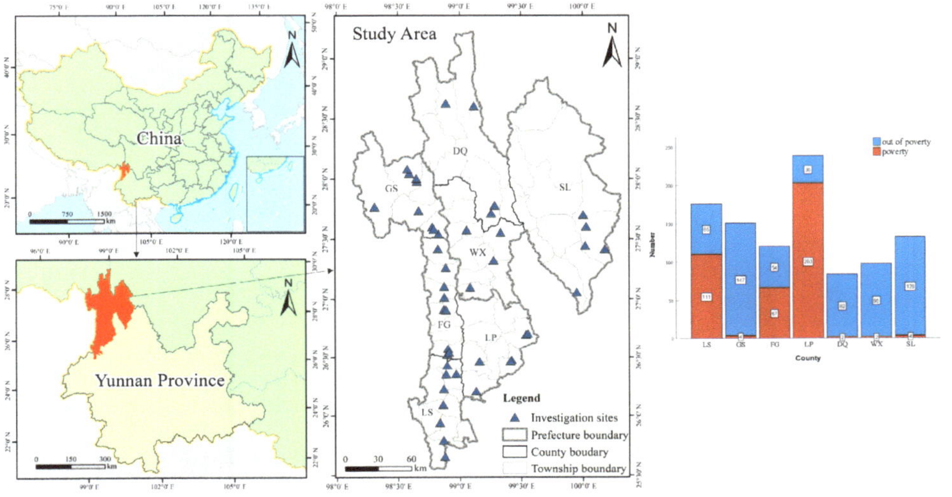

Figure 2. Location and basic condition of investigation sites Note: LS (Lushui City), GS (Gongshan County), FG (Fugong County), LP (Lanping County), DQ (Deqin County), WX (Weixi County), SL (Shangri-La City).

4. Results and Analysis

4.1. ACI

In the measurement of poverty elimination possibility, this study chose 15 family characteristic variables such as the proportion of population in compulsory education stage (ced), serious or long-term chronic patients (chr) as explanatory variables and chose the annual per capita income of rural households as the dependent variable to predict the future value, and calculated the probability that the annual per capita income of rural households in the next period is higher than the corresponding poverty line to judge the ability of resettled rural households to adapt to the new geographical environment. Yunnan Province used a net income per capita of CNY 4000 as the poverty line in 2020. Given that most of the resettled population lives in cities and towns and the living cost increases compared to the rural population, we used CNY 5000 as the poverty line (pl) to calculate the possibility of getting out of poverty. According to Formulas (1) to (12), we calculated the possibility of poverty elimination of 1002 resettled households in Eviews 9.0 software(HIS Global Inc., Irvine, CA, USA) and then summarized by county (city) and prefecture in the poverty-stricken areas of northwest Yunnan, as shown in Table 3.

Table 3. Geographical environment ACI of the resettled population in the study area.

Regions	ACI	Regions	ACI
Nujiang Prefecture	0.592	Diqing Prefecture	0.765
Gongshan County	0.461	Shangri-La City	0.896
Fugong County	0.476	Deqin County	0.741
Lushui City	0.585	Weixi County	0.674
Lanping County	0.657	Poverty-stricken areas of northwest Yunnan	0.660

The next step is to analyze the association between the possibility of poverty elimination of resettled population and family characteristic variables. We use the ACI as the dependent variable and the family characteristic variable as the explanatory variable and then use OLS to establish a multiple linear regression model of poverty elimination possibility:

$$AC = \beta_1 ced + \beta_2 chr + \beta_3 def + \beta_4 edu + \beta_5 hig + \beta_6 lntra + \beta_7 mla + \beta_8 non + \beta_9 pla + \beta_{10} sal + \beta_{11} sca + \beta_{12} wel + c \quad (17)$$

The results of regression analysis are shown in Table 4.

Table 4. Results of multiple linear regression analysis of ACI.

Variables	ced	chr	def	edu	hig	lntra
Coefficient (its t-value)	0.0023 (0.8784)	−0.0093 * (−8.7770)	−0.0497 * (11.2477)	0.0043 * (7.5935)	0.0243 * (6.2511)	0.0079 * (39.9053)
Variables	**mla**	**non**	**pla**	**sal**	**sca**	**wel**
Coefficient (its t-value)	0.0081 * (17.8760)	0.1688 * (58.9680)	0.0670 * (34.5145)	0.0189 * (12.3062)	−0.0039 * (−30.5103)	0.0284 * (30.6524)

Note: * indicates significant at the 1% level.

Among the explanatory variables, ced was not significant in the model, indicating that the possibility of poverty elimination has little to do with the proportion of the population in the compulsory education stage. The remaining family characteristic variables had a significant impact on AC, while non had the greatest impact on poverty elimination. Therefore, increasing income by out-migrant work is an important way to eliminate poverty. Sca, chr, def have a negative impact on AC. First, larger families often have a higher number of dependents and a smaller proportion of the labor force. This will lead to more labor constraints. Second, most families with disabled, seriously ill, or chronic patients have less labor force, higher medical expenses and lower per capita net income.

4.2. ALI

The AL of population to the geographical environment after relocation is affected by the AC of geographical environment, the implementation degree of relocation policy and other factors. We use the comprehensive index method to calculate the AL according to Equations (14)–(16). The calculation results are summarized by county (city) and prefecture, as shown in Table 5.

Table 5. Geographical environment adaptation level of resettled population in the study area.

Regions	ALI	Regions	ALI
Nujiang Prefecture	50.9	Diqing Prefecture	78.4
Gongshan County	53.1	Shangri-La City	86.5
Fugong County	43.4	Deqin County	76.0
Lushui City	65.2	Weixi County	63.8
Lanping County	44.7	Poverty-stricken areas of northwest Yunnan	61.2

4.3. AC and Its Regional Differentiation Pattern

4.3.1. Overall AC of Resettled Population

It can be seen from Table 4 that the geographical environment adaptive capacity of the resettled population in the poverty-stricken areas of northwest Yunnan is 0.660. This shows that the environment AC of the resettled population is weak. The probability that the expected per capita income is less than the poverty line (CNY 5000) is 34.0%. That is, there is a 34.0% risk of returning to poverty.

According to the field investigation and data analysis, the main reasons for the weak AC of the region's resettled population are as follows. First, the income level of the resettled family is low. The per capita income of the interviewed resettled households is only CNY

8629, which is not only lower than the rural per capita disposable income level of CNY 11,902 in Yunnan Province during the same period, but also a considerable number of resettled households have income that is on the edge of the poverty line. So, their ability to resist risks is poor. Second, the income structure is unreasonable, the proportion of wage income is low and the self-development ability of resettled households is insufficient. Third, the labor force quality is generally low and inherently vulnerable to environmental changes. The average years of education of the labor force in the resettled families were 4.7 years and the proportion of "uneducated or lower than primary school" was as high as 76.2%. Among the respondents, 37.7% could understand but could not speak Mandarin and 11.6% could not understand Mandarin at all. Fourth, the long-term regional occlusion has limited communication between the resettled population and the outside world. The labor force of the interviewed families accounted for 16.9% of the local workers and even fewer went out to work, accounting for only 6.5%. 76.6% of the labor force has been engaged in traditional agricultural production for a long time and has not undergone "training to adapt to the new environment". Fifth, the land transfer has not been kept up in time and the land operation income before the relocation has not been converted into the land property income after the relocation in time. More than 90% of the interviewed resettled households have no land transfer income and the average land transfer income accounts for only 0.2%. Sixth, the debts of some resettled households have lowered their real disposable income and weakened their AC to the environment. There are 22.5% of the interviewed households have debts. Thirty-two households have debts of CNY 50,000 to 100,000 accounting for 3.2%. Fourteen households have debts of more than CNY 100,000 accounting for 1.4% and the rest have debts below CNY 50,000.

4.3.2. Spatial Differentiation Pattern and Formation Mechanism of AC

At the prefecture level, the AC of the resettled population in Nujiang Prefecture was 0.592 and that in Diqing Prefecture was 0.765, with significant regional differentiations (Figure 3). It is mainly determined by factors such as policy arrangements, regional conditions and ethnic habits. As far as policy arrangements are concerned, Diqing Prefecture is a Tibetan area and enjoys the "three districts and three prefectures" poverty alleviation policy and the traditional support policies of Tibetan areas. In comparison, Nujiang Prefecture only enjoys the "three districts and three prefectures" poverty alleviation policy. Therefore, Diqing Prefecture is better than Nujiang Prefecture in terms of infrastructure and people's livelihood security. In addition, these two prefectures have different time schedules for poverty elimination and different levels of work progress, which also cause differences in AC. By the time of investigation, all three counties and cities in Diqing Prefecture had been lifted out of poverty. In contrast, only Gongshan County has achieved poverty elimination in Nujiang Prefecture. Lushui City, Fugong County and Lanping County plan to be lifted out of poverty by the end of 2020. In terms of regional conditions, Diqing also has a conspicuous advantage. The 214 National Road on the Yunnan-Tibet line crosses Diqing Prefecture and Shangri-La Airport has been in operation since 1999. In contrast, by 2020, the Nujiang Prefecture is still a rare "four noes" (no airports, railways, highways and inland waterways) area in China. The backward traffic causes regional blockages and the closure of people's minds. Furthermore, thanks to the integration of tourism areas with Lijiang City, Diqing Prefecture received 22.02 million tourists in 2019 and achieved tourism revenue of CNY 26.6 billion. Part of the resettled population in Diqing Prefecture is directly involved in tourism and their AC to the environment has been improved. Although Nujiang Prefecture has good tourism resource endowments, its tourism industry is far behind. The scale of the industry is about one-fifth of that of Diqing Prefecture and the participation of ordinary people is also low. As far as ethnic habits are concerned, the Tibetans in Diqing Prefecture are nomads. They are accustomed to regional migration and have strong AC to the geographical environment of the population. However, the Lisu, Nu and Dulong peoples of Nujiang Prefecture have lived in the mountains for generations and have little communication with the outside world. They are very sensitive to the change of geographical environment and their AC to the new environment is much lower.

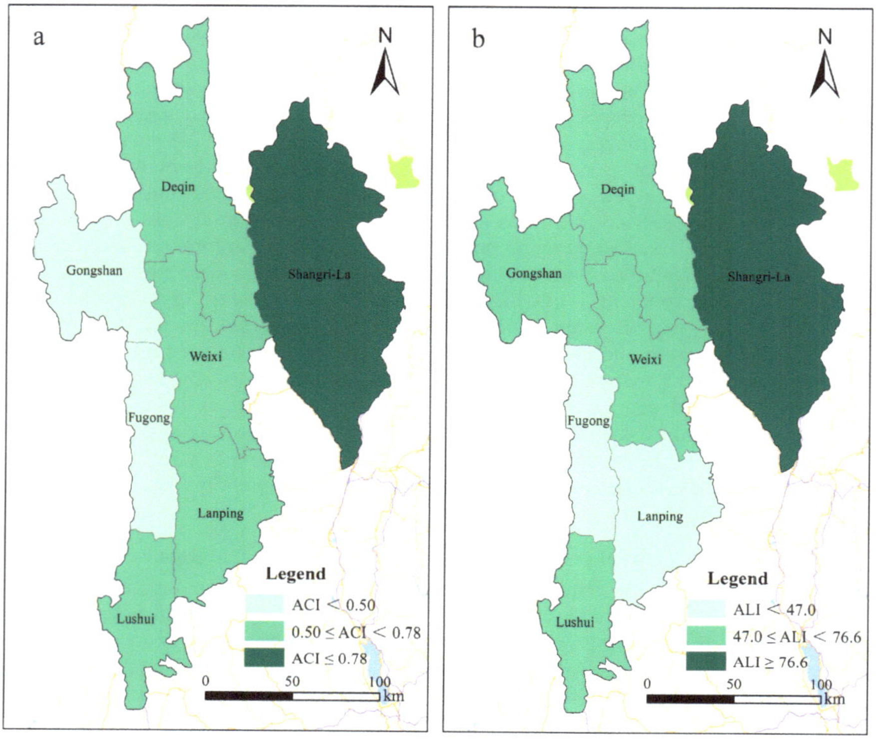

Figure 3. Spatial differentiation of ACI (**a**) and ALI (**b**).

The AC differences to the geographical environment of the resettled population were more significant at the county level. Shangri-La City had the largest AC, followed by Deqin County, Weixi County, Lanping County, Lushui City, Fugong County and Gongshan County. The formation mechanism of county-level differences in AC was almost the same as that at the prefecture-level above, but to different degrees. For example, the degree of occlusion in Gongshan County was much more serious than in other counties and cities. Before the Dulong River Tunnel opened in 2015, Dulong River Township in Gongshan County was isolated from the outside world for half a year due to heavy snow. Before the beautiful highway project in Nujiang Prefecture was completed in October 2019, it would take 12 h to drive from Gongshan County to the prefecture for a distance of 260 km. The closure of geographical space seriously restricts the enlightenment of the population's ideas and concepts, which is the main reason for the relatively weak ability of the local resettled population to adapt to the geographical environment.

4.4. AL and Its Regional Differentiation Pattern

4.4.1. Overall AL of Resettled Population

The geographical environment AL of the resettled population in the poverty-stricken areas of northwest Yunnan is 61.2. There is a very tight time frame to complete the site selection and construction of over 100 resettlement sites and the identification and relocation of 135 thousand of people from 2015 to 2019. Therefore, when implementing the relocation policy, governments at all levels focus on relocation organizations, such as relocation mobilization, settlement construction, relocation compensation, old house demolition, etc. The government's core task is to "immigrant out from the bad environment", but it lacks systematic planning for the employment and security of the resettled population and the disposal of their original means of production and pays relatively little attention to "obtaining stability" and "achieving prosperity". This also caused more than half of the resettled population to worry about their future life and have a low AL.

4.4.2. Spatial Differentiation Pattern and Formation Mechanism of AL

The AL of the resettled population in Nujiang Prefecture (50.9) was significantly lower than that in Diqing Prefecture (78.4), as can be seen in Figure 3. This is mainly because there are gaps in the following indicators: (1) In terms of "immigrant out of the bad environment", the completion of the relocation plan in Nujiang Prefecture is lower than that in Diqing Prefecture, while the proportion of households who have broken the contract and regretted moving out is much higher. By the time of the investigation, the relocation of Diqing Prefecture had almost ended and the contradictions and problems in the relocation had basically been effectively resolved. On the contrary, due to the late planning of poverty elimination and other special reasons in Nujiang Prefecture, its problem of "immigrant out of the bad environment" is still relatively prominent. The relocation in Nujiang Prefecture was still in progress and the relocation occupancy rate was less than 85%. Concerned about their future lives, about 6–7% of the population who have signed relocation agreements have decided to break the contract and refuse to relocate. 28.3% of the resettled households said they regretted their relocation. More than half of the resettled households indicated that they often returned to their original places of residence to facilitate agricultural production. (2) In terms of "obtaining stability", the per capita income of resettled households in Nujiang Prefecture was CNY 7520, while that in Diqing Prefecture was CNY 10,618, which is 41.2% higher than the former. The proportion of non-agricultural income of resettled households in Diqing was 82.7%, which is also 11.2% higher than that in Nujiang. At the same time, thanks to more policy dividends, the relocation households in Diqing Prefecture are more guaranteed. The coverage rate of public welfare posts, the proportion of low-income households and the coverage rate of security coverage in Diqing Prefecture are higher than those in Nujiang Prefecture. (3) In terms of "achieving prosperity", Diqing has better industrial support capacity and a more flexible employment pattern. In 2019, the per capita non-agricultural output value of the resident population in Diqing Prefecture was CNY 60,917.4, while that in Nujiang Prefecture was only CNY 29,954.8. The former is more than twice that of the latter. In terms of flexible employment, the number of out-migrant workers in the two prefectures is relatively small. But the proportion of the local labor force in Diqing prefecture is 25.8%, which is significantly higher than that in Nujiang prefecture, which is 12.4%.

At the county level, there are also significant differences in the actual adaptation levels of the resettled population. The ALI from high to low is Shangri-La City, Deqin County, Lushui City, Weixi County, Gongshan County, Lanping County and Fugong County. The formation mechanism of differentiations at the county level is almost the same as that at the prefecture level, except that some local factors are superimposed. For example, the Tibetan population in Deqin County is the largest. After relocation, there is almost no need for a transition period for ethnic and cultural integration and it is logically easy to adapt to the environment. There are many Christian believers in Fugong County. They are reluctant to accept government help and resist relocation, which has seriously affected the relocation progress and resulted in a low AL.

4.5. The Relationship between AC and AL

AC is an inherent determinant of AL. In theory, the two will show consistency, that is, if AC is weak, AL is also low. Through quantitative analysis, it was found that the linear correlation coefficient of the two indices was 0.833, indicating that there was a high positive correlation between the two indices, which was statistically significant. However, under the disturbance of external factors such as policies and national culture, the relationship between the two in some regions may also deviate from the overall trend. The AC and AL were divided into three grades with $\overline{K} \pm \delta_K$ as the classification mark. The AC and AL of the resettled population are consistent in Fugong County, Lushui City, Deqin County, Weixi County and Shangri-La City, while the two indicators of Gongshan County and Lanping County deviate from the overall trend: the AC of the resettled population in Gongshan County is "weak", but the AL is "medium", while Lanping County is the opposite, as shown in Figure 4.

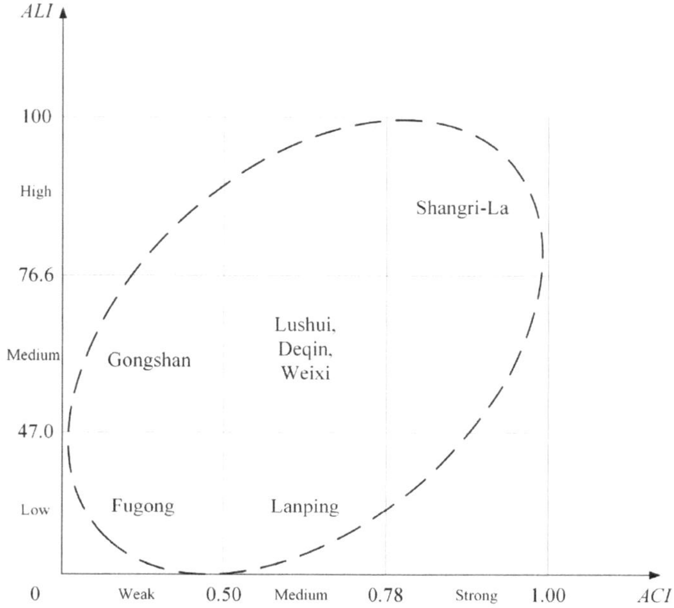

Figure 4. Consistency and difference of ACI and ALI. Notes: ($\overline{\text{ACI}} + \delta_{\text{ACI}} = 0.782, \overline{\text{ACI}} - \delta_{\text{ACI}} = 0.500$; $\overline{\text{ALI}} + \delta_{\text{ALI}} = 76.6$, $\overline{\text{ALI}} + \delta_{\text{ALI}} = 47.0$).

The AC of the resettled population in Gongshan County is weak, but the AL is medium. This is mainly because the implementation effect of the relocation policy is better, making up for the lack of AC of the resettled population to a certain extent. Gongshan County is the only county that took the lead in alleviating poverty in the poverty elimination plan of Nujiang Prefecture. The poverty alleviation work was carried out early and vigorously. Coupled with favorable factors such as a small population and light relocation tasks, the completion of relocation work was significantly higher than that of other counties and cities in the same prefecture. At the same time, Gongshan County has implemented the PAR policy more flexibly, with fewer problems and contradictions accumulated during the relocation process. For example, according to national policy, the per capita housing of resettled households cannot exceed 20 square meters. In this way, a 40-square-meter, one-bedroom house designed for a two-person family is unsuitable for special families such as father–daughter, mother—son, brother–sister and a house with a maximum of 140 square meters is also not suitable for a family with a particular large population. Gongshan County has effectively resolved the above-mentioned family's reluctance to relocate by building single-person apartments in some resettlement sites. In addition, the poverty alleviation of the Dulong people has received national attention, which has brought pressure to Gongshan County and favorable policies. It has effectively promoted the poverty alleviation work of the whole county and logically improved the actual AL of the resettled population.

The situation in Lanping County is much more complicated. Lanping is located in the east of Biluoxueshan Mountain, belonging to the Dali Cultural Circle. Its lead-zinc mines are world-famous and there are a large number of immigrants, so its degree of openness is relatively much higher. The overall quality and civilized degree of the resettled population in Lanping County are relatively high and the environment AC is also strong. The reason for the low AL of the resettled population to the geographical environment is that the relocation process is slow, the relocation work has not been completed at the beginning of 2020 and various contradictions and problems accumulated in the relocation process have not been effectively resolved. Second, the relocation is large in scale and heavy in tasks. Lanping County is located in the core area of the "Three Parallel Rivers" area, with complex natural and geographical conditions. It plans to relocate 44,000 people, accounting for 26% of the county's agricultural population and 45% of the prefecture's relocation tasks. It is the most important resettlement task in the county of the Nujiang Prefecture. Third, more than 70% of the resettled population in the county are resettled in the urban districts. The relocation distance is long and the living environment varies greatly, which increases the uncertainty of the future life of the resettled population and inevitably increases the difficulty of relocation. Fourth, the county's hydropower resettlement and PAR policies are not precisely connected. Some of the original hydropower resettled people included in the relocation plan refused to relocate because they thought they could not enjoy the relocation policy fairly.

5. Conclusions and Policy Implications

AL and AC are interrelated but distinctly different concepts, with the former indicating the objective state of adaptation and the latter reflecting the subjective adaptive capacity of relocated people to the new environment. Unlike sociological studies on the impact of individual factors such as climate, infrastructure and public services on the adaptation of the relocated population [55–58], this study provides a comprehensive evaluation and analysis of the relocated population's adaptive capacity and adaptation level to the new environment and their geographical differentiation based on a geographical perspective and the theory of man–land relations.

Through quantitative evaluation, it was found that the AC of the resettled population to the new environment was 0.660 and the AL was 61.2 in the poverty-stricken areas of northwest Yunnan, indicating that the resettled population in this area has obvious geographical environment adaptation obstacles and a high risk of returning to poverty. The geographical environment AC of the resettled population has significant regional differences. Diqing prefecture with better regional conditions, earlier time to eliminate poverty and lighter relocation task is better than Nujiang prefecture in terms of AC and AL. At the county and city level, Shangri-La City is in the first echelon of AC, Deqin County, Lanping County, Weixi County and Lushui City are in the second echelon and Fugong County and Gongshan County are in the third echelon. The three echelons of AL are almost the same, the difference is that the positions of Lanping County and Gongshan County have been reversed.

In general, out-migrant work, public welfare jobs, the size of the family labor force, the disabled and the sick and the population above high school are the key factors affecting the environment AC of the resettled population. Long-term regional occlusion and low population quality are the deep-seated reasons for the weak AC. The AL is the result of superimposing policy effects on the basis of AC. Next, it is necessary to consolidate the achievements of poverty alleviation and prevent the return of poverty from falling into a vicious circle. It is necessary to focus on Gongshan, Fugong, Lanping and other areas, make comprehensive plans and formulate long-term measures to promote the integration of the resettled population into the new geographical environment. In the short term, the first is to encourage the labor force to go out to work through skills training, material incentives, etc. The second is to continue to improve the industrial facilities of the relocation and resettlement sites and promote the employment of some laborers nearby. The third is to maintain the existing number of public welfare posts and strengthen the management of public welfare posts to solve the employment problem of the weak labor force. The fourth is to introduce social forces while the government is leading, revitalizing the contracted land, mountain forest land and homestead resources in the resettled area and finally increasing the property income of the resettled population. As a long-term measure, it is essential to concentrate on enhancing public services in the area of relocation, as well as the quality of the service level of education, health care, pensions and minimum living security. At the same time, it insists on carrying out the project of improving the overall quality of the resettled population. The resettled population will be encouraged to change their bad habits, adjust their ideas and generally improve their quality through ongoing Mandarin training, literacy training, home life training, meaningful cultural integration and home environment evaluation activities. We must acknowledge that good environmental adaptation is challenging to achieve overnight. It takes a generation or more. For example, while the "out-migrant work" is a decisive factor in the ACI as mentioned above, the bottleneck in the growth of the migrant population in Northwest Yunnan is due to the problems of primary education and skills training, which will take a decade or even a generation to solve. Therefore, it is necessary to scientifically compile and earnestly implement the follow-up development plan of the resettled population and do a good job in the three aspects of employment income increase, public service and bottom guarantee so that the resettled population can adapt to the new geographical environment and lifestyle as soon as possible.

However, there are still some limitations to this study. Firstly, we measured the geographic adaptation of the relocated population based on household attribute data in 2019 and 2020, with a short period and little change in farm households. Although the 2019 data are field research, the focus is on relocated farm households in medium and large resettlement sites. More attention should be paid to farm households in small relocated communities. Secondly, due to COVID-19, our team was unable to collect some data in 2020 by field investigation but has to rely on the local government to update them, which may impact the accuracy of the ACI and ALI. In the post-epidemic period, optimizing the sample structure and continuously following up on research and analysis are necessary.

Author Contributions: L.Q.: Conceptualization, original draft preparation, funding acquisition, designing the analytical framework; W.X.: investigation, review and editing, coordinating the research team, visualization; W.G.: data curation, validation, software, supervision. All authors have read and agreed to the published version of the manuscript.

Funding: This research was funded by The National Social Science Fund of China (Grant No. 18BMZ127).

Institutional Review Board Statement: Not applicable.

Informed Consent Statement: Not applicable.

Data Availability Statement: Not applicable.

Conflicts of Interest: The authors declare no conflict of interest.

References

1. Yang, Y.; de Sherbinin, A.; Liu, Y. China's poverty alleviation resettlement: Progress, problems and solutions. *Habitat Int.* **2020**, *98*, 102135. [CrossRef]
2. Wang, H.; Zhao, Q.; Bai, Y.; Zhang, L.; Yu, X. Poverty and Subjective Poverty in Rural China. *Soc. Indic. Res.* **2020**, *150*, 219–242. [CrossRef]
3. Fosu, A.K. Growth, inequality, and poverty reduction in developing countries: Recent global evidence. *Res. Econ.* **2017**, *71*, 306–336. [CrossRef]
4. Long, H.; Liu, Y. Rural restructuring in China. *J. Rural Stud.* **2016**, *47*, 387–391. [CrossRef]
5. Zhou, Y.; Li, Y.; Liu, Y. The nexus between regional eco-environmental degradation and rural impoverishment in China. *Habitat Int.* **2020**, *96*, 102086. [CrossRef]
6. Deng, Q.; Li, E.; Yang, Y. Politics, policies and rural poverty alleviation outcomes: Evidence from Lankao County, China. *Habitat Int.* **2022**, *127*, 102631. [CrossRef]

7. Guo, Y.; Liu, Y. Poverty alleviation through land assetization and its implications for rural revitalization in China. *Land Use Policy* **2021**, *105*, 105418. [CrossRef]
8. Fang, Y.; Zhang, F. The future path to China's poverty reduction—Dynamic decomposition analysis with the evolution of China's poverty reduction policies. *Soc. Indic. Res.* **2021**, *158*, 507–538. [CrossRef]
9. Sun, H.; Li, X.; Li, W.; Feng, J. Differences and Influencing Factors of Relative Poverty of Urban and Rural Residents in China Based on the Survey of 31 Provinces and Cities. *Int. J. Environ. Res. Public Health* **2022**, *19*, 9015. [CrossRef]
10. Liu, Y.; Guo, Y.; Zhou, Y. Poverty alleviation in rural China: Policy changes, future challenges and policy implications. *China Agric. Econ. Rev.* **2018**, *10*, 241–259. [CrossRef]
11. Leng, G.-X.; Feng, X.-L.; Qiu, H.-G. Income effects of poverty alleviation relocation program on rural farmers in China. *J. Integr. Agric.* **2021**, *20*, 891–904. [CrossRef]
12. Cernea, M.M. *The Economics of Involuntary Resettlement: Questions and Challenges*; World Bank Publications: Washington, DC, USA, 1999.
13. Li, X.; Yang, Y.; Liu, Y. Research progress in man-land relationship evolution and its resource-environment base in China. *J. Geogr. Sci.* **2017**, *27*, 899–924. [CrossRef]
14. Janssen, M.A.; Schoon, M.L.; Ke, W.; Börner, K. Scholarly networks on resilience, vulnerability and adaptation within the human dimensions of global environmental change. *Glob. Environ. Chang.* **2006**, *16*, 240–252. [CrossRef]
15. Shi, P.; Wang, J.; Chen, J. The future of human-environment interaction research in geography: Lessons from the 6th Open Meeting of IHDP. *Acta Geogr. Sin.* **2006**, *61*, 125.
16. Dadao, L. Theoretical studies of man-land system as the core of geographical science. *Geogr. Res.* **2002**, *21*, 135–145.
17. Fan, J. "Territorial system of human-environment interaction": A theoretical cornerstone for comprehensive research on for-mation and evolution of the geographical pattern. *Acta Geogr. Sin.* **2018**, *73*, 597–607.
18. Liu, S.; Ma, L.; Yao, Y.; Cui, X. Man-land relationship based on the spatial coupling of population and residential land–A case study of Yuzhong County in Longzhong Loess Hilly Region, China. *Land Use Policy* **2022**, *116*, 106059. [CrossRef]
19. Zhu, Z.; Kong, X.; Li, Y. Identifying the Static and Dynamic Relationships Between Rural Population and Settlements in Jiangsu Province, China. *Chin. Geogr. Sci.* **2020**, *30*, 810–823. [CrossRef]
20. Kitano, H. Systems Biology: A Brief Overview. *Science* **2002**, *295*, 1662–1664. [CrossRef]
21. Steward, J.H. *Theory of Culture Change: The Methodology of Multilinear Evolution*; University of Illinois Press: Champaign, IL, USA, 1972.
22. Tompkins, E.L.; Adger, W.N. Defining response capacity to enhance climate change policy. *Environ. Sci. Policy* **2005**, *8*, 562–571. [CrossRef]
23. Wall, E.; Marzall, K. Adaptive capacity for climate change in Canadian rural communities. *Local Environ.* **2006**, *11*, 373–397. [CrossRef]
24. Truelove, H.B.; Carrico, A.R.; Thabrew, L. A socio-psychological model for analyzing climate change adaptation: A case study of Sri Lankan paddy farmers. *Glob. Environ. Chang.* **2015**, *31*, 85–97. [CrossRef]
25. Nguyen, K.-A.; Liou, Y.-A.; Terry, J.P. Vulnerability of Vietnam to typhoons: A spatial assessment based on hazards, exposure and adaptive capacity. *Sci. Total Environ.* **2019**, *682*, 31–46. [CrossRef] [PubMed]
26. Adger, W.N. *Social Aspects of Adaptive Capacity. Climate Change, Adaptive Capacity and Development*; Imperial College Press: London, UK, 2003; pp. 29–49.
27. Cui, S.; Li, X.; Li, Y.; Li, F.; Huang, J. Review on adaptation in the perspective of global change. *Prog. Geogr.* **2011**, *30*, 1088–1098.
28. Zhou, L.; Li, H. Social adaptation, political trust and satisfaction of relocation policy-Based on the survey of relocated farmers in the concentrated contiguous destitute areas in Hunan Province. *Theory Pract. Financ. Econ.* **2020**, *41*, 86–93.
29. Zeng, L. Research on the Interaction between Government and Farmers' Professional Cooperatives in Poverty Governance—Taking H County in Guizhou Province as an Example. Bachelor's Thesis, Guizhou University of Finance and Economics, Guiyang, China, 2019.
30. Xiang, F.; Chen, X.; Wang, Y. The Practice of the Reconstruction of Migration Multiple Space in Relocation Poverty Alleviation: Based on Dejiang County Cross-regional Migration Research. *J. Huaihua Univ.* **2019**, *38*, 67–71.
31. Ma, L.; Chen, Q. Management relationship and optimization of the poverty-alleviation management of the immigrant resettlement community. *J. Yunnan Univ. Soc. Sci. Ed.* **2019**, *18*, 110–117.
32. Lyv, C. Study on the Coordinated Development Path of Poverty Alleviation Relocation and Citizenization of Relocated Pop-ulation in Guangxi. Bachelor's Thesis, Nanning Normal University, Nanning, China, 2019.
33. Pan, B.; Huang, Z.; Teng, F. Continued Efforts Made after Relocation for Poverty Alleviation—Experience and Implications of the "New Citizen" Plan of Qianxinan Prefecture of Guizhou Province. *Macroecon. Manag.* **2021**, *5*, 84–90.
34. Obokata, R.; Veronis, L.; McLeman, R. Empirical research on international environmental migration: A systematic review. *Popul. Environ.* **2014**, *36*, 111–135. [CrossRef]
35. Roland, H.B.; Curtis, K.J. The differential influence of geographic isolation on environmental migration: A study of internal migration amidst degrading conditions in the central Pacific. *Popul. Environ.* **2020**, *42*, 161–182. [CrossRef]
36. Dehcheshmeh, M.M.; Ghaedi, S. Climate Change and Ecological Migration: A Study of Villages in the Province of Khuzestan, Iran. *Environ. Res. Eng. Manag.* **2020**, *76*, 6–19. [CrossRef]
37. Llorca-Rodríguez, C.M.; Casas-Jurado, A.C.; García-Fernández, R.M. Tourism and poverty alleviation: An empirical analysis using panel data on Peru's departments. *Int. J. Tour. Res.* **2017**, *19*, 746–756. [CrossRef]

38. Wang, W.; Ren, Q.; Yu, J. Impact of the ecological resettlement program on participating decision and poverty reduction in southern Shaanxi, China. *For. Policy Econ.* **2018**, *95*, 1–9. [CrossRef]
39. Qiu, H.; Leng, G.; Feng, X.; Yang, S. Effects of the poverty alleviation relocation program on diet quality among low-income households. *China Agric. Econ. Rev.* **2020**, *13*, 397–417. [CrossRef]
40. Liu, M.; Feng, X.; Wang, S. Study on Poverty Vulnerability of the Poor Relocated Households. *Rural Econ.* **2019**, *3*, 64–72.
41. Ning, J.; Yin, H.; Wang, S.; Wang, Q. Does poverty alleviation relocation reduce poverty vulnerability: PSM-DID analysis based on the quasi-experimental study of the poverty alleviation relocation from 16 counties in 8 provinces. *China Popul. Resour. Environ.* **2018**, *28*, 20–28.
42. Hu, W.; Xie, Y.; Yan, S.; Zhou, X.; Li, C. The Reshaping of Neighboring Social Networks after Poverty Alleviation Relocation in Rural China: A Two-Year Observation. *Sustainability* **2022**, *14*, 4607. [CrossRef]
43. Liu, M.; Rao, D.; Yang, L.; Min, Q. Subsidy, training or material supply? The impact path of eco-compensation method on farmers' livelihood assets. *J. Environ. Manag.* **2021**, *287*, 112339. [CrossRef]
44. Liu, C.-L.; Xu, M.; Zhou, K.-Y.; Zeng, F.-C.; Liu, Z.-M. Coupling development mechanism and typical ways of targeted poverty alleviation and eco-compensation in China: Case analysis based on forestry. *J. Nat. Resour.* **2019**, *34*, 989–1002. [CrossRef]
45. Qin, B.; Yu, Y.; Ge, L.; Yang, L.; Guo, Y. Does Eco-Compensation Alleviate Rural Poverty? New Evidence from National Key Ecological Function Areas in China. *Int. J. Environ. Res. Public Health* **2022**, *19*, 10899. [CrossRef]
46. Maldonado, J.H.; del Pilar Moreno-Sánchez, R. Estimating the adaptive capacity of local communities at marine protected areas in Latin America: A practical approach. *Ecol. Soc.* **2014**, *19*, 16. [CrossRef]
47. Gillis, M.; Shoup, C.; Sicat, G.P. *World Development Report 2000/2001-Attacking Poverty*; The United Nations University World Institute for Development Economics Research (UNU-WIDER): Helsinki, Finland, 2001.
48. Vo, T.T. Household vulnerability as expected poverty in Vietnam. *World Dev. Perspect.* **2018**, *10*, 1–14. [CrossRef]
49. Gaiha, R.; Imai, K. *Measuring Vulnerability and Poverty Estimates for Rural India*; The United Nations University World Institute for Development Economics Research (UNU-WIDER): Helsinki, Finland, 2008.
50. Hoddinott, J.; Quisumbing, A. Methods for microeconometric risk and vulnerability assessment. In *Risk, Shocks, and Human Development*; Springer: Berlin/Heidelberg, Germany, 2010; pp. 62–100.
51. Zhou, J.; Zhang, Y.; Sha, Y.; Zhou, J.; Ren, H.; Shen, X.; Xu, H. The Effect of the "Triple-Layer Medical Security" Policy on the Vulnerability as Expected Poverty of Rural Households: Evidence from Yunnan Province, China. *Int. J. Environ. Res. Public Health* **2022**, *19*, 12936. [CrossRef] [PubMed]
52. Sun, H.; Li, X.; Li, W. The Nexus between Credit Channels and Farm Household Vulnerability to Poverty: Evidence from Rural China. *Sustainability* **2020**, *12*, 3019. [CrossRef]
53. Chaudhuri, S.; Jalan, J.; Suryahadi, A. *Assessing Household Vulnerability to Poverty from Cross-Sectional Data: A Methodology and Estimates from Indonesia*; Discussion paper no. 0102-52; Columbia University: New York, NY, USA, 2002.
54. Shapiro, S.S.; Wilk, M.B. An analysis of variance test for normality (complete samples). *Biometrika* **1965**, *52*, 591–611. [CrossRef]
55. Li, Y.; Gong, X.; Zhang, J.; Xiang, Z.; Liao, C. The Impact of Mobile Payment on Household Poverty Vulnerability: A Study Based on CHFS2017 in China. *Int. J. Environ. Res. Public Health* **2022**, *19*, 14001. [CrossRef]
56. Paavola, J. Livelihoods, vulnerability and adaptation to climate change in Morogoro, Tanzania. *Environ. Sci. Policy* **2008**, *11*, 642–654. [CrossRef]
57. Pandey, R.; Jha, S.K.; Alatalo, J.M.; Archie, K.M.; Gupta, A.K. Sustainable livelihood framework-based indicators for assessing climate change vulnerability and adaptation for Himalayan communities. *Ecol. Indic.* **2017**, *79*, 338–346. [CrossRef]
58. Liu, X.; Zeng, F. Poverty Reduction in China: Does the Agricultural Products Circulation Infrastructure Matter in Rural and Urban Areas? *Agriculture* **2022**, *12*, 1208. [CrossRef]

International Journal of
*Environmental Research
and Public Health*

MDPI

Article

The Effect of Stigma and Social Networks on Role Expectations among African Immigrants Living with HIV

Emmanuel F. Koku

Department of Sociology, Drexel University, 3201 Arch Street, Room 288, Philadelphia, PA 19104, USA; emmanuelkoku@drexel.edu

Abstract: This paper examines how African immigrants living with HIV negotiate and reconstruct their productive (i.e., educational and career opportunities), sexual, and reproductive identities. We used data from a mixed-methods study to explore how stigma and social networks in which participants were embedded shaped how they understood and negotiated their role expectations and responsibilities. Participants revealed how HIV not only changed their identities and limited their sex life, partner choices, and fundamental decisions about fertility and reproduction, but also presented them with the opportunity to reinvent/reshape their lives. Our analysis revealed that the cultural discourses about illness and HIV in participant's countries of origin, the acculturative and migratory stressors, and the competing influences and expectations from family and friends in their home and host countries shape their illness experience, and how they adjust to life with HIV. This paper builds on sociological understanding of illness experience as a social construct that shapes the ill person's identity, role, and function in society. Specifically, the paper contributes to discourses on how (i) participants' social location and identity (as transnational migrants adjusting to acculturative stressors associated with resettlement into a new country), (ii) cultural discourses about illness and HIV in their countries of origin, and (iii) embeddedness in transnational social networks influence health outcomes, including lived experiences with chronic illnesses and stigmatized conditions such as HIV.

Keywords: African immigrants; HIV stigma; social networks; sexual identity; reproductive decisions; role expectations; sub-Saharan Africa

Citation: Koku, E.F. The Effect of Stigma and Social Networks on Role Expectations among African Immigrants Living with HIV. *Int. J. Environ. Res. Public Health* **2024**, *21*, 782. https://doi.org/10.3390/ijerph21060782

Academic Editor: Paul B. Tchounwou

Received: 8 May 2024
Revised: 6 June 2024
Accepted: 11 June 2024
Published: 15 June 2024

1. Introduction

Fundamentally, illness is not only a biological condition, but also a socio-cultural phenomenon influencing an ill person's identity, role, and function in society. A rich line of sociological research has examined illness experience, the social forces shaping this experience, and how the ill individual copes and responds to illness [1–3]. Central to this theory is Bury's classic work "Chronic illness as a biographical disruption" [4], which examined the effect of chronic illness on a person's identity. Bury conceives of the onset of chronic illness as a disruptive event, fracturing a person's sense of self and identity, forcing them to either reconstruct a new identity or reinforce existing ones through the mobilization of resources to cope with the disruption.

Other scholars have critiqued, refined, and extended Bury's original conception of biographical disruption [5], by pointing out that chronic illnesses do not necessarily result in a disruption but the normalization of daily activities and lives. For example, people living with HIV or Ménière's disease experience shifts between disruption and normalization or what the authors called "biographical oscillation" in their lived experiences [5,6]. Such a process involves the integration of the new illness conditions into their pre-existing lives and selves [7]. Moreover, illnesses do not take place in a vacuum but are influenced and shaped by several processes, notably (a) the ill person's social demographic background—social class, aging, migratory history, and experience [8–10]—and (b) interactions and relationships with others.

Indeed, contemporary work has persistently linked social relationships to health outcomes [11–16]. As a social construct, illness experiences shape and are shaped by people's social networks. The onset of chronic illnesses in particular has been deemed a "network crisis" [17]. According to Pescosolido, such a crisis triggers the mobilization of (external) resources, "bringing individuals, their families, and wider social networks face to face with the character of their relationships in stark form, disrupting normal rules of reciprocity and mutual support" [18]. Thus, social networks have an enduring impact on the lived experiences, orientations, behaviors, and overall responses of the ill person to disruptive events, including living with HIV and other stigmatized conditions [19].

The continuing effort to understand biographical disruption and continuity is even more pertinent to the analysis of lived experiences of people living with HIV (PLWHA). With advances in antiretroviral therapy and treatment [20,21], HIV is now a manageable chronic condition, enabling people to live, renegotiate, and reconstruct their lives, despite the threats posed to their identity and life-chances by the illness [22–27]. In particular, how individuals living with chronic illnesses reimagine and renegotiate their lives and role expectations as women/men, spouses/partners, mothers/fathers, and productive members of society can further advance scholarly understanding of illness as a social construct that is subject to the vicissitudes of life course, cultural forces, and social network dynamics.

However, very few studies have examined these role expectations and transitions among those living with HIV, particularly among migrants whose lived experiences are shaped by their location at the intersection of the cultures of their home and host countries as well as the transnational networks in which they are embedded. Consequently, this paper examines (a) how African immigrants living with HIV negotiate and reconstruct their productive, sexual, and reproductive identities, and (b) how stigma and the structure and composition of the social networks in which they are embedded shape this identity negotiation and reconstruction.

2. Materials and Methods

2.1. Participant and Sample Selection

Data for this paper came from a larger study on HIV stigma and social networks among African immigrants in the Philadelphia region. In recent years, the region has become one of the main destinations of African immigrants, with an estimated population of 40 to 50,000 residing there [28]. More than half came from West African countries, with the largest concentrations from Liberia, Ghana, Nigeria, Sierra Leone, and Togo. African immigrants aged 18–65 years residing in the Philadelphia region were recruited between September 2016 and August 2019 to participate in a study examining the relationship between HIV stigma, social network characteristics, HIV risk, testing, and treatment adherence.

To be eligible for this study, participants had to be residents of the Philadelphia metropolitan region/area; aged 18 to 65 years; born in, self-identify with, or a citizen (at birth) of a sub-Saharan African country; able to read and speak English, French, or other local sub-Saharan African languages spoken within the African immigrant community; and must also be living with HIV. However, participants who were not from a sub-Saharan African region, those who were under 18 years of age, those who were non-residents of the Philadelphia region were excluded from this study.

For purposes of sampling, African immigrants could be considered a "hidden", "rare", and "elusive" [29] population partly because of the absence of a true sampling frame for the sub-population, and the documented difficulties in recruiting and engaging them in research [30,31], thereby compounding the challenges of selecting probability samples from the population [32]. Moreover, the practice of aggregating HIV surveillance data on African immigrants with that of African Americans makes it difficult to estimate the overall size and countries of origin of African immigrants living with HIV in many US jurisdictions [33–36]. Given the above considerations and challenges, this study used a purposive (non-probability) sampling method [37,38] to select participants.

2.2. Data Collection, Processing, and Analysis

This study employed a mixed-methods design involving quantitative and qualitative approaches. The quantitative component consisted of a computer-assisted personal interview (CAPI) with 265 respondents (n = 115 HIV-positive; n = 150 HIV-negative/unaware). The qualitative arm consisted of in-depth interviews with 48 participants (n = 20 HIV-positive; n = 23 HIV-negative/status-unaware) and three focus group sessions (one session with 5 HIV-positive participants; two sessions each with 8 participants who were HIV-negative/status unaware). Participants were purposively recruited from community settings (CBOs) and health centers. The primary author administered the CAPI and conducted all interviews and focus groups with the assistance of a trained research assistant and a community health nurse. These interviews and focus group discussions elicited the social meanings and construction of HIV/AIDS, HIV risk, and protective behaviors; the experiences of living with HIV(including responses to stigma, readjustments to life after diagnosis), treatment initiation, and adherence. A qualitative social network inventory was used to collect data on participant's network members (their socio-demographic characteristics, and their attitudes/behaviors and orientations towards PLWHA), the extent to which they experienced stigma or acceptance from network members, why they concealed/disclosed their status to specific network members, and how treatment and personal decisions related to their life with HIV varied by the characteristics of their social networks. The findings reported here were from the 25 HIV-positive participants who participated in the in-depth interviews and focus groups.

All interviews were audio-recorded and transcribed with any identifying details removed. Two graduate student research assistants (GRAs) checked each transcript for accuracy and, with the assistance of the primary research/author, separately reviewed and coded them [39]. The research team discussed the transcripts and resolved any discrepancies by consensus to enhance inter-coder reliability. To improve the trustworthiness of this study, we employed member checking strategies and external auditing, as recommended by [40]. Selected participants and community members with knowledge and experiences of living with HIV reviewed initial codes and findings and provided further suggestions that helped refine our interpretations. We employed thematic analysis [41] to link emerging themes to research questions and the analytical model. We used the software Dedoose 9.0 for data processing, coding, and analysis [42]. Those who completed this study received USD 35 in compensation in cash/gift cards. Ethical approval for this study was obtained from Drexel University and the Philadelphia Department of Public Health. To preserve anonymity, the names of study participants were replaced with pseudonyms assigned by the primary author/principal investigator.

3. Results

3.1. Background Characteristics of Participants

Table 1 presents the socio-demographic description of participants. Most were in their mid-30 s (range: 26–55 years) and were either married or in relationship. All (except 4) have children, and close to half (13 out of 25) do not plan to have any more. Almost all participants had attained at least a high school level of education and were also employed, full- or part-time. The average household income (when stated) was USD 30,000 per annum. Most had been in the US for about 10 to 15 years and can speak/understand English, although a few French speakers required interpreters to help them complete the interviews. All participants had families in sub-Saharan Africa, whom they routinely contacted or met in person during periodic visits. Some also had family members in the US and maintained active ties with them and other members of the broader African immigrant community. Almost all participants self-identified as heterosexuals, had been living with HIV for approximately 8 to 10 years, were on antiretroviral therapy, and reported undetectable viral loads.

Table 1. Socio-demographic characteristics of HIV-positive participants (N = 25).

	Men	Women	Total
Number of Participants	**10**	**15**	**25**
Region of Birth			
Southern Africa	0	3	3
West Africa	5	8	13
Central Africa	3	2	5
East Africa	2	2	4
Sexual Orientation			
Heterosexual (Straight)	8	15	23
Homosexual (Gay)	2	0	2
Number of Children			
No Children	1	3	4
1 Child	6	4	10
2 to 3 Children	2	5	7
4+ Children	1	3	4
Desire for More Children?			
Yes	6	2	8
No	2	11	13
Maybe	2	2	4
Marital Status			
Married/Domestic Partnership	4	7	11
Divorced/Separated/Widowed	2	3	5
Single (Never Married)	4	5	9
Highest Level of Education			
No Schooling Completed	1	1	2
Primary/High School	3	2	5
Some College/Associate Degree	3	7	10
Bachelor's Degree	1	4	5
Post-Graduate Degree	2	1	3
Employment Status			
Employed-Full/Part Time	4	8	12
Self-Employed	1	4	5
Not Employed	5	3	8
Religious Affiliation			
Protestant	2	6	8
Christian/Pentecostal	2	5	7
Catholic	1	2	3
Muslim	4	2	6
Traditional/No Affiliation	1	0	1
Age (Mean)	40	35	37.2
Years Living in USA (Mean)	11	10	10.5
Years Living with HIV(Mean)	6	8	7.5

3.2. Context of HIV Diagnosis

Our participants' experience and responses to HIV diagnosis and stigma need to be contextualized within their lives as transnational migrants. They arrived in the US via many routes: either as students, spouses, legal migrants, refugees, or undocumented. When asked to describe their current life conditions in the US, many were grateful for their success (in attaining education, health, and employment), but also reported varying acculturative stressors relating to poverty, housing, mounting family responsibilities, language barriers, and legal documentation concerns. In addition, African immigrants present with unique health needs: they have a disproportionately higher risk for HIV compared with US-born blacks and face stark barriers in access to HIV prevention, treatment, and other health services than do U.S.-born and other ethnic minorities residing in the country [33,36,43–47].

In the context of these stressors and challenges, the diagnosis of HIV became a major disruption in their migratory journey as they had to adjust to the reality of living with HIV, how/where they became infected, whether/how/to whom to disclose, and the implications of such a diagnosis on their present and future lives. Aside from disruptions associated with and resulting from diagnosis, regular clinic appointments, blood work, and the eventual initiation of antiretroviral therapy emerged as a secondary type of biographical disruption, as it required them to immerse themselves in and alter their schedules to meet treatment demands.

3.3. Adjustment to life with HIV: Stigma and Role Alteration

Regardless of the disruption from their diagnosis, interviewees tried to reestablish some sense of normalcy and continuity to their lives, a process that entailed a cognitive review of their current situation—their life goals, plans for family formation, employment, among others. To Bury, individuals tap into cognitive and material resources in their response to biographical disruption [4], including several restraints to cope with the impact of their diagnosis on themselves. Almost of all our respondents changed some salient aspects of their lives and gave up activities that may risk transmission of the virus, while they strived to forge new identities and restore and intensify existing ones through marriage, sexual relationships, parenting, employment, and other social/religious engagements.

3.3.1. African Discourses and Values: HIV, Family Responsibilities

Participants' responses to biographical disruption must be framed within their identities as Africans (with unique cultural values, beliefs, and practices), as well stigmatizing discourses that shape how they interpret their lived experiences with HIV. To be sure, African immigrants are differentiated by their national, linguistic, cultural, religious, and social backgrounds. Key elements of their culture and belief systems (e.g., social support) are protective from HIV risk, whereas others such as patriarchy, early marriage, fertility preferences, gender inequality, and concurrent sexual partnerships increase their vulnerability to HIV [48,49]. Within these cultures, HIV is framed by four predominant discourses: *mortality*, which sees HIV as a "death sentence"; *immorality*, which associates HIV with (sexual) promiscuity and deviance; *retribution*, which deems HIV as punishment for the contravention of religious edicts; and the discourse of *invisibility*, reflected in the generalized silence and discomfort about HIV as a taboo subject, often referenced with third-person pronouns such as "it", "thing", "this", or "the disease" [49–51]. Despite increased HIV knowledge and progress with stigma reduction programs in sub-Saharan Africa, these discourses continue to fuel negative attitudes towards HIV and PLWHA [52,53] in the region, survive through migration, and are reinforced through continuing contact by African immigrants with their countries of origin [48,54].

These discourses fueled stigma towards participants because of either a confirmed or suspected HIV status. The forms of stigma experienced varied, but they manifested mainly in the desire for physical and social distance by participants' network members and the wider African immigrant community. Some were judged and subjected to reprehensible gossip, while others lost friends and family because of their status. As a result, some participants anticipated stigma from kin and friends, though they were pleased (and, in some cases, pleasantly surprised) by the support they experienced after disclosure or breach of their statuses. All participants were vigilant about when/where/how they took their medications, while some traveled distances to see their HIV care providers and doctors. Their narratives also reflected high levels of internalized stigma, as they all had to cope, at various points, with the shame of having HIV.

These HIV-related discourses and experiences of stigma also take shape within the broader context of African cultural values and expectations about individual responsibilities to the welfare and sustenance of their families, communities and groups. African women and men are expected to fulfill specific role responsibilities through marriage and procreation to extend their lineage [55,56]. In many patrilineal societies for example, a man is considered a man only if he produces a child (particularly a male) to extend his lineage, while a woman is expected to marry, maintain a home, and bear children as a sign of respect and prestige not only to herself but also to her entire family [57]. In a similar vein, children are expected to undertake the necessary training (formal and informal education, apprenticeship) as they transition to adulthood to care for their own families, parents, and assume the mantle of leadership in their communities [58]. Any threat to the fulfillment of these expectations is a threat to their identity and "face" within their families and broader community networks [59,60]. As a result, participants negotiated their sexual relationships, decisions about whether to have children or not, responsibilities to their spouses and children, and other broader decisions about their lives in the context of these role expectations, while striving to avoid the stigma of living with HIV. One of these decisions relates to sexual relationships.

3.3.2. Negotiating Sexual Relationships

As men and women, sexual identity is one of the most intimate and salient aspects of one's identity that was not left unscarred by HIV. Participants who were not married or in a relationship at the time of diagnosis faced major challenges in initiating contact or engaging in sexual relationships due to stigma. For many, the decision to enter a relationship had to be weighed against the risk of disclosure and acceptance by their partners. Anella explained her dilemma: *"The last time, the doctor asked me 'how is your sex life'. I looked at that young man and asked myself, how do I answer?. He asked me 3 times. And he said, I have seen that you don't answer the question. But then he said he knows how I feel, but that you cannot punish yourself. So he encouraged me to go on a date. I told him I get dates, but I never wanted to go because I am afraid of stigma. I don't know how I would react if my partner does not accept me"* (Anella, a 46-year-old woman).

While Anella was interested in exploring and having intimate relationships, she was equally concerned about younger generations who were living with HIV and the longer-term impact it would have on their sexual lives: *"It has even made young girls or women not be intimate any longer. When I see the young ones, I wonder how they will live their life. They have to get married, get children. With stigma, this is difficult. How do you do this with a partner and you have to disclose. This woman in the [support] group told me 'this man is loving me, but I don't know what to do I am scared of the day I will tell him, I am afraid he will just leave me"*. In light of these restraints, other participants such as Tirida (a 38-year-old woman) became vigilant about when/how to negotiate disclosure, intimacy, and stigma: *"I got this boyfriend, did not want him to get it, this and that, I know. but I told him., oh my goodness, it was very frustrating. he didn't want to touch anything I touched... Oh my goodness! it took time for him to get it, that we can't just have sex like sex. I have to protect him"*.

To become involved in or maintain intimate relationships, some participants concealed their status from sexual partners while insisting on consistent condom use. Yaoko (a 47-year-old man), for example, did not disclose his status to his partner, because he did not feel "*close*" enough to reveal the secret, given the context of their relationship: *"I am here because I need papers. she marry me. I spend some night here. we get sex, but use condom. first she said no condom, but said i don't want no more children, so we use it. I don't tell her [that I have HIV], when I get my papers, is over. like a business"*. For a few, HIV infection signaled infidelity and the impending end of the marriage. Tirida stated: *"my relationship ended when I discovered that I had this (HIV) because I didn't know that I have it [from him] and when I had it, it made me realize... it made me terminate everything... a relationship that was built on lies"*. Other participants expected their partners to leave them following diagnosis and disclosure because becoming infected with HIV implied moral failure. Lamila (a 41-year-old woman), for instance, was deserted by her husband after diagnosis, although she was still torn between taking *"that risk to meet new people at her age"*, or *"just keep to my husband and convince him to come back and we live together"*.

Those who had or entered new relationships with serodiscordant partners required different role adjustments dictated by the need to protect and prevent exposure to HIV and other sexually transmitted infections. To maintain sexual fulfillment, some adopted several non-penetrative sexual practices, mutual masturbation, and intimate touching. Many, however, had to use condoms out of necessity to protect their partners (and themselves from secondary infections). For Karolina, it was the constraints around sexual intimacy and failure to experience what she defined as *"a real woman"* that depressed her: *"I miss sex. . .the normal sex, not condom sex, everything; with condom, not the same. . .like I am not a real woman."* (Karolina, 26-year-old woman). While some partners understood the necessity to engage in protected sex, others felt it deprived them from the pleasure and intimacy they desired, and sought pleasures elsewhere, usually with other seroconcordant partners, as Kanjobi (a 38-year-old man) explained: *"My woman friend—we meet when my woman travel. we don't know use condom. she is also married, but I think she also has it. We know we need to satisfy us, she does not like condom, and I also want to enjoy sex. . ."*.

3.3.3. Reproduction: A Dilemma

Negotiating protected or unprotected sex became even more challenging for those who want children and need to choose between the potential risk of HIV infection or fulfilment of fertility desires, leaving many participants to vacillate between two choices: to either have a child or not.

Decision to not have a child: The uncertainties about life with HIV, physical health, and concerns about the potential of transmitting the virus to their partner and unborn child led some participants to decide against having a child, contrary to societal and cultural expectations about reproduction. For instance, Kolifi (a 30-year-old man) has one child and would have loved to have more children, but he was petrified about exposing his wife and any other child to HIV; hence, he had to live what he calls "if only's" (regrets) over unfulfilled fertility desires. BoJonso (a 31-year-old woman) expressed fears of vertical transmission: *"Man, you know this stuff, you can give it. . ., I did not want to have any more kids—I put myself on birth control I don't want to put anyone in trouble"*. To Mansana (a 33-year-old woman), the dilemma was almost heartbreaking: *"I feel my HIV be is. . . big problem. The doctors tell my husband that we use condom. He like. . . like want children bad, and I not want him to get it. He want to do without condom. I refused then he start to use it"*. For BoJonso and Mansana, the availability of pre-exposure prophylaxis (PrEP) was a welcome option that could allow them to fulfill their fertility and sexual desires, while reducing the risk of HIV infection. But many participants were not aware of PrEP, and the few who did held inaccurate perceptions about its use and efficacy. Both BoJonso and Mansana discussed PrEP with their doctors; however, BoJonso was not willing to encourage her long-term boyfriend to use it, due to concerns about risk exposure: *"Yes, we discussed it with the doctor, but I can't ask him to take it. . ..maybe if he wants to take it. I think he is not interested. . .last time, he said he is ok, and doesn't want to discuss it. I also worry. If he forget to take it and get HIV and sick . . . so no more baby. . . we use condom"*. Mansana, on the other hand, was interested in and discussed PrEP with her husband extensively: *"Since he not like condom, I talk to doctor. She talk PrEP. . . to me and him* [my husband]. *But he refuse. . .say he cannot take medicine everyday. . . but we talk about it again . . . maybe he change mind"*.

Other participants such as Punda were not sure if anyone would accept or love them enough to have kids with them, so she decided not to have children: *"I mean due to the HIV, I don't know how it will work. hmm, you just feel like you know you can't, in my case I just feel like I can't have any friend any type of friend, relationship with anybody . . .—nothing is working for you, you're not gonna have kids- that's why I said I don't even know if I will. So, there's so many things. . . cause who's gonna go or like want to have sex with you if you have HIV and give you kids, you know? If you don't have money, you can't go to doctor to help have babies. . . Yeah, yeah you can do it but if you don't have money, no"* (Punda, a 34-year-old woman).

Decision to have a child: However, due to cultural considerations, other participants decided to have children, as a claim to normality and to deflect blame or stigma. In African contexts, certain identities such as that of a mother or father are so salient and culturally ingrained that a decision to not have a child raises suspicions about one's virility, fertility, and status as a respected member of the society. Thus, for some women and men living with HIV, having a child may be a way to avoid unwanted attention, mask, or divert attention from its related stigma [61,62]. For these participants, the prestige of continuing their family lineage, against the inherent stigma against infertility, was a strong motivator for having their own children, despite the fear of transmission. After years of refusal to get married or have children, Banito (a 41-year-old man) decided to throw in the towel. When probed, he explained: *"I need children, but I not trust if the woman can get it too. I was fearing... Mami [Mother] give me hard hard time, many questions she ask. I tell her I go to school, no time. One day she ask if I be a man, all ok 'down there'. I know I have to prove. If I no marry, get children, they think I like men* [as gay]. *With child, no question, I am man. I call him son... all ok... my brother!. Doctor* [Name withheld] *help big time"*.

As alluded to by Banito, almost all participants who were contemplating or concerned about having children discussed their plans with their providers and explored alternative reproductive options. Some participants such as Punda noted that they seriously considered in vitro fertilization (IVF) but were deterred by its cost, while others such as Erikus were grateful for partners who were willing to go on PrEP: *"I lucky... my woman is good...we want many babies* [laughs], *but I get HIV. She ok...no HIV, negative, nshalaa... we see doctor, she take medicine... we take together... so that help we get child now... nshalaa... she good woman..."*. For a few other respondents, the desire for children became so great that they separated from their existing discordant relationships (where they believed it was not possible to do so safely) in search for new partners.

For others, the need to secure the relationship with their partners was of paramount concern, as explained by Lila (a 31-year-old woman): *"Like my last child, husband forced that we have baby... he said he didn't care, and I want him to be for me, so we have her"*. Kanji (a 36-year-old woman) clarified the frustrations she was experiencing with her husband (who was HIV-negative) and his desire for more children. *"When we start, we said we get one child, it was ok, hmmm? He get one before we start, so ok? We get child, everyone happy, like we plan. Now he say he want one baby, every day, he say we get one more. I scare for baby that I give it to him too. Now he angry. I scare he get another woman"*.

Gay participants felt pressured to get married and conform to cultural expectations of masculinity and parenthood. Henrik (a 33-year-old gay man), for example, resisted repeated attempts by his family to set him up with a woman. To keep their families happy and be *"in-line"* with cultural expectations, some gay/bisexual PLWHA facing such pressures hid their status from family and potential partners, got married, lived on the "down-low", and had children. Explaining the basis of the pressure further, Henrik observed: *"our community is so steep!...I have a friend of mine, he's gay from [country-blinded] but he has to get married to a woman because he will never tell nobody that he like men or something like that... They will kill him."*

3.3.4. As a Parent (for Those with Children)

For participants with children, disclosure was an indirect indicator of past experiences and decisions they would rather want to keep secret from their children/family. Kabini (a 44-year-old man) was conflicted about if/when to disclose to his son: *"what can I tell my boy one day ...that Daddy was f**ing and not use condom...when I advise him do this and don't do that?"*. However, the degree of ambivalence felt by these participants depended on the degree of culpability they had for infection. While most of the men interviewed blamed themselves and (in a few cases their partners) for their risky sexual choices, the women on the other hand felt victimized by unfaithful partners and used disclosure to their children to explain and teach them lifelong lessons about sexual fidelity.

Ultimately, for most participants, disclosure/concealment became a duty to care and protect themselves and their kids from stigma and risky behaviors. To Susula, disclosure is important but timing matters: *"for me it is not good to hide it. if you hide it, you can be yourself. It is important for some people to know at the right time. Now I am 55. If God permits and I am 65, 70, I will call my children and tell them you know I have this for previous days. But I didn't tell you before because I don't know how you are going to react or how you feeling. so I have to tell you to protect yourself"* (Susula, a 55-year-old woman).

On the contrary, Erikus believed that it was not necessary to disclose. So long as he was in good health, it was better for his children to remain in the dark for their and his own peace of mind: "*I know I have to tell them. . .but it's not important, maybe one day. But I am doing good. I have good health, not sick. So, it's just like any other disease. If I tell them, they will think I am going to die. They will be worried about me. And I will be worried they will tell someone. . .so, I keep it to myself. . .better for me, better for them*" (Erikus, a 33-year-old man).

3.3.5. Productive Responsibilities

All participants reframed HIV diagnosis and the availability of treatment as a chance to reinvent their lives and give back to society. Mounting responsibilities from extended families abroad exerted added stressors on participants' adjustment and integration, demanding more of their attention. Fatubo (a 38-year-old woman) observed that: "*I have children, three children. Two girls, one boy. I taking care of first daughter [who] came here with husband and I living with them, taking care of their children. . . HIV is a big problem, but these bigger. HIV not the problem here*". As a result, many (re)-engaged in other productive activities (such as taking up education and other career opportunities) to fulfil family expectations and obligations, support extended family members within and outside the United States, and increase their social mobility while adjusting to life with HIV.

3.4. *Effect of Social Network and Cultural Contingencies*

These adjustments to "biographical disruptions" caused by HIV depend largely on the structure and composition of participants' transnational networks. In particular, a person's involvement and integration in community activities (as evidenced by regular attendance and visibility) increase their exposure to prevailing norms and attitudes. By the same token, integration into a transnational network of ties increases participants' awareness of cultural expectations around family lineage and procreation, an awareness that is reinforced by frequent contact with family members in their countries of origin. For participants such as Priestus (a 48-year-old man), the pressure to meet these expectations became so intense that he relented: "*my girlfriend here (negative will not have more children). I went home, my aunt arranged a girl for me, and we have a child . . .both my woman and my child are home and safe*".

Anelaka (a 31-year-old woman) went further: "*my mother wants grandchildren . . .she kept pressuring me. When I said I am not ready, she gets angry, and tries to get other people involved in my business, gives my number to men. . . eventually . . .you can't keep saying no to men. . .I pray for a good man" For these participants, as Beyeza-Kashesya aptly summarized: "The moral imperative may be to conform to the norms or risk being categorised as abnormal among one's social network.*" [63], as Priestus and Anelaka did.

Aside from integration, the composition of participants' networks (the knowledge and attitude of their network's members) has an important bearing on how they interpret and make sense of their cultural expectations, experiences of stigma, and its resultant role strain. Henrik has a network comprising people from different backgrounds, who accepted him without stigma, and exposed him to new and alternative means of resisting the pressure from his parents. Though his parents were not satisfied with his decision to not have children, he felt comfortable given the support he experienced from others in his network. Elaborating on the benefits of the diversity of his network, he explained:

"*Look on this list. oyibos* [slang for whites]: *HR28 and HR30 Whites; HR31, my girl from China; HR33 Indian; HR45 from South Africa—all from my work; they are good. They are different, they have no connection with my [African] people in the city, so I now relax, no rumors, gossips. We talk about HIV, they get tested too. Some of them know I have it [laughs]. I told them—HR45, HR31, HR28. some told me they have it. I know the stigma is here, but I don't feel it. You learn a lot more. But none of my African friends knows this. I only worry when I go shopping in the city. feel someone is looking at me. . . you know. Maybe is me. But I still have to be careful about who I hang around. Don't get me wrong. I love my people, I miss my community. . . . But being far away gives me options—who to invite, visit. I choose*" (Henrik, a 33-year-old gay man).

The fact that Henrik was not deeply integrated within his African network helped shield him from normative expectations regarding family formation. For others such as Anelaka, access to other participants who were similarly living with HIV moderated their experiences and provided them with alternative means of adjusting to their roles. She explained that the other PLWHA she met through an online support group provided her with a list of online dating sites for PLWHA, increasing her access to potential dates. To her, these homophilous ties (those who shared the same HIV status with her) were instrumental in helping ease her adjustment after diagnosis, and could also help her meet a suitable partner and start a family.

4. Discussion

This paper used data from a larger mixed-methods study to examine (1) how African immigrants living with HIV negotiated and reconstructed their productive, sexual, and reproductive identities, and (2) how stigma and the structure and composition of the social networks in which they are embedded shape this identity negotiation and reconstruction. We showed that participants' experience and responses to HIV diagnosis and stigma were shaped by their lives as transnational migrants. While some had increased their social mobility and educational attainment, others described their lives as characterized by precarity—unemployment/poverty, housing, mounting family responsibilities, language barriers, and legal documentation concerns—and other acculturative stressors.

In these contexts, diagnosis with HIV and the subsequent insertion into and initiation of treatment became a major disruption in their migratory journey as they had to adjust to the reality of living with HIV. Regardless of the disruption from their diagnosis, interviewees tried to reestablish some sense of normalcy and continuity to their lives, a process that entailed a cognitive review of their current situation—their life goals, plans for family formation, employment, among others. HIV not only affected them physically, in terms of their adjustments to the side-effects of their mediations, but it also shaped their sense of self—how they view themselves vis à vis others. These identity reappraisals were usually filtered through interactions with their social network ties, some of whom affirmed their identities (with support) while others stigmatized them.

In particular, participants observed that HIV has changed their self-identity and limited their sex life, partner choices, and fundamental decisions about fertility/reproduction in ways that were resonant with those observed among other groups [64–69]. For some PLWHA, having to come to and accept a decision to not have children was a rational response to (internalized) stigma, shame, and guilt about their reproductive potential, despite the promises of assisted and safer means of reproduction. For others, the decision to get married and/or have children was a strategic means of concealing their HIV status and/or deflecting attention from it [62]. As a form of biographical reinforcement [22], they were a means of maintaining their standing (or face) in the community and a source of renewed self-worth, conformity to social expectations around childbearing, and the continuity and reinforcement of parental identities held or expected before the disruption by HIV illness. For example, research has shown that women living with HIV often privilege and stress the primary importance of meeting their responsibilities as mothers and wives, regardless of the challenges posed by their HIV status, as some of our participants pointed out. They saw the disruption caused by an illness as an opportunity for biographical reinvention, and drew on resources, resilience, and other assets to transition to and maintain their new identities as non-smokers [70] or to reinvent their sense of self and future after the diagnosis of HIV [71].

To many partnered participants, HIV infection was the elephant in the room, the silent third-party that became more visible whenever their HIV-negative partner appeared to be seriously sick. The ever-present specter of risk increased their vigilance about the accidental exposure/transmission of HIV. At the same time, these adjustments were also a source of strength to many participants and demonstrated their love and support for each other and other network members (such as parents, children, intimate partners).

Those who remained in their relationships became more bonded over their shared desire to stay together and take care of their children or each other, regardless of their HIV status. A critical resource that participants leveraged was their social capital. While they recognized the social support available in their immigrant communities, they were also aware that these very communities reinforced stigmatizing discourses as well as normative expectations around family roles and responsibilities, and exerted pressure on PLWHA to come up with explanations about their role responsibilities and decisions, without disclosing their HIV status. To counter the stigma and expose themselves to countervailing norms, many PLWHA forged ties with network members outside the African immigrant community, including others living with HIV, for commiseration and further support. Almost all participants also turned or held to their religious faiths to cope with these changes and adjustments.

As a result of these challenges with reproductive choices and decisions about sexual intimacy, newer reproductive and HIV prevention technologies offered hope to PLWHA to meet their needs. Many participants have heard of the feasibility of assisted reproductive technologies (such as sperm washing, in vitro fertilization) but noted their inability to afford them. Other participants have also heard that PrEP (pre-exposure prophylaxis) and PEP (post-exposure prophylaxis) may offer new hopes for preventing HIV, especially among those who are in serodiscordant or other sexually risky relationships [72,73], but have little understanding of how it works, its availability, or how to overcome the stigma and other misconceptions surrounding its use [74–76]. Some participants pointed out that their doctors and other professionals became partners in helping them conceive and have children safely. In this vein, it is imperative to continue to provide education, information, and resources that address the reproductive and sexual needs of PLWHA in a culturally informed and respectful and receptive manner, using providers of appropriate age and gender, given the sensitivity of sex as a topic in African (immigrant) cultures [77,78].

5. Limitations and Strengths

There were limitations to this study, relating mainly to its design and recruitment of participants. This study used cross-sectional data collected purposively from a small sub-sample of African immigrants in the US. Thus, our findings may not be representative of the experiences of many other African immigrants in the country. Additionally, because we did not collect data from participants over time, we are unable to explore how their responses to role expectations and their reproductive desires changed with the entry and exit of friends, associates, and family members from their personal networks over their illness trajectory. However, some of our findings align with those reported in other studies on African immigrants and other groups [79–83]. Finally, given the sensitivity of HIV as a research subject, some community members were reluctant to participate in this study owing partly to documented concerns among African immigrants about participating in clinical studies [30,31]. Thus, we adopted a recruitment strategy (i.e., purposive sampling) to successfully reach participants in both community and clinical settings. However, participants recruited from clinical settings were likely those engaged in care, with different expectations and experiences of adjustment to life with HIV, introducing a possible recruitment bias.

Despite these limitations, our analysis contributes to theoretical work on biographical disruption and repair by showing that participants' responses and adjustments to life with HIV are shaped by experiences of stigma within their social networks. According to Pescosolido and Manago, stigma and its sequelae are "fundamentally tied to, negotiated in, and given meaning through the [crucible of] networked social interactions" [19]. An individual's social network—whom they know, whom they talk to and how often, and whom they confide in or disclose their HIV status to—are critical to shaping their adjustment to life with HIV and fulfillment of their role expectations and reproductive/productive desires.

Since 2019 when we concluded data collection for this project, the epidemiology of HIV has changed, with the wider availability of ARV(antiretroviral) medications and other treatment options, PrEP (pre-exposure prophylaxis), and PEP (post-exposure prophylaxis), leading to the gradual routinization of "treatment as prevention" or "undetectable = untransmittable" protocols [84]. These advances have increased the life expectancy of those living with HIV and their potential to live full and fulfilled lives, yet we know very little about how they have shaped the experiences and responses of PLWHA. As a result, it is imperative to collect more detailed data, using longitudinal and other appropriate designs, to illuminate how PLWHA adjust to the realities of living with a chronic condition, over their life course, in the context of changes in the epidemiology, treatment, and societal attitudes to HIV.

Our findings suggest the need for more support services for those living with HIV as they reconstruct their lives following diagnosis. Such services must include education about and the navigation to reproductive, sexual, and mental health resources to help participants cope with the challenges of living with HIV and attain and lead full productive lives. It is imperative to deliver these educational and related interventions in a culturally informed and respectful and receptive manner, using providers and health navigators of appropriate age and gender [85]. Above all, stigma reduction efforts must continue to stress the "normalcy" of HIV as a chronic condition to ensure wider accepting attitudes from the general public and participant's personal networks.

6. Conclusions

This paper explored how African immigrants living with HIV negotiated and 'repaired' the disruptions to their identities and role expectations and functions. Our analysis builds on and contributes to research that sees illness as a socio-cultural construct that not only disrupts an ill person's biography but also influences their identity and transforms their role expectations as women/men, spouses/partners, mothers/fathers, and productive members of society. These adjustments must be understood in the context of the ill person's cultural background and social location. For transnational migrants especially, the cultural discourses about illness and HIV in their countries of origin, acculturative stressors associated with their resettlement into a new country, and the competing influences and expectations from transnational social networks they maintain in their home and host countries differentiate and shape their illness trajectory, experience, and how they adjust to and negotiate the reality of life with HIV.

This paper contributes to the theoretical and scholarly discourse on how migrants' social location, identity, and embeddedness in transnational social networks influence health outcomes, including lived experiences with stigmatized illnesses such as HIV.

Funding: This research was supported by the National Science Foundation (Award Number: 1632751).

Institutional Review Board Statement: This study was conducted in accordance with the Declaration of Helsinki and approved by the Institutional Review Board (or Ethics Committee) of Drexel University (1807006494-R001; 8 July 2019) and the Philadelphia Department of Public Health (FWA00003616/2018-50; 1 October 2019).

Informed Consent Statement: Informed consent was obtained from all subjects involved in the study.

Data Availability Statement: The data presented in this study are available on request from the corresponding author.

Acknowledgments: I would like to acknowledge and thank all study participants who so generously shared their life narratives and time; research assistants (Marisa Felsher, Alexandra Eastus, Amna Khalafallah, Turo Boyiri, Rachael Deis, and Sabrina Gonzalez) who assisted with the design of research instruments, data collection, and processing; and the leadership and staff at the African Family Health Organization (AFAHO), African Cultural Alliance of North America (ACANA), and Health Centers of the Philadelphia Department of Public Health for their assistance with participant recruitment. I am grateful to the Department of Sociology at Drexel for their assistance with time and resources to undertake this study, and to other colleagues for their comments on earlier drafts of this paper.

Conflicts of Interest: The authors declare no conflicts of interest. The funders had no role in the design of the study; in the collection, analyses, or interpretation of data; in the writing of the manuscript; or in the decision to publish the results.

References

1. Bury, M.; Gabe, J. *The Sociology of Health and Illness: A Reader*; Routledge: London, UK, 2004.
2. Goffman, E. *Stigma: Notes on the Management of a Spoiled Identity*; Prentice-Hall: Englewood Cliffs, NJ, USA, 1963.
3. Strauss, A.L. Chronic illness and the quality of life. *AJN Am. J. Nurs.* **1976**, *76*, 82. [CrossRef]
4. Bury, M. Chronic Illness as Biographical Disruption. *Sociol. Health Illn.* **1982**, *4*, 167–182. [CrossRef] [PubMed]
5. Engman, A. Embodiment and the Foundation of Biographical Disruption. *Soc. Sci. Med.* **2019**, *225*, 120–127. [CrossRef] [PubMed]
6. Bell, S.L.; Tyrrell, J.; Phoenix, C. Ménière's Disease and Biographical Disruption: Where Family Transitions Collide. *Soc. Sci. Med.* **2016**, *166*, 177–185. [CrossRef] [PubMed]
7. Sanderson, T.; Calnan, M.; Morris, M.; Richards, P.; Hewlett, S. Shifting Normalities: Interactions of Changing Conceptions of a Normal Life and the Normalisation of Symptoms in Rheumatoid Arthritis. *Sociol. Health Illn.* **2011**, *33*, 618–633. [CrossRef] [PubMed]
8. Adamson, J.; Donovan, J. "Normal Disruption": South Asian and African/Caribbean Relatives Caring for an Older Family Member in the UK. *Soc. Sci. Med.* **2005**, *60*, 37–48. [CrossRef] [PubMed]
9. Richardson, J.C.; Ong, B.N.; Sim, J. Is Chronic Widespread Pain Biographically Disruptive? *Soc. Sci. Med.* **2006**, *63*, 1573–1585. [CrossRef] [PubMed]
10. Williams, S. Chronic Illness as Biographical Disruption or Biographical Disruption as Chronic Illness? Reflections on a Core Concept. *Sociol. Health Illn.* **2000**, *22*, 40–67. [CrossRef]
11. Bearman, P.S.; Moody, J.; Stovel, K. Chains of Affection: The Structure of Adolescent Romantic and Sexual Networks. *Am. J. Sociol.* **2004**, *110*, 44–91. [CrossRef]
12. Berkman, L.F.; Glass, T.; Brissette, I.; Seeman, T.E. From Social Integration to Health: Durkheim in the New Millennium. *Soc. Sci. Med. 1982* **2000**, *51*, 843–857. [CrossRef]
13. Kawachi, I.; Berkman, L.F. Social Cohesion, Social Capital and Health. In *Social Epidemiology*; Berkman, L.F., Ichiro, K., Eds.; Oxford University Press: New York, NY, USA, 2000; pp. 174–190.
14. Pescosolido, N.; Levy, J.A. The Role of Social Networks in Health, Illness and Disease and Healing: The Accepting Preseng, the Forgotton Past, and the Dangerous Potential for a Complacent Future. In *Social Networks and Health*; Levy, J.A., Pescosolido, B.A., Eds.; Elsevier Science: New York, NY, USA, 2002; pp. 3–25.
15. Smith, K.P.; Christakis, N.A. Social Networks and Health. *Annu. Rev. Sociol.* **2008**, *34*, 405–429. [CrossRef]
16. Valente, T.W. *Social Networks and Health: Models, Methods, and Applications*; Oxford University Press: New York, NY, USA, 2010.
17. Lipton, F.R.; Cohen, C.I.; Fischer, E.; Katz, S.E. Schizophrenia: A Network Crisis. *Schizophr. Bull.* **1981**, *7*, 144. [CrossRef] [PubMed]
18. Perry, B.L.; Pescosolido, B.A. Social Network Dynamics and Biographical Disruption: The Case of "First-Timers" with Mental Illness. *Am. J. Sociol.* **2012**, *118*, 134–175. [CrossRef]
19. Pescosolido, B.A.; Manago, B. *Getting Underneath the Power of "Contact": Revisiting the Fundamental Lever of Stigma as a Social Network Phenomenon*; Major, B., Dovidio, J.F., Link, B.G., Eds.; Oxford University Press: Oxford, UK, 2017; Volume 1.
20. Bor, J.; Fischer, C.; Modi, M.; Richman, B.; Kinker, C.; King, R.; Calabrese, S.K.; Mokhele, I.; Sineke, T.; Zuma, T.; et al. Changing Knowledge and Attitudes Towards HIV Treatment-as-Prevention and "Undetectable = Untransmittable": A Systematic Review. *AIDS Behav.* **2021**, *25*, 4209–4224. [CrossRef] [PubMed]
21. Yombi, J.C.; Mertes, H. Treatment as Prevention for HIV Infection: Current Data, Challenges, and Global Perspectives. *AIDS Rev.* **2018**, *20*, 131–140. [CrossRef] [PubMed]
22. Carricaburu, D.; Pierret, J. From Biographical Disruption to Biographical Reinforcement: The Case of HIV-positive Men. *Sociol. Health Illn.* **1995**, *17*, 65–88. [CrossRef]
23. Ciambrone, D. *Women's Experiences with HIV/Aids: Mending Fractured Selves*; Haworth Press: Binghamton, NY, USA, 2003.
24. Matovu, S.N.; La cour, K.; Hemmingsson, H. Narratives of Ugandan Women Adhering to HIV/AIDS Medication. *Occup. Ther. Int.* **2012**, *19*, 176–184. [CrossRef] [PubMed]
25. Pierret, J. An Analysis over Time (1990–2000) of the Experiences of Living with HIV. *Soc. Sci. Med.* **2007**, *65*, 1595–1605. [CrossRef] [PubMed]
26. Russell, S.; Seeley, J. The Transition to Living with HIV as a Chronic Condition in Rural Uganda: Working to Create Order and Control When on Antiretroviral Therapy. *Soc. Sci. Med.* **2010**, *70*, 375–382. [CrossRef]
27. Thorne, C.; Newell, M.L. Epidemiology of HIV Infection in the Newborn. *Early Hum. Dev.* **2000**, *58*, 1–16. [CrossRef]
28. Gambino, C.; Trevelyan, E.N.; Fitzwater, J.T. *The Foreign-Born Population from Africa: 2008–2012*; US Census Bureau: Washington, DC, USA, 2014.
29. Kish, L. Taxonomy of Elusive Populations. *J. Off. Stat.* **1991**, *7*, 339–347.
30. Commodore-Mensah, Y.; Turkson-Ocran, R.-A.; Nmezi, N.A.; Nkimbeng, M.; Cudjoe, J.; Mensah, D.S.; York, S.; Mossburg, S.; Patel, N.; Adu, E.; et al. Commentary: Engaging African Immigrants in Research Experiences and Lessons from the Field. *Ethn. Dis.* **2019**, *29*, 617–622. [CrossRef] [PubMed]

31. Kerani, R.; Narita, M.; Lipira, L.; Endeshaw, M.; Holmes, K.K.; Golden, M.R. Challenges in Recruiting African-Born, US-Based Participants for HIV and Tuberculosis Research. *J. Immigr. Minor. Health* **2019**, *21*, 533–539. [CrossRef] [PubMed]
32. Spring, M.; Westermeyer, J.; Halcon, L.; Savik, K.; Robertson, C.; Johnson, D.R.; Butcher, J.N.; Jaranson, J. Sampling in Difficult to Access Refugee and Immigrant Communities. *J. Nerv. Ment. Dis.* **2003**, *191*, 813–819. [CrossRef] [PubMed]
33. Kerani, R.P.; Kent, J.B.; Sides, T.; Dennis, G.; Ibrahim, A.R.; Cross, H.; Wiewel, E.W.; Wood, R.W.; Golden, M.R. HIV among African-Born Persons in the United States: A Hidden Epidemic? *J. Acquir. Immune Defic. Syndr.* **2008**, *49*, 102–106. [CrossRef] [PubMed]
34. Kerani, R.P.; Satcher Johnson, A.; Buskin, S.E.; Rao, D.; Golden, M.R.; Hu, X.; Hall, H.I. The Epidemiology of HIV among People Born outside the United States, 2010–2017. *Public Health Rep.* **2020**, *135*, 611–620. [CrossRef] [PubMed]
35. Kerani, R.P.; Lugg, A.; Berzins, B.; Gaye, O.; Lipira, L.E.; Bundy, C.; Kwakwa, H.; Holmes, K.K.; Golden, M.R. Post-Migration HIV Acquisition among African Immigrants in the U.S. *J. Immigr. Minor. Health* **2022**, *24*, 1459–1468. [CrossRef]
36. Koku, E.F.; Rajab-Gyagenda, W.M.; Korto, M.D.; Morrison, S.D.; Beyene, Y.; Mbajah, J.; Ashton, C. HIV/AIDS among African Immigrants in the U.S.: The Need for Disaggregating HIV Surveillance Data by Country of Birth. *J. Health Care Poor Underserved* **2016**, *27*, 1316–1329. [CrossRef] [PubMed]
37. Campbell, S.; Greenwood, M.; Prior, S.; Shearer, T.; Walkem, K.; Young, S.; Bywaters, D.; Walker, K. Purposive Sampling: Complex or Simple? Research Case Examples. *J. Res. Nurs.* **2020**, *25*, 652–661. [CrossRef] [PubMed]
38. LeCompte, M.D.; Schensul, J.J. *Designing and Conducting Ethnographic Research: An Introduction*; Rowman Altamira: Lanham, MD, USA, 2010; Volume 1.
39. Miles, M.B.; Huberman, A.M. *Qualitative Data Analysis: An Expanded Sourcebook*; Sage: Thousand Oaks, CA, USA, 1994; ISBN 0-8039-5540-5.
40. Creswell, J.W.; Poth, C.N. *Qualitative Inquiry and Research Design: Choosing among Five Approaches*; Sage Publications: Thousand Oaks, CA, USA, 2016; ISBN 1-5063-3019-3.
41. Braun, V.; Clarke, V. Using Thematic Analysis in Psychology. *Qual. Res. Psychol.* **2006**, *3*, 77–101. [CrossRef]
42. *Dedoose*, Version 9.2.012. Cloud Application for Managing, Analyzing, and Presenting Qualitative and Mixed Method Research Data. SocioCultural Research Consultants, LLC: Los Angeles, CA, USA, 2021.
43. Aidoo-Frimpong, G.; Agbemenu, K.; Orom, H. A Review of Cultural Influences on Risk for HIV and Culturally-Responsive Risk Mitigation Strategies Among African Immigrants in the US. *J. Immigr. Minor. Health* **2021**, *23*, 1280–1292. [CrossRef]
44. Blanas, D.A.; Nichols, K.; Bekele, M.; Lugg, A.; Kerani, R.P.; Horowitz, C.R. HIV/AIDS among African-Born Residents in the United States. *J. Immigr. Minor. Health* **2013**, *15*, 718–724. [CrossRef]
45. Commodore-Mensah, Y.; Himmelfarb, C.D.; Agyemang, C.; Sumner, A.E. Cardiometabolic Health in African Immigrants to the United States: A Call to Re-Examine Research on African-Descent Populations. *Ethn. Dis.* **2015**, *25*, 373–380. [CrossRef]
46. Cudjoe, J.; Nkimbeng, M.; Turkson-Ocran, R.-A.; Commodore-Mensah, Y.; Han, H.-R. Understanding the Pap Testing Behaviors of African Immigrant Women in Developed Countries: A Systematic Review. *J. Immigr. Minor. Health* **2021**, *23*, 840–856. [CrossRef] [PubMed]
47. Nmezi, N.A.; Turkson-Ocran, R.-A.; Tucker, C.M.; Commodore-Mensah, Y. The Associations between Depression, Acculturation, and Cardiovascular Health among African Immigrants in the United States. *Int. J. Environ. Res. Public. Health* **2022**, *19*, 6658. [CrossRef] [PubMed]
48. Airhihenbuwa, C.O.; Webster, J.D. Culture and African Contexts of HIV/AIDS Prevention, Care and Support. *Sahara-J. J. Soc. Asp. HIV/AIDS* **2004**, *1*, 4–13. [CrossRef]
49. Kalipeni, E.; Craddock, S.; Oppong, J.R.; Ghosh, J. *HIV and AIDS in Africa: Beyond Epidemiology*; Wiley-Blackwell: Malden, MA, USA, 2003.
50. Baxen, J.; Breidlid, A. *HIV/AIDS in Sub-Saharan Africa: Understanding the Implications of Culture & Context*; Juta and Company Ltd.: Cape Town, South Africa, 2009; ISBN 1-919895-18-3.
51. Taylor, J.J. Assisting or Compromising Intervention? The Concept of "culture" in Biomedical and Social Research on HIV/AIDS. *Soc. Sci. Med.* **2007**, *64*, 965–975. [CrossRef]
52. Mvilongo, P.T.N.; Vanhamel, J.; Siegel, M.; Nöstlinger, C. The "4th 90" Target as a Strategy to Improve Health-Related Quality of Life of People Living with HIV in Sub-Saharan Africa. *Trop. Med. Int. Health* **2022**, *27*, 1026–1043. [CrossRef] [PubMed]
53. Pantelic, M.; Shenderovich, Y.; Cluver, L.; Boyes, M. Predictors of Internalised HIV-Related Stigma: A Systematic Review of Studies in Sub-Saharan Africa. *Health Psychol. Rev.* **2015**, *9*, 469–490. [CrossRef]
54. Afulani, P.A.; Torres, J.M.; Sudhinaraset, M.; Asunka, J. Transnational Ties and the Health of Sub-Saharan African Migrants: The Moderating Role of Gender and Family Separation. *Soc. Sci. Med.* **2016**, *168*, 63–71. [CrossRef]
55. Awoniyi, S. African Cultural Values: The Past, Present and Future. *J. Sustain. Dev. Afr.* **2015**, *17*, 1–13.
56. Kyalo, P. A Reflection on the African Traditional Values of Marriage and Sexuality. *Int. J. Acad. Res. Progress. Educ. Dev.* **2012**, *1*, 84–92. [CrossRef] [PubMed]
57. Lesthaeghe, R.J. *Reproduction and Social Organization in Sub-Saharan Africa*; University of California Press: Berkeley, CA, USA, 2023; ISBN 978-0-520-33545-5.
58. Yaw, O.-K. *Children's Agency and Development in African Societies*; CODESRIA: Dakar, Senegal, 2017; ISBN 978-2-86978-718-6.

59. Yang, L.H.; Thornicroft, G.; Alvarado, R.; Vega, E.; Link, B.G. Recent Advances in Cross-Cultural Measurement in Psychiatric Epidemiology: Utilizing "What Matters Most" to Identify Culture-Specific Aspects of Stigma. *Int. J. Epidemiol.* **2014**, *43*, 494–510. [CrossRef] [PubMed]
60. Yang, L.H.; Kleinman, A. 'Face' and the Embodiment of Stigma in China: The Cases of Schizophrenia and AIDS. *Soc. Sci. Med.* **2008**, *67*, 398–408. [CrossRef]
61. Baumgartner, L.M. The Incorporation of the HIV/AIDS Identity into the Self over Time. *Qual. Health Res.* **2007**, *17*, 919–931. [CrossRef] [PubMed]
62. Pollard, R.; Saleem, H. Reproductive Identities Following an HIV Diagnosis: Strategies in the Face of Biographical Disruption. *Cult. Health Sex.* **2020**, *22*, 385–397. [CrossRef] [PubMed]
63. Beyeza-Kashesya, J.; Kaharuza, F.; Mirembe, F.; Neema, S.; Ekstrom, A.M.; Kulane, A. The Dilemma of Safe Sex and Having Children: Challenges Facing HIV Sero-Discordant Couples in Uganda. *Afr. Health Sci.* **2009**, *9*, 2–12. [PubMed]
64. Henny, K.D.; Nanin, J.; Gaul, Z.; Murray, A.; Sutton, M.Y. Gay Identity and HIV Risk for Black and Latino Men Who Have Sex with Men. *Sex. Cult.* **2018**, *22*, 258–270. [CrossRef] [PubMed]
65. Ho, L.P.P.; Goh, E.C.L. "I Have HIV but I'm Not the HIV"-the Experiences of Heterosexual Chinese Men Living with HIV in Singapore. *AIDS Care* **2020**, *32*, 296–301. [CrossRef]
66. Ho, V.T.; Levesque, L.L.; Rousseau, D.M. *Filling in the Blanks: How Social Networks Shape Psychological Contracts*; Graduate School of Industrial Administration, Carnegie Mellon University: Pittsburgh, PA, USA, 2003; p. 33.
67. Kanniappan, S.; Jeyapaul, M.J.; Kalyanwala, S. Desire for Motherhood: Exploring HIV-Positive Women's Desires, Intentions and Decision-Making in Attaining Motherhood. *AIDS Care* **2008**, *20*, 625–630. [CrossRef]
68. Saleem, H.T.; Surkan, P.J.; Kerrigan, D.; Kennedy, C.E. "If I Don't Have Children, They Will Know That I'm Sick": Fertility Desires of Women and Men Living with HIV in Iringa, Tanzania. *AIDS Care* **2019**, *31*, 908–911. [CrossRef] [PubMed]
69. Tan, R.K.J.; Lim, J.M.; Chan, J.K.W. "Not a Walking Piece of Meat with Disease": Meanings of Becoming Undetectable among HIV-Positive Gay, Bisexual and Other Men Who Have Sex with Men in the U = U Era. *AIDS Care* **2020**, *32*, 325–329. [CrossRef] [PubMed]
70. Ward, P.R.; Muller, R.; Tsourtos, G.; Hersh, D.; Lawn, S.; Winefield, A.H.; Coveney, J. Additive and Subtractive Resilience Strategies as Enablers of Biographical Reinvention: A Qualitative Study of Ex-Smokers and Never-Smokers. *Soc. Sci. Med.* **2011**, *72*, 1140–1148. [CrossRef] [PubMed]
71. Fauk, N.K.; Mwanri, L.; Gesesew, H.A.; Ward, P.R. Biographical Reinvention: An Asset-Based Approach to Understanding the World of Men Living with HIV in Indonesia. *Int. J. Environ. Res. Public Health* **2023**, *20*, 6616. [CrossRef] [PubMed]
72. Bazzi, A.R.; Leech, A.A.; Biancarelli, D.L.; Sullivan, M.; Drainoni, M.-L. Experiences Using Pre-Exposure Prophylaxis for Safer Conception Among HIV Serodiscordant Heterosexual Couples in the United States. *AIDS Patient Care STDs* **2017**, *31*, 348–355. [CrossRef]
73. Murchu, E.; Marshall, L.; Teljeur, C.; Harrington, P.; Hayes, C.; Moran, P.; Ryan, M. Oral Pre-Exposure Prophylaxis (PrEP) to Prevent HIV: A Systematic Review and Meta-Analysis of Clinical Effectiveness, Safety, Adherence and Risk Compensation in All Populations. *BMJ Open* **2022**, *12*, e048478. [CrossRef]
74. Aidoo-Frimpong, G.; Orom, H.; Agbemenu, K.; Collins, R.L.; Morse, G.D.; Nelson, L.E. Exploring Awareness, Perceptions, and Willingness to Use HIV Pre-Exposure Prophylaxis: A Qualitative Study of Ghanaian Immigrants in the United States. *AIDS Patient Care STDs* **2022**, *36*, 8–16. [CrossRef]
75. Coulibaly, K.; Bousmah, M.-A.-Q.; Ravalihasy, A.; Taéron, C.; Mbiribindi, R.; Senne, J.-N.; Gubert, F.; Gosselin, A.; Desgrées du Loû, A.; MAKASI Study Group. Bridging the Knowledge Gap of Biomedical HIV Prevention Tools among Sub-Saharan African Immigrants in France. Results from an Empowerment-Based Intervention. *SSM-Popul. Health* **2023**, *23*, 101468. [CrossRef]
76. Okoro, O.N.; Whitson, S.O. Sexual Health, HIV Care and Pre-Exposure Prophylaxis in the African Immigrant Population: A Needs Assessment. *J. Immigr. Minor. Health* **2020**, *22*, 134–144. [CrossRef]
77. Fauk, N.K.; Hawke, K.; Mwanri, L.; Ward, P.R. Stigma and Discrimination towards People Living with HIV in the Context of Families, Communities, and Healthcare Settings: A Qualitative Study in Indonesia. *Int. J. Environ. Res. Public Health* **2021**, *18*, 5424. [CrossRef]
78. Steiner, R.J.; Finocchario-Kessler, S.; Dariotis, J.K. Engaging HIV Care Providers in Conversations with Their Reproductive-Age Patients about Fertility Desires and Intentions: A Historical Review of the HIV Epidemic in the United States. *Am. J. Public Health* **2013**, *103*, 1357–1366. [CrossRef] [PubMed]
79. Dela Cruz, A.; Patten, S.; Abdulmalik, I.; Harrowing, J.; Hall, M.; Afzal, A.R.; Demeke Abate, T.; Carter, A.; Spies, P.; Mapfumo, S.; et al. Mandatory HIV Screening, Migration and HIV Stigma in Canada: Exploring the Experiences of Sub-Saharan African Immigrants Living with HIV in Western Canada. *Health Promot. Chronic Dis. Prev. Can. Res. Policy Pract.* **2020**, *40*, 38–46. [CrossRef] [PubMed]
80. Flowers, P.; Davis, M.; Hart, G.; Rosengarten, M.; Frankis, J.; Imrie, J. Diagnosis and Stigma and Identity amongst HIV Positive Black Africans Living in the UK. *Psychol. Health* **2006**, *21*, 109–122. [CrossRef]
81. Hachfeld, A.; Darling, K.; Calmy, A.; Ledergerber, B.; Weber, R.; Battegay, M.; Wissel, K.; Di Benedetto, C.; Fux, C.A.; Tarr, P.E.; et al. Why Do Sub-Saharan Africans Present Late for HIV Care in Switzerland? *HIV Med.* **2019**, *20*, 418–423. [CrossRef] [PubMed]
82. Heus, L. "There Is No Love Here Anyway." Sexuality, Identity and HIV Prevention in an African Sub-Culture in Amsterdam, The Netherlands. *Sex. Health* **2010**, *7*, 129–134. [CrossRef] [PubMed]

83. Nevin, P.E.; Frey, S.; Lipira, L.; Endeshaw, M.; Niemann, L.; Kerani, R.P.; Rao, D. "You Are Always Hiding. It's the Worst Way to Live." Exploring Stigma in African Immigrants Living with HIV in a Large Northwest U.S. Metropolitan Area. *J. Assoc. Nurses AIDS Care* **2018**, *29*, 417–425. [CrossRef] [PubMed]
84. Wells, N.; Richman, B.; Grace, D.; Riley, B.; Hui, C.; Vojnov, L.; Stackpool-Moore, L.; Ong, J.J.; Dowell-Day, A.; Allan, B. 2023 Undetectable = Untransmittable Global Policy Roundtable Report: A Multistakeholder Perspective on Undetectable = Untransmittable Research and Policy Priorities. *Sex. Health* **2024**, *21*, SH24017. [CrossRef]
85. McMahon, T.; Ward, P.R. HIV among Immigrants Living in High-Income Countries: A Realist Review of Evidence to Guide Targeted Approaches to Behavioural HIV Prevention. *Syst. Rev.* **2012**, *1*, 56. [CrossRef]

International Journal of
Environmental Research and Public Health

MDPI

Article

Network Diversity and Health Change among International Migrants in China: Evidence from Foreigners in Changchun

Wenbin Wang *,† and Yang Cao ‡

Sociology Department, Jilin University, Changchun 130012, China
* Correspondence: wangwb@jlu.edu.cn; Tel.: +86-13604309307
† Wenbin Wang is a professor and doctoral supervisor in the Department of Sociology, Jilin University. His research interests include studies of foreigners in China, social capital and social networks.
‡ Yang Cao is currently a PhD candidate in the Department of Sociology, Jilin University. His research interests include studies on foreigners in China and the health of immigrants.

Abstract: Objective: Is the migration process likely to lead to sustained changes in individual social networks and health status? There are many controversies about the relationship between migrants' networks and migrants' health. An important reason may be that the constraints of specific social contexts on immigrant networks and health consequences are neglected. This study distinguished two types of social networks of international immigrants to China—their Chinese networks (Chinese-Net) and home-country networks (Motherland-Net). In addition, the study investigated the construction basis of immigrant social networks and health effects based on the Chinese context. Method: A cross-sectional survey was conducted in 2017, 2018, and 2019. The survey was carried out by an on-site questionnaire survey of foreigners in China in the entry-exit hall of the National Immigration Administration. The survey asked foreigners about their immigration experience, labor and employment, social networks, and access to health care. Results and conclusions: Immigrants from more developed countries are more likely to succeed in establishing Chinese-Net and reduce the dependence on Motherland-Net. The Japanese and South Korean immigrants tended to be associated with their home-country compatriots, excluding the Chinese from social contacts and immigration networks. The mixed residence of non-home-country immigrants reduces both the Motherland-Net and Chinese-Net of international immigrants. From the perspective of the health effect, the establishment and expansion of Chinese-Net did not present the "bright side" of encouraging immigrants to reach a better health status. In contrast, Motherland-Net has a stronger explanatory power for the health changes in immigrants.

Keywords: health change; immigration network; international immigration in China; destination-country networks; home-country networks

Citation: Wang, W.; Cao, Y. Network Diversity and Health Change among International Migrants in China: Evidence from Foreigners in Changchun. *Int. J. Environ. Res. Public Health* **2022**, *19*, 16227. https://doi.org/10.3390/ijerph192316227

Academic Editors: Maria De Jesus and Ernesto Castañeda

Received: 22 September 2022
Accepted: 2 December 2022
Published: 4 December 2022

1. Introduction

Driven by globalization and the adjustment of immigration policies, China, as a traditional migrant-sending country, is increasingly becoming the destination of many international migrants [1]. According to the seventh national census of the National Bureau of Statistics of China, there are approximately 850,000 foreigners living in the Chinese mainland, mainly coming to China for business, employment, and study (See http://www.gov.cn/xinwen/2021-05/11/content_5605792.htm (accessed on 30 September 2022); considering that illegal immigrants were not included, the number is likely to be underestimated). China is not a traditional country of immigrants, and the history of immigrants coming to China is relatively recent. Therefore, there are very few special studies on international immigrants in China, and the majority of these studies focus on African immigrants in Pearl River Delta, in south China (such as Guangzhou or Foshan) [2–4]. However, studies have pointed out that a broader group of immigrants in other Chinese cities exhibit different life patterns from the typical African immigrants in Pearl River Delta [5].

Many studies have shown that the link between migration networks and social adaptation is a key issue for migration research in all countries, but health consequences are often excluded. Migration is not only regarded as an economic process, but also as a social process, in which immigrant networks and embedded immigrant social capital play a continuous role. Migration networks are considered to positively affect the social adaptation of migrants, including increasing economic and educational opportunities, maintaining family integrity, and accelerating upward integration [6–8]. However, although the positive or negative impact of social networks and social interactions on health has been widely emphasized, its function in migrant networks is little investigated [9,10]. The drastic change in living environment often leads to the weakening of formal social support, leading to the deterioration of the health status of migrants compared with native residents [11], and the impact of their migration network on their health status is also important.

Recent studies have noted that migration networks are not always consistent or positive. Personal ties to immigrants in the home-country and the destination-country population may play completely different roles in immigrants' subsequent survival and development [9–11]. For one, the different statuses of various individuals in the social context may lead them to develop immigrant networks with varying qualities and quantities of social capital [12,13]. Therefore, we should not ignore internal distribution differences and potential health consequences of migration networks.

As China has a limited history of receiving immigrants during the modern era, what influence the Chinese context might have on the social network and health effect of immigrants is largely unknown. Different from developed countries, most of which are traditional destinations for immigrants, and the south–north migration of traditional immigrant waves, China started its unique immigrant reception process only after entering the new century. First, thanks to its continuous rapid economic growth and its important position in the global division of labor, China continues to attract immigrants from both developing and developed countries, forming two new waves of migration: South–south migration and north–south migration. Second, due to its long cultural tradition and recent immigration history, the Chinese native culture represented by Confucianism is still in an absolutely dominant position, which may have different behavioral influences on immigrants with different cultural backgrounds and relations to it (such as countries inside and outside the Confucian cultural circle). Finally, China maintains a pragmatic and prudent immigration policy, expecting immigrants to contribute to social development, but also concerned about the risks of introducing large numbers of immigrants. Except for a few cities with developed international trade (such as Guangzhou and Yiwu), immigrants are dominated by international students and foreign employees of enterprises. They are allowed to come to China only after being strictly screened by local schools and enterprises and receiving an invitation. After coming to China, they usually live in a certain area under the arrangement and assistance of their schools or enterprises. This residential area contains not only immigrants of their own ethnic background, but also immigrants from other countries.

On the basis of the above characteristics, this study focused on the following two issues: 1. How will these factors, which are unique to immigrants in the Chinese context, affect their construction of immigrant networks? 2. On this basis, what are the impacts of various migration networks on immigrants' health changes?

1.1. Health Change and Migration Networks

The social determinants of health model argue that a person's health is the result of a combination of multiple factors. The first is personal characteristics and lifestyle (gender, age, race, etc.), the second is the macro-socioeconomic and cultural background, and the third is the community and social network of the individual [14–17]. When migrants leave their home society and enter a new and unfamiliar one, they undergo an adaptation process filled with health risks. The social determinants of migrants' health, such as language and work skills, social attitudes, and cultural orientations, and the composition of social networks, all change with the process of migration, bringing new challenges and pressures to the health status of migrants. The very limited evidence from Chinese society also points to this challenge, African immigrants in Pearl River Delta often face significant barriers to access to health care and are not satisfied with the services they receive [18]. The migration process is one of the important driving forces leading to the change (usually deterioration) of the health status of individuals [19,20]. Although contrary results suggest that the health status of migrants may be better than local residents, this is generally regarded as being explained by the "healthy migrant" hypothesis: Only healthier people can withstand the health pressures of migration and complete the migration process [21].

As an intermediate mechanism in regard to migration and social adaptation, migration networks are often mentioned. However, there are many controversies about the relationship between migration networks and migrant health. Supporters of the migration network and cumulative causality theory assume that the migration network is a dynamic process connecting the origin and destination. Therefore, it promotes the continuous self-maintenance and diffusion of immigration waves [14]. However, how do migration networks affect the survival of migrants once they make it to their destination? In the positive view, social networks and social capital can help them access other resources, improve their social support and health knowledge, help them find a suitable job, reduce the burden of work and life, and provide emotional protection for immigrants to cope with the cultural pressure imposed by the destination society. Therefore, these factors would have a positive effect on the physical and mental health of migrants [22–24]. However, a small number of negative views suggest that social networks could also have a negative impact on health; for example, they could promote the spread of negative emotions among different immigrant groups [25,26]. Although not everyone agrees on how immigrant social networks affect health, they almost all agree that these networks are important for immigrant health, in conjunction with cultural, economic, and other factors.

These studies tend to treat health and migration networks more as established outcomes than as changing ones [27]. While migrants inevitably face greater health risks when entering unfamiliar societies, they differ in how they respond to health challenges. After the completion of migration, immigrants will try to establish and maintain a stable reciprocal relationship with a new environment to help them avoid becoming victims in the new social and cultural system [28], in a process called social adaptation. Addressing health challenges is also an important part of this social adaptation process. However, subsequent studies have suggested that the adaptation process of immigrants is not linear, but full of selection and segregation, caused by incompatibilities between individual characteristics and social environment [29–31]. Since formal support is absent or unstable, individuals' social behaviors are more dependent on informal social support, represented by social networks, which then have a greater impact on their health. The communication objects of immigrants are no longer limited to their relatives or fellow citizens, who are homogeneous and have a strong connection; instead, they will also involve residents and immigrants from other countries in the place of migration. The composition of the immigration network includes interpersonal contact with residents and other immigrants, which may lead to different health consequences [24]. In addition, the focus on the process of health change allows us to eliminate the "health migration" hypothesis and gain a better understanding of the health consequences of the migration process.

In the same way, not all social networks of immigrants can be viewed as constituting forms of social capital. Moreover, it is highlighted that networks and health among individuals are continuously evolving and self-adjusting, with high correlation to the social context and social structure [32]. There are two orientations to social capital based on their different levels: The collective level [33] and the individual level [34]. The individual level of social capital comprises the social resources contained in social networks, which determine the value of "capital." Social network theory typically divides networks into strong and weak ties, with these different types of ties associated with different types of social capital. Bonding social capital is the closed social bond between people, characterized by connections among family members, close friends, neighbors, or members of the same ethnic group [35]. This social capital, based on close family and friendship bonds, serves the self-interest of individuals or small groups. In contrast, bridging social capital tends to be open and inclusive, covering people from different social groups and backgrounds, thus forming broader social connections and cohesion [36]. If bonding social capital is suitable for a satisfactory life, then bridging social capital should be crucial to helping individuals to become successful in life [35].

Using this distinction, in many cases, immigrant networks are only regarded as solid connections with relatives or people of the same nationality. Moreover, the social capital generated is closer to bonding social capital emphasized by Putnam [23,37]. International immigrants have more resources for social communication in "post-migration" social adaptation. In addition to expanding strong links and bonding social capital with ethnic groups in their home countries, it is possible to seek bridging social capital. This is more open and heterogeneous, functioning through weak connections with residents. The various types of immigrant networks, especially the different compositions of motherland immigrants and residents in the immigrant network will have varying effects on the health change in the immigrant network owner [24,25].

Migration network distribution and function in different environments and the crowd is not necessarily consistent [38]. For immigrants entering the Chinese context, they are likely to maintain ties with their native ethnic group as well as establish ties with Chinese residents. However, their different positions in the Chinese social context may drive them to make different choices, which will have an impact on their health change. Drawing on the research above, this study splits immigration networks into two: Social networks with native Chinese residents (Chinese-Net), more suitable for bridging social capital, and social networks with motherland migrant (Motherland-Net), more suitable for bonding social capital. In this study, in the Chinese context, the construction and influences of two different networks were investigated based on social structure.

1.2. International Migrants' Network Construction in China

There are noticeable differences among various immigrant groups in China, which cannot be neglected when we examine international immigration in China. This study focused on the structural characteristics of immigrants in the context of Chinese society. It investigated three dimensions: Economic background, cultural concept, and mixed living pattern.

1.2.1. Economic Background

The ethnic origins of immigrants are often different in various societies. In the Changchun sample, interviewees come from 143 different countries and regions, among which 84.15% are from developing countries, and 15.85% are from developed countries. Among developing countries, India (12.72%) and Pakistan (8.84%) had the highest proportion, whereas, among developed countries, South Korea (7.89%), the United States (2.54%), and Japan (1.34%) had the highest proportion. There is no "typical" ethnic group, with absolute superiority in number, and ethnic groups with different economic and cultural backgrounds are evenly distributed among international immigrants in Changchun. Due to China's short history of welcoming immigrants, most international immigrants to China are first-generation immigrants; accordingly, they are still significantly influenced by their origin countries.

The economic gap between the source and destination countries of immigrants is regarded as the basis for the generation of immigration waves by classical immigration theories, such as New Economics of Migration and Dual Labor Market theories, which entails that migrants will choose to migrate from their home country to a more developed country to spread family risks and gain financial rewards. However, these theories on international migration overwhelmingly rely on the South-to-North Flows [39], failure to assess migration consequences that may arise when the economic background of the source country is similar to or better than the destination country. Some evidence has shown that about a third of all international migratory flows occur between developing countries [40]; China's important position in the global industrial division of labor has not only attracted immigrants from developing countries, but also became a work migration destination for junior staffs and senior managers of multinational enterprises in some developed countries.

Therefore, the link between the economic background of the source country and the construction of the migration network becomes more differentiated. In the initial stage of entering a foreign society, migrants generally need to build a home-country network through ethnic ties to obtain basic support [16]. Immigrants from more developed countries usually have better economic resources and human capital, which can help them in the achievement of greater value in the labor market. Due to their economic value, the receiving units then pay more attention and support to them, and they also find it easier to obtain the welcome of residents in Chinese society. Therefore, individuals' needs for ethnic affiliation decrease, and this also reduces the ethnic norms that restrict their interactions [30]. Relatively speaking, immigrants from more developed countries are less dependent on the Motherland-Net, thus limiting the expansion of their Motherland-Net. Simultaneously, advantageous flow options from north to south and a more mature intermediary and support system help them take more initiative in contact with Chinese society, thus building a broader Chinese-Net. On this basis, the hypothesis regarding the economic background is proposed:

Hypothesis 1. *The migration network of international immigrants in China varies due to the different economic backgrounds.*

Hypothesis 1.1. *Compared with immigrants from developing countries, immigrants from more developed countries have a higher proportion of Chinese-Net.*

Hypothesis 1.2. *Compared with immigrants from developing countries, immigrants from more developed countries have a lower proportion of Motherland-Net.*

1.2.2. Cultural Concept

In addition to economic factors, the cultural concept perspective is often neglected by existing studies. The East Asian ethnic group is a particular cultural group appearing in Chinese society. According to the World Values Survey (WVS), Japanese, South Korean, and Chinese societies have similar cultural backgrounds. At the same time, they collectively constitute the Confucian cultural circle, which has certain characteristics that distinguish it from other cultures. The similarity and closeness of East Asian cultures also shows its strength in their social networks and social capital. Although the level of social capital varies widely across countries, social ties have been improved to be rather strong and networks rather closed in East Asia, which cause strong ties to be more preferred and more powerful. As a result, East Asia has markedly less bridging social capital than Western Europe or North America, for instance [41,42].

When Japanese and Korean immigrants, who also belong to East Asian societies, meet Chinese residents in a Chinese context, due to the similarity and closeness of cultural concepts, which characteristic will dominate the construction of the immigration network of Japanese and Korean immigrants? The question may hinge on whether Chinese residents are likely to be these migrants' "own people". If similarity dominates, Chinese, Japanese, and Korean residents are more familiar with each other's customs, cultural concepts, and even languages based on the long history of cultural exchanges. This may help Japanese and South Korean immigrants to regard Chinese residents as more suitable friends and communicate more with Chinese residents [31] (Data from www.worldvaluessurvey.org (accessed on 30 September 2022). The countries and regions belonging to the "Confucian cultural circle" are Japan, South Korea, Mainland China, Taiwan, Macau, Mongolia and Hong Kong. With the exception of Japan and South Korea, the Changchun sample does not include immigrants from other regions and countries). In turn, they will be less dependent on ethnic ties and home-country networks.

However, it is also found that immigrant groups consisting of Chinese, Japanese, and Koreans tend to have stronger family and ethnic identities after entering a foreign society. This closeness may be helpful for school education and lead to economic success but will constrain individual social interaction choices [23,31]. For example, when East Asian ethnic groups seek partners, closed ethnic ties may play a more important role, driving them to seek partners from their own ethnic group and reject external partners. For Japanese and South Korean immigrants, although Chinese residents are similar to "us," they are still "others" with whom we have no ethnic ties or strong ties. East Asian ethnic groups tend to maintain the Motherland-Net and reject the Chinese-Net. On the basis of previous research on the prevalence of social networks in East Asian ethnic groups, we hypothesize that closeness may play a more important role; therefore, the following hypothesis regarding the cultural concept is proposed:

Hypothesis 2. *The migration networks of international immigrants in China vary due to different cultural concepts.*

Hypothesis 2.1. *The proportion of Chinese-Net in East Asian ethnic groups is lower than non-East Asian ethnic groups.*

Hypothesis 2.2. *Compared with non-East Asian ethnic groups, East Asian ethnic groups have a higher proportion of Motherland-Net.*

1.2.3. Mixed Living Pattern

Residential assistance provided by receiving units may profoundly impact the network construction of international migrants. The international immigrants in Changchun are mainly technical personnel from enterprises and students at college. These embedded international migrants can receive close help from their units, including financial support, accommodation arrangements, and assistance with relevant procedures. Compared with African businesspeople in Pearl River Delta, who struggle alone and find it difficult to obtain formal social support, the help provided by receiving units makes up for the gap in social support for international immigrants in Changchun. It effectively reduces the difficulties international immigrants face in Changchun due to entering a foreign society. Moreover, the residence forms related to the receiving units are factors shaping the differences in the social networks of international immigrants in Changchun.

For safety and convenience, centralized residence is directly provided to international immigrants in Changchun as part of social support. For example, the university provides alternative student apartments for international students, and enterprises offer rental assistance for foreign technical personnel on the premise of respecting their wishes. The international immigrant settlement in Changchun is different from the spontaneous gathering of traditional immigrants from bottom to top; instead, it is realized in the centralized system arrangement from top to bottom. Under this institutional arrangement, the residential boundaries of international immigrants in different regions, skin colors, and languages are broken, and the heterogeneity and internationalization degree of international immigrant settlements are enhanced. The international immigrant settlements in Changchun are "international villages." This mixed pattern may help international migrants break free from the strong constraints of their home-country networks, but it may also further isolate them from Chinese society and residents. On this basis, the hypothesis from the destination is proposed:

Hypothesis 3. *The network construction of international immigrants in China is affected by the mixed form of the destination.*

Hypothesis 3.1. *The more non-home-country immigrants live in Changchun, the lower the proportion of the Chinese-Net will be.*

Hypothesis 3.2. *The more non-home-country immigrants live in Changchun, the lower the proportion of the Motherland-Net will be.*

1.3. Health Effects of Disparate Migration Networks

Regarding the heterogeneity of migration networks, it is worth considering whether different types of migration networks are conducive to the health change in international migrants in China. In particular, which social network is more likely to help immigrants to China deal with their apparent health challenges? In fact, the effects of both Chinese-Net and Motherland-Net on health are considered positive by most studies, although some studies believe that the two types of social networks have no direct relationship with health or have negative effects [43]. However, the influences of Chinese-Net and Motherland-Net on the health change in Chinese immigrants have never been compared. They follow different possible influence paths, and the resulting health consequences may also be different.

Theoretically, there are two potential pathways for the positive effects of social networks and social capital on health. One is the information and resource pathway. Social networks are helpful for individuals to obtain more information about health behaviors and a healthy life. When individuals are faced with medical service needs, the existence of their social network improves the accessibility of medical services and health facilities, and avoids the possibility of health damage as early as possible. The second path is the emotional and normative path. High level of social interaction and mutual trust in social relationships provide sufficient emotional support, which can reduce the impact of migration stress on physical and mental health. Trusting social group interactions can lead to a sense of mastery and responsibility for oneself and one's group. Individuals are more likely to accept and follow group norms of behavior and curb unhealthy behaviors, such as smoking, alcohol, and substance abuse [44,45]. At the same time, group interaction may also attract individuals to participate in more health promotion or disease prevention behaviors, such as physical exercise.

The positive roles of Chinese-Net and Motherland-Net for health are present along different paths: Chinese-Net may be more conducive to the information and resources pathway, while Motherland-Net deals more with the emotional and normative pathway. Due to the large social and cultural differences between immigrants and local residents, the Chinese-Net usually contains more heterogeneous information and resources, which may be more favorable for international migrants to obtain necessary medical and health information. For example, when international migrants are sick and need treatment, if they have the help of Chinese friends, they can enjoy better medical services in Chinese society [5]. In contrast, homogeneity information from Motherland-Net may not help international immigrants improve their access to medical resources, but based on the tight-knit, trustful Motherland-Net, migrants receive a large amount of emotional support to cope with the psychological shock and loneliness of entering a strange society. Under the group norms of Motherland-Net, migrants are more likely to maintain their old lifestyles without interference, avoid self-marginalization under Chinese social pressures, and have more health-boosting opportunities to participate in group activities and physical exercise with home-country compatriots [44,46].

Considering the relatively good health status of Chinese international migrants and the stable support provided by their employers, we believe that Motherland-Net may be a more important factor affecting the health of Chinese international migrants than Chinese-Net. The effects of Motherland-Net and Chinese-Net on health changes are essentially a discussion of the resources and emotional dimensions behind health changes. Although health facilities providing international care are scarce and expensive [47], the majority of high-quality healthcare resources in China are concentrated in public hospitals and open to the whole society. Due to the relatively good health status of international migrants to China, their demand for medical resources is relatively low. Moreover, when there is a need for medical services, immigrants can also seek help from their units through formal channels, rather than relying on the information advantages provided by Chinese-Net. The influence of Chinese-Net on their health changes may also be limited. The emotional support and group norms provided by Motherland-Net, through prolonged contact in daily life, are difficult to replace for international migrants. Trust and dependence on Motherland-Net by international migrants may have a more sustained impact on their lifestyle and health behaviors. On this basis, the hypotheses of health change effects are proposed:

Hypothesis 4. *Motherland-Net affects international migrants' health change more than Chinese-Net.*

Hypothesis 4.1. *Regardless of Chinese-Net value, the health of international migrants does not change significantly.*

Hypothesis 4.2. *The higher the Motherland-Net, the healthier the international migrants become.*

2. Methods

2.1. Changchun Sample

On the basis of Changchun sample of Survey of Foreigners in China (SFRC), Changchun is used as a study sample to represent a new pattern of immigration composition in Chinese society. Compared with the Pearl River Delta samples, which have attracted more attention, the composition of Changchun samples is more diverse. Moreover, as Changchun is located in the geographic center of Northeast Asia, and has geo-cultural ties with Korea and Japan, the Japanese and Korean ethnic groups have become relatively distinct and important among Changchun foreigners. This makes it convenient to examine the influence of the economic background and cultural concept of immigrants.

In terms of location, due to the lack of sufficiently developed international trade in Changchun, the proportion of businesspeople among immigrants is lower and the proportion of international students and foreign employees of enterprises is higher. Immigrants are most commonly supported and assisted by local schools and enterprises, and a mixed living pattern is more typical. More importantly, with the improvement in the degree of opening up to the outside world and the internal transfer of industrial clusters, inland cities with a large number of people but less developed international trade have also began to attract immigrants. The Changchun sample, which is dominated by international students and corporate employees, although smaller in number, is likely to represent a more general pattern of immigration composition in Chinese society in the future: Immigrants present a diversified economic background and cultural concept from the source country, and form a centralized mixed residence mode with interracial immigrants with the help and support of schools and enterprises.

2.2. Data Sources

The data in this study were obtained from the Survey of Foreigners in China (SFRC), which was launched by the Institute of National Governance of Sun Yat-sen University in Guangzhou in 2016 and subsequently expanded to six cities, including Changchun, Hangzhou, Xi'an, Lanzhou, Yiwu, and Xuzhou. The author's research team conducted the Changchun survey in September and October 2017, 2018, and 2019. The survey was carried out by an on-site questionnaire survey of foreigners in China in the entry-exit hall of the National Immigration Administration. Before the survey, relevant ethical approval and informed consent were obtained. Each participant voluntarily participated in the survey on the premise of being informed of the research objectives and data confidentiality policy regarding social-demographic characteristics of the participants, including gender, age, education level, and marital status. Moreover, the survey asked foreigners about their immigration experience, labor and employment, social networks, and access to health care. After questionnaire screening and data cleaning, 1624 samples were finally used for analysis, which is the largest sample size and the most extensive thematic survey data for international immigrants in Northeast China.

2.3. Main Variables

The dependent variables included migration network and health change. Two migration networks with different characteristics were generated based on the network scale. The opportunity structure of intergroup interactions is strongly influenced by the relative group size. The fewer the people of the same nationality, the less likely they are to have friends of the same nationality [31]. The variables above were generated by relative quantity rather than absolute quantity to avoid the influence of chance structure on network characteristics. First, we measured the number of Chinese residents, the number of people from their home countries, and the number of immigrants from other countries known by respondents in Changchun, as three continuous variables. Second, the total size of the network was obtained by adding the number of Chinese, motherland immigrants, and other immigrants. Finally, we divided the number of Chinese and the number of motherland immigrants by the total size of the network, respectively to obtain the Chinese-Net (mean = 0.306, STD = 0.260) and the Motherland-Net (mean = 0.307, STD = 0.246). The generated variable is a continuous proportional variable between 0 and 1. For explanation, we took the percentage and scaled it to produce a continuous variable from 0 to 100. As other migrants' networks were usually recreational [48], they were not examined further here. Depending on the network size, an ideal network structure for a foreigner in Changchun might be similar to Figure 1.

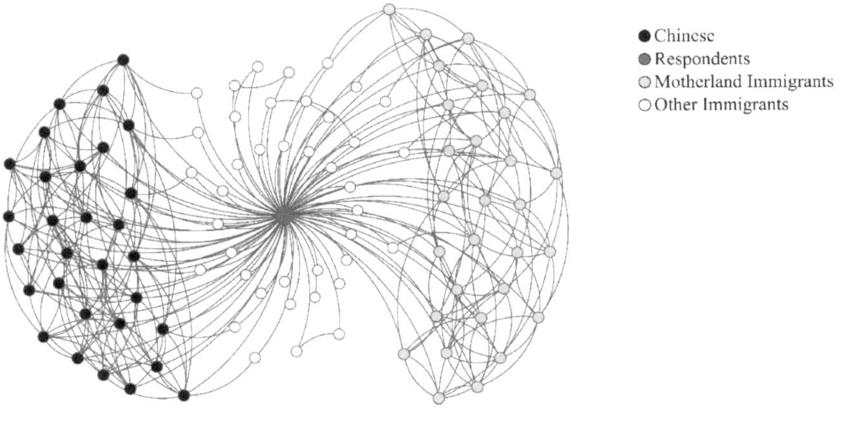

Figure 1. The ideal network structure for a foreigner in Changchun.

Health change comes directly from the questions in the questionnaire. We asked participants to indicate changes in their health status after coming to China. Originally a five-level scale was used; we reduced it to "Same or became unhealthier than before" and "became healthier than before."

Independent variables included economic background, cultural concept, and mixed living pattern. The Human Development Index (HDI) was used to assess the economic background of immigrants' original country. This is a more comprehensive and nuanced assessment than considering developing vs. developed countries, with migrants classified as coming from high-HDI countries (higher than China), mid-HDI countries (similar to China), or low-HDI countries (lower than China). Then, immigrants from East Asian vs. non-East Asian groups (0 = immigrants from East Asia) were distinguished to measure the influence of cultural concepts. The variable of residence form was generated according to the distribution of non-home-country immigrants in the place of residence (0 = no or few non-home-country immigrants live in the place of residence).

In addition, we further controlled for survey years, age, sex, years of education, marital status, Chinese proficiency, residence duration, Engel's coefficient, and motherland of immigrants in the place of residence. Meanwhile, in the health change model, we further controlled current self-rated health to better investigate the health change effect.

3. Results

Table 1 shows a multivariable linear regression model with Chinese-Net and Motherland Net as dependent variables. We introduced variables related to economic background, cultural concept, and mixed living pattern, respectively.

Table 1. Multivariable linear regression model of migration network differences (N = 1624).

	Model 1	Model 2	Model 3	Model 4
VARIABLES	Chinese-Net	Chinese-Net	Motherland-Net	Motherland-Net
Control variables	Controlled	Controlled	Controlled	Controlled
High-HDI countries (base)				
Mid-HDI countries	−7.599 ***	−7.344 ***	9.769 ***	10.053 ***
	(2.482)	(2.472)	(1.948)	(1.954)
Low-HDI countries	−12.215 ***	−12.139 ***	15.797 ***	15.881 ***
	(2.051)	(2.044)	(1.350)	(1.342)
Cultural groups (0 = non-East Asian groups, 1 = East Asian groups)	−5.674 **	−6.462 **	19.191 ***	18.314 ***
	(2.688)	(2.711)	(2.065)	(2.075)
Residence form (0 = not living with many non-home immigrants, 1 = many non-home immigrants live together)		−3.580 ***		−3.983 ***
		(1.335)		(1.215)
Constant	25.931 ***	27.321 ***	17.388 ***	18.808 ***
	(6.192)	(6.219)	(5.578)	(5.616)
R-squared	0.116	0.120	0.140	0.146

Note: 1. Robust standard errors in parentheses; 2. *** $p < 0.01$, ** $p < 0.05$; 3. The control variables included survey years, age, sex, years of education, marital status, Chinese proficiency, residence duration, Engel's coefficient, motherland immigrants in the place of residence.

Models 1 and 2 are the influencing factor models of Chinese-Net. The Chinese-Net of immigrants higher-HDI countries is significantly higher than the immigrants from lower-HDI countries, which supports Hypothesis 1.1. In comparison, the Chinese-Net of East Asian groups is significantly lower than the non-East Asian groups, which supports hypotheseis 2.1. Moreover, the Chinese-Net of international immigrants who live together with more immigrants from other countries is significantly lower, supporting Hypothesis 3.1.

Models 3 and 4 are the influencing factor models of the Motherland-Net. The results revealed that the Motherland-Net of immigrants from higher-HDI countries is significantly lower than the lower-HDI countries. The Motherland-Net of East Asian groups is significantly higher than the non-East Asian groups, supporting hypotheses 1.2 and 2.2. The Motherland-Net of international migrants, with more non-home migrants living in their residential areas, is significantly lower, supporting Hypothesis 3.2.

To verify the robustness of the above findings, in Table 2, we took the original ratio of Chinese-Net and Motherland-Net (i.e., the continuous ratio between 0 and 1 without percentage enlargement) as the dependent variable and constructed a proportional logistic regression model. The model settings are consistent with Table 1. The results revealed that the international immigrants from higher-HDI countries have significantly higher Chinese-Net and significantly lower Motherland-Net. For international migrants from East Asian groups, the proportion of Chinese-Net and Motherland-Net in their migration network both are significantly lower. When more non-home immigrants live in the same area, the proportion of Chinese-Net and Motherland-Net in their migration network is significantly lower. In summary, the data findings above are consistent with those in Table 1.

Table 2. Robustness test of migration network differences (N = 1624).

	Model 5	Model 6	Model 7	Model 8
VARIABLES	**Chinese-Net**	**Chinese-Net**	**Motherland-Net**	**Motherland-Net**
Control variables	Controlled	Controlled	Controlled	Controlled
High-HDI countries (base)				
Mid-HDI countries	0.722 ***	0.730 ***	1.843 ***	1.869 ***
	(0.079)	(0.080)	(0.209)	(0.212)
Low-HDI countries	0.577 ***	0.578 ***	2.456 ***	2.466 ***
	(0.052)	(0.052)	(0.207)	(0.207)
Cultural groups (0 = non-East Asian groups, 1 = East Asian groups)	0.790 **	0.760 **	2.887 ***	2.765 ***
	(0.094)	(0.091)	(0.313)	(0.302)
Residence form (0 = not living with many non-home immigrants, 1 = many non-home immigrants live together)		0.841 ***		0.824 ***
		(0.055)		(0.049)
Constant	0.386 ***	0.414 ***	0.192 ***	0.206 ***
	(0.108)	(0.116)	(0.051)	(0.055)

Note: 1. Robust standard errors in parentheses; 2. *** $p < 0.01$, ** $p < 0.05$; 3. The control variables are the same as in Table 1.

Note: 1. The coefficient is the odds ratio. Standard errors are robust standard errors; 2. To avoid very small coefficients, the original values are used here for Chinese-Net and Motherland-Net rather than the percentage values expanded to equal proportions. 3. *** $p < 0.01$, ** $p < 0.05$, * $p < 0.1$; 4. On the basis of Table 1, the control variables further add self-rated health.

To compare different effects of Motherland-Net and Chinese-Net on immigrants' health change, we constructed a logistic model of the impact of the two immigrant networks on health change, as shown in Figure 2.

The results in Model 9 indicated that the occurrence ratio of Chinese-Net on health change is less than 1 and that it is not significant. In Model 10, although the coefficient of Chinese-Net is greater than 1, it is still not significant. The impact of Chinese-Net on the health change in immigrants tends to be not very positive. In contrast, the impact of Motherland-Net on the health change in immigrants tends to be positive. In Model 10, it can be found that Motherland-Net has a significant positive influence on whether they have become healthier after entering China. Hypothesis 4 is supported by the data.

In summary, after considering the Chinese context characteristics of immigrants, we distinguished two different types of immigration networks, Chinese-Net and Motherland-Net, and constructed a model to investigate its health effectiveness from the perspective of the process of dynamic changes.

According to our data results, the economic background, cultural concept, and mixed residence pattern have a significant impact on the difference in the migration network of international immigrants in China. Specifically, compared with immigrants from less-developed countries, immigrants from more developed countries are more likely to succeed in establishing Chinese-Net with the advantages of economic background provided by their home countries, and reduce the dependence on ethnic ties and Motherland-Net. Despite cultural similarities with Chinese society, the preference of East Asian cultural concepts for strong ties and closet networks indicated that the Japanese and South Korean immigrants tended to be associated with their home-country compatriots, excluding the Chinese from social contacts and immigration networks. The mixed residence of non-home-country immigrants reduces the Motherland-Net of international immigrants and further blocks their contact with Chinese society, which is not conducive to the establishment of a Chinese-Net.

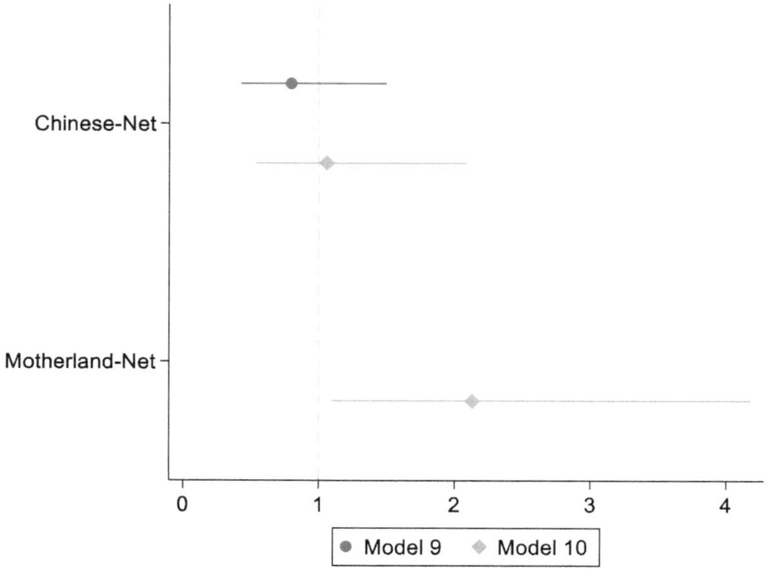

Figure 2. Logistic model for health change analysis of immigrant networks (N = 1624).

From the perspective of the health effect, the establishment and expansion of Chinese-Net did not present the "bright side" of encouraging immigrants to reach a better health status, as we often hypothesize. This appears to be a departure from previous findings based on the same survey but with different samples, which found that interaction with natives, as measured by immigrants' education in China, may have a significant positive health effect on immigrants [5]. We suspect that this may be related to different sample characteristics. In the Changchun sample, a higher proportion of international migrants have organizations that can help them, such as businesses and schools. The information and resources from organizations may replace the advantages of information and resources provided by Chinese-Net, thus weakening their health utility. In contrast, Motherland-Net has a stronger explanatory power for the health changes in immigrants. People with more Motherland-Net are more likely to resist the health risks of immigration, and maintain and improve their health status in the unfamiliar society.

4. Discussion

Drawing on Putnam's distinction between two types of social capital, health and social networks are viewed as dynamic processes rather than predetermined results, and these dynamic processes are constrained by both migration processes and social situations in China. There have been numerous studies suggesting a strong association between social networks, social capital, and health [24], but the focus on immigrant groups, especially those in emerging destinations, is still very limited. This is not only the neglect of an expanding group, but also the exclusion of migration processes that can have a significant impact on the construction of social networks and the health status of migrants. The data and findings of this study partially confirm the positive effect of social networks on helping migrants cope with post-migration health risks, but this effect is more reflected in Motherland-Net, which has strong connection and homogeneity. Close and trusting interpersonal relationships can provide adequate emotional support, shape healthy life patterns of immigrants, and provide long-term health promotion effects for immigrants. Although Chinese-Net is more likely to provide sufficient information, the construction of this network is more difficult for immigrant groups, especially those from developing countries and Japan and South Korea, and is further limited by the mixed residence mode. In addition, since more international migrants can receive health service assistance from their employers in the Chinese context, their dependence on Chinese-Net has decreased, and the health utility brought by Chinese-Net is also limited.

Through our analysis of the largest sample for international immigrants in Northeast China, in addition to providing new insights for research on international migrants in China, we emphasize the importance of the Chinese social context in the study of international migration. The number of immigrants in Changchun is significantly less than the cities in Pearl River Delta, such as Guangzhou and Foshan. However, it represents a different, maybe more widespread immigration pattern in Chinese society compared with cities in Pearl River Delta, where migrants are mostly from African ethnic groups, lack formal social supports, and often have legitimacy crises. The characteristics of immigrants elsewhere in China are significantly different. Under China's practical and prudent immigration policy, people with diverse economic backgrounds and cultural concepts are welcomed by the Chinese society, but they need to undergo strict screening and are subject to continuous attention from Chinese society. This study generally contributes to the existing literature on international migration by applying an approach that tries to show the power of the Chinese social context in shaping the living conditions of immigrants to China. More importantly, we emphasize the influence of East Asian cultural concepts and the Chinese social immigration governance system on the construction of immigrant networks and health effectiveness. The inherent heterogeneity and inequality bring great complexity and flexibility to immigration networks and social capital, which leads to different social consequences.

Unfortunately, due to data limitations, we cannot satisfactorily consider the possibility of endogeneity in some of our models. In either case, the data are cross-sectional and do not support a causal argument; we can only limit our conclusions to correlations at present. For the rapidly expanding number of immigrants to China, who are only beginning to enter the academic horizon, high-quality tracking data are undoubtedly necessary in the future.

Scholars interested in continuing this line of research should consider the following. First, time is a dimension worth considering. We place equal importance on the source factor and the destination factor for first-generation immigrants. However, as first-generation immigrants stay longer and more second-generation immigrants join the international immigrant community in China, not only is the influence of destination factors likely to increase, but structural factors affecting the survival of international migrants in Chinese society may also change. Moreover, China's reform and opening-up policy is still being constantly adjusted; it will be essential to trace the resonances between international immigrant networks and Chinese society.

Second, due to the lack of an available sampling frame, we could not achieve strict random sampling of respondents. This might have increased some inherent bias. However, as a result of China's strict visa censorship, nearly all foreigners need to pass through the Exit and Entry Administration formalities periodically. Therefore, the time limit may be extended by further investigation. It may expand the sample size to alleviate these problems. The use of respondent-driven sampling may also be helpful for future surveys.

Third, interpersonal differences and health consequences need to be explored further through qualitative study. As our study found, the complex origins and residence status of international migrants in China reveal the differential consequences of social interaction. Since our study is based on quantitative analysis, a qualitative study on international immigrants in China involving representative individuals may be a supplement to find mediating mechanisms linking individual differences with adaptive consequences.

Finally, it is necessary to consider the potential impact of COVID-19, which may change the way people interact socially and the functioning of social capital. Some social networks may be more functional, while others may be weaker [34]. Accordingly, the foundation and functions of the international migration networks in China will also change. Data from SFRC collected after COVID-19 will enable us to explore the impact of COVID-19 on migrant networks in the future.

To provide improved answers to the aforementioned questions, we have launched a new and improved survey in 2022. This survey, with its extended time limits, has been initiated in July, with a plan to terminate it in December. Although the current survey was often interrupted due to COVID-19, presumably it aided in increasing our visitors' representation. Furthermore, to counter the disruptions of the epidemic, we created an electronic version of the questionnaire and highly distributed it based on a respondent-driven strategy. In the questionnaire, we included more questions for measuring mindsets and behavioral patterns, pre- and post-COVID-19. At the end of the survey, we might be able to provide further insights into foreigners in China, and how their health status changed before and after the epidemic.

Furthermore, our findings have substantial implications for policy. If the goal of migrant governance is to promote their survival and development in China, it will be crucial to promote interactions between international migrants in China and the local society. Although the Chinese government continues to improve international immigration policies and laws, it pays more attention to management than to services and lacks an accurate understanding of the characteristics of immigrant groups. The practical effects of these measures have been limited or even the reverse of what was intended. On the basis of our findings, potential measures for improving the situation of international migrants in China may include providing refined service strategies for different ethnic groups, creating open mixed communities, and improving the international service level of the hospital.

5. Conclusions

The study investigated the construction and health change effect of different network types. The results indicated that an economic background from more developed countries improves the Chinese-Net and reduces the Motherland-Net, whereas the cultural concept of East Asia reduces the Chinese-Net and improves the Motherland-Net. A mixture of immigrants from different countries will reduce both the Motherland-Net and the Chinese-Net. Regarding the health change effect, the motherland network plays a positive role in helping immigrants to reach a better health status after coming to China, while the Chinese network has no clear positive effect on the health change in immigrants.

Author Contributions: Conceptualization, Y.C. and W.W.; methodology, Y.C.; software, W.W.; validation, Y.C. and W.W.; formal analysis, Y.C.; investigation, Y.C.; resources, W.W.; data curation, W.W.; writing—original draft preparation, W.W.; writing—review and editing, Y.C. and W.W.; visualization, Y.C.; supervision, W.W.; project administration, W.W.; funding acquisition, W.W. All authors have read and agreed to the published version of the manuscript.

Funding: This research is supported by "the Fundamental Research Funds for the Central Universities", China (grant number 2022CXTD16).

Institutional Review Board Statement: All procedures performed in studies involving human participants were in accordance with the ethical standards of the institutional and/or national research committee, and with the 1964 Helsinki declaration and its later amendments, or comparable ethical standards.

Informed Consent Statement: Informed consent was obtained from all subjects involved in the study.

Data Availability Statement: The data presented in this study are available upon request from the corresponding author.

Conflicts of Interest: The author declares no conflict of interest.

References

1. Liang, Z.; Song, Q. Migration in China. In *International Handbooks of Population*; Springer: Dordrecht, The Netherlands, 2016; pp. 285–309. [CrossRef]
2. Bork-Hüffer, T.; Rafflenbeul, B.; Kraas, F.; Li, Z. Global change, national development goals, urbanisation and international migration in China: African migrants in Guangzhou and Foshan. In *Megacities*; Springer: Dordrecht, The Netherlands, 2014; pp. 135–150.
3. Liang, Y. The causal mechanism of migration behaviors of African immigrants in Guangzhou: From the perspective of cumulative causation theory. *J. Chin. Sociol.* **2014**, *1*, 2. [CrossRef]
4. Song, G.; Liu, L.; He, S.; Cai, L.; Xu, C. Safety perceptions among African migrants in Guangzhou and Foshan, China. *Cities* **2020**, *99*, 102624. [CrossRef]
5. Fan, X.; Yan, F.; Yan, W. Better choice, better health? Social integration and health inequality among international migrants in Hangzhou, China. *Int. J. Environ. Res. Public Health* **2020**, *17*, 4787. [CrossRef] [PubMed]
6. Davis, B.; Stecklov, G.; Winters, P. Domestic and international migration from rural Mexico: Disaggregating the effects of network structure and composition. *Popul. Stud.* **2002**, *56*, 291–309. [CrossRef]
7. Martinez, R., Jr.; Lee, M.T.; Nielsen, A.L. Segmented assimilation, local context and determinants of drug violence in Miami and San Diego: Does ethnicity and immigration matter? *Int. Migr. Rev.* **2004**, *38*, 131–157. [CrossRef]
8. Massey, D.S.; Aysa-Lastra, M. Social capital and international migration from Latin America. *Int. J. Popul. Res.* **2011**, *2011*, 834145. [CrossRef]
9. Kim, D.; Kawachi, I.U.S. State-Level social capital and health-related quality of life: Multilevel evidence of main, mediating, and modifying effects. *Ann. Epidemiol.* **2007**, *17*, 258–269. [CrossRef]
10. Panagopoulos, C.; Fraser, T.; Aldrich, D.P.; Kim, D.; Hummel, D. Bridging the Divide: Does Social Capital Moderate the Impact of Polarization on Health? *Pol. Res. Q.* **2022**, *75*, 875–891. [CrossRef]
11. Park, H.; Pappalardo, A.A. Invited perspective: Call to action-reduce immigrants' disparities in environmental exposures and health. *Environ. Health Perspect.* **2022**, *130*, 91301. [CrossRef]
12. Aguilera, M.B.; Massey, D.S. Social capital and the wages of Mexican migrants: New hypotheses and tests. *Soc. Forces.* **2003**, *82*, 671–701. [CrossRef]
13. Tegegne, M.A. Immigrants' social capital and labor market performance: The effect of social ties on earnings and occupational prestige. *Soc. Sci. Q.* **2015**, *96*, 1396–1410. [CrossRef]
14. Massey, D.S.; Arango, J.; Hugo, G.; Kouaouci, A.; Pellegrino, A.; Taylor, J.E. Theories of international migration: A review and appraisal. *Popul. Dev. Rev.* **1993**, *19*, 431. [CrossRef]
15. Brody, E.B. Migration and adaptation: The nature of the problem. *Am. Behav. Sci.* **1969**, *13*, 5–13. [CrossRef]
16. Zhou, M. Segmented assimilation: Issues, controversies, and recent research on the new second generation. *Int. Migr. Rev.* **1997**, *31*, 975–1008. [CrossRef] [PubMed]
17. Fong, E.; Verkuyten, M.; Choi, S.Y.P. Migration and identity: Perspectives from Asia, Europe, and North America. *Am. Behav. Sci.* **2016**, *60*, 559–564. [CrossRef]
18. Lin, L.; Brown, K.B.; Yu, F.; Yang, J.; Wang, J.; Schrock, J.M.; Bodomo, A.B.; Yang, L.; Yang, B.; Nehl, E.J.; et al. Health care experiences and perceived barriers to health care access: A qualitative study among African migrants in Guangzhou, Guangdong Province, China. *J. Immigr. Minor. Health* **2015**, *17*, 1509–1517. [CrossRef]
19. Castañeda, H.; Holmes, S.M.; Madrigal, D.S.; Young, M.E.; Beyeler, N.; Quesada, J. Immigration as a social determinant of health. *Annu. Rev. Public Health* **2015**, *36*, 375–392. [CrossRef]
20. Maimaitijiang, R.; He, Q.; Wu, Y.; Bouey, J.Z.H.; Koné, A.; Liang, Y.; Hao, C.; Tu, J.; Gu, J.; Hao, Y. Assessment of the health status and health service perceptions of international migrants coming to Guangzhou, China, from high-, middle- and low-income countries. *Global. Health.* **2019**, *15*, 9. [CrossRef]
21. Chiswick, B.R.; Lee, Y.L.; Miller, P.W. Immigrant selection systems and immigrant health. *Contemp. Econ. Policy.* **2008**, *26*, 555–578. [CrossRef]
22. Portes, A.; Rumbaut, R.G. *Legacies. The Story of the Immigrant Second Generation*; University of California Press: Berkeley, CA, USA, 2001.
23. Zilberberg, M.D. The clinical research enterprise: Time to change course? *JAMA* **2011**, *305*, 604–605. [CrossRef]
24. Bamford, J.; Klabbers, G.; Curran, E.; Rosato, M.; Leavey, G. Social capital and mental health among black and minority ethnic groups in the UK. *J. Immigr. Minor. Health* **2021**, *23*, 502–510. [CrossRef] [PubMed]
25. Arthur, T. The role of social networks: A novel hypothesis to explain the phenomenon of racial disparity in kidney transplantation. *Am. J. Kidney Dis.* **2002**, *40*, 678–681. [CrossRef] [PubMed]
26. Christakis, N.A.; Fowler, J.H. The spread of obesity in a large social network over 32 years. *N. Engl. J. Med.* **2007**, *357*, 370–379. [CrossRef] [PubMed]
27. Xu, T. The effect of health change on long-term settlement intentions of international immigrants in new destination countries: Evidence from Yiwu city in China. *Int. J. Environ. Res. Public Health* **2022**, *19*, 7574. [CrossRef]
28. Paul, A.M. Stepwise international migration: A multistage migration pattern for the aspiring migrant. *Am. J. Sociol.* **2011**, *116*, 1842–1886. [CrossRef]
29. Zeng, Z.; Xie, Y. A preference-opportunity-choice framework with applications to intergroup friendship. *Am. J. Sociol.* **2008**, *114*, 615–648. [CrossRef]

30. Williams, N.E.; Hughes, C.; Bhandari, P.; Thornton, A.; Young-DeMarco, L.; Sun, C.; Swindle, J. When does social capital matter for migration? A study of networks, brokers, and migrants in Nepal. *Int. Migr. Rev.* **2020**, *54*, 964–991. [CrossRef]
31. Hurh, W.M.; Kim, K.C. Social and occupational assimilation of Korean immigrants in the United States. *Korea J.* **1979**, *19*, 4–14.
32. Bian, Y.; Miao, X.; Lu, X.; Ma, X.; Guo, X. The emergence of a COVID-19 related social capital: The case of China. *Int. J. Sociol.* **2020**, *50*, 419–433. [CrossRef]
33. Putnam, R.D. Bowling alone: America's declining social capital. *J. Democr.* **1995**, *6*, 65–78. [CrossRef]
34. Lin, N. *Social Capital: A Theory of Social Structure and Action*; Cambridge University Press: New York, NY, USA, 2001.
35. Putnam, R.D. *Bowling Alone: The Collapse and Revival of American Community*; Simon & Schuster: New York, NY, USA, 2000.
36. Parker, D.; Song, M. Ethnicity, social capital and the Internet: British Chinese Websites. *Ethnicities* **2006**, *6*, 178–202. [CrossRef]
37. Evergeti, V.; Zontini, E. Introduction: Some critical reflections on social capital, migration and transnational families. *Ethn. Racial Stud.* **2006**, *29*, 1025–1039. [CrossRef]
38. Garip, F. Social capital and migration: How do similar resources lead to divergent outcomes? *Demography* **2008**, *45*, 591–617. [CrossRef] [PubMed]
39. Freier, L.F.; Holloway, K. The impact of tourist visas on intercontinental South-South migration: Ecuador's policy of "open doors" as a quasi-experiment. *Int. Migr. Rev.* **2019**, *53*, 1171–1208. [CrossRef]
40. Abel, G.J.; Sander, N. Quantifying global international migration flows. *Science* **2014**, *343*, 1520–1522. [CrossRef] [PubMed]
41. Horak, S.; Taube, M.; Yang, I.; Restel, K. Two not of a kind: Social network theory and informal social networks in East Asia. *Asia Pac. J. Manag.* **2019**, *36*, 349–372. [CrossRef]
42. Lee, D.; Jeong, K.-Y.; Chae, S. Measuring social capital in East Asia and other world regions: Index of social capital for 72 countries. *Glob. Econ. Rev.* **2011**, *40*, 385–407. [CrossRef]
43. Wellman, B.; Wortley, S. Different strokes from different folks: Community ties and social support. *Am. J. Sociol.* **1990**, *96*, 558–588. [CrossRef]
44. Folland, S. An economic model of social capital and health. *HEPL* **2008**, *3*, 333–348. [CrossRef]
45. Lin, N.; Simeone, R.S.; Ensel, W.M.; Kuo, W. Social support, stressful life events, and illness: A model and an empirical test. *J. Health Soc. Behav.* **1979**, *20*, 108–119. [CrossRef]
46. Lin, N.; Woelfel, M.W.; Light, S.C. The buffering effect of social SupportSubsequent to an important life event. *J. Health Soc. Behav.* **1985**, *26*, 247–263. [CrossRef] [PubMed]
47. Yu, M.; He, S.; Wu, D.; Zhu, H.; Webster, C. Examining the multi-scalar unevenness of high-quality healthcare resources distribution in China. *Int. J. Environ. Res. Public Health* **2019**, *16*, 2813. [CrossRef] [PubMed]
48. Bochner, S.; McLeod, B.M.; Lin, A. Friendship patterns of overseas students: A functional model. *Int. J. Psychol. J. Int. Psychol.* **1977**, *12*, 277–294. [CrossRef]

International Journal of
Environmental Research and Public Health

Article

Leaving the Homestead: Examining the Role of Relative Deprivation, Social Trust, and Urban Integration among Rural Farmers in China

Wentao Si, Chen Jiang and Lin Meng *

School of Public Administration, Shandong Normal University, Jinan 250014, China
* Correspondence: menglin@sdnu.edu.cn

Abstract: Actively promoting the orderly and voluntary withdrawal of idle rural house bases and effectively activating "sleeping" land assets are considered important measures to accelerate the modernization of agriculture and rural areas, as well as promoting the integrated development of urban and rural areas. However, few studies have focused on the superimposed effects of negative psychological and social environmental factors on the willingness of farmers to withdraw from their homestead. Therefore, we conducted this study in order to clarify the logical ideas of rural home base withdrawal, analyze the factors that influence the decision of home base withdrawal behavior of interest subjects, and provide a scientific decision basis for promoting rural home base withdrawal and accelerating the process of transferring citizens of agricultural population in terms of policies, measures, and paths, so as to design and develop an incentive mechanism for home base withdrawal of citizens of agricultural transfer population. The results of the study show that: (1) the findings indicate that social deprivation, economic deprivation, and emotional deprivation all significantly and negatively affect farmers' willingness to withdraw from their homesteads; (2) social trust plays a mediating role between relative deprivation and farmer homestead withdrawal behavior; and (3) urban integration plays a moderating role between social and emotional deprivation and the social trust of farmers, but does not have a significant moderating role in the relationship between economic deprivation and social trust. Furthermore, it plays a moderating role between all deprivation factors (i.e., economic, social, and emotional deprivation) and farmer homestead withdrawal behavior. This study aims to provide useful guidance and policy suggestions for optimizing policies related to farmer homestead withdrawal behaviors, and for scientifically designing the homestead withdrawal mechanism and policy system.

Keywords: relative deprivation; social trust; urban integration; homestead; willingness to withdraw; Jinan

Citation: Si, W.; Jiang, C.; Meng, L. Leaving the Homestead: Examining the Role of Relative Deprivation, Social Trust, and Urban Integration among Rural Farmers in China. *Int. J. Environ. Res. Public Health* **2022**, *19*, 12658. https://doi.org/10.3390/ijerph191912658

Academic Editors: Maria De Jesus and Ernesto Castañeda

Received: 19 August 2022
Accepted: 29 September 2022
Published: 3 October 2022

1. Introduction

The root cause of the lagging process regarding the urban citizenship of the agricultural migrant population is considered to be the "umbilical cord" relationship between farmers and rural residential bases [1]. With the continuous promotion of new types of urbanization, a large number of migrant agricultural workers are expected to flow into cities, with a total of 292.51 million migrant workers in China by 2021 [2]. According to statistics, by the end of 2021, the urbanization rate of China's resident population had reached 64.72%, but the urban household registration rate was only 46.7% [3]. The current registered residence system in China divides the household registration into urban household registration and rural household registration according to the relationship of blood inheritance and geographical location. This urban–rural "amphibious" living pattern of rural laborers has created a dilemma, in which the rigid demand for urban land co-exists with the wasteful use of rural land [4]. According to data from the Ministry of Agriculture and Rural Development, the rural labor force has been living in rural areas for more than

20 years. According to the data of the Ministry of Agriculture and Rural Affairs, the area of rural house bases is 168 million mu, accounting for 48.62% of the collective construction land area. According to the relevant data, there are 261 million migrant workers and their accompanying family members who have become permanent residents in urban areas, and the idle rate of rural residential bases is as high as 17.6% [5]. This large number of unused rural residential bases not only leads to a waste of land resources and various safety hazards, but also seriously affects the improvement of the rural living environment and the promotion of rural urbanization [6]. In order to resolve the dilemma of idle and inefficient use of residential bases, in 2004, the State Council already pointed out in the Central Document No. 28 that it advocates the moderate adjustment of rural construction land, and the moderate increase of urban construction land should be linked with the moderate reduction of rural construction land. In 2008, the State Council clearly put forward the policy of "urban-rural linkage increase/decrease" in the "Management Measures of Urban-Rural Construction Land Increase/Decrease Pilot". In 2016, the State Council issued "Several Opinions on Deepening the Construction of a New Type of Urbanization" (No.8 Document of State Council [2016]), which pointed out that "exploring the mechanism of voluntary and compensated withdrawal of farmers' rights to land contract, use homestead and collective income distribution". In 2022, the No. 1 document of "the Central Committee of the Communist Party of China (CPC) and the State Council on the key work of comprehensive promotion of rural revitalization in 2022" further emphasized "prudently promote the pilot reform of the rural homestead system, and standardize the registration of housing land as one of the homestead rights". It points out the direction for regulating rural construction land, promoting the voluntary and compensated withdrawal of rural land rights and interests of the agricultural transfer population, and implementing the withdrawal mechanism of rural homestead in the context of citizenship. The newly amended Land Management Law in 2019 stipulates that the state will allow rural villagers who have settled in cities to withdraw from their residential bases voluntarily and be compensated, according to the law. However, the results of a large number of surveys regarding the willingness to withdraw from residential bases have shown that the percentage of farmers who settle in cities and are unwilling to withdraw from their residential bases is 50–70% [7]. As the voluntary principle is the basis for the implementation of the homestead withdrawal system [8], it is of great practical significance to study the influencing mechanisms of the decision to withdraw from residential bases by farmers who have settled in cities in depth, in order to scientifically design the mechanism for voluntary and paid withdrawal from residential bases, thus encouraging farmers who have settled in cities to withdraw from their residential bases voluntarily and steadily promoting the reform of the rural residential base system.

In the existing relevant literature, scholars have mainly focused on value perception [9], risk expectation [10], ownership [11], local attachment [12], and so on, and have explored the various influences on the willingness of urban farmers to withdraw from their residential bases. The decision to voluntarily withdraw from residential bases is based on a rational analysis of the trade-off between pros and cons; however, as there is no uniform standard for the judgment of pros and cons, this judgment may be highly subjective [13]. The decision of farmers to voluntarily withdraw from their residential land is based on rational analysis, instinctive psychological factors (e.g., internal emotions, desires, and perceptions), and their external social environment [14]. Therefore, in this study, we analyze the interactions between and influence of emotional, psychological, and social environment factors on the willingness of farmers in cities to withdraw from their homestead bases.

From the perspective of the armer's own internal psychological factors, 55.98% of farmers subjectively believe that homestead bases are privately owned by the farmers [4]. However, from the perspective of legal system, the ownership of rural homestead in China belongs to the collective, and farmers only have the right to use the homestead. This is because rural homestead assume a variety of functions, such as production, living, and emotional belonging, to which farmers assign higher value expectations [15]. Withdrawal from the rural homestead is a major problem, which entails the loss of these functions and rights. Therefore, farmers will repeatedly make psychological trade-offs when withdrawing from their homesteads, which makes farmers have a strong sense of relative deprivation which, in turn, inhibits their homestead withdrawal behavior [16]. The relative dispossession of farmers arises from their sense of dispossession. The sense of relative deprivation in farmers originates from a loss of functional dependence on the homestead, which also reflects their concerns regarding access to material resources, social relations, and development opportunities after losing the functional rights and interests carried by the homestead under the conditions of relatively institutionalized social inequality [17].

An individual's life situation is no longer confined to the private world but is increasingly influenced by the broader social context and social structure. In other words, the relative sense of deprivation produced by social comparison of individuals is not only related to their own conditions, but also, to some extent, is the result of the social environment. In terms of the factors that influence the willingness of farmers to withdraw from their homestead, the following two aspects are the most important.

First, the behavior of farmers will be influenced by external social environment factors (i.e., social trust). With the implementation of the rural revitalization strategy and the construction of rural civilization, the social trust among farmers has been enhanced. Social trust relationships reflect an individual's rights and obligations to others or social organizations to honor the relationship. So, does the level of social trust affect the homestead withdrawal behavior of farmers? Does the level of social trust play a mediating role in the relative sense of deprivation on their willingness to withdraw from their homestead? Does the sense of relative deprivation lead to a decrease in trust in the government, which in turn has an impact on the willingness of rural residents to withdraw from their homestead? These questions are worth exploring in depth. Second, homestead withdrawal requires farmers to complete urban integration into a new place. Urban integration does not only involve economic integration, in terms of labor and employment, economic income, and living conditions but, more importantly, it involves a higher level of integration in social and psychological aspects. This is mainly reflected in the conceptual acceptance and recognition of urban culture, such as the customs, behavioral norms, and values in cities. This cultural and psychological urban integration status reflects the degree of attachment and psychological distance of urban farmers to the city and influences their behavior and decision making. Urban integration can lead to a positive interaction between individual development and social development. Therefore, in this paper, we incorporate urban integration into the considered analytical framework and explore the moderating effect of urban integration on the homestead withdrawal behavior of farmers.

Based on this, we conducted this study in order to clarify the logical ideas of rural home base withdrawal, analyze the factors that influence the decision of home base withdrawal behavior of interest subjects, and provide a scientific decision basis for promoting rural home base withdrawal and accelerating the process of transferring citizens of agricultural population in terms of policies, measures and paths, so as to design and develop an incentive mechanism for home base withdrawal of citizens of agricultural transfer population. We selected some urban migrants for empirical research. The urban migrant group studied in this paper refers to those who move from rural to urban areas for a long period of time, referred to as "rural migrants". This concept breaks through the limitations of the concept of "migrant workers" used in earlier studies, based on the background of the urban–rural dual structure, and is consistent with the trend characteristics of the rural population moving to the city to work and live, in the context of accelerating the citizenship of the migrant agricultural population in the new urbanization construction stage. The concept of "migrant workers" has been widely used in academic circles, as it is in line with the trend of long-term, family-oriented, and sedentary living of the rural population in the context of accelerating the citizenship of the agricultural transfer population in the new urbanization stage. Our empirical study investigates the intrinsic mechanisms of relative deprivation that influence the withdrawal of rural households from their homestead and identifies the mediating effect of social trust and the moderating effect of urban integration.

2. Literature Review and Research Hypothesis

2.1. Connotation Definition

2.1.1. Connotation of Relative Deprivation

The sense of relative deprivation is a subjective perception that individuals or groups find themselves in a disadvantaged position through comparison, which includes not only cognitive components of social comparison, but also emotional components such as anger and dissatisfaction, and even behavioral components such as complaints, conflicts, and revenge. Disadvantaged individuals may experience a sense of deprivation of basic rights during the process of social comparison, and this sense of deprivation easily leads to negative effects on their psychological and behavioral adaptation. Relative deprivation can lead to a variety of negative problem behaviors [18]. As a negative subjective experience, the sense of relative deprivation—as an evaluation of one's deprived rights and low social status—can easily produce frustration and depression, thus increasing the risk of externalizing problem behaviors [19]. Based on the multiple functions of homestead, the relative deprivation of farmers can be divided into economic deprivation, social deprivation, and emotional deprivation [20–22]. Previous studies have taken the hypothesis of rational economic man of farmers as the premise of the study and so could not comprehensively understand the homestead withdrawal decision behaviors of farmer, and cannot explain the fact why many farmers are still reluctant to withdraw from their homestead, even after their human capital situation (e.g., education and employment) has been improved. Recent studies in sociology, psychology, or consumer behavior fields have found that, when individuals or groups experience a sense of relative deprivation, obtaining corresponding psychological compensation is their fundamental core demand [23]. This is also the solution to promoting the voluntary withdrawal from residential bases of urban farmers.

2.1.2. The Connotation of Homestead to Farmers

Residential land is the land used by farmers to build houses, buildings, and facilities related to residential life [24]. The main characteristics of the Chinese residential land system can be described as: "collective ownership, use by members, free of land price, and long-term occupation" [25]. Although the current law stipulates that residential bases are collectively owned, in practice they have been occupied and used by different farmers separately, and the concept of ownership of residential bases by farmers has long been rather vague, or the concept of thinking that they own them has not fundamentally changed [26]. A homestead is land for living acquired by farmers, as members of collective economic organizations without compensation, thus having the nature of welfare distribution. When they own a residential base, farmers not only live there and store crops and farming tools, but also generate other productive collateral benefits, such as the convenience of growing fruits and vegetables on the residential base, handicraft workshop production, and so on [27]. At the same time, the sense of security brought by having a place to live and the psychological satisfaction of building a relationship with the surrounding environment are also important components of family welfare for farmers, which are shared by family members [28]. From this perspective, the relationship between farmers and their homestead is not only economic, but also embedded with socio-cultural and psycho-emotional factors, which determines the complexity of homestead withdrawal decisions. Therefore, when farmers choose to withdraw from their homestead, it means that these benefits attached to the homestead will also be lost [29]. Thus, the homestead is currently an important place for a significant majority of farmers to live and survive, and the choice to withdraw from the homestead or not will affect the overall welfare of their households.

2.1.3. The Connotation of Urban Integration

The urban integration of migrant farmers refers to the process by which farmers establish their economic status in the city, adapt to urban social norms and security, and finally achieve urban psychological identity [30,31]. In this study, we analyze the urban integration of migrant farmers in three dimensions: Economic integration, social integration, and psychological integration. Economic integration refers to the integration of farmers into the economic conditions of urban life when they move from rural to urban areas, which is the basis of urban integration of migrant farmers [30,32]. Social integration refers to the establishment of positive social networks with people around them (e.g., colleagues, leaders, neighbors) and the creation of continuous interactive behaviors [33]. Psychological integration emphasizes the acceptance and recognition of the city by the farmers; that is, the farmers have a sense of belonging to the city, are more willing to live in urban areas, and have a sense of citizenship in the city. The completion of psychological integration is the completion of the process of transforming farmers from rural to urban people, thus realizing urban integration in the true sense [34].

2.1.4. The Connotation of Social Trust

Social trust is formed between members of society based on a combination of morality and interest and can be viewed as a psychological contract of mutual expectation, mutual trust, and interdependence. Social trust, as a systemic trust, is also an important influential factor affecting the social mindset of farmers [35]. Social trust is an implicit commitment among, is practiced by, and its benefits act on all members of society, thus having the properties of public goods. When every member of the society remembers the promise of "all for one, one for all" and imparts general trust to the society, the cost of interaction is reduced and the efficiency of interaction is improved, helping to build a stable cooperation rule and reciprocity mechanism, thus improving the efficiency of cooperation [36]. From a sociological perspective, this study views social trust as a social phenomenon based on jurisprudence (regulatory system) or ethics (social and cultural norms). On this basis, two different types of social trust are distinguished: juridical social trust and ethical social trust. The former originates from the regulatory system [37], while the latter is based on moral norms and values [38]. Specifically, the social trust of urban farmers also includes the following two levels: legal social trust (i.e., trust in government and law) and moral social trust (i.e., trust in the urban environment and social justice) [37–40].

2.2. Theoretical Assumptions and Analysis

2.2.1. The Direct Effect of Relative Deprivation on Farmer Homestead Withdrawal Behavior

Although the institutional arrangements for the collectivization of homestead ownership are becoming clearer at the legal system level, the long-term factual possession and "monopoly" use of homesteads by farmers have not changed their "quasi-ownership" of homesteads, due to policy changes [41]. This causes farmers to assign higher value expectations to these functions, and withdrawal from the homestead means the loss of these functional rights and interests. Longitudinal comparison before and after the withdrawal causes farmers to have a strong sense of relative deprivation [14] which, in turn, generates negative perceptions and discourages farmers from withdrawing from their homesteads.

Based on the above analysis, the following hypotheses are proposed.

H1. *Relative deprivation has a negative effect on the willingness of farmers to withdraw from their homesteads.*

H1a. *The sense of economic deprivation has a negative effect on the willingness of farmers to withdraw from their homesteads.*

H1b. *Social deprivation has a negative effect on the willingness of farmers to withdraw from their homesteads.*

H1c. *Affective deprivation has a negative effect on the willingness of farmers to withdraw from their homesteads.*

2.2.2. The Mediating Effect of Social Trust

(1) The direct effect of relative deprivation on social trust.

From the perspective of population mobility, the sense of relative deprivation acts as a disincentive to labor mobility. For incoming urban farmers, the sense of relative deprivation reduces their social trust and increases the social cost of citizenship, to a certain extent [42]. Farmers are rational, mostly risk-averse, and conservative, such that a higher sense of relative deprivation reduces their expectations of future employment, income, and a better life, which adversely affects their willingness to withdraw from the homestead [43]. Related to this, the satisfaction of farmers with their socio-economic status affects their evaluation of the performance, management, and governance ability of government departments which, in turn, affects their level of social trust; that is, an individual's sense of individual deprivation, and the resulting negative emotional reactions and adverse social perceptions, may trigger their distrust of the legitimacy of institutional norms [44]. From the above, we can hypothesize that:

H2. *The higher the relative deprivation of farm households, the lower the level of their social trust.*

H2a. *The higher the sense of economic deprivation of farmers, the lower their level of social trust.*

H2b. *The higher the sense of social deprivation of farmers, the lower their level of social trust.*

H2c. *The higher the emotional deprivation of farmers, the lower their level of social trust.*

(2) The direct influence of social trust on farmer homestead withdrawal behavior.

The higher the degree of social trust of farm households, the lower their expectation of opportunistic behavior of others, and the lower the expectation of risk of loss they face. The specific impact paths are described as follows: (1) An increase in social trust can enhance the trust of farmers in the government's commitment, thus reducing their worries about various risks after homestead withdrawal [45]. (2) In the implementation of homestead withdrawal policies, farmers often do not have a direct dialogue with the government and, instead, are represented by village cadres or township cadres to carry out the policy. (3) After moving into the city, if the social trust of the farmers is high, they will believe that the relevant government departments can give equal civil and social rights to the migrant population, eliminate institutional exclusion, and give priority to solving their work injury insurance and medical protection for major diseases, as well as gradually solving the problem of pension protection [46].

H3. *Social trust has a positive effect on the willingness of farmers to withdraw from their homesteads.*

(3) The mediating effect of relative deprivation between the effect of social trust and farmer willingness to withdraw from their homestead.

The decrease in trust in society triggered by the sense of relative deprivation, in turn, has an impact on the willingness of farmers to withdraw from their homestead. The functions of local governments are closely related to the productive and living activities of rural residents, and directly affect the rational distribution of social resources, social equity, and justice [47]. The sense of relative deprivation means that rural households have not been provided with social resources within a reasonable expectation within the institutionalized environment [48], which will lead to the farmers doubting the credibility of the government, in turn affecting the willingness of farmers to withdraw from their homestead.

Accordingly, the following research hypotheses were formed.

H4. *Social trust mediates the relationship between relative deprivation perception and the willingness of farmers to withdraw from their homestead.*

H4a. *Social trust mediates the relationship between feelings of economic deprivation and the willingness of farmers to withdraw from their homestead.*

H4b. *Social trust mediates the relationship between feelings of social deprivation and the willingness of farmers to withdraw from their homestead.*

H4c. *Social trust mediates the relationship between feelings of emotional deprivation and the willingness of farmers to withdraw from their homestead.*

2.2.3. Moderating Effects of Urban Integration

(1) The moderating role of urban integration in the relationship between the sense of relative deprivation and willingness to withdraw from their homestead.

According to neoclassical economic theory, farmers, as "rational economic agents", are willing to give up their homesteads only when the risk is within the tolerable range and the total benefit of land withdrawal is significantly higher than the total cost [49]. The purpose of withdrawal is to maximize economic and social returns. High-quality urban integration can promote equal opportunities in employment, housing, medical care, and education, as well as reducing the loneliness associated with discrimination and exclusion from citizenship and rights [50]. Thus, it weakens the negative impact of relative deprivation of farmers, in economic, social, and emotional terms, on their homestead withdrawal behavior, thus compensating for the relative deprivation in the sense of loss of functional rights and interests regarding the homestead. Thus, it can be hypothesized that urban integration plays an important moderating role in the effect of relative deprivation on farmer homestead withdrawal behavior.

Therefore, the following hypotheses are proposed.

H5. *Urban integration has a positive moderating effect on the relative sense of deprivation affecting the homestead withdrawal behavior of farmers.*

H5a. *Urban integration has a positive moderating effect on the sense of economic deprivation affecting the homestead withdrawal behavior of farmers.*

H5b. *Urban integration has a positive moderating effect on the sense of social deprivation affecting the homestead withdrawal behavior of farmers.*

H5c. *Urban integration has a positive moderating effect on the sense of emotional deprivation affecting the homestead withdrawal behavior of farmers.*

(2) The moderating role of urban integration in the relationship between relative deprivation and social trust.

When farmers become urban workers and perform the same work as urban workers, they still do not enjoy the same social security benefits as urban workers, thus creating multiple compensation systems. China's current social security system, such as pension insurance, unemployment insurance and medical insurance, requires a local registered residence, which obviously only protects the urban population and excludes the vast rural population. Migrant workers in the cities cannot enter the relatively complete urban social security system, they do not have minimum subsistence money and unemployment protection, and if they cannot work or do not have a job, they can only starve or go back to the countryside [51]. In the comparison with urban workers, the group of rural migrants moving to urban areas have a sense of "relative deprivation", which not only makes them feel distrustful and lack a sense of identity with urban areas, but also restricts the flow of labor and affects the effective allocation of labor resources.

The social trust relationship involves the cashing in of the rights and obligations of the individual urban migrant to others or social organizations [52]. Social trust is based on the norm of mutual benefit and reciprocity, which means that interest relationships are important factors affecting the operation of trust [53]. Such interest relationships include economic, social and psychological aspects. The interactions between farmers and urbanites, their feelings during such interactions, and the information they obtain about the society provide an important basis for building social trust [54]. Therefore, the following hypothesis was proposed:

H6. *Urban integration has a positive moderating effect on the relationship between relative deprivation and social trust.*

In summary, in this paper, we attempt to incorporate the sense of relative deprivation, social trust, urban integration, and homestead withdrawal willingness into the same analytical framework (Figure 1), thus constructing a theoretical model of farmer homestead withdrawal willingness in order to provide a new perspective for the study of farmer homestead withdrawal in the context of homestead system reform. The model better utilizes the explanatory framework of psychological factors of farmers to analyze how the willingness of farmers to withdraw from their homesteads is generated. The model consists of three parts: The first part considers the role of relative deprivation on the willingness of farmers to withdraw from their homesteads; the second part considers the mediating role of social trust between relative deprivation and the willingness to withdraw; and the third part considers the moderating role of urban integration between relative deprivation and willingness to withdraw, also considering the moderating role of urban integration in the relationship between relative deprivation and social trust (see Figure 1).

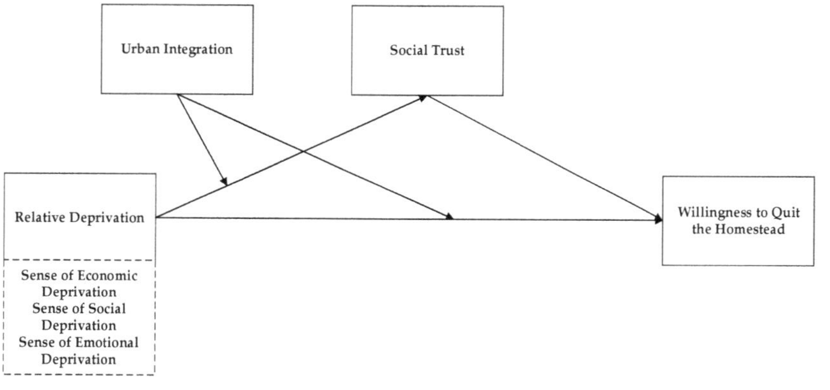

Figure 1. Theoretical framework of the study.

3. Study Design

3.1. Research Methodology

The Amos 21.0 (IBM, New York, USA) software was applied to analyze the effect of each dimension of relative deprivation on the willingness to withdraw behavior. Each latent variable was measured through multiple entries in the scale. To further validate the mediating effect of perceived benefits, the Bootstrap moderated mediation test method approach was used to validate the mediating effect of social trust, while the moderating effect of urban inclusion was tested using multi-variate cascade regression.

3.2. Variable Selection

3.2.1. Independent Variable: Sense of Relative Deprivation

With reference to Smith [55], Osborne [56], and Xiong M. [57], we designed a measure of farmer relative deprivation including nine indicators. Among them, economic deprivation indicators included changes in perceptions of agricultural production, new house acquisition, and production costs before and after retirement; social deprivation indicators included changes in perceptions of employment, pension, and urban treatment before and after retirement; and emotional deprivation indicators included changes in perceptions of belonging, loneliness, and local attachment before and after retirement. The indicators were all on a 5-point Likert scale, with 1 indicating "strongly disagree" and 5 indicating "strongly agree". The higher the score, the greater the relative deprivation of the farmers (Table 1).

Table 1. Relative deprivation evaluation index.

Dimension	Indicators	Average Value	Standard Deviation
Sense of economic deprivation	1. I think it is inconvenient for agricultural production after withdrawing from the house base	3.46	1.228
	2. I think it costs too much to buy a new house after withdrawing from the house site	3.38	1.275
	3. I think the cost of living increases a lot after withdrawing from the residential land	3.35	1.184
Sense of social deprivation	4. I think employment is a problem after withdrawing from the homestead	3.61	1.119
	5. I think it's a problem to retire after withdrawing from the homestead	3.69	1.114
	6. I don't think I can enjoy the same urban treatment after withdrawing from the residential base	3.71	1.065
Sense of emotional deprivation	7. I feel that I don't have a sense of belonging in the new environment after withdrawing from my homestead	3.12	1.266
	8. I feel that after I quit my homestead, I will feel lonely because I have fewer neighbors to interact with	3.11	1.321
	9. I think I will stay in my original village life after I quit the house site	3.13	1.236

3.2.2. Mediating Variable: Social Trust

Specifically for migrant workers, social trust includes at least two levels: legal social trust (i.e., trust in government and law) [58–60] and moral social trust (i.e., trust in the urban environment and social justice) [61]. The four dimensions of trust were measured by the eight questions described in Table 2. These indicators were also on a 5-point Likert scale, with 1 indicating "strongly disagree" and 5 indicating "strongly agree". Again, the higher the score, the greater the relative deprivation of the farmers (Table 2).

Table 2. Social trust evaluation index.

Dimension	Indicators	Average Value	Standard Deviation
Government Trust	1. I believe the government can protect us wage earners	2.23	1.101
	2. If you are infringed by the rights and interests, find the government can be used	2.43	1.18
Legal Trust	3. I believe that my rights and interests can be protected through legal means	2.46	1.015
	4. I believe that the law does not protect only the powerful and rich people	2.45	1.097
Urban Environmental Trust	5. There are still more good people in the city	2.44	1.074
	6. I like the urban environment	2.49	1.082
Social Equity Trust	7. I believe that as long as I work hard, working people can also be very successful	2.43	1.149
	8. I believe that this society is still very fair	2.38	1.098

3.2.3. Moderating Variable: Urban Integration

With reference to Li, H.B. et al. [62], Tian, M. [63], and Zhao, Q. [64], the indicators to measure the urban integration of migrant workers were selected from three dimensions: Economic integration, social integration, and psychological integration. A total of nine measurement questions were used (see Table 3), which were measured on a 5-point Likert scale, with 1 indicating "strongly disagree" and 5 indicating "strongly agree". The higher the score, the greater the degree of urban integration of rural households (Table 3).

Table 3. Urban integration evaluation index.

Dimension	Indicators	Average Value	Standard Deviation
Economic Integration	1. I have a satisfactory employment situation	3.3	1.165
	2. I have the financial ability to accept city price levels	3.29	1.182
	3. I have satisfactory living conditions	3.33	1.241
Social Inclusion	4. I get along with local people	3.35	1.265
	5. I am willing to solve problems with other residents if there are problems affecting the whole neighborhood	3.34	1.207
	6. I understand the difference in social rules between urban and rural areas	3.33	1.246
Psychological integration	7. I have urban identity	3.31	1.211
	8. I wish to contribute to the development of the city	3.3	1.146
	9. I feel at home locally	3.32	1.142

3.2.4. Dependent Variable: Willingness to Withdraw from the Homestead

Willingness to withdraw from the homestead is a psychological state. With reference to Kwong Fo-yeon [65], Huang Yanxin [66], Peng Changsheng [67], and other scholars, the following three questions were chosen to measure willingness to withdraw: "I am willing to exchange my homestead for a government-unified resettlement house", "I am willing to exchange my homestead for a commercial house of the same area", and "I am willing to exchange my homestead for financial compensation". The indicators were measured on a 5-point Likert scale, with 1 indicating "strongly disagree" and 5 indicating "strongly agree". The higher the score, the stronger the willingness to withdraw from the residential base (Table 4).

Table 4. Homestead withdrawal intention evaluation index.

Dimensional	Indicators	Average Value	Standard Deviation
Willingness to withdraw	1. I am willing to exchange my homestead for a government-unified resettlement house	2.35	0.978
	2. I am willing to exchange my homestead for a commercial house of the same size	2.37	0.987
	3. I am willing to exchange my homestead for financial compensation	2.41	0.962

3.3. *Study Area and Data Acquisition*

The data used in this paper came from a sample survey of farmers moving into the city of Jinan, conducted by the subject group. Jinan, one of the 15 sub-provincial cities in China, has been one of the major inflow areas for migrant population in the country. In April 2020, Jinan introduced the "Measures to Deepen the Reform of Household Registration System and Accelerate the Gathering of Talents", which completely abolished the restrictions on settling in urban areas and townships for foreigners who are willing to work and live in Jinan. Thus, Jinan became the third provincial capital in China, after Shenyang and Nanchang, to have "zero threshold" for settling down. The urbanization rate of the resident population in Jinan reached 74.2%, 10.48 percentage points higher than the national average. The existing urbanized farmers in Jinan are mainly distributed in six major industries: manufacturing; transportation, warehousing, and postal services; construction; accommodation and catering; wholesale and retail; and residential services and repair [68]. Therefore, the findings from the case study of Jinan City are considered to be representative of the urban integration and willingness to withdraw from residential bases in large- and medium-sized cities across China, in terms of the number and employment patterns of urban migrant farmers.

The data for the empirical study in this paper were obtained from a survey questionnaire. In order to collect data, we formulated the "Study on the Willingness of Farmers in Jinan to Withdraw from Homesteads" which involved a total of 37 survey items and set up a survey team of 30 students. For some migrant workers who could not understand the content of the questionnaire correctly, we used the method of dictating the questionnaire questions to the respondents and recording the answers. In addition, in order to reduce the influence of social expectation bias, we explained to respondents in the introduction section of the questionnaire that this survey is anonymous and that the data will only be used for academic research. We used a combination of stratified sampling and random sampling to distribute and research the questionnaire. The principles of quotas were as follows: Firstly, districts were used as primary sampling units in Jinan city, and five districts—namely, Lixia district, Shizhong district, Licheng district, Huaiyin district, and Changqing district—were selected as sample survey areas, according to the regional economic development indicators. Among them, Lixia district is the district with the highest level of economic development in Jinan city; Shizhong district, Licheng district, and Huaiyin district are in the middle level; and Changqing district presents relatively weak economic development. Secondly, we selected 240–360 farmers in each district who moved to the city (120–180 in commercial complexes, 72–108 in construction projects, and 48–72 in factories). Next, two commercial complexes, two construction projects, and two factories were randomly selected in each district and we conducted the survey in the form of one-on-one questionnaire interviews. From the perspective of the industries engaged in by migrant workers, the number of people engaged in the secondary industry accounts for about 50.56%, of which the manufacturing industry accounts for about 19.45% and the construction industry accounts for about 31.11%. The tertiary industry accounts for about 49.44%, and these migrant workers mainly work in six major industries, namely manufacturing, transportation, warehousing and postal services, construction, accommodation and catering, wholesale and retail, and resident service repair.

The urban farmers studied were those who had a rural household registration and a rural residential base, but who had left their hometown to work in a non-agricultural industry in Jinan, including domestic workers, maintenance workers, restaurant chefs, hotel waiters, laborers, construction workers, store salesmen, and take-away courier workers. In addition, in order to reduce the influence of social expectation bias, the introduction of the questionnaire explained to the respondents that this was an anonymous survey and that the data would only be used for academic research. The data collection was divided into two stages: A pre-survey and a formal survey. A total of 100 questionnaires were returned in the pre-survey stage from May to June 2021, and some items were improved after reliability and validity analyses (Table 5).

Table 5. Descriptive Statistics of Samples.

Subjects' General Information	Category	Frequency	Percentage
Gender	Male	621	47
	Female	699	53
Age	19–30 years old	208	15.8
	31–40 years old	317	24
	41–50 years old	344	26.1
	51–60 years old	238	18
	61 years old and above	213	16.1
Current Residence Address	Lixia District	251	19
	Licheng District	331	25.1
	Changqing District	199	15.1
	Samuel District	212	16.1
	Zhangqiu District	327	24.8
Monthly income	Under 3500 RMB	103	7.8
	3500–4500 RMB	331	25.1
	4500–5500 RMB	449	34
	5500–6500 RMB	265	20.1
	6500 RMB and above	172	13

Table 5. *Cont.*

Subjects' General Information	Category	Frequency	Percentage
Academic qualifications	Undergraduate	106	8
	College	212	16.1
	High school or junior college	383	29
	Junior High School	423	32
	Elementary school and below	196	14.8
How did you get your current job?	Apply for the job yourself	647	49
	Referral from friends, relatives, or acquaintances	251	19
	Introduction of intermediary organizations	422	32
Your current housing type	Unit allocation	199	15.1
	Government low-cost housing	133	10.1
	Individual Rental	727	55.1
	Individual purchase	261	19.8
Work Unit	Manufacturing	199	15.1
	Transportation, storage, and postal industry	195	14.8
	Construction	302	22.9
	Accommodation and Catering	245	18.6
	Wholesale and retail trade	168	12.7
	Residential service repair industry	211	16

4. Empirical Tests and Analysis of Results

4.1. Structural Equation Model Testing

4.1.1. Reliability and Validity Tests

The Cronbach's alpha values for sense of economic deprivation, social deprivation, emotional deprivation, social trust, urban integration, and willingness to withdraw were 0.850, 0.897, 0.905, 0.930, 0.954, and 0.835, respectively, all of which were greater than 0.7. It is evident that the questionnaire scale used in this study had good reliability. In addition to this, the CITC (corrected item total correlation) between the observed variables and their latent variables met the requirement of being greater than 0.5, indicating that the questionnaire reliability was good for each latent variable, with a good set of question items.

In order to determine the structural validity of the measurement scale for each latent variable, we used the SPSS 21 software to conduct exploratory factor analysis for each dimensional composition. The initial test results showed that the KMO test value for the survey data was 0.943, which was greater than 0.70, indicating that the questionnaire was suitable for factor analysis. The Bartlett's sphericity test showed that the approximate chi-square value was 28,856.003, with a significance level of 0.000 ($p < 0.01$). Therefore, the scale was suitable for factor analysis and, therefore, had a good validity.

In the results of the validity test for the overall questionnaire, six factors with eigenvalues greater than one were extracted in the factor analysis, including a factor with an eigenvalue of 5.915, explaining 20.291% of the variance; an "emotional deprivation" factor with an eigenvalue of 1.758, explaining 8.681% of the variance; and a "social deprivation" factor with an eigenvalue of 1.454, explaining 7.778% of the variance. The cumulative explained variance of these six factors was 74.547%, which was greater than the general standard of 60%, such that the validity of the scale was considered good. The loadings of each measure were higher than 0.5, and there were no cases of high loadings for both factors. The measurement items under each dimension were aggregated together, according to the theoretical distribution, indicating that the questionnaire also had good content validity.

To judge whether the validated factor analysis model was valid, we considered various fitting indicators. In particular, the X^2/df value was 3.216, which is greater than 3; and the RMSEA was 0.041, less than the standard level of 0.08, indicating a good fit. Furthermore, gfi = 0.943, agfi = 0.932, nfi = 0.960, ifi = 0.972, cfi = 0.972, and TLI = 0.969, such that all goodness-of-fit indicators met the general criteria, indicating that the validated factor analysis model developed in this study was valid and matched well with the recovered data (Table 6).

Table 6. Factor analysis results.

Variables	Measurement Topics	Estimate	SE	CR	p	CR	AVE
Sense of economic deprivation	A1	0.831					
	A2	0.83	0.032	32.065	***	0.851	0.656
	A3	0.767	0.03	29.593	***		
Sense of social deprivation	A4	0.885					
	A5	0.887	0.024	42.419	***	0.898	0.745
	A6	0.816	0.023	37.448	***		
Sense of emotional deprivation	A7	0.858					
	A8	0.913	0.026	42.105	***	0.906	0.762
	A9	0.846	0.025	38.421	***		
Social Trust	B1	0.886					
	B2	0.8	0.025	38.1	***		
	B3	0.71	0.024	31.228	***		
	B4	0.748	0.025	33.879	***	0.931	0.628
	B5	0.791	0.023	37.348	***		
	B6	0.739	0.025	33.273	***		
	B7	0.771	0.025	35.657	***		
	B8	0.877	0.022	45.589	***		
City Integration	C1	0.818					
	C2	0.826	0.028	35.988	***		
	C3	0.847	0.029	37.383	***		
	C4	0.856	0.03	38.005	***		
	C5	0.839	0.029	36.876	***	0.954	0.697
	C6	0.841	0.03	37.008	***		
	C7	0.844	0.029	37.18	***		
	C8	0.824	0.028	35.868	***		
	C9	0.818	0.028	35.46	***		
Willingness to withdraw	D1	0.818					
	D2	0.796	0.033	29.406	***	0.836	0.629
	D3	0.765	0.033	28.315	***		

Note: ***, $p < 0.001$, CR, critical ratio (i.e., the t-value corresponding to each item loading); SE, standard error.

As can be seen from the above table, the standardized factor loadings of each question item ranged from 0.71 to 0.913, which were all greater than 0.5, and the standard error values of SE were all less than the standard value of 0.5, indicating that each question item could explain its dimension well, which echoed the results of exploratory factor analysis and further proved that the validity of the questionnaire was good. The combined reliability CR was greater than 0.7, indicating that all the items in each latent variable could consistently explain the latent variable. The AVE values were all above the standard value of 0.5, indicating that the scale used in this paper had good convergent validity.

4.1.2. Structural Equation Model Fitting Index

The validity of the structural equation model is mainly measured in terms of various fitting indicators. Here, the X^2/df value was 1.368, which was less than 3; and the RMSEA was 0.034, less than the standard level of 0.08, indicating a good fit. Furthermore, gfi = 0.917, agfi = 0.9, nfi = 0.919, ifi = 0.977, cfi = 0.977, and TLI = 0.974, such that all goodness-of-fit indicators met the general criteria, indicating that the structural equation model developed in this study was valid and fit the recovered data well.

4.2. Analysis of Data Results

The AMOS 21.0 (IBM, New York, NY, USA) software was used to conduct the structural equation model path analysis, from which we obtained the structural equation model path coefficient values and CR values shown in Table 7. The path coefficients reflect the relationships and degree of influence between variables, while the critical ratio (CR) can determine whether the regression coefficients are significant or not; generally speaking, the CR value should be greater than or equal to 1.96, which indicates a significant difference at the 0.05 significance level (Table 7).

Table 7. Path analysis results.

Hypothetical Path			Estimate	SE	CR	p
Social Trust	<–	Sense of economic deprivation	−0.416	0.032	−13.888	***
Social Trust	<–	Sense of social deprivation	−0.329	0.033	−11.309	***
Social Trust	<–	Sense of emotional deprivation	−0.18	0.024	−7.119	***
Willingness to withdraw	<–	Sense of economic deprivation	−0.226	0.034	−5.92	***
Willingness to withdraw	<–	Sense of social deprivation	−0.309	0.033	−8.539	***
Willingness to withdraw	<–	Sense of emotional deprivation	−0.198	0.023	−6.557	***
Willingness to withdraw	<–	Social Trust	0.142	0.033	3.508	***

Note: ***, $p < 0.001$.

4.2.1. Path Analysis of the Influence of Relative Deprivation Feeling on the Willingness to Withdraw

The standardized path coefficient of economic deprivation on withdrawal intention was −0.226 (t-value = −5.92; $p = 0.000 < 0.001$), indicating that economic deprivation had a significant negative effect on withdrawal intention. Therefore, 2a is valid. The standardized path coefficient of social deprivation on withdrawal intention was −0.309 (t-value = −8.539; $p = 0.000 < 0.001$), indicating that social deprivation had a significant negative influence on the willingness to withdraw. Thus, H2b is valid. The standardized path coefficient of emotional deprivation on the willingness to withdraw was −0.198 (t-value = −6.557; $p = 0.000 < 0.001$), indicating that emotional deprivation had a significant negative influence on the willingness to withdraw. Therefore, H2c is valid.

4.2.2. Path Analysis of the Influence of Social Trust on the Willingness to Withdraw

The standardized path coefficient of social trust on withdraw intention was 0.142 (t-value = 3.508; $p = 0.000 < 0.001$), indicating that social trust has a significant positive effect on withdrawal intention. Thus, H3 holds.

4.2.3. Path Analysis of the Influence of Relative Deprivation Feeling on Social Trust

The standardized path coefficient of economic deprivation on social trust was −0.416 (t-value = −13.888; $p = 0.000 < 0.001$), indicating that economic deprivation had a significant negative effect on social trust. Thus, H1a is valid. The standardized path coefficient of social deprivation on social trust was −0.329 (t-value = −11.309; $p = 0.000 < 0.001$), indicating that social deprivation had a significant negative influence on social trust. Therefore, H1b is valid. The standardized path coefficient of emotional deprivation on social trust was −0.18 (t-value = −7.119 ; $p = 0.000 < 0.001$), indicating that emotional deprivation had a significant negative influence on social trust. Thus, H1c is valid.

4.2.4. Analysis of the Mediating Effect of Social Trust

To verify whether there exists a mediating role of social trust in the path of relative deprivation's influence on willingness to withdraw, a mediating effects test was conducted using the Bootstrap method in the AMOS software, with 2000 replicate samples and 95% confidence intervals. The results of the analysis are shown in Table 8.

Table 8. Bootstrap method mediating effects test results.

Effect Path	Effect Type	Effect Value	SE	95% Confidence Interval		p	Effectiveness Ratio
				Lower Interval	Upper Interval		
Sense of economic deprivation–Social trust–Willingness to withdraw	Total effect	−0.285	0.034	−0.35	−0.218	0.001 **	-
	Direct effect	−0.226	0.046	−0.316	−0.133	0.001 **	79.3%
	Indirect effects	−0.059	0.027	−0.111	−0.006	0.027 *	20.7%
Sense of social deprivation–Social trust–Willingness to withdraw	Total effect	−0.356	0.034	−0.427	−0.29	0.001 **	-
	Direct effect	−0.309	0.041	−0.392	−0.227	0.001 **	86.8%
	Indirect effects	−0.047	0.021	−0.088	−0.005	0.027 *	13.2%
Sense of emotional deprivation–Social trust–Willingness to withdraw	Total effect	−0.223	0.035	−0.291	−0.158	0.001 **	-
	Direct effect	−0.198	0.037	−0.271	−0.125	0.001 **	88.8%
	Indirect effects	−0.026	0.011	−0.047	−0.003	0.023 *	11.2%

Note: *, $p < 0.05$; **, $p < 0.01$.

In the mediated path of economic deprivation–social trust–willingness to withdraw, the total effect value was −0.285, the 95% confidence interval was negative and did not contain 0, and the p-value was less than 0.05, indicating that the total effect existed. The direct effect value was −0.226, the 95% confidence interval was negative and did not contain 0, and the p-value was less than 0.05. The indirect effect value was −0.059, the 95% confidence interval was negative and did not contain 0, and the p-value was less than 0.05. Therefore, the indirect effect existed, accounting for 20.7% of the total effect, and H4a is valid.

In the mediated path of social deprivation–social trust–willingness to withdraw, the total effect value was −0.356, the 95% confidence interval was negative and did not contain 0, and the p-value was less than 0.05, indicating that the total effect existed. The direct effect value was −0.309, the 95% confidence interval was negative and did not contain 0, and the p-value was less than 0.05. The indirect effect value was −0.047, the 95% confidence interval was negative and did not contain 0, and the p-value was less than 0.05. Therefore, the indirect effect existed, accounting for 13.2% of the total effect, and H4b is valid.

In the mediated path emotional deprivation–social trust–willingness to withdraw, the total effect value was −0.223, the 95% confidence interval was negative and did not contain 0, and the p-value was less than 0.05, indicating that the total effect existed. The direct effect value was −0.198, the 95% confidence interval was negative and did not contain 0, and the p-value was less than 0.05. The indirect effect value was −0.026, the 95% confidence interval was negative and did not contain 0, and the p-value was less than 0.05. Therefore, the indirect effect existed, accounting for 11.2% of the total effect, and H4c is valid.

4.2.5. Analysis of the Moderating Effect of Urban Integration

(1) Test of the moderating role of urban integration in the relationship between relative deprivation and social trust.

The test of the moderating effect was mainly conducted using multiple cascade regression, mainly involving the construction of two multiple regression models. The second model introduces the independent and moderating variables, in order to determine whether the independent and moderating variables affect the dependent variable and determine the explanatory power of the model; that is, to judge the model R^2. The third model introduces the independent and moderating variables and their interaction terms. If the regression coefficient of the interaction term is significant and the R^2 value is significantly higher, it means that the moderating variables have a significant effect (Table 9).

Table 9. The moderating effect of urban integration between perceived economic deprivation and social trust.

Variables	Model 1		Model 2	
	B	t	β	t
Sense of economic deprivation	−0.600 ***	−27.162	−0.600 ***	−27.15
Urban Integration	0.044 *	1.988	0.039 *	1.741
Sense of economic deprivation × Urban integration	-	-	0.036 *	1.612
R^2	0.370		0.371	
Adjusted R^2	0.369		0.370	
ΔR^2	-		0.001	
F	387.146 ***		259.277 ***	

Note: ***, $p < 0.001$; *, $p < 0.05$.

As shown in the table above, Model 1 was a multiple regression model with economic deprivation and urban integration as independent variables and social trust as a dependent variable, while Model 2 was a multiple regression model with economic deprivation, urban integration, and the interaction term economic deprivation × urban integration as independent variables and social trust as a dependent variable. In Model 1, the independent variable economic deprivation had a significant negative effect on social trust (β = −0.600; t = −27.162; $p < 0.001$). In Model 2, the regression coefficient of the interaction term between the independent variable and the moderating variable was 0.036 (t = 1.612; $p > 0.05$), indicating that the interaction term did not have a significant effect on social trust. The R^2 of Model 1 was 0.370 and that for Model 2 was 0.371, which did not change significantly. Therefore, the moderating variable—urban integration—does not play a significant moderating role in the relationship between the effect of economic deprivation and social trust. Thus, H5a is not valid.

1) Testing the moderating role of urban integration in the relationship between social deprivation and social trust.

As shown in the table above, Model 1 was a multiple regression model with economic deprivation and urban integration as independent variables and social trust as a dependent variable, while Model 2 was a multiple regression model with economic deprivation, urban integration, and the interaction term economic deprivation × urban integration as independent variables and social trust as a dependent variable. In Model 1, the independent variable economic deprivation has a significant negative effect on social trust (β = −0.600; t = −27.162; $p < 0.001$). In model 2, the regression coefficient of the interaction term between the independent variable and the moderating variable was 0.036 (t = 1.612; $p > 0.05$), indicating that the interaction term did not have a significant effect on social trust. The R^2 of Model 1 is 0.370 and that for Model 2 was 0.371, which did not change significantly. Therefore, it the moderating variable urban integration does not have a significant moderating role in the relationship between the effect of economic deprivation and social trust. Therefore, H5a is not valid (Table 10).

Table 10. Test of the moderating effect of urban integration between perception of social deprivation and social trust.

Variables	Model 1		Model 2	
	β	t	β	t
Sense of economic deprivation	−0.600 ***	−27.162	−0.600 ***	−27.15
Urban Integration	0.044 *	1.988	0.039 *	1.741
Sense of economic deprivation × Urban integration	-	-	0.036	1.612
R^2	0.370		0.371	
Adjusted R^2	0.369		0.370	
ΔR^2	-		0.001	
F	387.146 ***		259.277 ***	

Note: ***, $p < 0.001$; *, $p < 0.05$.

2) Test of the moderating role of urban integration in the relationship between social deprivation and social trust.

As shown in the table above, Model 1 was a multiple regression model with social deprivation and urban integration as independent variables and social trust as a dependent variable, while Model 2 was a multiple regression model with social deprivation, urban integration, and the interaction term social deprivation × urban integration as independent variables and social trust as a dependent variable. In Model 1, the independent variable social deprivation has a significant negative effect on social trust ($\beta = -0.594$; $t = -26.378$; $p < 0.001$). In Model 2, the regression coefficient of the interaction term between the independent variable and the moderating variable was 0.097 ($t = 4.370$; $p < 0.001$), indicating that the interaction term had a significant positive effect on social trust. The R^2 of Model 1 was 0.357, and that for Model 2 was 0.366, which was significantly higher, indicating the enhanced explanatory power of the model. Therefore, the moderating variable—urban integration—has a significant positive moderating effect in the relationship between social deprivation and social trust. In particular, urban integration weakens the negative relationship between social deprivation and social trust, and so, H5b is valid (Table 11, Figure 2).

Table 11. Test of the moderating effect of urban integration between perception of social deprivation and social trust.

Variables	Model 1		Model 2	
	β	t	β	t
Sense of social deprivation	−0.594 ***	−26.378	−0.593 ***	−26.522
Urban Integration	0.020	0.876	0.004 **	0.185
Social deprivation × Urban integration	-	-	0.097 ***	4.370
R^2	0.357		0.366	
Adjusted R^2	0.356		0.365	
ΔR^2	-		0.009	
F	365.784 ***		253.571 ***	

Note: *** $p < 0.001$, ** $p < 0.01$.

3) Test of the moderating role of urban integration in the relationship between emotional deprivation and social trust.

As shown in the table above, Model 1 was a multiple regression model with emotional deprivation and urban integration as independent variables and social trust as a dependent variable, while Model 2 was a multiple regression model with emotional deprivation, urban integration, and the interaction term emotional deprivation × urban integration as independent variables and social trust as a dependent variable. In Model 1, the independent variable emotional deprivation had a significant negative effect on social trust ($\beta = -0.160$; $t = -18.543$; $p < 0.001$). In Model 2, the regression coefficient of the interaction term between the independent variable and the moderating variable was 0.053 ($t = 2.148$; $p < 0.001$), indicating that the interaction term had a significant positive effect on social trust. The R^2 of model 1 was 0.221 and that for Model 2 was 0.224, comprising a significant improvement, indicating the enhanced explanatory power of the model. Therefore, it the moderating variable urban integration has a significant positive moderating effect on the relationship between emotional deprivation and social trust. Thus, urban integration weakens the negative relationship between emotional deprivation and social trust, and so, H5c is valid (Table 12, Figure 3).

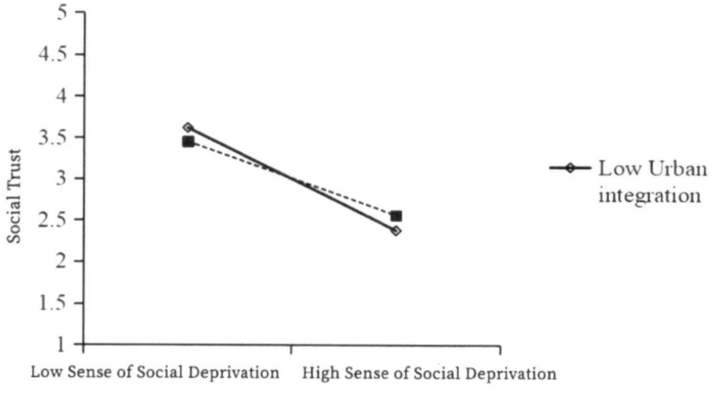

Figure 2. Graph of the moderating effect of urban integration in the relationship between the sense of social deprivation and social trust.

Table 12. Test of the moderating effect of urban integration on the relationship between emotional deprivation and social trust.

Variables	Model 1		Model 2	
	β	t	β	t
Sense of emotional deprivation	−0.460 ***	−18.543	−0.458 ***	−18.481
Urban Integration	0.041	1.647	0.033 *	1.301
Emotional deprivation × Urban integration	-	-	0.053 *	2.148
R^2	0.221		0.224	
Adjusted R^2	0.220		0.222	
ΔR^2	-		0.003	
F	186.690 ***		126.339 ***	

Note: ***, $p < 0.001$; *, $p < 0.05$.

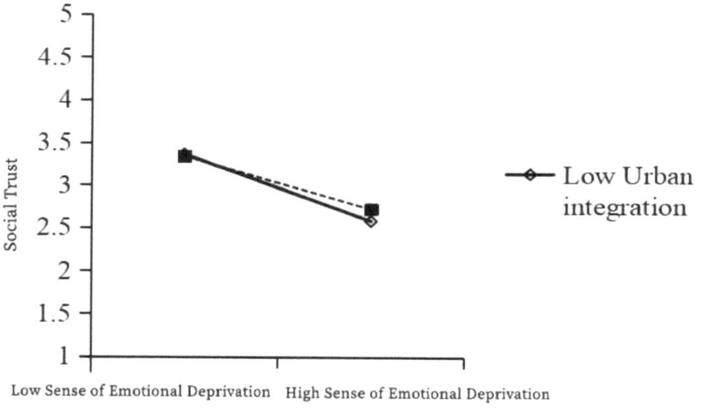

Figure 3. The moderating effect of urban integration on the relationship between emotional deprivation and social trust.

(2) Test of the moderating role of urban integration in the relationship between relative deprivation and willingness to withdraw.

1) Testing the moderating role of urban integration in the relationship between the sense of economic deprivation and the willingness to withdraw.

As shown in the table above, Model 1 was a multiple regression model with sense of economic deprivation and urban integration as independent variables and withdrawal intention as a dependent variable, while Model 2 was a multiple regression model with sense of economic deprivation, urban integration, and the interaction term sense of economic deprivation × urban integration as independent variables and withdrawal intention as a dependent variable. In Model 1, the independent variable economic deprivation had a significant negative effect on withdrawal intention (β = −0.455; t = −18.911; $p < 0.001$). In Model 2, the regression coefficient of the interaction term between the independent variable and the moderating variable was 0.126 (t = 5.313; $p < 0.001$), indicating that the interaction term has a significant positive effect on withdrawal intention. The R^2 of Model 1 was 0.256 and that of Model 2 was 0.271, presenting a significant improvement, indicating the enhanced explanatory power of the model. Therefore, the moderating variable—urban integration—had a significant positive moderating effect on the relationship between economic deprivation and the willingness to withdraw. In particular, urban integration weakens the negative relationship between the feeling of economic deprivation and the willingness to withdraw, and so, H6a is valid (Table 13, Figure 4).

Table 13. The moderating effect of urban integration on the relationship between economic deprivation and willingness to withdraw.

Variables	Model 1		Model 2	
	β	t	β	t
Sense of economic deprivation	−0.455 ***	−18.911	−0.453 ***	−19.021
Urban Integration	0.164 ***	6.835	0.146 ***	6.082
Sense of economic deprivation × Urban integration	-	-	0.126 ***	5.313
R^2	0.256		0.271	
Adjusted R^2	0.254		0.270	
ΔR^2	-		0.016	
F	226.039 ***		163.217 ***	

Note: ***, $p < 0.001$.

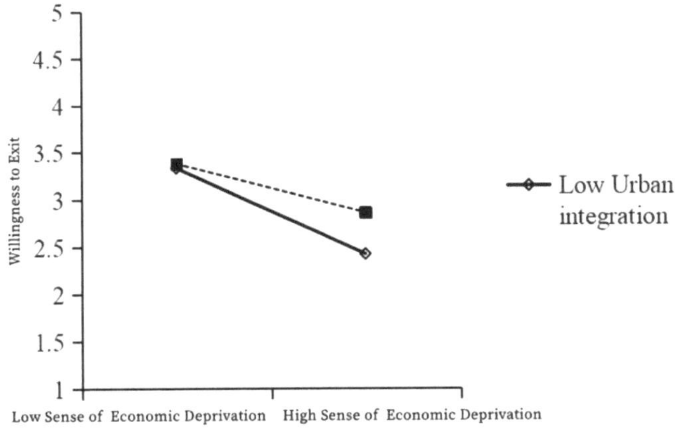

Figure 4. Moderating effect of urban integration between the sense of economic deprivation and willingness to withdraw.

2) Test of the moderating effect of urban integration between the sense of social deprivation and the willingness to withdraw.

As shown in the table above, Model 1 was a multiple regression model with social deprivation and urban integration as independent variables and withdrawal intention as a dependent variable, while Model 2 was a multiple regression model with social deprivation, urban integration, and the interaction term social deprivation × urban integration as independent variables and withdrawal intention as a dependent variable. In Model 1, the independent variable social deprivation had a significant negative effect on withdrawal intention (β = −0.507; t = −21.6; $p < 0.001$). In Model 2, the regression coefficient of the interaction term between the independent variable and the moderating variable was 0.172 (t = 7.523; $p < 0.001$), indicating that the interaction term had a significant positive effect on withdrawal intention. The R^2 of Model 1 was 0.301 and that of Model 2 was 0.330, presenting a significant improvement and indicating the enhanced explanatory power of the model. Therefore, the moderating variable—urban integration—has a significant positive moderating effect on the relationship between social deprivation and the willingness to withdraw. In particular, urban integration weakens the negative relationship between social deprivation and willingness to withdraw, and so, H6b is valid (Table 14, Figure 5).

Table 14. The moderating effect of urban integration on the relationship between social deprivation and willingness to withdraw.

Variables	Model 1		Model 2	
	β	t	β	t
Sense of social deprivation	−0.507 ***	−21.6	−0.505 ***	−21.99
Urban Integration	0.135 ***	5.755	0.108 ***	4.623
Sense of social deprivation × Urban integration			0.172 ***	7.523
R^2	0.301		0.330	
Adjusted R^2	0.300		0.328	
ΔR^2	-		0.029	
F	283.573 ***		215.895 ***	

Note: ***, $p < 0.001$.

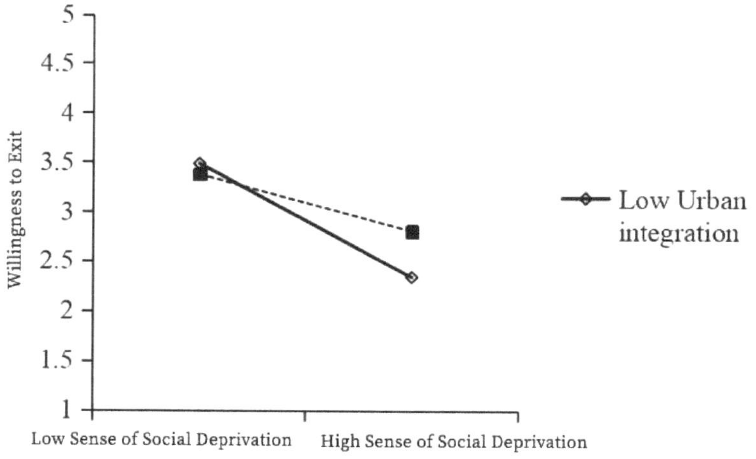

Figure 5. Moderating effect of urban integration between the sense of social deprivation and willingness to withdraw.

3) Test of the moderating role of urban integration between emotional deprivation and willingness to withdraw.

As shown in the table above, Model 1 was a multiple regression model with emotional deprivation and urban integration as independent variables and withdrawal intention as a dependent variable, while Model 2 was a multiple regression model with emotional deprivation, urban integration, and the interaction term emotional deprivation × urban integration as independent variables and withdrawal intention as a dependent variable. In Model 1, the independent variable emotional deprivation had a significant negative effect on withdrawal intention (β = −0.409; t = −16.429; $p < 0.001$). In Model 2, the regression coefficient of the interaction term between the independent variable and the moderating variable was 0.083 (t = 3.373; $p < 0.001$), indicating that the interaction term has a significant positive effect on withdrawal intention. The R^2 of Model 1 was 0.214 and that of Model 2 was 0.221, showing a significant improvement, indicating the enhanced explanatory power of the model. Therefore, the moderating variable—urban integration—has a significant positive moderating effect on the relationship between emotional deprivation and willingness to withdraw. In particular, urban integration weakens the negative relationship between emotional deprivation and willingness to withdraw, and so, H6c is valid (Table 15, Figure 6).

Table 15. Test of the moderating effect of urban integration on the relationship between emotional deprivation and willingness to withdraw.

Variables	Model 1		Model 2	
	β	t	β	t
Sense of emotional deprivation	−0.409 ***	−16.429	−0.406 ***	−16.364
Urban Integration	0.15 ***	6.013	0.137 ***	5.449
Emotional deprivation × Urban integration	-	-	0.083 **	3.373
R^2	0.214		0.221	
Adjusted R^2	0.213		0.219	
ΔR^2	-		0.007	
F	179.702 ***		124.537 ***	

Note: ***, $p < 0.001$; **, $p < 0.01$.

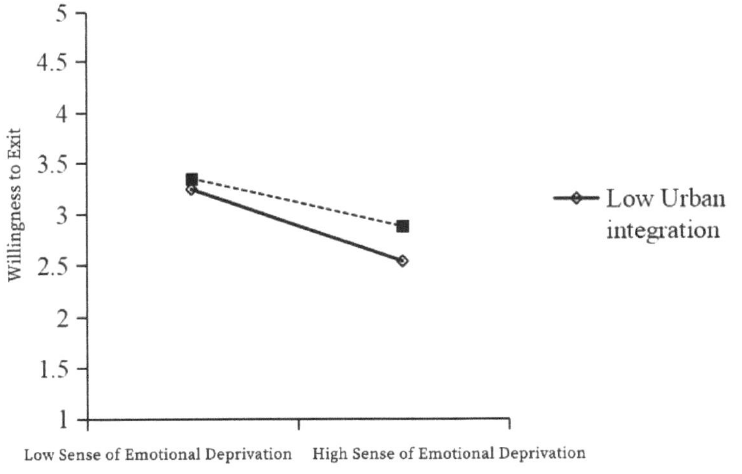

Figure 6. Moderating effect of urban integration between the sense of emotional deprivation and willingness to withdraw.

5. Discussion

Compared with previous studies, this study has more comprehensive considerations. Using the research data of 1320 households in Jinan, we analyzed the interaction and influence of the emotional psychological factors and social environmental factors of the peasants who entered the city on their willingness to withdraw from the homestead. We divided the relative deprivation of farmers into economic deprivation, social deprivation and emotional deprivation innovatively. At the same time, we empirically explored the internal mechanism of the impact of various dimensions of relative deprivation on farmers' homestead withdrawal and differentiated the intermediary effect of social trust and the regulatory effect of urban integration.

First, we found that relative deprivation has a significant negative effect on the homestead withdrawal behavior of farmers, which inhibits them from withdrawing from their homesteads. Second, social trust was found to play a mediating role in all dimensions of relative deprivation on the homestead withdrawal behavior of farmers. Third, urban integration was found to play a positive moderating role in inhibiting the homestead withdrawal behavior of farmers: the higher the degree of urban integration, the weaker the inhibiting effect of relative deprivation on the withdrawal behavior. Urban integration was also found to play a positive moderating role in inhibiting the effects of social deprivation and emotional deprivation on social trust, such that an increase in the urban integration degree can weaken the influence of emotional deprivation on the homestead withdrawal behavior of farmers.

As a member of the rural collective, the homestead is a source of income. As a necessary place for rural collective members to live and use without compensation for an indefinite period of time, the homestead guarantees the survival needs of members of the collective. Therefore, the homestead also assumes part of the function of social security [12]. However, when farmers move to the city, it is difficult for them to get a home and to enjoy the same treatment as urban residents, in terms of employment, pension, education, and medical care, such that withdrawal from their homesteads may induce a loss of social security function rights and interests [8]. Therefore, the implementation of urban farmer homestead withdrawal may generate a strong sense of social deprivation, considering the loss of their social security function and rights. This sense of social deprivation that inhibits their willingness to withdraw from their homestead bases. At the same time, the local society has endowed the homestead with the function of emotional inheritance, carrying the farmer's love for the land and emotional attachment [69]. When farmers are faced with the problem of withdrawing from their homestead base, it may bring about an expectation of loss of emotional functional rights and interests, thus generating a strong sense of emotional deprivation, which will inhibit their homestead withdrawal behavior. Although relative deprivation is unavoidable, people can resolve and prevent it in certain ways. Improving farmers' social trust is one of the effective ways to alleviate the sense of relative deprivation.

Regarding H1, these results supported H1a–H1c. The results are consistent with the results of Pierce, J.L. et al. (2001) [70], Niu, X. F. et al. (2021) [71] and Morewedge, C. K. et al. (2009) [72]. First, the homestead base not only facilitates agricultural production activities and the development of yard economy for farmers but, also, with the state's emphasis on the usufruct rights of homestead bases, the economic property attributes of the homestead bases are increasingly obvious. Therefore, this will raise the expectation regarding the economic functional value of the homestead, and the expected loss of economic functional rights and interests brought by the withdrawal of the homestead will generate a strong sense of economic deprivation which, in turn, will inhibit the willingness to withdraw from the homestead [38,72].

Regarding H2, these results supported H2a–H2c. The results are consistent with the results of Hooghe, M. et al. (2017) [73] and Fischer, J.A.V. et al. (2013) [74].Generally speaking, individuals who are successful in socio-economic life are more likely to trust state institutions [73]. Then, relative to the rural residents who are in a disadvantaged position, the generation of a sense of relative deprivation affects their degree of trust in social, organizational, power, management, and governance systems [74]. Although a sense of relative deprivation is unavoidable, it can be resolved and prevented in certain ways, providing a means to enhance the social trust of farmers. Social trust is one of the means with which the sense of relative deprivation can be hedged.

Regarding H3, these results supported H3. The results are consistent with the results of Beaudoin, C.E. et al. (2004) [45], Meng, T. et al. (2014) [75] and Jiang, J. et al. (2021) [47]. (1) Good social trust can enhance their courage to withdraw from their homestead bases and eliminate their fear of the unknown risks that may be brought about by the homestead reform [75]. In turn, this can enhance their willingness to withdraw from their homestead bases [35]. (2) The higher the trust of farmers in village cadres or councils, the stronger the guarantee mechanism of village cadres or councils and the more confidence they have in the household registration commitment, compensation commitment, and policy commitment being true and credible, which plays an important role in overcoming the psychological "uncertainty in homestead withdrawal" of farmers. Thus, farmers will be motivated to choose to withdraw from their homestead bases. (3) It is believed that judicial, administrative, and legislative bodies will protect the legal rights and interests of the rural-to-urban migrant workers and provide legal support for them to live and work in the city. In this way, the social trust of the urban migrant population can be enhanced, which, in turn, will enhance the willingness of farm households to withdraw from their homesteads.

Regarding H4, these results supported H4a–H4c. The results are consistent with the results of Shen, S. et al. (2022) [47] and Xu, Z. et al. (2020) [51]. The specific impact paths of relative deprivation and governmental trust on the willingness of farmers to withdraw can be described as follows: (1) The negative emotional reactions and cognitive changes derived from relative deprivation, as well as the frustration generated by social comparison, lead some members of society with an avoidance mentality to adopt outward attribution. This will, to a certain extent, reduce their trust in the government and promote their recourse to extra-institutional means of benefit protection, which has a negative impact on their willingness to withdraw from their homestead [76]. (2) The local government is the main government organization related to the distribution of social benefits and the implementation of policies and measures for rural residents [77]. A sense of relative deprivation will lead to dissatisfaction in the social living standard and social status of rural residents, which will lead them to question the performance of the local government or the competence of its staff [48]. This will affect the trust of rural residents in the grassroots government, thus affecting the willingness of rural households to withdraw.

Regarding H5, these results supported H5b and H5c, but not supported H5a. Regarding H5a, the results are not consistent with the results of Chen, Z. et al. (2019) [32]. Theoretically, urban integration can alleviate the economic pressure or reduce the various forms of material deprivation of retiring farmers by providing stable employment, a livable environment and complete public services, thus weakening the negative influence of the sense of economic deprivation on farmers' homestead withdrawal behavior. However, from the current data, there is no significant impact. It may be because: migrant workers only consider the city as a place to work, and do not consider themselves as part of the city, and they do not obtain the corresponding emotional support and sense of value, which will reduce their willingness to integrate into the local city. This results in an involutional identity of migrant workers, which increases the social distance between migrant workers and the city, thus causing the migrant worker group to voluntarily choose to form their own community network and create a deep separation from the urban society, thus affecting their trust level in the city. [32]. Regarding H5b and H5c, the results are consistent with the results of Sun, X. et al. (2022) [31] and Wang, W.W. et al. (2012) [34]. Firstly, urban integration can expand an individual's options to participate in political and community activities by giving them various opportunities for social participation, thus enhancing their social rights and abilities through participation in social interactions and, consequently, weakening the negative influence of the sense of social deprivation on the homestead withdrawal behavior of farmers [31]. Secondly, urban integration involves achieving integration into urban culture and identifying oneself as an "urbanite". Having a psychologically comfortable urban life can only be achieved when the psychological integration of urban farmers is completed [34]. Psychological integration will motivate farmers to choose to settle in the city, significantly weakening their cultural and emotional attachment to the homestead, such that they will be more willing to give up their old homes in the countryside and better realize their settlement in the city using the property gains from the withdrawal from their homestead. In other words, psychological integration affects the negative influence on the homestead withdrawal behavior of farmers by weakening their sense of emotional deprivation.

Regarding H6, these results supported H6. The results are consistent with the results of Xu, D. et al. (2020) [78] and Xu, Y. et al. (2021) [51]. In general, rural societies are acquaintance-oriented societies, while urban societies are stranger-oriented societies. As urban farmers leave the society of acquaintances and come to the city to make a living, the anonymity and fickleness of human interactions are strong, and it becomes more and more difficult to establish social trust [79]. The reason for the social distrust of urban migrant farmers is that they are disadvantaged in the distribution of social resources, due to institutional and policy constraints [78]; that is, therefore, it can be hypothesized that high-quality urban integration can enhance social identity and sense of belonging by improving the quality of life, forming solidarity and stable values, and thus weakening the negative effects of emotional deprivation.

6. Conclusions

In the context of the accelerated development of new urbanization, exploring and establishing a mechanism for the paid withdrawal from rural residential bases is considered a general trend for rural residential base system reform in the future, which is of great significance to revitalize the inefficiently utilized land resources in rural areas, activate the dormant land assets in rural areas, increase the property income of farmers, optimize the land structure and spatial layout of urban and rural areas, and promote rural revitalization. The following aspects should be considered in such processes.

(1) The government should pay attention to and helping farmers to rationalize the property rights of residential bases. On one hand, although the legal level clearly defines that the ownership of residential bases belongs to the collective, most farmers have conducted a de facto "blurring" of the concept of "collective", such that it is necessary to further clarify and standardize the meaning and scope of "collective. For this reason, publicity and popularization should be carried out by building an information platform regarding residential base policy, in order to gradually weaken the misperception of "possession means ownership" in the traditional thinking of farmers. On the other hand, clarifying property rights relationships and the registration of rights is fundamental. Government should speed up the process of issuing real estate property rights certificates, as well as further deepening the knowledge and understanding of farmers in the process of confirming and issuing certificates.

(2) Weakening the sense of relative deprivation in farmers. First, we need to accelerate the improvement of the market price formation mechanism for rural residential bases. In order to achieve the reasonableness and fairness of the withdrawal compensation and value-added income, the withdrawal cost of farmers should be shared through realization of the property value of residential bases, which will help to weaken their sense of economic deprivation. Second, focus should be placed on the livelihood and development of farmers after their withdrawal from residential bases; improving social acceptance; and achieving fair rights, fair opportunities, and fair distribution in the construction of social security, in order to alleviate the worries of farmers who have withdrawn from their residential bases and weaken their sense of social deprivation. The third is to improve the ability of migrant workers to integrate into society. Governments should focus on designing inclusive development policies to promote the social integration of urban farmers. Link government performance with inclusive governance to improve the government's incentive for inclusive governance. At the same time, encourage social organizations to synergize with government departments and play a complementary function to ensure the equalization of public services. Attention should also be paid to building a socially inclusive environment with equal opportunities and shared outcomes, eliminating various forms of social exclusion and weakening their sense of emotional deprivation.

(3) Improve and enhance the level of social trust of farming households. Given that social trust has a good external effect, society should actively advocate the concept of equal pay for equal work and equal rights in the same city, guarantee the citizenship of the rural-to-urban migrant workers, and improve the trust level in the rural-to-urban migrant workers. The government, society, and enterprises are the protagonists of social trust building, and these three parties need to coordinate and cooperate in order to effectively promote the social integration of the rural-to-urban migrant workers. The government plays the role of coordination, supervision, and management, with a focus on balancing the social rights of the rural-to-urban migrant workers and granting them equal citizenship

rights when designing policies. Society should enhance the city's inclusive and pluralistic character, adopting an accepting attitude toward the rural-to-urban migrant workers and improving urban governance. Employers should treat foreigners equally, take social responsibility, provide vocational training and benefits to foreigners, and promote professional integration. Only in this way can urban society achieve long-lasting peace and stability, in the process of which the rural-to-urban migrant workers can truly achieve welfare growth and social integration.

First, village and township cadres should effectively perform their duties, reach out to the masses, and respond to needs of farmers and win their trust. Second, construction of residential base withdrawal mechanisms should be conducted differently, according to the local conditions and orderly promotion of residential base withdrawal. Due to the large differences in the locations of homesteads and farm buildings, different family planning patterns, and different levels of social trust, in order to avoid various social risks and contradictions in the process of homestead withdrawal, it is necessary to develop differentiated policies which are applicable to different groups of farmers and avoid one-sided "one-size-fits-all" practices, which may cause adverse social consequences. Third, the social integration capacity of farmers should be improved, through designing inclusive development policies to promote the social integration of farmers into cities. In this context, the performance of the government should be integrated in an inclusive manner to improve the government's incentive for inclusive governance; second, social organizations should be encouraged to synergize with government departments, playing a complementary function to ensure the equality of public services; and, finally, a socially inclusive environment with equal opportunities and shared results to eliminate various forms of social exclusion should be built up, thus innovating social participation and improving social empowerment.

Author Contributions: Conceptualization, W.S. and L.M.; methodology, W.S. and L.M.; software, W.S.; validation, L.M.; formal analysis, W.S.; investigation, W.S.; resources, W.S.; data curation, W.S.; writing—original draft preparation, W.S. and L.M.; writing—review and editing, W.S., C.J. and L.M.; visualization, W.S. and L.M.; supervision, W.S. and L.M.; project administration, W.S.; funding acquisition, W.S. All authors have read and agreed to the published version of the manuscript.

Funding: This research was funded by Social Science Planning and Research Project of Shandong, China (Grant NO. 22DGLJ32) and Philosophy and Social Science Project of Jinan, China (Grant NO. JNSK22C101).

Institutional Review Board Statement: Not applicable.

Informed Consent Statement: Informed consent was obtained from all subjects involved in the study.

Data Availability Statement: Not applicable.

Conflicts of Interest: The authors declare no conflict of interest.

References

1. Liu, R.; Yu, C.; Jiang, J.; Huang, Z.; Jiang, Y. Farmer differentiation, generational differences and farmers' behaviors to withdraw from rural homesteads: Evidence from Chengdu, China. *Habitat Int.* **2020**, *103*, 102231. [CrossRef]
2. State Statistical Bureau. Monitoring and Investigation Report of Migrant Workers in 2021. Available online: www.stats.gov.cn/xxgk/sjfb/zxfb2020/202204/t20220429_1830139.html (accessed on 29 April 2022).
3. State Statistical Bureau, Statistical Bulletin of National Economic and Social Development in 2021. Available online: http://www.stats.gov.cn/xxgk/sjfb/zxfb2020/202202/t20220228_1827971.html (accessed on 28 February 2022).
4. Yuan, Z.; Fu, C.; Kong, S.; Du, J.; Li, W. Citizenship Ability, Homestead Utility, and Rural Homestead Transfer of "Amphibious" Farmers. *Sustainability* **2022**, *14*, 42067. [CrossRef]
5. National Agricultural and Rural Sector.Notice on the Active and Steady Development of Rural Idle House Bases and Idle Residential Inventory and Utilization. Available online: http://www.moa.gov.cn/nybgb/2019/201910/202001/t20200109_6334695.htm (accessed on 9 January 2020).
6. Liang, F.; Wang, Z.; Lin, S.-H. Can Land Policy Promote Farmers' Subjective Well-Being? A Study on Withdrawal from Rural Homesteads in Jinjiang, China. *Int. J. Environ. Res. Public Health* **2022**, *19*, 7414. [CrossRef] [PubMed]
7. Han, W.L.; Liu, L. Tenure awareness, resource endowment, and willingness to quit the homestead. *Agric. Econ. Issues* **2020**, *3*, 31–39. (In Chinese)

8. Chen, H.; Zhao, L.; Zhao, Z. Influencing factors of farmers' willingness to withdraw from rural homesteads: A survey in Zhejiang, China. *Land Use Policy* **2017**, *68*, 524–530. [CrossRef]
9. Liu, R.; Jiang, J.; Yu, C.; Rodenbiker, J.; Jiang, Y. The endowment effect accompanying villagers' withdrawal from rural homesteads: Field evidence from Chengdu, China. *Land Use Policy* **2021**, *101*, 105107. [CrossRef]
10. Liang, F.; Lin, C.; Lin, S.H. Farmers' livelihood, risk expectations, and homestead withdrawal policy: Evidence on JinJiang pilot of China. *Int. J. Strateg. Prop. Manag.* **2022**, *26*, 56–71. [CrossRef]
11. Lu, X.; Peng, W.; Huang, X.; Fu, Q.; Zhang, Q. Homestead management in China from the "separation of two rights" to the "separation of three rights": Visualization and analysis of hot topics and trends by mapping knowledge domains of academic papers in China National Knowledge Infrastructure (CNKI). *Land Use Policy* **2020**, *97*, 104670. [CrossRef]
12. Liu, R. Incomplete Urbanization and the Trans-Local Rural-Urban Gradient in China: From a Perspective of New Economics of Labor Migration. *Land* **2022**, *11*, 282. [CrossRef]
13. Dong, G.; Zhang, W.; Xu, X.; Jia, K. Multi-Dimensional Feature Recognition and Policy Implications of Rural Human-Land Relationships in China. *Land* **2021**, *10*, 1086. [CrossRef]
14. Dong, G.; Ge, Y.; Cao, H.; Zhai, R. Withdrawal and Transformation of Rural Homesteads in Traditional Agricultural Areas of China Based on Supply-Demand Balance Analysis. *Front. Environ. Sci.* **2022**, *10*, 570. [CrossRef]
15. Cao, Q.; Sarker, M.N.I.; Sun, J. Model of the influencing factors of the withdrawal from rural homesteads in China: Application of grounded theory method. *Land Use Policy* **2019**, *85*, 285–289. [CrossRef]
16. Qin, W.; Xu, L.; Wu, S.; Shao, H. Income, Relative Deprivation and the Self-Rated Health of Older People in Urban and Rural China. *Front. Public Health* **2021**, *9*, 658649. [CrossRef] [PubMed]
17. Lu, P.; Yu, M.; Hu, Y. Contradictions in and improvements to urban and rural residents' housing rights in China's urbanization process. *Habitat Int.* **2020**, *97*, 102101. [CrossRef]
18. Jin, L. Migration, Relative Deprivation, and Psychological Well-Being in China. *Am. Behav. Sci.* **2016**, *60*, 750–770. [CrossRef]
19. Kafle, K.; Benfica, R.; Winters, P. Does relative deprivation induce migration? Evidence from Sub-Saharan Africa. *Am. J. Agric. Econ.* **2020**, *102*, 999–1019. [CrossRef]
20. Visser, M.; Gesthuizen, M.; Scheepers, P. The Impact of Macro-Economic Circumstances and Social Protection Expenditure on Economic Deprivation in 25 European Countries, 2007-2011. *Soc. Indic. Res.* **2014**, *115*, 1179–1203. [CrossRef]
21. Ayala, L.; Jurado, A.; Perez-Mayo, J. Multidimensional deprivation in heterogeneous rural areas: Spain after the economic crisis. *Reg. Stud.* **2021**, *55*, 883–893. [CrossRef]
22. Hannum, E.; Hu, W.; Park, A. Home, School, and Community Deprivations: A Multi-Context Approach to Childhood Poverty in China. *J. Contemp. China* **2019**, *28*, 864–882. [CrossRef]
23. Yuan, Y.; Xu, M.; Cao, X.; Liu, S. Exploring urban-rural disparity of the multiple deprivation index in Guangzhou City from 2000 to 2010. *Cities* **2018**, *79*, 1–11. [CrossRef]
24. Zhang, L.; Fan, W. Rural Homesteads Withdrawal and Urban Housing Market: A Pilot Study in China. *Emerg. Mark. Financ. Trade* **2020**, *56*, 228–242. [CrossRef]
25. Wu, Y.; Mo, Z.; Peng, Y.; Skitmore, M. Market-driven land nationalization in China: A new system for the capitalization of rural homesteads. *Land Use Policy* **2018**, *70*, 559–569. [CrossRef]
26. Gao, J.; Song, G.; Liu, S. Factors influencing farmers' willingness and behavior choices to withdraw from rural homesteads in China. *Growth Chang.* **2022**, *53*, 112–131. [CrossRef]
27. Huang, X.; Li, H.; Zhang, X.; Zhang, X. Land use policy as an instrument of rural resilience—The case of land withdrawal mechanism for rural homesteads in China. *Ecol. Indic.* **2018**, *87*, 47–55. [CrossRef]
28. Kong, X.; Liu, Y.; Jiang, P.; Tian, Y.; Zou, Y. A novel framework for rural homestead land transfer under collective ownership in China. *Land Use Policy* **2018**, *78*, 138–146. [CrossRef]
29. Liu, R.; Jia, Y. Resilience and Circularity: Revisiting the Role of Urban Village in Rural-Urban Migration in Beijing, China. *Land* **2021**, *10*, 1284. [CrossRef]
30. Zou, J.; Deng, X. To inhibit or to promote: How does the digital economy affect urban migrant integration in China? *Technol. Forecast. Soc. Chang.* **2022**, *179*, 121647. [CrossRef]
31. Sun, X.; Chen, J.; Xie, S. Becoming Urban Citizens: A Three-Phase Perspective on the Social Integration of Rural-Urban Migrants in China. *Int. J. Environ. Res. Public Health* **2022**, *19*, 5946. [CrossRef]
32. Chen, Z. How the choice of reference group matters: Economic integration of rural-to-urban migrants in China. *J. Ethn. Migr. Stud.* **2019**, *47*, 4428–4456. [CrossRef]
33. Wang, M.; Ning, Y. The Social Integration of Migrants in Shanghai's Urban Villages. *China Rev. Interdiscip. J. Greater China* **2016**, *16*, 93–120.
34. Wang, W.W.; Fan, C.C. Migrant Workers' Integration in Urban China: Experiences in Employment, Social Adaptation, and Self-Identity. *Eurasian Geogr. Econ.* **2012**, *53*, 731–749. [CrossRef]
35. Huhe, N.; Chen, J.; Tang, M. Social trust and grassroots governance in rural China. *Soc. Sci. Res.* **2015**, *53*, 351–363. [CrossRef] [PubMed]
36. Li, F.; Loyalka, P.; Yi, H.; Shi, Y.; Johnson, N.; Rozelle, S. Ability tracking and social trust in China's rural secondary school system. *Sch. Eff. Sch. Improv.* **2018**, *29*, 545–572. [CrossRef]

37. Chen, D.; Liu, X.; Wang, C. Social Trust and Bank Loan Financing: Evidence from China. *Abacus-A J. Account. Financ. Bus. Stud.* **2016**, *52*, 374–403. [CrossRef]
38. Lyon, F.; Porter, G. Market institutions, trust and norms: Exploring moral economies in Nigerian food systems. *Camb. J. Econ.* **2009**, *33*, 903–920. [CrossRef]
39. Kim, P.H.; Li, M. Seeking Assurances When Taking Action: Legal Systems, Social Trust, and Starting Businesses in Emerging Economies. *Organ. Stud.* **2014**, *35*, 359–391. [CrossRef]
40. Rapp, C. Moral opinion polarization and the erosion of trust. *Soc. Sci. Res.* **2016**, *58*, 34–45. [CrossRef]
41. Su, K.; Wu, J.; Yan, Y.; Zhang, Z.; Yang, Q. The Functional Value Evolution of Rural Homesteads in Different Types of Villages: Evidence from a Chinese Traditional Agricultural Village and Homestay Village. *Land* **2022**, *11*, 903. [CrossRef]
42. Liu, Q.; Pan, H. Investigation on Life Satisfaction of Rural-to-Urban Migrant Workers in China: A Moderated Mediation Model. *Int. J. Environ. Res. Public Health* **2020**, *17*, 2454. [CrossRef]
43. Huhe, N. Understanding the Multilevel Foundation of Social Trust in Rural China: Evidence from the China General Social Survey. *Soc. Sci. Q.* **2014**, *95*, 581–597. [CrossRef]
44. Cho, J. Will Social Media Use Reduce Relative Deprivation? Systematic Analysis of Social Capital's Mediating Effects of Connecting Social Media Use with Relative Deprivation. *Int. J. Commun.* **2014**, *8*, 2811–2833.
45. Beaudoin, C.E.; Thorson, E. Social capital in rural and urban communities: Testing differences in media effects and models. *J. Mass Commun. Q.* **2004**, *81*, 378–399. [CrossRef]
46. Jiang, J.; Li, Q.; Kang, R.; Wang, P. Social Trust and Health: A Perspective of Urban-Rural Comparison in China. *Appl. Res. Qual. Life* **2020**, *15*, 737–756. [CrossRef]
47. Shen, S.; Quan, Q. Rural tourism development perceived by involved local farmers: Evidences from Gaochun County of China. *J. Tour. Cult. Chang.* **2022**, *20*, 196–220. [CrossRef]
48. Yao, Y.; Lu, S.; Wang, H. Relative Deprivation and Farmers' Willingness to Participate in Village Governance: Evidence from Land Expropriation in Rural China. *Asian Surv.* **2021**, *61*, 917–941. [CrossRef]
49. Ma, Y.; Koondhar, M.A.; Liu, S.; Wang, H.; Kong, R. Perceived Value Influencing the Household Waste Sorting Behaviors in Rural China. *Int. J. Environ. Res. Public Health* **2020**, *17*, 6093. [CrossRef]
50. Li, F.; Sun, Y.; Zhang, Y.; Zhang, W. Research on Multi-Dimensional Influencing Factors Regarding the Perceived Social Integration of New Urban Immigrants: An HLM Analysis Based on Data from 58 Large- and Medium-Sized Cities in China. *Int. J. Environ. Res. Public Health* **2022**, *19*, 7017. [CrossRef]
51. Xu, Y.; Li, B.; Huang, X. Outsiders to urban-centric growth: The dual social exclusion of migrant tenant farmers in China. *Third World Q.* **2021**, *42*, 1314–1328. [CrossRef]
52. James, S.C. The Foundations of Social Theory; Fang, D. , *Translator*; Social Science Literature Press: Beijing, China, 1992. (In Chinese)
53. Fukuyama, F.; Bangli, L.; Shengli, W. *The Great Schism: Human Nature and the Reconstruction of Social Order*; China Social Science Press: Beijing, China, 2002. (In Chinese)
54. Huang, X. The Chinese Dream: Hukou, Social Mobility, and Trust in Government. *Soc. Sci. Q.* **2020**, *101*, 2052–2070. [CrossRef]
55. Smith, H.J.; Pettigrew, T.F.; Pippin, G.M.; Bialosiewicz, S. Relative Deprivation: A Theoretical and Meta-Analytic Review. *Personal. Soc. Psychol. Rev.* **2012**, *16*, 203–232. [CrossRef]
56. Osborne, D.; Smith, H.J.; Huo, Y.J. More Than a Feeling: Discrete Emotions Mediate the Relationship Between Relative Deprivation and Reactions to Workplace Furloughs. *Personal. Soc. Psychol. Bull.* **2012**, *38*, 628–641. [CrossRef] [PubMed]
57. Xiong, M.; Ye, Y.R. Relative deprivation: Concept, measurement, influencing factors and role. *Adv. Psychol. Sci.* **2016**, *24*, 438–453. (In Chinese) [CrossRef]
58. Lee, Y. Government for Leaving No One Behind: Social Equity in Public Administration and Trust in Government. *Sage Open* **2021**, *11*, 1–11. [CrossRef]
59. Vitale, D. A Trust Network Model for Social Rights Fulfilment. *Oxf. J. Leg. Stud.* **2018**, *38*, 706–732. [CrossRef]
60. Sun, W.; Wang, X. Do government actions affect social trust? Cross-city evidence in China. *Soc. Sci. J.* **2012**, *49*, 447–457. [CrossRef]
61. Nikitas, A.; Avineri, E.; Parkhurst, G. Understanding the public acceptability of road pricing and the roles of older age, social norms, pro-social values and trust for urban policy-making: The case of Bristol. *Cities* **2018**, *79*, 78–91. [CrossRef]
62. Li, H.B.; Zhang, Y.J. The impact of urban residential welfare of migrant workers on their urban integration—An empirical analysis based on structural equation modeling. *Urban Dev. Res.* **2020**, *27*, 11–14+25. (In Chinese)
63. Tian, M.; Bao, J.L. A comparative study of migrant urban integration with principal component analysis. *Hum. Grography* **2014**, *29*, 43–48. (In Chinese)
64. Zhao, Q. Residential spatial differentiation and its impact on urban integration of suburban landless farmers—Based on research data from Fenggang County, Guizhou Province. *Agric. Econ. Issues* **2015**, *36*, 71–78+111–112. (In Chinese)
65. Kuang, F.Y.; Chen, M.K. The influence of risk expectation and livelihood capital on farmers' willingness to quit their homesteads and their intergenerational differences—Based on 456 farmers' survey data in Jiangxi Province. *J. Agric. For. Econ. Manag.* **2021**, *20*, 92–101. (In Chinese)
66. Huang, Y.X. The way to solve the problem of reforming the rural house base system[J]. *Agric. Econ. Issues* **2021**, *8*, 83–89. (In Chinese)

67. Peng, C.H. Influence of farmers' home base property rights perception status on their willingness to quit their home bases–an empirical analysis based on a questionnaire survey of 1413 farm households in six counties of Anhui Province. *China Rural. Obs.* **2013**, *1*, 21–33+90–91. (In Chinese)
68. Jinan Bureau of Statistics. Statistical Bulletin of National Economic and Social Development of Jinan City in 2021.2022-03-04. Available online: http://jntj.jinan.gov.cn/art/2022/3/4/art_18254_4745381.html (accessed on 10 September 2022).
69. Li, B.; Mi, Z.; Zhang, Z. Willingness of the New Generation of Farmers to Participate in Rural Tourism: The Role of Perceived Impacts and Sense of Place. *Sustainability* **2020**, *12*, 766. [CrossRef]
70. Pierce, J.L.; Kostova, T.; Dirks, K.T. Toward a theory of psychological ownership in organizations. *Acad. Manag. Rev.* **2001**, *26*, 298–310. [CrossRef]
71. Niu, X.F.; Yang, Y.Z. Measurement and influencing factors of Endowment Effect of Homestead. *Econ. Problems* **2021**, *4*, 96–103. (In Chinese) [CrossRef]
72. Morewedge, C.K.; Shu, L.L.; Gilbert, D.T.; Wilson, T.D. Bad riddance or good rubbish? Ownership and not loss aversion causes the endowment effect. *J. Exp. Soc. Psychol.* **2009**, *45*, 947–951. [CrossRef]
73. Hooghe, M.; Marien, S.; Oser, J. Great expectations: The effect of democratic ideals on political trust in European democracies. *Contemp. Politics* **2017**, *23*, 214–230. [CrossRef]
74. Fischer, J.A.V.; Torgler, B. Do positional concers destroy social capital: Evidence from 26 countries. *Econ. Inq.* **2013**, *51*, 1542–1565. [CrossRef]
75. Meng, T.; Chen, H. A multilevel analysis of social capital and self-rated health: Evidence from China. *Health Place* **2014**, *27*, 38–44. [CrossRef]
76. Xu, Z.; Sun, B. Influential mechanism of farmers' sense of relative deprivation in the sustainable development of rural tourism. *J. Sustain. Tour.* **2020**, *28*, 110–128. [CrossRef]
77. McNicholl, D.; McRobie, A.; Cruickshank, H. Characteristics of Stakeholder Networks Supporting Local Government Performance Improvements in Rural Water Supply: Cases from Ghana, Malawi, and Bolivia. *Water Altern. -Interdiscip. J. Water Politics Dev.* **2017**, *10*, 541–561.
78. Cao, W.; Zhou, S.; Wu, S.; Song, C. Factors influencing farmers' intentions for urban-rural harmony in metropolitan fringes and regional differences therein. *Pap. Reg. Sci.* **2020**, *99*, 201–224. [CrossRef]
79. Xu, D.; Yong, Z.; Deng, X.; Zhuang, L.; Qing, C. Rural-Urban Migration and its Effect on Land Transfer in Rural China. *Land* **2020**, *9*, 81. [CrossRef]

International Journal of
Environmental Research and Public Health

MDPI

Review

A Systematic Review of Evidence-Based Family Interventions for Trauma-Affected Refugees

Chansophal Mak * and Elizabeth Wieling

Department of Human Development and Family Science, College of Family and Consumer Science, University of Georgia, Athens, GA 30602, USA; ewieling@uga.edu
* Correspondence: makchansophal@uga.edu

Abstract: Family connections are crucial for trauma-affected refugees from collectivistic cultures. Evidence-based family interventions are consistently promoted to support a host of mental and relational health needs of families exposed to traumatic stressors; however, there is still limited research focused on cultural adaptation and the testing of the effectiveness of these interventions on some of the most disenfranchised populations in the aftermath of forced displacement. This systematic review was conducted to examine the reach of existing evidence-based family interventions implemented with newly resettled refugees globally. Studies included in this review include those testing the effectiveness of a systemic treatment with pre and post intervention evaluation, studies with or without control groups, and studies that include at least one family member in addition to the target participants. Twelve studies met the inclusion criteria. Barriers to conducting randomized control trials with displaced refugee populations are discussed. Recommendations are made for future studies to include a focus on scientifically rigorous multi-method designs, specific cultural adaptation frameworks, and the integration of relational aspects rather than focusing only on individual adjustment. Global displacement continues to rise; therefore, it is imperative that the mental health and wellbeing of displaced populations be treated with a comprehensive, multi-level framework.

Keywords: family; mental health; refugees; traumatic stress; culture; displacement; intervention

Citation: Mak, C.; Wieling, E. A Systematic Review of Evidence-Based Family Interventions for Trauma-Affected Refugees. *Int. J. Environ. Res. Public Health* **2022**, *19*, 9361. https://doi.org/10.3390/ijerph19159361

Academic Editors: Paul B. Tchounwou, Ernesto Castañeda and Maria De Jesus

Received: 5 May 2022
Accepted: 27 July 2022
Published: 30 July 2022

1. Introduction

Forced displacement estimates exceeded 89.3 million people globally by end of 2021 and is expected to be even higher in the future with new and ongoing global conflicts [1]. The full impact of the COVID-19 pandemic on displacement is yet to be determined. United Nations High Commissioner for Refugees (UNHCR) data showed that arrivals of new refugees and asylum-seekers were sharply down in most regions, which is likely a reflection of how many people were stranded as a result of the pandemic. Forcibly displaced and stateless people are among the most adversely affected groups around the world and continue to face increased food and economic insecurity as well as challenges in accessing health and protection services [1]. Climate change is also driving displacement and increasing the vulnerability of these populations [2]. Many are living in climate "hotspots" where they typically lack the resources to adapt to an increasingly inhospitable environment. The dynamics of poverty, food insecurity, climate change, conflict, and displacement are increasingly interconnected and mutually reinforcing, driving an increasing number of people to search for safety and security [3]. It is also important to note that children account for an estimated 41 per cent of all forcibly displaced people [1].

Forced displacement disrupts the entire community and family structure of migrant and refugee populations [4]. Exposure to multiple traumatic stressors and life adversities are often unavoidable before and during the process of migration [4]. After resettlement in a new country, cumulative daily stressors, additional exposures to traumatic stress over time, poverty, and acculturation stress place refugee families at risk for serious negative mental health outcomes and relational challenges [5–7]. The overwhelming consequences of exposure to displacement and traumatic stressors demand multilevel systemic interventions that are culturally responsive while also addressing individual, family relational, and community health needs [8].

Most refugees belong to collectivistic societies that value family connection and interdependence [9]. Family unity and cohesion represent an important indicator of individual mental and relational health in collectivistic cultures [8]. Where there is forced displacement because of human rights violations, organized violence, natural disasters, and climate change in their home countries, refugee families are stripped from their natural contexts and resources and face multiple and enduring losses [8].

The COVID-19 pandemic further exacerbated existing mental and relational health issues; specifically, it created more barriers for refugee families to stay connected when they were geographically separated [10]. Resettlement communities around the world have a sociopolitical and moral responsibility to create infrastructures to support these families. Most importantly, mental health professionals have a critical role in developing and testing interventions to effectively address the mental and relational health of various refugee populations. Despite the overwhelming challenges to survival, these communities have tremendous resilience, and we know historically that when families are provided with opportunities to heal, they recover and thrive in their new countries of resettlement [8].

In 2015, Slobodin and de Jong published a systematic review of family interventions for refugees [4]. This work documented the impact of traumatic stress on individual mental health, the need to interrupt the intergenerational transmission of psychopathology and violence related to trauma exposure, and the need to support family and community healing [4]. Slobodin and de Jong's study [4] reported that only six experimental studies met their inclusion criteria of family-based interventions, with four being school-based interventions and two being multifamily support groups. They went on to underscore the shortage of research in this area and discussed the challenges of drawing clear conclusions regarding the effectiveness of family interventions for trauma-affected immigrants and refugees. They also called for future trials to go beyond individual-level Post traumatic Stress Disorder (PTSD) treatments and called for a greater focus on family-level processes that incorporate relationships, communication, and resilience. With the increased crisis of global displacement, the focus of this paper is to return to the literature and conduct a follow-up systematic review to further examine studies that test the effectiveness of evidence-based family interventions among trauma-affected refugees globally, as well as to examine cultural adaptation processes and implementation and dissemination strategies utilized across empirical studies. Our purpose was to raise awareness and create a call to action in support of prevention and intervention studies focused on supporting refugee families after resettlement. It is important to evaluate the effectiveness of these family-based programs in terms of scientific rigor and cultural fit for various refugee communities. Specifically, to evaluate the effectiveness of an evidence-based intervention, in addition to measuring clinical outcomes, it is important to examine program implementation and dissemination outcomes to see if there is evidence of promoting or protecting health and preventing ill health in a particular population [11].

1.1. Working with Displaced and Minoritized Refugee Families

Displacement can be life threatening for refugee families. Three common stages of migration (i.e., premigration, during, and post migration) are often linked with the development of cumulative traumatic stress among forcibly displaced communities [4,12] often resulting in deleterious mental health and relational maladjustments [13,14]. In premigration, severe traumatic events such as political turmoil leading to mass violence, wars, genocide, human rights violations, as well as natural disasters and climate change have forced people to migrate and seek safety [2,15,16]. During migration, refugees often continue to be exposed to traumatic events through forced displacements both inside and outside their home countries for years [3]. Refugees continue to live in harsh conditions in refugee camps and have to deal with uncertainty and the ambiguity of hope during migration. In post migration, refugees arrive in resettled countries with additional stressors such as family separation, a lack of social support, a lack of employment and language skills, transportation difficulties [17], and limited support from local authorities [14,18]. Additional migration experiences include acculturation stress, severe poverty, living in high crime neighborhoods, and most importantly, living with untreated mental health after exposure to severe adversities before and during their resettlement [19–21]. Cumulative traumatic stress at premigration, during, and post migration is associated with psychological and relational consequences such as depression, anxiety disorders, adjustment disorders, PTSD, complicated grief, psychosis, suicide [5–7,13,20,22–27], the comorbidity of mental health disorders [13,14], the comorbidity of mental health and physical health issues, substance abuse, the disruption of family functioning (e.g., the disruption of couple relationships and parent–child relationships) [6,17,25,28–31], and the intergenerational transmission of traumatic stress among refugee families [32–34].

Mental health professionals working with refugees need to be aware that refugees encounter multiple stressors across all system levels (i.e., individual, family, and community) over prolonged periods of time [8] and suffer from mental health complications due to their comorbid nature [6,13,14,17,25,28,31,35]. At the individual subsystem, exposure to traumatic events during migration leads to extreme stress responses in the brain of affected refugees [36–40]. The amygdala dominates brain functioning and leads to the fragmentation of memory systems as the brain is wired to activate the implicit sensory, physiological, cognitive, and emotional aspects of the traumatic events (associated with the amygdala) without connecting those memories to the context, time, space, and chronology of the events (associated with the hippocampus) that are processed in the prefrontal cortex of the brain [36–38]. This fragmentation of memory systems often results in posttraumatic stress symptoms. Individual symptoms of PTSD include re-experiencing, arousal, avoidance, and negative cognitive and affective changes after experiencing life-threatening events or witnessing the life-threatening events of significant others [41]. Trauma-affected individuals tend to isolate themselves, be on guard and hypervigilant, and utilize fear-based coping and avoidance in their daily functioning and relationships [42]. Moreover, trauma survivors may continue to be impaired emotionally, behaviorally, cognitively, biologically, and spiritually long after experiencing the traumatic events [43].

At the family subsystem, exposure to trauma and prolonged family separation during migration disrupts refugees' family processes [44,45]. Traumatic stress affects not only individuals, but also their families and communities [46–48]. The adversities experienced in one system level affects all others as they are interrelated in an ecosystem [8]. These horrifying experiences often impair the individual's ability to maintain healthy relationships with their family, especially with people who are close to them such as their partners and children [48].

In couple relationships, traumatic stress affects the intimacy and marital satisfaction of trauma-affected individuals. The inability to control one's emotional and behavioral reactions in response to traumatic memories can lead to anger outbursts [42,49] and all forms of family violence [50–53]. Specifically, anger outbursts experienced by trauma-affected partners frequently result in intimate partner violence [42,49,54]. This violence is harmful to their relationship as a couple and can be transmitted to subsequent generations as well [55].

In parent–child relationships, trauma-affected parents may employ corporal punishment as a form of child discipline; however, they may not be able to differentiate between punishment as discipline and punishment resulting from their inability to control their anger outbursts [56]. These relational patterns between parent and child are pathways to the intergenerational transmission of traumatic stress among refugee families [32–34,44,51,55,57,58]. Having limited to no access to trauma treatment and parenting supports, trauma-affected parents cannot perform their parenting roles adequately [58,59]. As a result, their children are at risk of adverse mental health and relationship consequences such as aggression, low self-esteem, low emotional adjustment, and impulsivity [56,60–62], as well as poor school performance, poor peer relationships, violence and delinquency, substance abuse, anxiety, depression, and PTSD [51–53,63]. This intergenerational transmission continues to pass on if there are no proper interventions to disrupt its cycle.

Notably, not only do family members, and particularly parents, children, and spouses, influence each other through their adverse experiences; they also influence each other through their strengths and resilience [46,63,64]. Family bonding, a form of family resilience through shared values and interdependence, is a powerful resource for trauma treatment [65]. Moreover, fostering resilience at multi-system levels (i.e., individual, family, and community) is crucial in trauma treatment since resilience in one level affects the other levels too [66,67]. Thus, involving family members in individual and relational trauma treatment is strongly recommended [46–48,68].

At the community subsystem level, the resources and support offered by resettlement countries define how fast refugee individuals and their families recover from adversities and cumulative traumatic stress [14]. Local authorities usually fail to provide multi-systemic mental health support to newly resettled refugees [14,18]. Specifically, schools, the main social organizations that work directly with refugee children, often underestimate the complexity of daily stressors that affect their ability to learn and acquire knowledge [69]. At home, witnessing harsh labor conditions, poverty, emotional dysregulation, anger outbursts, and domestic violence between their parents and other family members disrupts the development of refugee children. Child labor is also very common among refugee children and youth, because their labor is often necessary to sustain family functioning. At school, refugee children are prone to being victims of and/or a part of gang violence and delinquency, experiencing discrimination, substance abuse, and a lack of study motivation, and have a lack of educational role models and supports [8,52,69]. All these factors underscore the need for specific systemic interventions to be effectively developed and deployed across all system levels within resettled refugee communities.

1.2. Family Interventions Implemented with Trauma-Affected Refugees

A few notable evidence-based family interventions have been adapted for implementation with trauma-affected displaced populations. The interventions have focused on parenting [59,70–73], multifamily groups [74–77], and school-based approaches [78–82]. Family-based interventions have proven to be effective in treating traumatic stress and disrupting the intergenerational transmission of traumatic stress among various contexts, but it is difficult to track broad-based effectiveness among refugee populations due to the paucity of family interventions [4]. Most importantly, there is still a lack of culturally adapted or tailored interventions for different ethnic minority refugee populations since most of the evidence-based interventions are based on western and white Euro-American populations [43,47,83].

2. Materials and Methods

2.1. Search Strategy

We followed the guidelines for systematic reviews suggested by the Preferred Reporting Items for Systematic Review and Meta-Analyses (PRISMA) to identify the studies for inclusion in our systematic review [84]. Our review was registered through PROSPERO as a systematic review with the registration number CRD42022316665. Consistent with the previous systematic review on this topic [4], we also tried to search the Cochrane Central Register of Controlled Trials (CENTRAL), CINAHL, EMBASE, ERIC, Entrez-Pubmed, APA PsycArticles, APA PsycInfo, and the Psychology and Behavioral Sciences Collection. However, because the University of Georgia Library does not have access to EMBASE and Entrez-Pubmed, we replaced EMBASE with the Social Sciences Citation Index and Entrez-Pubmed with PubMed after consulting with the university librarian. As a result, our systematic search sources were APA PsycArticles, APA PsycInfo, the Social Sciences Citation Index, the Psychology and Behavioral Sciences Collection, CINAHL,

ERIC, and PubMed. We searched for keywords such as traumatic stress/PTSD, family, prevention/intervention, culture/refugees/immigrants, and displacement/resettlement. Additionally, we incorporated studies included in a previous review article with a similar focus [4]. The search started in June 2013 (when the previous review paused their search) and ended in February 2022.

2.2. Criteria for Inclusion and Exclusion

The initial search was conducted by collapsing all of our key terms in each database thus producing a very limited number of articles with the additional limiters of academic peer review, English language, and publication date June 2013 to February 2022. This first search generated 69 articles for screening: four from APA PsycArticles, fifteen from APA PsycInfo, five from the Psychology and Behavioral Science Collection, four from CINAHL, three from PubMed, zero from ERIC, and thirty-eight from the Social Sciences Citation Index. The hand search recommended by the second author who is the expert in the field including the six articles of the previous review by Slobodin and de Jong in 2015 resulted in eleven studies. Table 1 is a brief description of the search procedures.

Table 1. Description of search procedures.

Keywords	Databases	Articles Found
We entered into each database with similar set of keywords:	APA PsycArticles	4
	APA PsycInfo	15
	Social Sciences Citation Index	38
"Traumatic stress" OR "PTSD", AND "Family",	Psychology and Behavioral Science Collection	5
AND "Prevention" OR "Intervention",	CINAHL	4
AND "Culture" OR "Refugees" OR "Immigrants",	ERIC	0
AND "Displacement" OR "Resettlement"	PubMed	3
	TOTAL	69
	Other sources: Articles that met criteria for inclusion and articles from the previous review by Slobodin and de Jong (2015) [4]	11

Because the purpose of this review was to examine the effectiveness of evidence-based family interventions to address traumatic stress among refugee families worldwide, we developed inclusion and exclusion criteria. Our inclusion criteria were: (1) studies that described family-based interventions designed to address individual and relational functioning after trauma exposure and displacement, including pre and post intervention assessments; (2) studies that used Randomized Control Treatment (RCT) designs, non-experimental designs, and feasibility studies that prepared the stage for RCTs; (3) studies that involved more than one family member during the intervention (i.e., not just the target participants); (4) studies that targeted refugees who were affected by traumatic stress (not necessary meeting the PTSD criteria) prior to, during, and after migration; (5) studies that included refugees of all ages; and (6) studies that included interventions that were delivered both in community settings (e.g., refugee camps, schools) and clinical settings (e.g., mental health agencies, hospitals).

The exclusion criteria were: (1) studies that did not target the treatment of traumatic stress symptoms; (2) studies that addressed traumatic stress symptoms among refugee children and youth, but did not involve their caregivers (e.g., parents, grandparents, older siblings, and other family members) during the treatment; and (3) studies that did not examine the effectiveness of a relational intervention, did not address traumatic stress symptoms, or did not intervene at a family level.

3. Results

3.1. Study Selection

The initial search resulted in eighty articles, but only twelve met the full inclusion criteria, including the six articles from the previous systematic review conducted by Slobodin and de Jong (2015). Figure 1 is the summary of our study selection process following PRISMA (2020) guidelines.

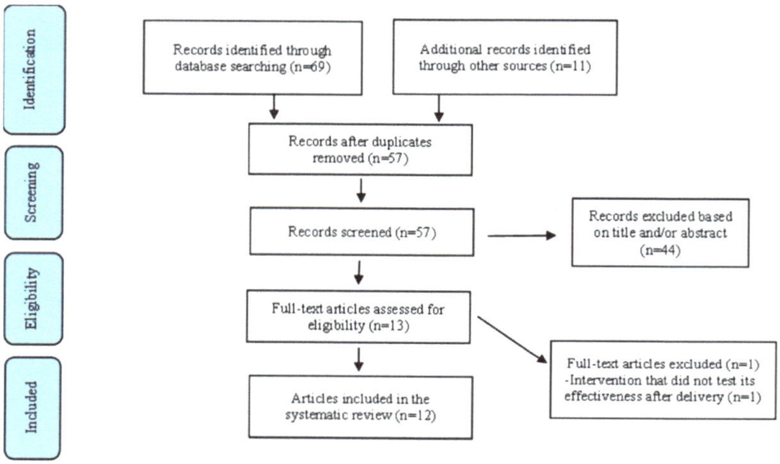

Figure 1. Study Selection Flow Diagram.

3.2. Study Designs

Four studies were identified as being in the feasibility testing phase and included assessments and/or qualitative interviews at both baseline and post intervention stages [70,72,74,77]. Five studies were non-experimental and included evaluations at baseline and post intervention without a control group [75,78–80]. Three studies were experimental and included assessments at pre and post intervention, and a control group [73,76,81]. One study used a quasi-experimental design by including a control group along with pre and post intervention evaluations [82]. Appendix A demonstrates. Table A1 is a summary description of studies included in this review.

3.3. Types of Interventions

3.3.1. Parenting Interventions

Three studies used parenting interventions [70,72,73]. The first study was part of a working group that adapted GenerationPMTO for the context of traumatic stress. The first feasibility study of this adapted parenting intervention was conducted with trauma-affected Acholi mothers in Northern Uganda and demonstrated both acceptability, usability, and limited effectiveness within that population [59]. The working group adapted the intervention for feasibility testing with Karen refugees (from the country of Myanmar) in the U.S. This intervention was grounded in the human ecological model, the social interaction learning theory, and social justice principles [70,71]. GenerationPMTO is an evidence-based parenting intervention adapted in the context of traumatic stress among displaced populations to assist parents in managing their children's misbehavior. The intervention included nine parenting group sessions for mothers of children ages 5–13. Assessments were conducted with parents and children at pre intervention, post intervention, and at a 3-month follow-up.

The second study used a brief parenting intervention program called Strong Family with the purpose of improving mothers' parenting skills, mothers' perceptions of their children, and child behavior [72]. Strong Family is a brief family intervention that consists of three sessions. The total participation time is no more than five hours. In the first week, a one-hour pre group session was conducted among 10–12 caregivers. In the second and third weeks, caregivers and their children first attended separate groups (i.e., a parent's group and a children's group) for one hour. Immediately after that, both caregivers and children attended one hour of a family group to conclude the program. The intervention was conducted among 25 Afghanistan refugee families (twenty mothers and five fathers of participating children whose age was between 8–15 years) resettled in Serbia. Assessments were conducted at pre test (t1 at baseline), post test (t2 two weeks after), and follow-up (t3 six weeks after completion) to evaluate the effectiveness of the intervention.

The third study used a parenting and family skills training intervention called Happy Families, adapted from the Strengthening Families Program [73]. The intervention was conducted among 479 Burmese migrant families (i.e., 513 caregivers and 479 children aged 7–15) in 20 communities in Thailand. Happy Families consisted of 12 group sessions. Each session lasted 2.5 h. Caregivers and children attended parallel group sessions followed by joint family sessions. Standardized assessments were conducted at pre and post intervention to evaluate the effectiveness of the intervention through parent–child relationships and family functioning. The follow-up assessments were conducted a month after the intervention for both control and treatment groups, and again six months after the intervention for treatment groups only.

3.3.2. Multifamily Interventions

Four studies employed multifamily group interventions [74–77]. In 2003 and 2008, Weine and colleagues conducted two studies using multifamily group interventions (i.e., TAFES: Tea and Family Education and Support and CAFES: Coffee and Family Education and Support) that included therapy, psychoeducation, and coping skills for individual and family members in the context of Post Traumatic Stress Disorder among 42 Kosovar refugee families [77] and among 197 Bosnian refugee families resettled in Chicago [76]. Both interventions consisted of nine sessions over 16 weeks. The interventions were grounded in family strength and resilience approaches. The purpose was to assess the effectiveness of the intervention in increasing access to mental health services and decreasing depression. Standardized assessments were conducted prior to and 3 months following the interventions [77], while similar standardized assessments were conducted four times in the 2008 study (at baseline, 6 months, 12 months, and 18 months) [76].

A recent study conducted by Betancourt et al. used a home visiting intervention, the Family Strengthening Intervention for Refugees (FSI-R), that included ten 90-min weekly home-visit sessions among 40 Somali Bantu and 40 Bhutanese refugee families [74]. Similar to the two studies of Wein et al. [76,77], the invention used family strength and resilience approaches grounded in ecological and systemic theories. Standardized assessments were conducted at pre and post intervention to examine the traumatic stress reaction and depression symptoms in children as well as family functioning.

Another recent study conducted by Gotseva-Balgaranova et al. utilized an Evidence-Based Trauma Stabilization (EBTS) that included five psychodrama sessions with children and parent dyads (i.e., 15 children and 16 parents), and four psychoeducation sessions for parents about traumatic stress symptoms and their impact on child development [75]. This study was conducted among seven Iraqi, three Afghan, and five Syrian refugees resettled in Germany and Bulgaria. Psychological assessments were conducted at pre and post intervention to examine the effectiveness of the intervention in reducing PTSD symptoms and depression in both parents and children.

3.3.3. School-Based Interventions

Five studies employed school-based interventions that included caregiver group sessions prior to or/and along with children and youth's individual and group sessions [78–82]. The first study used the Cultural Adjustment and Trauma Services (CATS) intervention that included relationship building between classroom teachers and CATS staff, outreach services involving cultural brokers as assessors for mental health issues, and clinical services involving psychoeducation, therapy, and family services [78]. CATS is grounded in the Family, Adult, and Child Engagement Services model [79] designed for trauma-affected refugee children and funded by National Child Traumatic Stress Network. The study was conducted among 1049 multiethnic refugee children (only 894 received outreach services, and 149 enrolled in clinical services) from 29 countries resettled in New Jersey in the U.S. Two standardized assessments were conducted at baseline and every 3 months during a three-year period to examine the effectiveness of the intervention in decreasing the symptoms of PTSD and improving functioning.

The second study used International Family, Adult, and Child Enhancement Services (FACES) that included mental health assessment, therapy (individual, group, family), psychiatric services, and support services (e.g., translation/interpretation, travel/transportation) [79]. FACES was initially developed in 1976, and specifically designed for Southeast Asian refugees fleeing Vietnam. The study was conducted with mixed groups of refugee children and youth resettled in the U.S. At the beginning, 97 children and youth participated and only 68 remained at the end of the program, which was conducted over a three-year period. Standardized assessments were conducted longitudinally from December 2003 to August 2005.

The third study used the Trauma Healing Club (THC) intervention adapted from the evidence-based Cognitive Behavioral Interventions for Trauma in Schools (CBITS) [80]. The THC included 12 sessions (i.e., ten CBITS sessions and two drumming sessions in response to the cultural values of African refugees) along with psychoeducation about adverse childhood experiences and their impact on child development for parents and students throughout the intervention implementation. The study was conducted among 88 students and their caregivers who were African refugees resettled in the U.S. Standardized assessments were conducted at pre and post intervention to examine the effectiveness of the intervention in decreasing trauma-related symptoms and increasing coping skills and school performance outcomes.

The fourth study used the Mental Health for Immigrants Program (MHIP) that included eight CBT group sessions for children and youth, two multifamily group sessions for parents along with a child-based intervention, and training about the symptoms and effects of trauma on immigrant children for classroom teachers [81]. The study was conducted among 198 Latinx immigrant children from the third to eighth grade who were diagnosed with trauma-related depression and/or PTSD symptoms. Standardized assessments were conducted at pre and post intervention, and at a 3-month follow-up to evaluate the improvement of PTSD and depressive symptoms.

The fifth study used a multimodal program that included psychoeducation for parents, creative techniques (painting, playing, acting), and relaxation techniques in individual, family and group sessions [82]. The program consisted of twelve sessions over 12 weeks: two information sessions, two diagnostic sessions, six group sessions, two to four individual sessions, and one family session. The study was conducted among 10 Kosovar refugee youth and their parents resettled in Germany. Standardized assessments were conducted at pre and post intervention to examine the effectiveness of the intervention in reducing emotional distress and improving psychosocial functioning among trauma-affected refugee children and adolescents.

We would also like to note an important study that did not meet our inclusion criteria but is directly related to our systematic review. Erdemir conducted a Preschool Education Program (PEP) with the aim of promoting holistic development and boosting school readiness skills before starting primary school among Syrian refugee children resettled in

Turkey [85]. The program operated for nine weeks in two schools. The findings showed an improvement in mother–child relationships, positive changes in child behaviors and the mothers' concepts of their children, as well as positive parenting practices at the end of the program, based on the interviews with the mothers.

3.4. Effectiveness of the Interventions/Results of the Studies

Not all interventions in this systematic review measured the same outcomes of PTSD among refugee populations. Six studies reported a reduction in PTSD symptoms (i.e., intrusion, arousal, depression, dissociation, traumatic stress reaction) in children/youth and caregivers at post intervention [74,75,78,80–82] in comparison to a control group [80]. Four studies reported the improvement in social functioning among the participants at post intervention [78–80,82]. Two studies reported an increase in mental-health-seeking behaviors among participants after completing the program [76,77]. Four studies included family variables (i.e., family hardiness, family problem solving, family comfort in discussing trauma, family arguing, family functioning, and family communication) and they reported positive changes in all family variables [73,74,76,77]. Three studies reported more positive parent–child relationships, especially in parent–child relationship quality, discipline practices (i.e., teaching, directions, emotional regulation, child compliance), and family functioning among participants at post intervention [70,72,73].

3.5. Cultural Adaptation Processes

Cultural adaptation is referred to as a process that enhances the fit between the intervention and the target population through the modification, tailoring, and adaptation of intervention elements, while still following the guidelines that contribute to the fidelity and effectiveness of the intervention [86]. There are numerous frameworks to guide the cultural adaptation of an intervention, but these frameworks usually fall into two main categories: (1) the adaptation of intervention content (what to adapt?), and (2) the adaptation process (how/when to adapt, and who should be involved in decision making?). Among the thirteen studies included in this review, only two studies employed cultural adaptation frameworks. The first study, conducted by Ballard et al. [70], used the ecological validity cultural adaptation model developed by Bernal et al. [87]. The cultural adaptation of the evidence-based parenting intervention, GenerationPMTO, also included qualitative needs assessments among stakeholders in the community, intervention development and adaptation focusing on eight ecological dimensions (i.e., language, persons, metaphors, content, concepts, goals, methods, and context), and intervention delivery conducted by trained therapists, intervention coaches, and trained Karen interpreters.

The second study was conducted by Elswick et al. [80], and it used the three steps of cultural adaptation of the intervention (THC) from the original CBITS in response to the needs and cultural values of African refugee families resettled in the U.S. First, African drumming was added into each session to offer emotional regulation during the sessions. Second, the researchers added a pyramid mentoring process developed to foster cultural socialization, cultural identity, and cognitive development through modeling and social support. Third, the original 10-session CBITS was extended to the 12-session THC to ensure the fidelity of the evidence-based intervention despite the additional cultural value of drumming.

Seven studies included in this review did not reference any specific model for the cultural adaptation of the intervention, but focused on different aspects of the relevant culture such as the use of cultural brokers, interpreters, and facilitators who were bilingual and members of immigrant populations [76–78,82], observations in their natural setting by program staff to tackle the need for mental health services among refugee children and youth [79], the use of a community-based participatory research approach (CBPR) [77], and the use of initial qualitative interviews to inform the adaptation of the intervention [73].

Three studies did not employ any specific model for the cultural adaptation of the intervention, nor any aspects of the relevant culture. The studies focused on the involvement of parents and teachers in addition to group sessions among students [81], the involvement of parents in four psychoeducation sessions about trauma and five parent–child interaction sessions [75], and the claim that the intervention was already culturally adapted among the population [72].

3.6. Implementation and Dissemination Strategies

Implementation science is referred to as methods that help to ensure the accurate translation of research findings and evidence-based practices into community settings with the purpose of improving the quality of health care (i.e., effectiveness, reliability, safety, appropriateness, equity, efficacy) [88]. In other words, implementation science focuses on moving research into practice by incorporating contextual factors and by using multi-systemic perspectives. Therefore, implementation and dissemination strategies consider factors that affect the adoption, implementation, and sustainability of a specific intervention in normal settings. According to Fixen et al., the core components of implementations are: (1) staff selection, (2) preservice and in-service training, (3) ongoing coaching and consultation, (4) staff performance assessment, (5) decision-supporting data systems, (6) facilitative administrative supports, and (7) systems interventions [89].

All twelve studies in this review incorporated most of the main components of implementation described by Fixen et al. [89]. Specifically, seven studies conducted preservice training, ongoing consultation and supervision, and regular performance evaluations. For example, the first study, conducted by Ballard et al., included interventionists who were culturally informed intervention coaches and trained therapists committed to working with war-affected and displaced populations [70]. The interventionists adapted the intervention core elements and protocol in response to the needs of the ethnic minority population they worked with by incorporating their cultural values, language, and meaning-making process in the context of displacement. The second study, by Betancourt et al., had a highly trained intervention team consisting of experts in the field (i.e., research assistants, interventionists, licensed clinical social workers, clinical supervisors) and trained staff from two refugee communities [74].

In the third study, by Puffer et al., the intervention team consisted of 40 lay facilitators including staff and non-staff from the implementation organization [73]. The facilitators worked in pairs (one staff and one non-staff), and received an 11-day training. During implementation, staff conducted observation sessions to supervise non-staff. Observers used standardized checklists to evaluate facilitation skills and to determine how much supervision non-staff needed.

In the fourth and fifth studies, led by Weine et al., the intervention team were members of the immigrant populations [76,77]. They received 20 h of implementation training, weekly group and individual supervision, and monthly videotaping of the TAFES and CAFES sessions by an experienced family therapist. In the sixth study, conducted by Birman et al., the intervention team was composed of program assistants who were trained by scale developers, clinicians composed of a doctoral or master level psychologist, an art therapist, a dance therapist, an occupational therapist, a child psychiatrist, and practicum students supervised by licensed staff [79]. Lastly, in the seventh study, by Kataoka et al., the intervention team was composed of school clinicians, educators, and researchers who received 16 h of MHIP intervention training, 2 h of weekly supervision with a psychologist, and 1 h of weekly supervision from an onsite clinical supervisor [80].

Two studies included preservice and in-service training, but did not say much about on-going supervision and performance evaluation during the process of intervention implementation. For example, Beehler et al. developed an intervention team that relied on refugee resettlement staff who were trained in mental health treatments, and CATS clinicians who were bilingual and trained by intervention developers [78]. In the study conducted by El-Khani et al., the intervention team involved two research assistants who were trained by the program developers, and interpreters who were community members [72].

Three studies did not include the delivery of preservice and in-service training among their interventionist team. For example, in the study conducted by Elswick et al., the intervention team was composed of researchers and a clinician, and no other details were provided [80]. In the study conducted by Mohlen et al., the intervention team consisted of a child psychiatrist who led a diagnostic session, a trained medical student who provided therapy, and a Kosovo-Albanian interpreter [82]. Lastly, in the study by Gotseva-Balgarannova et al., the intervention team consisted of trained researchers, EBTS leaders, and an interpreter [75].

4. Discussion

This systematic review identified twelve studies that tested the effectiveness of evidence-based family interventions for displaced and trauma-affected refugees. Three studies examined parenting interventions; four studies examined multifamily group interventions; and five studies examined school-based interventions. In terms of study design, only three studies were RCTs and the remaining were non-experimental (i.e., four nonexperimental, one quasi-experimental, and four feasibility studies). No studies compared the effectiveness between individual-based and family-based treatments. Most importantly, only two studies specified the cultural adaptation frameworks they employed while the others simply referred to incorporating exploratory qualitative interviews, cultural brokers, bilingual research teams, and interpreters. The lack of elaboration on cultural adaptation/tailoring and specific dissemination and implementation approaches to target displaced populations points to a shortage of scientifically rigorous and culturally responsive research designs to support individual and relational health among displaced refugees of an ethnic minority.

We would like to frame this discussion as a call to action for those in the mental health field regarding the serious dearth of relational interventions designed and tested to promote healing among refugees following trauma exposure and displacement. It is concerning that despite the knowledge that we face alarming and growing rates of global displacement, we as a prevention and intervention field have not ethically and responsively addressed the mental and relational health of refugee communities. In 2010, the National Institutes of Health assembled a panel to conduct an extensive Delphi study to identify grand challenges in global mental health [90].

The report advanced the following goals: (a) identify root causes, risks, and protective factors; (b) advance the prevention and implementation of early interventions; (c) improve treatments and expand access to care; (d) raise awareness of the global burden; (e) build human resource capacity; and (f) transform health systems and policy responses. Effectively meeting these goals would simultaneously expedite the mental health treatment of refugee communities around the globe. Over a decade has passed since that report was released, yet sustained evidence of growth across those targeted goal areas is missing. We continue to struggle to address the needs of one of the most vulnerable segments of the global population, forcibly displaced refugees.

Known Barriers to Advancing Mental Health and Systemic Treatments

Design challenges have been pervasive in developing and testing both individual and relational treatments within displaced communities. Gold standards inherent in RCT designs (e.g., control groups, recruitment, blind assignment, statistical power, retention/attrition, dose levels), also create challenges to the effectiveness and superiority of trials and often slow behavioral-based translational sciences. There have been increasing calls to expand our conceptualization of the scientific process to encompass more critical and ethically informed frames that also include deep collaboration with members of the targeted communities [91]. For example, Critical Participatory Action Research (PAR) models specifically incorporate social justice, empowerment, and liberation as part of the scientific endeavor [91–93]. The adoption of culturally tailored multi-informant and multi-method research (quantitative, qualitative, and mixed-method approaches) would expand our capacity for developing, implementing, and testing interventions with greater potential for uptake and sustainability within displaced refugee communities [94–97]. Key researchers in this review also recommended including qualitative studies such as case study methods [79], ethnographic methods [76,77], and community-based participatory research methods [74] along with RCT designs in future research to enhance the effectiveness of family interventions that address mental health and family functioning among diverse displaced refugee families.

Another barrier is the poor resettlement infrastructure in host countries. Considering that the largest percentages of displaced people (86 percent of refugees worldwide) resettled into middle- and low-income countries, limited and often inadequate public and mental health institutions are available to support the resettlement process [3]. Similarly, inadequate infrastructure is also part of the refugee experience in high-income countries [43]. A lack of state policies to systematically assess mental health needs and provide support to resettled families significantly compromises successful family adjustment. For example, a national study conducted by Shannon et al. in the U.S. with 44 refugee health coordinators exploring the mental health training of refugee health coordinators and the systematic screening of refugee mental health reported that they believed it was possible to administer a brief mental health screening during early resettlement meetings; however, only half of the coordinators had received any mental health training [98]. These coordinators identified PTSD and major depression as their top concerns related to refugee mental health and requested training on the mental health needs of arriving refugees. They linked mental health screening with positive referral outcomes for refugee populations. Similarly, a lack of training and awareness of professionals in primary and secondary educational institutions, along with a lack of trained mental health professionals and community health workers, exacerbates concerns and a lack of healing post resettlement. Among the studies reviewed in this paper, Mohlen et al. also highlighted the need to train professionals (i.e., social workers and teachers) who work directly with refugees [82] while Puffer et al. suggested training lay providers who are community members to ensure the sustainability of intervention implementation [73]. Beyond individual assessment and mental health, other studies [59,60,71] documented the broad need for parental support post resettlement as parents feel poorly equipped to navigate new legal, educational, and labor systems.

In addition to the need for greater emphasis on both evidence-based and practice-based interventions for resettled refugee communities (e.g., parenting groups, relational health, peer support), an emphasis on institutional programs that enhance professional capacity, the trauma-focused training of health providers, and community-based refugee centers would go a long way in promoting successful adjustment [99]. Slobodin and de Jong highlighted the need for the implementation of intervention in community settings such as schools, women's health clinics, or primary care clinics, rather than solely clinical settings, in order to increase the accessibility and cultural responsiveness of mental health services among trauma-affected and displaced refugee families [4].

Most studies in traumatic stress treatment have primarily focused on symptom reduction rather than other aspects of human relationships, such as parent–child relationships, couple relationships, sibling relationships, and both familial and community relationships. Specifically, trauma-affected refugees experience complicated grief and other comorbidities related to mental and relational issues [43], so we advocate for trauma treatments that incorporate multiple systemic factors (i.e., relationship, identity, meaning-making, and community supports) that affect refugee families during resettlement [100]. Several key researchers in this review suggested the inclusion of additional variables in future research in the area of family intervention implementation science: (1) family mental health and functioning along with individual treatment [72]; (2) the cultural components of specific ethnic minority refugees [80]; and (3) timing (e.g., developmental time, family life cycle, time since exposure to trauma, and time of resettlement) [76].

5. Conclusions

All studies included in this systematic review report that their programs are somewhat effective in either improving family functioning or reducing PTSD symptoms by comparing the intervention groups and control group or by comparing the pre and post test of the intervention groups. Findings also highlight that culturally adapted, evidence-based family interventions are needed for specific ethnic minority refugee populations to provide multi-systemic support after resettlement. These treatments should also incorporate the specific refugee histories of displacement, traumatic experiences, cultural values, and ethnic identities as part of a broader culturally responsive agenda for resettlement.

Author Contributions: Conceptualization, C.M. and E.W.; methodology, C.M. and E.W.; software, C.M.; validation, C.M. and E.W.; formal analysis, C.M. and E.W.; investigation, C.M. and E.W.; resources, C.M.; data curation, C.M. and E.W.; writing—original draft preparation, C.M.; writing—review and editing, C.M.; visualization, C.M.; supervision, E.W.; project administration, C.M.; funding acquisition, E.W. All authors have read and agreed to the published version of the manuscript.

Funding: This research received no external funding.

Institutional Review Board Statement: Not applicable.

Informed Consent Statement: Not applicable.

Data Availability Statement: Not applicable.

Acknowledgments: We would like to thank the expert librarian, Sandra Elain Riggs, at the University of Georgia for her assistance in the systematic literature search and references throughout the process of this review.

Conflicts of Interest: The authors declare no conflict of interest.

Appendix A

Table A1. Description of studies included in the review.

	Study	Design	Intervention	Aims of the Intervention	Were the Aims Achieved?	Culturally Adaptation Process	Implementation and Dissemination Strategies
1.	Beehler et al. (2012) [78]	Nonexperimental	School-based	Reduce PTSD symptoms Improve social functioning	Yes	Not specified	Refugee staff
2.	Birman et al. (2008) [79]	Nonexperimental	School-based	Improve social functioning	Yes	Not specified	Scale developer/therapist/ psychiatrist/graduate students
3.	Kataoka et al. (2003) [81]	RCT	School-based	Reduce PTSD symptoms	Yes	Not specified	School clinicians/ educators/psychologist
4.	Mohlen et al. (2005) [82]	Quasi-experimental	School-based	Reduce PTSD symptoms Improve social functioning	Yes	Use of native translator	Psychiatrist/Medical student/translator
5.	Elswick et al. (2021) [80]	Nonexperimental	School-based	Reduce PTSD symptoms Improve social functioning	Yes	Including drumming	Not specified
6.	Weine et al. (2008) [76]	RCT	Multifamily group	Increase mental health seeking Improve family functioning	Yes	Use of native facilitators	Refugee staff

Table A1. *Cont.*

	Study	Design	Intervention	Aims of the Intervention	Were the Aims Achieved?	Culturally Adaptation Process	Implementation and Dissemination Strategies
7.	Wein et al. (2003) [77]	Feasibility	Multifamily group	Increase mental health seeking Improve family functioning	Yes	Use of native facilitators	Refugee staff
8.	Betancourt et al. (2020) [74]	Feasibility	Multifamily group	Reduce PTSD symptoms Improve family functioning	Yes	Community participatory research approach (CBPR)	Refugee staff/social workers
9.	Gotseva-Balgaranova et al. (2020) [75]	Nonexperimental	Multifamily group	Reduce PTSD symptoms	Yes	Not specified	EBTS leaders/interpreter
10.	Ballard et al. (2017) [70]	Feasibility	Parenting	Improve parent–child relationships and family functioning	Yes	Ecological validity model	Trained therapists/Intervention Coaches
11.	Puffer et al. (2017) [73]	RCT	Parenting	Improve parent–child relationships and family functioning	Yes	Not specified	Trained lay facilitators
12.	El-Khani et al. (2021) [72]	Feasibility	Parenting	Improve child behaviors, family functioning	Yes	Not specified	Trained research assistants/translators

References

1. UNHCR. Refugee Data Finder. Available online: https://www.unhcr.org/refugee-statistics/ (accessed on 20 July 2022).
2. Wilmsen, B.; Webber, M. What can we learn from the practice of development-forced displacement and resettlement for organised resettlements in response to climate change? *Geoforum* **2015**, *58*, 76–85. [CrossRef]
3. UNHCR. Global Trends. Available online: https://www.unhcr.org/flagship-reports/globaltrends/ (accessed on 2 May 2022).
4. Slobodin, O.; De Jong, J.T.V.M. Family interventions in traumatized immigrants and refugees: A systematic review. *Transcult. Psychiatry* **2015**, *52*, 723–742. [CrossRef] [PubMed]
5. Birman, D.; Tran, N. Psychological distress and adjustment of Vietnamese refugees in the United States: Association with pre- and postmigration factors. *Am. J. Orthopsychiatry* **2008**, *78*, 109–120. [CrossRef] [PubMed]
6. Mollica, R.F.; McInnes, K.; Pool, C.; Tor, S. Dose-effect relationships of trauma to symptoms of depression and post-traumatic stress disorder among Cambodian survivors of mass violence. *Br. J. Psychiatry* **1998**, *173*, 482–488. [CrossRef]
7. Wieling, E.; Utržan, D.S.; Witting, A.B.; Seponski, D.M. Global mental health, traumatic stress, and displaced families. In *The Handbook of Systemic Family Therapy: Systemic Family Therapy and Global Health Issues*; Wampler, K.S., Rastogi, M., Singh, R., Eds.; Wiley Blackwell: London, UK, 2020; Volume 4, pp. 215–241.
8. Landau, J.; Mittal, M.; Wieling, E. Linking Human Systems: Strengthening Individuals, Families, and Communities in the Wake of Mass Trauma. *J. Marital Fam. Ther.* **2008**, *34*, 193–209. [CrossRef]
9. Whyte, M.U.D.L.O. Cultural Differences in Conflict Styles: Vietnamese Refugees and Established Residents. *Howard J. Commun.* **1998**, *9*, 57–68. [CrossRef]
10. Rees, S.; Fisher, J. COVID-19 and the Mental Health of People from Refugee Backgrounds. *Int. J. Health Serv.* **2020**, *50*, 415–417. [CrossRef]
11. Rychetnik, L.; Frommer, M.; Hawe, P.; Shiell, A. Criteria for evaluating evidence on public health interventions. *J. Epidemiol. Commun. Health* **2002**, *56*, 119–127. [CrossRef]
12. Bhugra, D.; Gupta, S. *Migration and Mental Health*; Cambridge University Press: Cambridge, UK, 2011; ISBN 978-0-52119-077-0.
13. Shannon, P.; Im, H.; Becher, E.; Simmelink, J.; Wieling, E.; O'Fallon, A. Screening for War Trauma, Torture, and Mental Health Symptoms Among Newly Arrived Refugees: A National Survey of U.S. Refugee Health Coordinators. *J. Immigr. Refug. Stud.* **2012**, *10*, 380–394. [CrossRef]
14. Shannon, P.J.; Wieling, E.; McCleary, J.S.; Becher, E. Exploring the Mental Health Effects of Political Trauma with Newly Arrived Refugees. *Qual. Health Res.* **2014**, *25*, 443–457. [CrossRef]
15. Schmeidl, S. Exploring the causes of forced migration: A pooled time-series analysis, 1971–1990. *Soc. Sci. Q.* **1997**, *78*, 284–308.
16. Black, R.; Adger, W.N.; Arnell, N.W.; Dercon, S.; Geddes, A.; Thomas, D. The effect of environmental change on human migration. *Glob. Environ. Change* **2011**, *21*, S3–S11. [CrossRef]

17. Berthold, S.M.; Kong, S.; Mollica, R.F.; Kuoch, T.; Scully, M.; Franke, T. Comorbid Mental and Physical Health and Health Access in Cambodian Refugees in the US. *J. Community Health* **2014**, *39*, 1045–1052. [CrossRef]
18. Shannon, P.J.; Wieling, E.; Simmelink-McCleary, J.; Becher, E. Beyond Stigma: Barriers to Discussing Mental Health in Refugee Populations. *J. Loss Trauma* **2014**, *20*, 281–296. [CrossRef]
19. Bogic, M.; Njoku, A.; Priebe, S. Long-term mental health of war-refugees: A systematic literature review. *BMC Int. Health Hum. Rights* **2015**, *15*, 29. [CrossRef]
20. Kim, W. Beyond Trauma: Post-resettlement Factors and Mental Health Outcomes among Latino and Asian Refugees in the United States. *J. Immigr. Minor. Health* **2015**, *18*, 740–748. [CrossRef]
21. Sangalang, C.C.; Becerra, D.; Mitchell, F.M.; Lechuga-Peña, S.; Lopez, K.; Kim, I. Trauma, Post-Migration Stress, and Mental Health: A Comparative Analysis of Refugees and Immigrants in the United States. *J. Immigr. Minor. Health* **2018**, *21*, 909–919. [CrossRef]
22. Carlson, E.B.; Rosser-Hogan, R. Trauma experiences, posttraumatic stress, dissociation, and depression in Cambodian refugees. *Am. J. Psychiatry* **1991**, *148*, 1548–1551. [CrossRef]
23. Fazel, M.; Wheeler, J.; Danesh, J. Prevalence of serious mental disorder in 7000 refugees resettled in western countries: A systematic review. *Lancet* **2005**, *365*, 1309–1314. [CrossRef]
24. Kirmayer, L.J.; Narasiah, L.; Munoz, M.; Rashid, M.; Ryder, A.G.; Guzder, J.; Hassan, G.; Rousseau, C.; Pottie, K. Common mental health problems in immigrants and refugees: General approach in primary care. *Can. Med. Assoc. J.* **2010**, *183*, E959–E967. [CrossRef]
25. Mollica, R.F.; Wyshak, G.; Lavelle, J. The psychosocial impact of war trauma and torture on Southeast Asian refugees. *Am. J. Psychiatry* **1987**, *144*, 1567–1572. [CrossRef] [PubMed]
26. Murray, K.E.; Davidson, G.R.; Schweitzer, R.D. Review of refugee mental health interventions following resettlement: Best practices and recommendations. *Am. J. Orthopsychiatry* **2010**, *80*, 576–585. [CrossRef] [PubMed]
27. Tracy, M.; Norris, F.H.; Galea, S. Differences in the determinants of posttraumatic stress disorder and depression after a mass traumatic event. *Depress. Anxiety* **2011**, *28*, 666–675. [CrossRef] [PubMed]
28. Berthold, S.M.; Loomis, A.M.; Kuoch, T.; Scully, M.; Hin-McCormick, M.M.; Casavant, B.; Buckley, T. Social Disconnection as a Risk Factor for Health among Cambodian Refugees and Their Offspring in the United States. *J. Immigr. Minor. Health* **2018**, *21*, 290–298. [CrossRef]
29. Cohen, J.A.; Perel, J.M.; Debellis, M.D.; Friedman, M.J.; Putnam, F.W. Treating Traumatized Children: Clinical implications of the psychobiology of posttraumatic stress disorder. *Trauma Violence Abuse* **2002**, *3*, 91–108. [CrossRef]
30. Hinton, D.; Ba, P.; Peou, S.; Um, K. Panic disorder among Cambodian refugees attending a psychiatric clinic. *Gen. Hosp. Psychiatry* **2000**, *22*, 437–444. [CrossRef]
31. Hinton, D.E.; Nickerson, A.; Bryant, R.A. Worry, worry attacks, and PTSD among Cambodian refugees: A path analysis investigation. *Soc. Sci. Med.* **2011**, *72*, 1817–1825. [CrossRef]
32. Pears, K.C.; Capaldi, D.M. Intergenerational transmission of abuse: A two-generational prospective study of an at-risk sample. *Child Abuse Negl.* **2001**, *25*, 1439–1461. [CrossRef]
33. Rowland-Klein, D.; Dunlop, R. The Transmission of Trauma across Generations: Identification with Parental Trauma in Children of Holocaust Survivors. *Aust. N. Z. J. Psychiatry* **1998**, *32*, 358–369. [CrossRef]
34. Yehuda, R.; Halligan, S.L.; Grossman, R. Childhood trauma and risk for PTSD: Relationship to intergenerational effects of trauma, parental PTSD, and cortisol excretion. *Dev. Psychopathol.* **2001**, *13*, 733–753. [CrossRef]
35. Hinton, D.; Barlow, D.H.; Reis, R.; de Jong, J. A transcultural model of the centrality of "thinking a lot" in psychopathologies across the globe and the process of localization: A Cambodian refugee example. *Cult. Med. Psychiatry* **2016**, *40*, 570–619. [CrossRef]
36. Arnsten, A.F.T. Stress signalling pathways that impair prefrontal cortex structure and function. *Nat. Rev. Neurosci.* **2009**, *10*, 410–422. [CrossRef]
37. Elbert, T.; Schauer, M.; Ruf, M.; Weierstall, R.; Neuner, F.; Rockstroh, B.; Junghöfer, M. The Tortured Brain: Imaging neural representations of traumatic stress experiences using RSVP with affective pictorial stimuli. *J. Psychol.* **2011**, *219*, 167–174. [CrossRef]
38. Kozlowska, K.; Walker, P.; McLean, L.; Carrive, P. Fear and the Defense Cascade: Clinical implications and management. *Harv. Rev. Psychiatry* **2015**, *23*, 263–287. [CrossRef]
39. Schauer, M.; Elbert, T. Dissociation following traumatic stress: Etiology and treatment. *J. Psychol.* **2010**, *218*, 109–127. [CrossRef]
40. van der Kolk, B.A. *The Body Keeps the Score: Brain, Mind, and Body in the Healing of Trauma*; Penguin Books: New York, NY, USA, 2015; pp. 51–89.
41. American Psychiatric Association. *Diagnostic and Statistical Manual of Mental Disorders*, 5th ed.; American Psychiatric Publishing: Washington, DC, USA, 2013.
42. Monson, C.M.; Taft, C.T.; Fredman, S.J. Military-related PTSD and intimate relationships: From description to theory-driven research and intervention development. *Clin. Psychol. Rev.* **2009**, *29*, 707–714. [CrossRef]
43. Hanson-Bradley, C.; Wieling, E. Mental health. In *Immigrant and Refugee Families: Global Perspectives on Displacement and Resettlement Experiences*, 2nd ed.; Ballard, J., Wieling, E., Solheim, C., Dwanyen, L., Eds.; University of Minnesota Libraries Publishing: Minneapolis, MN, USA, 2020; pp. 99–124.

44. Catani, C. Krieg im Zuhause—Ein Überblick zum Zusammenhang zwischen Kriegstraumatisierung und familiärer Gewalt. *Verhaltenstherapie* **2009**, *20*, 19–27. [CrossRef]
45. Walsh, F. Traumatic loss and major disasters: Strengthening family and community resilience. *Fam. Process* **2007**, *46*, 207–227. [CrossRef]
46. McIlwaine, F.; O'Sullivan, K. 'Riding the Wave': Working Systemically with Traumatised Families. *Aust. N. Z. J. Fam. Ther.* **2015**, *36*, 310–324. [CrossRef]
47. Nickerson, A.; Bryant, R.A.; Brooks, R.; Steel, Z.; Silove, D.; Chen, J. The familial influence of loss and trauma on refugee mental health: A multilevel path analysis. *J. Trauma. Stress* **2011**, *24*, 25–33. [CrossRef]
48. Weine, S.; Muzurovic, N.; Kulauzovic, Y.; Besic, S.; Lezic, A.; Mujagic, A.; Muzurovic, J.; Spahovic, D.; Feetham, S.; Ware, N.; et al. Family Consequences of Refugee Trauma. *Fam. Process* **2004**, *43*, 147–160. [CrossRef] [PubMed]
49. Taft, C.T.; Schumm, J.A.; Panuzio, J.; Proctor, S.P. An examination of family adjustment among Operation Desert Storm veterans. *J. Consult. Clin. Psychol.* **2008**, *76*, 648–656. [CrossRef] [PubMed]
50. Ballard, J.; Witham, M.; Mittal, M. Intimate partner violence among immigrants and refugees. In *Immigrant and Refugee Families: Global Perspectives on Displacement and Resettlement Experiences*, 2nd ed.; Ballard, J., Wieling, E., Solheim, C., Dwanyen, L., Eds.; University of Minnesota Libraries Publishing: Minneapolis, MN, USA, 2020; pp. 125–150.
51. Catani, C.; Jacob, N.; Schauer, E.; Kohila, M.; Neuner, F. Family violence, war, and natural disasters: A study of the effect of extreme stress on children's mental health in Sri Lanka. *BMC Psychiatry* **2008**, *8*, 33. [CrossRef]
52. Catani, C.; Schauer, E.; Elbert, T.; Missmahl, I.; Bette, J.-P.; Neuner, F. War trauma, child labor, and family violence: Life adversities and PTSD in a sample of school children in Kabul. *J. Trauma. Stress* **2009**, *22*, 163–171. [CrossRef] [PubMed]
53. Catani, C.; Schauer, E.; Neuner, F. Beyond Individual War Trauma: Domestic Violence against Children in Afghanistan and Sri Lanka. *J. Marital Fam. Ther.* **2008**, *34*, 165–176. [CrossRef]
54. Morgan, E.; Wieling, E.; Hubbard, J.; Kraus, E. The Development and Implementation of a Multi-Couple Therapy Model with Torture Survivors in the Democratic Republic of the Congo. *J. Marital Fam. Ther.* **2017**, *44*, 235–247. [CrossRef]
55. Siegel, J.P. Breaking the Links in Intergenerational Violence: An Emotional Regulation Perspective. *Fam. Process* **2013**, *52*, 163–178. [CrossRef]
56. Gershoff, E.T. Corporal punishment by parents and associated child behaviors and experiences: A meta-analytic and theoretical review. *Psychol. Bull.* **2002**, *128*, 539–579. [CrossRef]
57. Beardslee, W.R.; Gladstone, T.R.G.; Wright, E.J.; Cooper, A.B. A Family-Based Approach to the Prevention of Depressive Symptoms in Children at Risk: Evidence of Parental and Child Change. *Pediatrics* **2003**, *112*, e119–e131. [CrossRef]
58. Gewirtz, A.; Forgatch, M.; Wieling, E. Parenting Practices as Potential Mechanisms for Child adjustment Following Mass Trauma. *J. Marital Fam. Ther.* **2008**, *34*, 177–192. [CrossRef]
59. Wieling, E.; Mehus, C.; Möllerherm, J.; Neuner, F.; Achan, L.; Catani, C. Assessing the Feasibility of Providing a Parenting Intervention for War-Affected Families in Northern Uganda. *Fam. Community Health* **2015**, *38*, 252–267. [CrossRef]
60. Ferguson, C.J. Spanking, corporal punishment and negative long-term outcomes: A meta-analytic review of longitudinal studies. *Clin. Psychol. Rev.* **2013**, *33*, 196–208. [CrossRef]
61. Slep, A.M.S.; O'Leary, S.G. Multivariate models of mothers' and fathers' aggression toward their children. *J. Consult. Clin. Psychol.* **2007**, *75*, 739–751. [CrossRef]
62. Smith, J.R. Correlates and Consequences of Harsh Discipline for Young Children. *Arch. Pediatr. Adolesc. Med.* **1997**, *151*, 777–786. [CrossRef]
63. Catani, C.; Gewirtz, A.H.; Wieling, E.; Schauer, E.; Elbert, T.; Neuner, F. Tsunami, War, and Cumulative Risk in the Lives of Sri Lankan Schoolchildren. *Child Dev.* **2010**, *81*, 1176–1191. [CrossRef]
64. Carlson, E.B.; Dalenberg, C.J. A Conceptual Framework for the Impact of Traumatic Experiences. *Trauma Violence Abuse* **2000**, *1*, 4–28. [CrossRef]
65. Walsh, F. A Family Resilience Framework: Innovative Practice Applications. *Fam. Relat.* **2002**, *51*, 130–137. [CrossRef]
66. Masten, A.S. Resilience in developmental systems: Principles, pathways, and protective processes in research and practice. In *Multisystemic Resilience: Adaptation and Transformation in Contexts of Change*; Ungar, M., Ed.; Oxford University Press: London, UK, 2021; pp. 113–134.
67. Ungar, M. Resilience, Trauma, Context, and Culture. *Trauma Violence Abuse* **2013**, *14*, 255–266. [CrossRef]
68. Wieling, E. Family Interventions for Populations Exposed to Traumatic Stress Related to War and Violence. *J. Marital Fam. Ther.* **2017**, *44*, 189–192. [CrossRef]
69. Paat, Y.-F. Working with Immigrant Children and Their Families: An Application of Bronfenbrenner's Ecological Systems Theory. *J. Hum. Behav. Soc. Environ.* **2013**, *23*, 954–966. [CrossRef]
70. Ballard, J.; Wieling, E.; Forgatch, M. Feasibility of Implementation of a Parenting Intervention with Karen Refugees Resettled from Burma. *J. Marital Fam. Ther.* **2017**, *44*, 220–234. [CrossRef]
71. Ballard, J.; Wieling, E.; Dwanyen, L. Parenting Practices in the Karen Refugee Community. *Int. J. Fam. Ther.* **2019**, *42*, 95–107. [CrossRef]
72. El-Khani, A.; Haar, K.; Stojanovic, M.; Maalouf, W. Assessing the Feasibility of Providing a Family Skills Intervention, "Strong Families", for Refugee Families Residing in Reception Centers in Serbia. *Int. J. Environ. Res. Public Health* **2021**, *18*, 4530. [CrossRef] [PubMed]

73. Puffer, E.S.; Annan, J.; Sim, A.; Salhi, C.; Betancourt, T.S. The impact of a family skills training intervention among Burmese migrant families in Thailand: A randomized controlled trial. *PLoS ONE* **2017**, *12*, e0172611. [CrossRef] [PubMed]
74. Betancourt, T.S.; Berent, J.M.; Freeman, J.; Frounfelker, R.L.; Brennan, R.T.; Abdi, S.; Maalim, A.; Abdi, A.; Mishra, T.; Gautam, B.; et al. Family-Based Mental Health Promotion for Somali Bantu and Bhutanese Refugees: Feasibility and Acceptability Trial. *J. Adolesc. Health* **2020**, *66*, 336–344. [CrossRef] [PubMed]
75. Gotseva-Balgaranova, K.; Popivanov, I.D.; Mutafchieva, M. Impact evaluation of the evidence-based trauma stabilisation programme for refugee, asylum seeking and immigrant families. *Zeitschrift für Psychodrama und Soziometrie* **2020**, *19*, 147–160. [CrossRef]
76. Weine, S.; Kulauzovic, Y.; Klebic, A.; Besic, S.; Mujagic, A.; Muzurovic, J.; Spahovic, D.; Sclove, S.; Pavkovic, I.; Feetham, S.; et al. Evaluating A Multiple-Family Group Access Intervention for Refugees with PTSD. *J. Marital Fam. Ther.* **2008**, *34*, 149–164. [CrossRef]
77. Weine, S.M.; Raina, D.; Zhubi, M.; Delesi, M.; Huseni, D.; Feetham, S.; Kulauzovic, Y.; Mermelstein, R.; Campbell, R.T.; Rolland, J.; et al. The TAFES multi-family group intervention for Kosovar refugees: A descriptive study. *J. Nerv. Ment. Dis.* **2003**, *191*, 100–107. [CrossRef]
78. Beehler, S.; Birman, D.; Campbell, R. The Effectiveness of Cultural Adjustment and Trauma Services (CATS): Generating Practice-Based Evidence on a Comprehensive, School-Based Mental Health Intervention for Immigrant Youth. *Am. J. Community Psychol.* **2011**, *50*, 155–168. [CrossRef]
79. Birman, D.; Beehler, S.; Harris, E.M.; Everson, M.L.; Batia, K.; Liautaud, J.; Frazier, S.; Atkins, M.; Blanton, S.; Buwalda, J.; et al. International Family, Adult, and Child Enhancement Services (FACES): A community-based comprehensive services model for refugee children in resettlement. *Am. J. Orthopsychiatry* **2008**, *78*, 121–132. [CrossRef]
80. Elswick, S.; Washington, G.; Mangrum-Apple, H.; Peterson, C.; Barnes, E.; Pirkey, P.; Watson, J. Trauma Healing Club: Utilizing Culturally Responsive Processes in the Implementation of an After-School Group Intervention to Address Trauma Among African Refugees. *J. Child Adolesc. Trauma* **2021**, *15*, 155–166. [CrossRef]
81. Kataoka, S.H.; Stein, B.D.; Jaycox, L.H.; Wong, M.; Escudero, P.; Tu, W.; Zaragoza, C.; Fink, A. A School-Based Mental Health Program for Traumatized Latino Immigrant Children. *J. Am. Acad. Child Adolesc. Psychiatry* **2003**, *42*, 311–318. [CrossRef]
82. Möhlen, H.; Parzer, P.; Resch, F.; Brunner, R. Psychosocial Support for War-Traumatized Child and Adolescent Refugees: Evaluation of a Short-Term Treatment Program. *Aust. N. Z. J. Psychiatry* **2005**, *39*, 81–87. [CrossRef]
83. Mollica, R.F.; Cui, X.; Mcinnes, K.; Massagli, M.P. Science-based policy for psychosocial interventions in refugee camps: A Cambodian example. *J. Nerv. Ment. Dis.* **2002**, *190*, 158–166. [CrossRef]
84. Page, M.J.; McKenzie, J.E.; Bossuyt, P.M.; Boutron, I.; Hoffmann, T.C.; Mulrow, C.D.; Shamseer, L.; Tetzlaff, J.M.; Akl, E.A.; Brennan, S.E.; et al. The PRISMA 2020 statement: An updated guideline for reporting systematic reviews. *J. Clin. Epidemiol.* **2021**, *134*, 178–189. [CrossRef]
85. Erdemir, E. Transactional relations and reciprocity between refugee mothers and their children: Changes in child, parenting, and concept of child. *Eur. Early Child. Educ. Res. J.* **2020**, *29*, 547–568. [CrossRef]
86. Cabassa, L.J.; Baumann, A.A. A two-way street: Bridging implementation science and cultural adaptations of mental health treatments. *Implement. Sci.* **2013**, *8*, 90. [CrossRef]
87. Bernal, G.; Bonilla, J.; Bellido, C. Ecological validity and cultural sensitivity for outcome research: Issues for the cultural adaptation and development of psychosocial treatments with Hispanics. *J. Abnorm. Child Psychol.* **1995**, *23*, 67–82. [CrossRef]
88. Powell, B.J.; Proctor, E.K.; Glass, J.E. A Systematic Review of Strategies for Implementing Empirically Supported Mental Health Interventions. *Res. Soc. Work Pract.* **2013**, *24*, 192–212. [CrossRef]
89. Fixsen, D.L.; Blase, K.A.; Naoom, S.F.; Wallace, F. Core Implementation Components. *Res. Soc. Work Pract.* **2009**, *19*, 531–540. [CrossRef]
90. Collins, P.Y.; Patel, V.; Joestl, S.S.; March, D.; Insel, T.R.; Daar, A.S.; Bordin, I.A.; Costello, E.J.; Durkin, M.; Fairburn, C.G.; et al. Grand challenges in global mental health. *Nature* **2011**, *475*, 27–30. [CrossRef] [PubMed]
91. van der Velde, J.; Williamson, D.L.; Ogilvie, L.D. Participatory Action Research: Practical Strategies for Actively Engaging and Maintaining Participation in Immigrant and Refugee Communities. *Qual. Health Res.* **2009**, *19*, 1293–1302. [CrossRef] [PubMed]
92. O'Neill, M.; Hubbard, P. Walking, sensing, belonging: Ethno-mimesis as performative praxis. *Vis. Stud.* **2010**, *25*, 46–58. [CrossRef]
93. Pittaway, E.; Bartolomei, L.; Hugman, R. Stop Stealing Our Stories: The Ethics of Research with Vulnerable Groups. *J. Hum. Rights Pract.* **2010**, *2*, 229–251. [CrossRef]
94. Barrera, M.; Berkel, C.; Castro, F.G. Directions for the Advancement of Culturally Adapted Preventive Interventions: Local Adaptations, Engagement, and Sustainability. *Prev. Sci.* **2016**, *18*, 640–648. [CrossRef] [PubMed]
95. Rodríguez, M.M.D.; Baumann, A.; Schwartz, A.L. Cultural Adaptation of an Evidence Based Intervention: From Theory to Practice in a Latino/a Community Context. *Am. J. Community Psychol.* **2010**, *47*, 170–186. [CrossRef] [PubMed]
96. Kumpfer, K.; Magalhães, C.; Xie, J. Cultural Adaptation and Implementation of Family Evidence-Based Interventions with Diverse Populations. *Prev. Sci.* **2016**, *18*, 649–659. [CrossRef]
97. Powell, B.J.; Beidas, R.S.; Lewis, C.C.; Aarons, G.A.; McMillen, J.C.; Proctor, E.K.; Mandell, D.S. Methods to Improve the Selection and Tailoring of Implementation Strategies. *J. Ment. Health Adm.* **2015**, *44*, 177–194. [CrossRef]
98. Shannon, P.; McCleary, J.; Wieling, E.; Im, H.; Becher, E.; O'Fallon, A. Exploring Mental Health Screening Feasibility and Training of Refugee Health Coordinators. *J. Immigr. Refug. Stud.* **2015**, *13*, 80–102. [CrossRef]

99. Weisz, J.R.; Jensen-Doss, A.; Hawley, K. Evidence-based youth psychotherapies versus usual clinical care: A meta-analysis of direct comparisons. *Am. Psychol.* **2006**, *61*, 671–689. [CrossRef]
100. Palic, S.; Elklit, A. Psychosocial treatment of posttraumatic stress disorder in adult refugees: A systematic review of prospective treatment outcome studies and a critique. *J. Affect. Disord.* **2011**, *131*, 8–23. [CrossRef]

International Journal of
Environmental Research and Public Health

Article

The Implications of Health Disparities: A COVID-19 Risk Assessment of the Hispanic Community in El Paso

Carina Cione [1], Emma Vetter [2], Deziree Jackson [3], Sarah McCarthy [4] and Ernesto Castañeda [5,*]

1 Center for Latin American and Latino Studies, American University, Washington, DC 20016, USA
2 Department of Sociology & Anthropology, George Mason University, Fairfax, VA 22030, USA
3 Department of Sociology, Indiana University Bloomington, Bloomington, IN 47405, USA
4 Department of Sociology, State University of New York at Albany, Albany, NY 12222, USA
5 Department of Sociology, Center for Latin American and Latino Studies, Immigration Lab, Center for Health, Risk, and Society, American University, Washington, DC 20016, USA
* Correspondence: ernesto@american.edu; Tel.: +1-(202)-885-2412

Abstract: Since the outbreak of the COVID-19 pandemic in the United States, Latinos have suffered from disproportionately high rates of hospitalization and death related to the virus. Health disparities based on race and ethnicity are directly associated with heightened mortality and burden of illness and act as underlying causes for the staggering impacts of COVID-19 in Latin communities in the United States. This is especially true in the city of El Paso, Texas, where over 82% of the population is Hispanic. To ascertain the level of danger that COVID-19 poses in El Paso, we constructed a point-in-time risk assessment of its Latin population and assessed a Latin individual's likelihood of hospitalization or death related to COVID-19 by comparing relevant health profiles with high-risk co-morbidities that the Centers for Disease Control (CDC) identified in 2020. Data for this risk assessment come from 1152 surveys conducted in El Paso. The assessment included comprehensive demographic, socioeconomic, and health data to analyze disparities across Hispanic sub-populations in the city. Results revealed that around 49.3% of Hispanics in the study had been previously diagnosed with a high-risk co-morbidity and therefore have an increased likelihood of hospitalization or death related to COVID-19. Additional factors that led to increased risk included low income, homelessness, lack of U.S. citizenship, and being insured. The findings from this study additionally demonstrate that structural inequality in the U.S. must be addressed, and preventive measures must be taken at local and state levels to decrease the mortality of pandemics. Baseline population health data can help with both of these goals.

Keywords: health equity; COVID pandemic; Hispanic health; immigrant; minority health

Citation: Cione, C.; Vetter, E.; Jackson, D.; McCarthy, S.; Castañeda, E. The Implications of Health Disparities: A COVID-19 Risk Assessment of the Hispanic Community in El Paso. *Int. J. Environ. Res. Public Health* **2023**, *20*, 975. https://doi.org/10.3390/ijerph20020975

Academic Editor: Paul B. Tchounwou

Received: 15 November 2022
Revised: 30 December 2022
Accepted: 1 January 2023
Published: 5 January 2023

1. Introduction

Existing health disparities have been exacerbated by COVID-19 [1,2]. Long before the pandemic, race and ethnicity were proven to be associated with life expectancy, mortality, and the burden of illness in the United States [3]. Communities of color consistently lack access to care, proper treatment, care provider diversity, and the resources that exist in high-income and White-populated areas of the country [3]. These disparities cause and prolong poor health in minority communities and result in higher-risk individuals with multiple risk factors beyond old age [2]. This is echoed by public health professionals who observe Black and Hispanic individuals die at higher rates because of an increased likelihood of underlying health conditions and structural barriers to healthcare [1]. Gaps in healthcare increase the vulnerability of groups of people, and their existence springs from discrimination, inequality, and structural racism.

Institutions that place lesser value on the lives of Black and Hispanic people not only turn a blind eye to health disparities but restrict minorities to riskier jobs where they work in dangerous conditions. Research in the United States, Canada, and Europe shows that immigrants and other minority communities bear higher rates of work-related accidents, illnesses, and deaths because of their over-representation in high-risk occupations [4]. Because of these factors and being less likely to work remotely, they came into contact with COVID-19 before other racial groups and experienced its impacts earlier in the pandemic.

This article examines COVID-19 risk factors in the context of the Hispanic-majority border city of El Paso, Texas. To ascertain the level of danger that COVID-19 poses for the Hispanic community in El Paso, we constructed a point-in-time risk assessment of its Latin population. We assessed a Latin individual's likelihood of hospitalization or death related to COVID-19 by comparing relevant health profiles with high-risk co-morbidities that the Centers for Disease Control (CDC) identified in 2020 [5]. El Paso is an important research site on health disparities, as proven by prior research documenting that the border city's Hispanic population faces compounded structural inequalities, high risk of morality, and poor health outcomes [6,7].

Our study contributes to understanding how racial, ethnic, socioeconomic, and other intersectional experiences are predictive of health outcomes within regional and historical contexts. First, we provide a brief overview of how the COVID-19 pandemic has unfolded in El Paso and its "sister city" of Ciudad Juárez, Mexico. Then, we describe the methodology employed in gathering comprehensive survey data on Hispanics living in El Paso and compiling our risk assessment. The subsequent section analyzes significant demographic, socioeconomic, and health factors that encompass essential determinants of health and risk associated with COVID-19. These measures allowed us to predict Hispanic El Pasoans' high risks of hospitalization and death related to COVID-19 before the pandemic struck El Paso, and thus demonstrate the foreseen impact of COVID-19 on the Latin community in the U.S. [8–11]. In doing so, we also acknowledge and explore structural forms of discrimination and violence against communities of color, particularly Latinos, that contribute to health disparities.

In the early months of 2020, cities and entire regions around the world declared public health emergencies while COVID-19, also known as coronavirus, stole millions of lives and disabled many more [12]. Its arrival in the United States was swift. Former President Donald Trump, who dissolved the White House pandemic response team in 2018, assumed a perilously disinterested approach to information about the virus spreading in Asia. Reuters estimated a COVID-19 death count of at least 69,457 in the United States on 5 May 2020 [13]. This number continued to rise, reaching 92,038 on 20 May. This marked the United States as the country with the highest COVID-19 death toll in the world [13]. The number of lives lost to COVID-19 exceeded that of the United Kingdom, then the country with the second-highest mortality rate, by over 57,000 [13]. In 2020, the total estimated number of cases in the U.S. was also the highest across the globe at 1,189,198, outnumbering China by more than 1 million cases, despite China's population being approximately four times larger [13]. However, not all geographical areas were impacted at the same time. For example, the pandemic reached New York City many months before El Paso, Texas.

The great loss that the U.S. experienced in 2020 was also reflected in local cities' rates of hospitalization and death related to COVID-19, which tracked demographic data and allowed researchers to glimpse the differences in rates across ethno-racial groups. In New York, the Bureau of Communicable Disease Surveillance System reported that, as of 16 April 2020, the death rates for Blacks were 92.3 per 100,000 people, and 74.3 per 100,000 for Latinos [14]. In comparison, the White and Asian death rates were 45.2 and 34.5 per 100,000 people, respectively [14]. Just two months later, the mortality and infection rates skyrocketed. At least 5322 Latinos had died from COVID-19, the majority of whom were ages 65 and above [15]. This was the highest number of lab-confirmed deaths of a racial group in New York City, exceeding that of the White population by almost 1000 [15]. Even so, these numbers were understood to be low estimates since the data cover only lab-confirmed cases, effectively excluding asymptomatic and non-lab-confirmed cases.

As the COVID-19 pandemic continued to unfold and healthcare workers fought to save lives, a familiar pattern arose that concerned researchers and advocates: Black and Hispanic individuals were not only suffering from more infections but also dying at incredibly higher rates than White and Asian people [14,15].

2. El Paso, Texas

El Paso is city in the western corner of Texas, bordering Las Cruces, New Mexico, and directly to the south, Ciudad Juarez, Mexico. El Paso City's population was around 649,000 in 2010 and 679,000 in 2020 and El Paso County has over 800,000 residents. El Paso is around 83% Hispanic. El Paso is a majority Latin city, with over 24% of the population being foreign-born [16]. It also includes Hispanics who have been in the area for decades and many generations, thus making it a great place to study the impact of health disparities within the same ethno-racial category. Poverty is directly related to health; this is visible in the U.S.–Mexico border [17].

El Paso experienced mounting pressure as time passed in the first months of the pandemic. Sixty-five people were hospitalized in El Paso in the first week of May 2020, and 17 were put on ventilators [18]. Local public health officials worried El Paso would suffer from limited resources, as the county only had 285 licensed ICU hospital beds [18]. Unfortunately, the City Director of Public Health, Robert Resendes, resigned on 4 May, and his replacement had not been selected at the time of his departure. The city insisted that his resignation would not negatively impact preventative action since the Office of Emergency Management handles public health crises, but the community continued to buzz with concern given that Texas was one of the top ten most infected states, with over 32,954 cases in 2020 [19,20].

Ciudad Juárez, which sits on the Mexican side of the border right next to El Paso, was also grappling with an upward trajectory of COVID-19 cases. El Paso and Ciudad Juárez are sister cities that are economically and socially intertwined. The first case of COVID-19 in the Mexican state of Chihuahua was confirmed in Ciudad Juárez on 17 March 2020, not long after cities in the U.S. began issuing public health mandates, mandatory quarantines, and other lockdown procedures [21]. Since then, the official response paralleled somewhat that of the U.S. because of the lax approach that President Andrés Manuel López Obrador took to prepare for outbreaks. He refused to close the Mexican border to visitors, instead allowing Americans and foreign tourists into the country, even though the U.S. imposed major entry restrictions at its legal entry points [22].

The border cities of Tijuana and Juárez, where Mexican and U.S. nationals travel to and from every day, and the popular destination of Cancún, had the three highest rates of documented COVID-19 cases in Mexico between January and May 2020 [23]. Things grew so dire that Armando Cabada, mayor of Ciudad Juárez, wrote to the foreign affairs secretary to ask that they block Americans from filtering into the city and spreading the coronavirus [22]. Another significant factor that the Mexican government had to consider was the Migrant Protection Protocols, or "Remain-in-Mexico", U.S. program. As a result, Juárez served as a temporary shelter for more than 19,000 Central American and Mexican migrants awaiting decisions on their U.S. asylum applications [24–26]. The foreign affairs secretary, however, did not fulfill Cabada's wishes, and U.S. citizens continued to pass into Mexico. Consequently, hospitals saw a massive influx of patients. Cemeteries were hosting as many as six burials each day, and the cost to bury a loved one increased by some USD 600 [27]. Unlike in El Paso, people living on the urban periphery of Ciudad Juárez had limited access to clean water and could not practice as effectively the CDC-recommended hygienic practices to counter COVID-19 [21]. They also faced other health barriers, such as the lack of COVID-19 testing sites, which increased the number of cases and deaths in the region [22].

3. Data and Methods

The data used in this study were collected through ethno-surveys, which provided close-ended and open-ended data regarding health, employment, socioeconomic status, housing, transborder habits, and citizenship. These surveys were conducted in 2011–2012, nine years before the start of the pandemic, as part of a study funded by the National Institutes for Health (NIH) conducted by Dr. Ernesto Castañeda and research teams who trained for several months as part of a research methods course. The sample consisted of 1152 Hispanic respondents aged 18 and over residing in El Paso, Texas. All surveys were conducted and recorded in Spanish and/or English (at the preference of the respondent) in a variety of locations in El Paso, such as at individual's homes, shelters, and workplaces. Only close-ended questions from the ethno-surveys are referenced in this study. All researchers who participated in data collection were certified to work with human subjects, and the project had IRB approval from the University of Texas, El Paso. The NIH's National Institute on Minority Health and Health Disparities further reviewed and approved the project before releasing funds.

The risk assessment comprises several analyses conducted using the IBM SPSS 27 statistical package. Notably, we used purposeful sampling techniques [28] that specifically considered the heterogeneity of respondents, such as education levels, profession, housing status, and age, to construct an adequate representation of El Paso's geographic neighborhoods. Furthermore, we stopped data collection when saturation of responses was reached and we had a sample large and diverse enough to generalize to the Hispanic population of the whole city. No exclusionary criteria were identified when recruiting participants beyond self-identification as Hispanic, Latino, Mexican American, Chicano, Mexican, or of Latin American or Caribbean origin [6].

Undocumented Hispanics and those experiencing housing insecurity were over-sampled because of their relative exclusion across census counts and research studies [29]. Therefore, to take these differential selection probabilities into account and adjust to the El Paso demographic, weighted data were utilized to account for this over-sampling in the dataset. Throughout the following sections, we provide descriptive analyses to present various differences in the distributions of citizenship status, social class, and medical insurance coverage, among other factors, across the sample of Hispanic El Pasoans. Pearson's chi-squared tests determined bivariate associations.

The data precede the COVID pandemic, but when we embarked on this analysis, we wondered whether they could be used as a baseline to calculate population risks before the pandemic struck El Paso. It is safe to assume that most of the people who participated in the survey still reside in El Paso and that the demographic and health profile has not changed much; if anything, it may have worsened as the people in the sample have aged, but this also depends on the health status of the younger generations for whom comparative data do not exist. Health data are seen as a personal attribute, and patients' data are protected by HIPA. Even if hospitals engage in big data analysis with their anonymized patient data, they do not have access to all types of populations in a city; thus, the importance of databases such as this.

4. Latinos and High-Risk Populations

4.1. Race and Ethnicity

Risk is not only related to physiological factors but also socioeconomic, cultural, racial, and ethnic ones. The CDC distinguishes racial and ethnic minorities, as well as people who are currently homeless, pregnant, and breastfeeding, as individuals who are "high-risk" for COVID-19 [5]. This is because Latin communities across the U.S. have suffered disproportionately high rates of hospitalization and death caused by the virus compared to other racial and ethnic groups. According to the City of New York and the CDC, Black and Latin communities had borne the brunt of virus-related deaths [14]. In a weekly report, the CDC revealed that although 18% of the U.S. population is Black, 33% of hospitalized COVID-19 cases were among Black people in May 2020 [14].

The Latin population in the United States has received relatively little attention in relation to the pandemic despite its vulnerability to COVID-19. This is especially true in the city of El Paso, Texas, where Hispanics constitute over 83% of the population and have suffered disproportionately from the pandemic's damage [16]. On 28 May 2020, the city recorded 1029 cases and 22 deaths [18]. Over a year later, the cumulative number of infections surpassed 111,000 and the death toll across El Paso had skyrocketed to 1651 lives lost. Hispanic individuals comprised the vast majority of COVID-related deaths at this time, at 91.25% of the population [30].

4.2. Essential and Frontline Workers

The Hispanic community is an integral part of the U.S. labor force. In 2018, 17% of the national labor force was comprised of documented Hispanic citizens, 61% of whom were Mexican [31]. However, this percentage does not include undocumented workers, who constitute upwards of an estimated 5.1% of the U.S. workforce [32]. This is supported by our data gathered in El Paso, as reported in Table 1, which show that 53.5% of undocumented Hispanics in 2011 were employed. The way the data were obtained means that the unemployed may be students, homemakers, or retired.

Table 1. Employment by Citizenship Status among Hispanics in El Paso, TX in 2011–2012.

Status	Citizen	Resident	Undocumented	Visa	Total
Unemployed	33.6% 138,083	46.5% 36,477	46.5% 8232	19.2% 2530	35.6% 185,322
Employed	66.4% 273,471	53.5% 41,990	53.5% 9461	80.8% 10,655	64.4% 335,577

Note: $p < 0.001$.

Furthermore, the CDC reports that at least 25% of the Hispanic population in the U.S. is employed in the service industry, including hospitality, transportation/travel, delivery, food, healthcare, and education services [33]. Unfortunately, these industries severely struggled under COVID-19 restrictions and regulations, and nonessential businesses laid off millions of workers across the country as a result of forced closures [34]. This was particularly worrisome for undocumented immigrants because they could not file for unemployment insurance and did not qualify for Pandemic Unemployment Assistance (PUA), which was passed in the Coronavirus Aid, Relief, and Economic Security (CARES) Act [35].

Then, there are those who were considered "essential" employees, including people working in grocery stores, mail services, agriculture, city maintenance, and construction, in addition to the service industries mentioned earlier, who were legally required to work in person during the pandemic. Laws surrounding "essential and emergency employees" require that such employees continue working through national emergencies, including those who are immunocompromised or have pre-existing health conditions [36]. This makes it difficult for frontline workers to receive unemployment benefits if they prefer not to work because one must be fired or laid off in order to collect unemployment insurance [37]. Employees who quit during the pandemic were disqualified from unemployment claims, a policy that jeopardizes their financial stability for the sake of maintaining their health. Therefore, "essential" workers were forced to engage with customers and coworkers in close quarters, as before COVID-19 regulations, and thus ran a higher risk of contracting and spreading the virus.

4.3. Prison, Jail, and Juvenile Delinquent Centers

Incarcerated populations in prisons, jails, and juvenile delinquent centers are also at higher risk of severe illness related to COVID-19. The close quarters, shared spaces, and lack of comprehensive medical care in correctional institutions create a breeding ground for the virus. The Marshall Project reports that there were at least 9437 cases of positive COVID-19 diagnoses in state and federal prisons across the U.S. as of 25 April 2020 [38]. As a result, 131 incarcerated individuals and seven prison employees died [38]. The deaths of prisoners rapidly increased throughout the spring months, eventually amounting to 496 dead inmates by 4 June 2020 [39]. There was no testing protocol for individual states at that time, and many refused to release information regarding the number of prisoners who were tested. The Federal Bureau of Prisons even went so far as to report lower numbers compared to state correctional facilities [40].

In the second year of the pandemic, the institution's reporting habits had not improved. The Federal Bureau released information indicating that 799 federal inmates tested positive for the virus, along with 319 staff members. Although no staff member was among the deceased, 27 inmates died from virus-related complications. Furthermore, three inmates died at Fort Worth Federal Medical Center alone, and all federal prisons in Texas currently had at least one positive diagnosis within the facility [40]. The Marshall Project, however, defines these numbers as "almost certainly an undercount" [38].

This puts racial and ethnic minorities at further risk, given the mass incarceration of communities of color. In the U.S., Hispanics are imprisoned at a rate 1.4 times higher than that of Whites [41]. In 2016, approximately 61% of state prisoners in New Mexico were Hispanic, although approximately 49.1% of people living in New Mexico were Hispanic [42]. The ratio of Black and Hispanic prisoners exceeds that of incarcerated Whites across the country, but the disparities are widest in Texas and other southern states. For example, ranking second only to the number of incarcerated Black individuals, 541 per 100,000 prisoners in Texas are Hispanic [41]. The state's ratio of Hispanic to White prisoners is 2:1, and its neighbor, Arizona, has the highest number of Hispanic prisoners in the U.S. [41].

Juvenile delinquent centers incarcerating children ages 10 to 17 share similar demographic trends with adult correctional institutions. The Department of Justice revealed that Latino youth in the U.S. have a 65% higher chance of being detained and incarcerated than their White counterparts [43]. This profound disparity also exists in Texas, where juvenile prisoners are 1.47 times more likely to be Latino than White [43]. Disproportionate imprisonment because of higher policing and stricter sentencing is also one of the reasons that Black, Hispanic, and other minority communities in the U.S. were contracting, spreading, and dying from COVID-19 at higher rates than White Americans.

4.4. Medical Insurance and Citizenship

Immigration status dramatically impacts an individual's access to healthcare and medical treatment. Our data revealed that the likelihood of being medically insured increased with the stability of immigration status, as detailed in Table 2. In 2011, 89.3% of undocumented Hispanics living in El Paso lacked medical insurance, followed by 66% of lawful permanent residents.

Table 2. Medical Insurance by Citizenship among Hispanics in El Paso, TX in 2011–2012.

Status	Citizen	Resident	Undocumented	Visa	Total
Does not have medical insurance	43.1% 177,533	66.0% 52,188	89.3% 15,792	40.2% 5046	48.0% 250,559
Has medical insurance	56.9% 234,673	34% 26,914	10.7% 1900	59.8% 7515	52% 271,002

Note: $p < 0.001$.

These data were obtained before the Affordable Care Act was passed. Still, the Affordable Care Act does not provide coverage for all immigrants and excludes the undocumented community from nonemergency services [44]. Recipients of Deferred Action for Childhood Arrivals (DACA) have been denied both Medicaid and ACA benefits since 2012, and children of undocumented parents must be lawful residents or citizens in order to qualify for Medicaid or Children's Health Insurance Program (CHIP) services [44]. Despite the implementation of the Affordable Care Act, undocumented individuals have not experienced any major improvement in access to healthcare, so it is unlikely that these figures have changed significantly as a result of the Act.

Upon assessment of Hispanics who fulfilled the CDC criteria for individuals at high risk of severe illness related to COVID-19, our data, as shown in Table 3, revealed that only those insured by Medicaid and Medicare were over-represented in the high-risk category.

Table 3. Health Insurance Plan and High Risk of COVID-19 Complications.

Health Insurance Type	Not at Risk for COVID	At Risk for COVID	Total
Private healthcare plan	51.9% 70,011	43.6% 60,104	47.7% 130,115
Medicaid	8.3% 11,254	12.3% 16,991	10.4% 28,245
Medicare	2.3% 3125	9.5% 13,134	6.0% 16,259
VA	0.9% 1250	2.3% 3135	1.6% 4385
Tricare	6.0% 8125	3.6% 5010	4.8% 13,135
Unspecified healthcare plan	28.7% 38,758	26.8% 36,985	27.8% 75,743
Government employee healthcare	0.9% 1250	0.5% 625	0.7% 1875
Foreign insurance	0.9% 1250	1.4% 1875	1.1% 3125

Note: $p < 0.001$.

4.5. Homelessness

The U.S. struggles to provide affordable housing and address homelessness. In 2019, over 500,000 people were estimated to have been homeless on any given night nationwide [45]. People experiencing homelessness are at high risk of severe illness related to COVID-19 for multiple reasons. There are almost no isolated or private spaces in shelters, encampments, and other congregate housing settings that homeless individuals occupy [46]. People are in close proximity to one another, which makes it challenging to maintain the six feet of distance that medical professionals recommend to inhibit the spread of COVID-19. The Council of Economic Advisers found that around 200,000 people sleep in unsheltered places, such as cars, parks, sidewalks, and abandoned buildings. Those who may not sleep in the presence of others must still interact with people at social service facilities [45].

People experiencing housing instability are also less likely to have access to masks, gloves, and other materials that prevent the spread of the virus. This also includes basic hygienic facilities and necessities, such as soap [46]. They can also rely on public transportation and facilities, such as bathrooms and water fountains. Interacting without precautionary measures increases the possibility of exposure to COVID-19. According to our data collected in El Paso, housing instability lessens the likelihood of having medical insurance. In 2011, only about one-quarter (24.7%) of homeless Hispanics in El Paso were medically insured, which is a much lower percentage than for those who were housed (see Table 2).

Additionally, Hispanics experiencing housing instability constituted only 0.3% of those with a high-risk medical condition. However, they are still considered particularly vulnerable because of their heightened likelihood of contracting COVID-19 and limited access to medical providers. Individuals and families experiencing homelessness who are uninsured have a decreased likelihood of being tested for COVID-19 and adequately treated for potentially fatal symptoms (see Table 4). Furthermore, people who have not sought a visit to a medical clinic or provider are unaware of their health status and may be living with an illness that has gone undiagnosed. So, although our data only show 1% of Hispanics experiencing homelessness as "high risk," the reality is that unhoused people may not know enough about their health to provide information that can assess their level of risk [6].

Table 4. Disease Prevalence among Hispanics Experiencing Homelessness.

Health Condition	Percent	*N*
Smoking	22.5%	469
Obesity	18.5%	438
High Blood Pressure	8.1%	219
High Cholesterol	4.3%	117
Diabetes	4.0%	107
Asthma	3.4%	92
Hepatitis or Cirrhosis	2.8%	76
Heart Attack/Stroke	1.9%	51
Kidney Disease	1.5%	31
Cancer	0.5%	10
Tuberculosis	0.5%	10
Emphysema	0.4%	10
HIV/AIDS	0.4%	10
		1640

Note: Unweighted data was used to include all of the oversampled unhoused respondents.

Altogether, experiencing homelessness can almost guarantee poorer health outcomes. Compared to housed individuals, people who have ever experienced homelessness are more likely to face health issues, have unmet healthcare needs, and be subject to accelerated health erosion [47–49]. Their obstructed access to basic hygienic amenities, isolated spaces, and medical care makes it challenging for homeless individuals to protect themselves from COVID-19.

4.6. Socioeconomic Status

Of the total sample, 52.1% could be classified as low-income and 7.1% as high-income. Racial and ethnic minorities who are low-income are at heightened risk of severe illness related to COVID-19. As shown in Table 5 below, Hispanics with a lower SES are more likely to have a pre-existing high-risk illness that renders them physiologically vulnerable to COVID-19.

Table 5. Hispanics with High-Risk Pre-Existing Health Conditions by Socioeconomic Status.

Socioeconomic Status	High-Risk
Low SES	53.8% 146,205
Medium SES	45.0% 95,793
High SES	37.4% 13,790

Note: $p < 0.001$.

It is vital to analyze the risks associated with socioeconomic status, race, ethnicity, and pre-existing health conditions because they are often co-occurring factors that influence an individual or community's well-being and life expectancy. Similarly, among immigrants, income and employment are intimately associated with citizenship, immigration status, and health insurance. The same is true for people experiencing homelessness, who are typically low-income and vulnerable to COVID-19 [46].

5. Latinos and High-Risk Pre-Existing Health Conditions

In May 2020, the CDC stated that "older adults and people of any age who have serious underlying medical conditions" are at highest risk of severe illness from COVID-19 [5]. It defines severe illness as "hospitalization, admission to the ICU, intubation or mechanical ventilation, or death" that is caused or exacerbated by the contraction of COVID-19 [50]. Furthermore, the umbrella term of "serious underlying medical conditions" refers to people with chronic lung diseases, severe asthma, heart conditions, obesity, diabetes, immunocompromising illnesses (including, but not limited to chemotherapy/radiation or organ/bone marrow transplantation, HIV/AIDS, or prolonged use of corticosteroids), liver disease, and those undergoing dialysis for chronic kidney disease [5]. The CDC Morbidity and Mortality Weekly Report released on 17 April 2020 disclosed that 89.3% of people hospitalized due to COVID-19 had at least one of the following underlying health conditions: hypertension (49.7%), obesity (48.3%), chronic lung disease (34.6%), type 2 diabetes mellitus (28.3%), or cardiovascular disease (27.8%) [51]. Table 6 shows the distribution of our sample according to our created risk categories.

Table 6. Number of Pre-Existing Health Conditions Associated with Severe Illness Related to COVID-19 among Hispanics in El Paso in 2011–2012.

Risk Assessment	Percent	*N*
No risk factors	50.70%	266,383
1 risk factor	31.90%	167,396
2 risk factors	15.50%	81,278
3 or more risk factors	2.00%	10,264
		525,321
Not at-risk	50.70%	266,383
At-risk	49.30%	258,938
		525,321
Deaths (as of 22 April 2021)		2506
El Paso County pop. 2019		839,238
Death rate	0.3% of the population	
U.S. Death rate	0.00%	
Global Death rate	~0.4%	

Sources: Reuters Graphics [12,13], U.S. Census Bureau [16].

In the section below, we outline a set of analyses that explore the prevalence of high-risk pre-existing health conditions as they relate to medical insurance status, socioeconomic status, medication, age, and homelessness. We included data on medical insurance, socioeconomic status, and age for all conditions. We included information on medication and homelessness only when the findings were at least statistically significant at $p < 0.01$ or significantly exceeding the average percentage of the sample population.

Table 7 below reflects the prevalence of high-risk health conditions and diseases in the Hispanic community of El Paso in 2011–2012.

Two variables were created to paint a clearer picture of Hispanics' COVID-19 risk profiles. Individuals who had been diagnosed with one or more of the above diseases were categorized into an "at-risk" group, and then further sorted according to their pre-existing condition. Those with two or more, as well as three or more, conditions were grouped into their respective categories because of their compounded physiological vulnerabilities to severe illness related to COVID-19. Emphysema, tuberculosis, and HIV/AIDS were not included in these variables, and because their prevalence is very low, this does not have a significant effect on the results. The table below outlines the percentage of the Hispanic population of El Paso in 2011–2012 that is considered high-risk according to an individual's number of pre-existing conditions (see Table 8).

Table 7. High-Risk Illness and Disease Prevalence among Hispanics in El Paso.

Health Condition	Percent	N
Obesity	26.2%	95,818
Smoking	17.7%	92,989
High Blood Pressure	16.0%	83,980
High Cholesterol	12.9%	67,629
Asthma	7.6%	40,100
Diabetes	7.3%	38,235
Heart Attack/Stroke	2.6%	13,810
Kidney Disease	2.3%	11,905
Hepatitis or Cirrhosis	2.2%	11,326
Cancer	1.4%	7510
Emphysema	1.3%	6885
Homelessness	0.5%	2707
Tuberculosis	0.2%	1260
HIV/AIDS	<0.1%	10

Table 8. High-Risk Pre-Existing Health Conditions Associated with Severe Illness Related to COVID-19 Among Hispanics.

Health Condition	Percent	N
Obesity (only)	17.4%	45,000
High Blood Pressure (only)	11.3%	29,389
Diabetes (only)	3.9%	9999
Asthma (only)	7.2%	18,754
Heart Attack/Stroke (only)	0.7%	1875
Kidney Disease (only)	0.7%	1875
Cancer (only)	0.5%	1250
Smoking (only)	21.3%	55,043
Homelessness (only)	1.6%	4203
2 of the above	31.4%	81,278
3 or more	4.0%	10,264

Obesity, hypertension, asthma, and type 2 diabetes were the most common illnesses to render Hispanics at high risk. Most notably, however, is that the majority of Hispanic individuals had been diagnosed with one or more health conditions that put them at risk of dying from COVID. Altogether, those with compounded risk comprised about one-third of the total Hispanic population of El Paso at the time that the survey was taken. This indicates poor widespread health outcomes in the community overall and the importance of extreme public health precautions in dealing with respiratory pandemics.

Additionally, differences in disease prevalence arose when risk was cross-analyzed with place of birth. In Table 9, those with at least one pre-existing health condition were considered higher risk, and those with no pre-existing health condition were categorized as lower risk. Native-born Hispanics made up a slightly smaller portion of high-risk individuals, revealing a lesser likelihood of being diagnosed with a high-risk pre-existing health condition if they had been born in the U.S. These data suggest that birthplace is statistically associated with an individual's risk of contracting COVID-19. Hispanic immigrants in El Paso showed a collectively higher risk profile.

Table 9. Hispanics Diagnosed with High-Risk Pre-Existing Health Conditions by Birthplace.

At Risk for COVID-19	Born in the U.S.	Foreign Born	Total
Higher risk	47.4% 146,417	52.0% 112,521	50.7% 266,383
Lower risk	52.6% 162,588	48.0% 103,795	49.3% 258,893

Note: $p < 0.001$.

These disparate health outcomes were more closely examined by separating each specific illness according to individuals' birthplaces, shown below in Table 10. Hispanics born outside of the U.S. bore the brunt of type 2 diabetes, hypertension, kidney disease, and cancer diagnoses. Foreign-born Hispanics were also slightly more likely to have two high-risk pre-existing health conditions. On the other hand, U.S.-born individuals reported higher rates of asthma and smoking, indicating that immigrant Hispanics and U.S.-born Hispanics struggle with different health concerns in El Paso.

Table 10. Pre-Existing Health Conditions Associated with High Risk of Severe Illness Related to COVID-19, According to Birthplace.

Health Condition	Born in the U.S.	Foreign-Born
Obesity (only)	18.4%	16.1%
High Blood Pressure (only)	11.1%	11.7%
Diabetes (only)	2.1%	6.1%
Asthma (only)	9.4%	4.4%
Heart Attack/Stroke (only)	0.4%	1.1%
Kidney Disease (only)	0.0%	1.7%
Cancer (only)	0.0%	1.1%
Smoking (only)	22.6%	19.5%
Homelessness (only)	1.0%	2.4%
2 of the above	30.5%	32.5%
3 or more	4.4%	3.4%

Note: $p < 0.001$.

These findings challenge previous research on what scholars have labeled the "Immigrant Paradox". A close cousin of the Hispanic Health Paradox, this contradiction arose when researchers began seeing an unexpected pattern in the health outcomes of foreign-born people in the U.S. In general, the Paradox asserts that immigrants exhibit significantly better physical and mental health compared to their native-born counterparts, even within racial and ethnic subgroups of the country's population [52–55]. Our data, however, reflect the opposite: Hispanic immigrants were more likely than those born on U.S. soil to be diagnosed with a range and multiplicity of chronic illnesses, all of which are associated with severe sickness upon contraction of COVID-19.

5.1. High Blood Pressure

In El Paso, 16.0% of Hispanics reported a high blood pressure diagnosis, and 59.5% of them were low-income. High blood pressure, also known as hypertension, has been coined the "silent killer" given the absence of symptoms that accompany it. Many people go unaware of their high blood pressure, which can lead to the development of kidney disease, cardiovascular diseases, or fatal cardiac events, such as heart attack or stroke [56]. According to our data, 23.2% of adult Hispanics had never had their blood pressure checked. These numbers are concerning because the contraction of COVID-19 is especially dangerous for people with hypertension. The CDC reported that 49.7% of people hospitalized due to virus-related complications had hypertension in March 2020 [51]. Given the high number of those who had never checked their blood pressure, this analysis only accounted for Latin individuals who were aware of their blood pressure status, in addition to a large subsample whose blood pressure was measured as part of the study, as we discuss elsewhere [6].

Although high blood pressure is a cause of serious health conditions, medical coverage varied greatly among those with diagnoses. Our analysis revealed that 33.7% of Hispanics were aware of their high blood pressure but were not medically insured. Even though these individuals knew of their diagnosis, they either chose not to enroll in medical insurance or could not because of cost or citizenship status.

5.2. Cholesterol

High cholesterol was almost equally as common as hypertension within our sample, as 12.9% of Hispanics reported being diagnosed by a health professional. Similar to high blood pressure, people are often unaware of their cholesterol levels until a serious or fatal event occurs. High cholesterol is a predicting factor of heart disease, hypertension, and type 2 diabetes [57]. Low-lipid cholesterols increase plaque growth in the arteries that flow to the brain and heart, eventually accumulating to the point where blood struggles to pass [58]. Heart attack (myocardial infarction) and stroke occur when plaque buildup has completely obstructed the blood from flowing through the arteries [57]. Both are extremely dangerous health conditions that exhibit little to no symptoms, and the lack of knowledge regarding residents' blood pressure and cholesterol status might render them especially susceptible to health complications caused by COVID-19.

This analysis showed that 28.8% of those diagnosed with high cholesterol did not have medical insurance at the time. More than half (52.8%) of those who had been diagnosed were low-income, whereas 10.2% were high-income. Because of these disparate figures, it is possible that socioeconomic status plays a role in the stress and diet, both of which impact cholesterol levels of Hispanic El Pasoans. Age was also an important factor in analyzing cholesterol, as the majority of cases occurred among people between the ages of 46 and 65.

5.3. Asthma

The study revealed that 7.6% of Hispanics reported asthma diagnoses. When treated and closely monitored, asthma is not life-threatening. However, if someone with asthma has an asthma attack and lacks access to an inhaler or ventilator, then it can be fatal. An attack is caused by severe inflammation that constricts and narrows the air passages that lead to the lungs [59]. Communicable diseases, such as the flu or an upper respiratory infection, can trigger an asthma attack [59]. It is dangerous to be unaware of the condition because those with asthma are at higher risk of complications or death after contracting a communicable illness. Although it is unknown whether COVID-19 induces asthma attacks, shortness of breath and dry cough are common symptoms of the virus that alter the flow of breath through the airways [60]. Severe symptoms and difficulty breathing might trigger an asthma attack, so medical professionals warn individuals with asthma to take caution. Nonetheless, there has been no information that distinguishes asthma attacks from common symptoms of COVID-19. Because of this, virus-related symptoms may be mistaken as a routine asthma attack and deter individuals with asthma from seeking medical attention.

Out of this portion of the Hispanic population in El Paso, approximately half (51.7%) did not have medical insurance to help them manage their asthma diagnosis prior to the Affordable Care Act. An individual's socioeconomic status also informed the likelihood of receiving an asthma diagnosis, given that 56.3% of Hispanic residents with asthma were low-income and 42.1% middle-income.

5.4. Heart Attack/Stroke

A small percentage (2.6%) of Latin individuals in El Paso reported a previous heart attack or stroke. Given the significance of socioeconomic status and medical insurance in the previous analyses, it is perhaps unsurprising that 27.4% were not medically insured, and an overwhelming percentage (72.8%) were low-income. Socioeconomic status was also associated with the use of medication to treat heart attack or stroke, as half (50.2%) of low-income Latin individuals who received this diagnosis reported being on medication compared to 83.2% of middle-class Hispanics.

When examining the age groups most affected by these conditions, our data showed that 27.2% of heart attacks or strokes were reported by people between the ages of 60 and 80. Deaths caused by COVID-19 are highest among those over the age of 64, so Latin individuals in this age group who have suffered a heart attack or stroke have compounded risk factors that render them disproportionately vulnerable to COVID-19-related complications [61].

Heart attack and stroke are often caused by high cholesterol, as the low-lipid cholesterols create buildups of plaque that block proper blood flow to the heart and brain [57]. A heart attack is defined as a form of cardiovascular disease by itself, but it may also be an indicator of heart diseases such as arteriosclerosis, diabetes, or coronary artery disease [57]. Further, the CDC reported that 27.8% of COVID-related hospitalizations were among people with cardiovascular disease [51]. Heart attack and stroke are both potentially fatal health events that affect an individual for the rest of their life. For example, Cione's father experienced three heart attacks before receiving a diagnosis of arteriosclerosis. He was prescribed multiple pharmaceuticals that altered his metabolism, sleep quality, mood, energy levels, and ability to eat. His diet changed drastically, and he must regulate his consumption of cholesterol-rich foods for the remainder of his life.

The physiological processes leading to stroke are similar to those that result in heart attacks, although the life-long impacts may differ greatly. Depending on the part of the brain that was depleted of blood, stroke can cause paralysis, memory loss, changes in behavior, speech issues, and/or vision impairment. In extreme cases, individuals lose entirely the ability to speak or move their body [62]. Those who are medically uninsured and have experienced one or both of these health events are at higher risk of other health complications, such as an additional heart attack or stroke, if they do not receive proper follow-up care.

5.5. Emphysema

A minority (1.3%) of survey participants had received an emphysema diagnosis. Emphysema is a chronic lung disease that heightens one's susceptibility to severe illness [51]. Smoking tobacco is the most common cause of emphysema, but air pollution and respiratory infections can also cause or aggravate it. It is defined as a chronic obstructive pulmonary disease (COPD), and people can live with emphysema for years before symptoms develop [63]. Medical treatment typically involves medications, surgery, and oxygen therapy, but it is typical for those with emphysema to forgo these costly treatments [63,64].

Our data revealed that about one-quarter (27.4%) of those who were diagnosed with emphysema was not medically insured. Furthermore, emphysema was associated with lower socioeconomic status, as 54.5% of those with emphysema were low-income, whereas none were high-income. Regarding age, emphysema most commonly affected people ages 60–85, an age group that has been classified as particularly susceptible to severe illness or death related to COVID-19 [5].

5.6. Hepatitis or Cirrhosis

A total of 2.2% of the Hispanic population of El Paso reported a diagnosis of hepatitis, cirrhosis, or both. All hepatitis infections (A, B, C, D, and E) are inflammatory and occur in the liver, as well as cirrhosis, as cirrhosis is technically the progression of any liver disease [65]. Hepatitis B and C are the most common causes of cirrhosis, and those who are most at risk of contracting B, C, and D are injection drug users and those who practice unsafe sex [65]. While Hepatitis A is curable, all its other types are not [65]. Injection drug use and unsafe sex are risk factors also associated with the contraction of HIV, and any HIV-positive person who contracts hepatitis is at severe risk of health complications [66].

Of those who received a diagnosis, 33.6% are not medically insured. This diagnosis was distributed unequally across socioeconomic classes, given that low-income Hispanics once again constituted the majority at 77.8%, which is also the highest percentage across the illnesses in this risk assessment. Clearly, hepatitis and cirrhosis diagnoses are impacted by an individual's financial and social standing. This diagnosis also happened to almost exclusively strike young people between the ages of 18 and 30, indicating that younger people may be more susceptible to contracting hepatitis or developing cirrhosis.

5.7. Kidney Disease

Around 2.3% of Hispanic study participants reported kidney disease, of whom 42.2% did not have medical insurance and therefore struggled to receive regular care. Many of those with kidney disease diagnoses were middle-income (52.8%) and low-income (41.3%). Kidney disease is an illness that does not exhibit symptoms until the occurrence of a potentially fatal event, such as kidney failure. It is intimately linked with heart disease, diabetes, high blood pressure, and certain forms of cardiovascular disease known to cause or evolve into kidney disease. Further, it is a chronic disease, meaning that the kidneys are permanently damaged and cannot properly filter blood. Unless the patient immediately changes their diet and seeks medical treatment, their condition will worsen with time [67]. A share of 36.4% of Hispanics in El Paso with kidney disease are above the age of 60, which adds another layer of risk in the case of a positive COVID-19 diagnosis.

5.8. Cancer

Those with cancer diagnoses amounted to 1.4% of the Hispanic population, which is approximately equal to the proportions of kidney disease and heart attack/stroke. The ethno-surveys also revealed that 16.8% of Hispanic residents of El Paso who had cancer were uninsured, one of the lowest rates of lacking medical insurance across this report. This could be because the culture surrounding cancer in the United States is serious and fearful, which encourages people to remain insured after a diagnosis. People who are nearing remission, are in remission, or may have been diagnosed as a child are also among those who are likely to be insured.

Approximately half of the Hispanic residents diagnosed with cancer at some point in the past are of low socioeconomic status (50.1%), whereas 40.9% are considered middle-class. However, the ages of people who reported cancer diagnoses at one point in their lives varied greatly: 8.3% were ages 18–25, 16.6% were ages 31–35, and 8.3% were ages 46–50. Ultimately, the highest rates were reported by people between the ages of 51 and 65, who constituted 58.2% of the diagnosed population. This is significant because people ages 65 and older are considered "high risk" by the CDC for COVID-19. Hispanics who also have cancer are more likely to be negatively impacted by COVID-19. Nonetheless, this overall assessment shows how uncommon it is for older Hispanic people in El Paso to have cancer.

5.9. HIV/AIDS

The unweighted sample with over-representation of people experiencing homelessness has a 0.2% HIV rate. In our survey, 100% of those with HIV/AIDS were homeless at the time of the survey. Given the high-risk status associated with being homeless and having a positive HIV/AIDS diagnosis, respectively, this portion of the Latin population is extremely vulnerable to health complications or death related to COVID-19.

The percentage of those with HIV/AIDS in our weighted data constitutes about 0.00002% of all Hispanics living in El Paso, which is significantly lower than the 2019 national percentage of 0.34% [66,68]. However, the stigma surrounding HIV/AIDS makes people wary of getting tested and learning about prevention methods. It is estimated that 1 in 7 people living with HIV/AIDS in the United States are unaware of their positive status [66]. Therefore, it is likely that there are other HIV/AIDS-positive Latin people living in the region.

None of the HIV/AIDS-positive Hispanic residents in the sample were medically insured. Although the number of HIV/AIDS-positive people in the data is small, it is nonetheless worrisome, considering that HIV/AIDS killed over 37,000 people in the U.S. in 2018 [69]. The year before, 53% of new known HIV cases were diagnosed in the South, 21% of which were among Hispanics/Latinos. Although numbers have gradually decreased over the past few years, the rate of new cases in Texas was 15.4 per 100,000 in 2019 [69]. Care for the HIV/AIDS-positive community in the region is also subpar. Recently, the U.S. South reported the lowest number of HIV-positive people who received medical care and had a suppressed viral load from being treated with antiretroviral therapy [69].

Similarly, according to our data, only half of the Hispanic residents with HIV/AIDS were on medication in 2011. Whether the medication being taken was antiretroviral therapy is unknown, so it is possible that even fewer were being treated for HIV/AIDS.

5.10. Tuberculosis

The rates of tuberculosis are falling 2% each year globally, but it is still one of the top 10 leading causes of death worldwide [70]. A quarter of the global population has the tuberculosis bacteria lying dormant in their system, so others in the Hispanic community in El Paso may have contracted the bacteria as well. Only 5–15% of these people are estimated to fall ill with tuberculosis, but those with compromised immune systems and pre-existing conditions are at high risk of developing the illness. For instance, HIV/AIDS-positive people are 19 times more likely to die from tuberculosis, which causes further concern that many HIV/AIDS-positive people lack medical insurance [70].

The prevalence of tuberculosis is low in the El Paso community. Only 0.2% of the Hispanic community of El Paso reported having tuberculosis at one point in their lives, approximately half (49.6%) of whom have medical insurance. This is concerning because all of the tuberculosis diagnoses occurred among Hispanic people of low socioeconomic status who might not be able to afford the proper treatment or medicines without pharmaceutical or medical insurance coverage. Individuals over the age of 45 recalled no previous bouts of tuberculosis—instead, almost half of the reported diagnoses occurred among people aged 18–25.

5.11. Diabetes

According to our survey data, 7.3% of Hispanics in El Paso reported a diabetes diagnosis, 60.1% and 3.3% of whom were low-income and high-income, respectively. More than half (65.5%) had medical insurance, but 34.5% were not insured. According to the CDC, diabetes puts one at considerably higher risk of severe health complications related to COVID-19 given that nearly half (49.7%) of people hospitalized with severe virus-related illness as of 30 March 2020 had a previous diabetes diagnosis [51].

Low insulin adherence, which puts individuals in danger of unregulated and dangerous blood sugar levels, can be attributed to multiple factors such as access, affordability, willingness, and guidance on self-administered injection. This was a concern with our sample because only 31.2% of Hispanics with diabetes took insulin at least once. Positive diabetes diagnoses varied considerably according to age, and Hispanics over the age of 60 constituted 29.3% of total cases. This presents evidence that an insulin adherence barrier affected multiple different age groups. Previous research has drawn connections between low insulin usage and depression, embarrassment, a busy schedule, and travel among people living with type 2 diabetes [71,72]. Patients have also reported fears associated with insulin-related weight gain and accidental hypoglycemia, or low blood sugar, induced by an overproduction or excessive dosage of insulin [73]. In a study conducted by Hu et al., Hispanic immigrants with type 2 diabetes conflated insulin therapy with a death sentence, calling it a "last resort" and expressing that they feared injections because the insulin itself might cause further damage [74]. Many participants, especially women, cited a lack of positive family support and access to syringes as barriers to proper insulin use [74].

The survey data draw awareness to a persistent problem affecting the Hispanic community's well-being. Individuals with diabetes who are not receiving proper insulin treatment, if receiving any at all, will likely be hit harder by a positive COVID-19 diagnosis than those who follow regular schedules and guidelines outlined by a health provider. These are significant findings that reveal the disproportionately poor health experienced by Hispanic individuals living with chronic diseases and inform us of who might be especially vulnerable to COVID-19.

5.12. Obesity

Just over one-quarter (26.2%) of survey participants were considered obese, of whom 3.4% were considered severely obese with a Body Mass Index (BMI) of 40 or higher [51]. Almost half of obese Hispanics lived without medical coverage, and 58.2% of those diagnosed as obese were low-income. Over one-third (38.3%) received a diagnosis between the ages of 18 and 30, although 10.8% of obese Hispanics were ages 61 and older.

Obesity, characterized by a body mass index of 30 or higher, increases a person's vulnerability to severe illness related to COVID-19 [51]. The CDC reported that 48.3% of individuals hospitalized for virus-related health complications were obese in March 2020 [51]. Before COVID-19, obesity was regarded as a public health issue for the U.S. Hispanic population. In 2019, an estimated 80.4% of Hispanics living in the United States were overweight or obese and were more likely to be obese than White adults [75,76]. These trends are concerning because obesity is associated with many health conditions, including type 2 diabetes, hypertension, stroke, coronary heart disease, sleep apnea, certain cancers, and gallbladder disease [77]. Some of these conditions, as previously discussed, increase the risk of complications from COVID-19.

6. Conclusions

Throughout this paper, we dissect the socioeconomic factors that tie into health and well-being and their detrimental effect on racial and ethnic minorities. The COVID-19 pandemic, albeit unexpected, further exposed and reproduced health disparities that were previously less discernible to the general public. The Hispanic community across the United States is already at higher risk of COVID-19 because of institutional discrimination across the sectors of employment, housing, and health. In El Paso, where more than half of Hispanics were of low socioeconomic status, and 48% lacked medical insurance a decade before, their chances of suffering from severe illness related to COVID-19 are even higher. This is particularly dangerous for those with pre-existing health conditions, such as type 2 diabetes, cardiovascular disease, HIV/AIDS, and cancer. It remains unclear whether more Hispanics living in the U.S. will die from COVID-19 than other racial and ethnic groups, as the pandemic has not run its full course. However, preventive measures must be taken in order to protect the Hispanic community in El Paso from tragedy, including the proper allocation of health resources and financial support for low-income, homeless, undocumented, and medically uninsured individuals.

Although discussion of racial disparities is critical, it is just the tip of the iceberg. Health disparities explain how communities of color disproportionately suffer from poor health, but not why state and federal institutions do not properly allocate health resources. The heart of the problem lies in systemic racism, discrimination, and state-sanctioned violence against minorities. Given that communities of color face many structural inequalities, such as poverty, residential segregation, racism, and access to healthcare, they are not to blame for pre-existing or virus-related health disparities [78]. We should take caution in our reporting of racial and ethnic inequities to ensure that data are contextualized within a critical understanding of structural factors that cause disproportionate COVID-19 rates among minority groups.

In this study, we have outlined how it is not a coincidence that infection and death rates of COVID-19 among Native American, Black, and Hispanic populations in the U.S. have been among the highest in the world since the beginning of the pandemic. Structural inequalities incurred by institutional racism have created, and continue to create, underlying medical conditions and enable increased exposure to the virus, which puts Native American, Black, and Hispanic citizens in far more vulnerable positions regarding COVID-19 than their non-Hispanic White counterparts. When assessing preventative and recovery measures, policymakers and public health officials should consider pre-existing health disparities and their heightened likelihood of working essential or frontline jobs [31,32]. Cities and towns with higher numbers of working-class Latin people should be prepared to conduct extensive community-based health education and outreach through *promotoras de salud* and provide referrals to critical medical care for sub-populations at higher risk. In addition, further research should investigate the lasting effects of COVID-19 infection and "long-COVID" on these groups.

The dataset used to assess the risk that the population of a city had to COVID was collected much before the pandemic started. Nonetheless, this paper shows how similarly detailed data about a city or population can and should be used by public health officials in a preventive fashion to reduce deaths. Public health data should not be limited to prevalence rates, and epidemiology, but should also include social variables and cultural and sociological insights to include the role of beliefs and ideas in health-seeking behavior and the role of socioeconomic factors in producing different health outcomes between and among ethnic and racial groups. Migration and immigration status are essential determinants of health and well-being. Longitudinal health and social data of large and diverse samples that oversample minority, immigrant, and unhoused individuals are an important tool in creating a healthy population.

Author Contributions: Conceptualization, C.C. and E.C.; methodology, C.C. and E.C.; software, C.C.; validation, C.C., E.V., D.J., S.M. and E.C.; formal analysis, C.C., D.J.; investigation, C.C.; resources, C.C., E.C.; data curation, C.C.; writing—original draft preparation, C.C.; writing—review and editing, C.C., E.V., D.J., S.M. and E.C.; visualization, C.C., E.V. and D.J.; supervision, E.C.; project administration, E.C.; funding acquisition, E.C. All authors have read and agreed to the published version of the manuscript.

Funding: The data was gathered as part of the project "Social Determinants of Physical and Mental Health of Migrant and Transient Populations: Health Disparities amongst Hispanics in El Paso", which was supported by Award Number P20MD00287-04 from the National Institute on Minority Health and Health Disparities to UTEP's Hispanic Health Disparities Research Center. The content is solely the responsibility of the authors and does not necessarily represent the official views of the National Institute on Minority Health and Health Disparities or the National Institutes of Health.

Institutional Review Board Statement: The study was conducted in accordance with the Declaration of Helsinki and approved by the Institutional Review Board of the University of Texas, El Paso, IRB reference numbers: 271104-1 and 271104-2.

Informed Consent Statement: Informed consent was obtained from all subjects involved in the study.

Acknowledgments: Abby Ferdinando, Jhamiel Prince, and Kai Wasson helped with previous versions of this paper.

Conflicts of Interest: The authors declare no conflict of interest. The funders had no role in the design of the study; in the collection, analyses, or interpretation of data; in the writing of the manuscript, or in the decision to publish the results.

References

1. Lovelace, B. White House Officials Worry the Coronavirus Is Hitting African Americans Worse than Others. Available online: https://www.cnbc.com/2020/04/07/white-house-officials-worry-the-coronavirus-is-hitting-african-americans-worse-than-others.html (accessed on 28 April 2021).
2. Nania, R. Blacks, Hispanics Hit Harder by the Coronavirus, Early U.S. Data Show. Available online: https://www.aarp.org/health/conditions-treatments/info-2020/minority-communities-covid-19.html (accessed on 28 April 2021).
3. Barr, D. *Health Disparities in the United States: Social Class, Race, Ethnicity, and Health*, 2nd ed.; Johns Hopkins University Press: Baltimore, MD, USA, 2014.
4. Premji, S.; Duguay, P.; Messing, K.; Lippel, K. Are Immigrants, Ethnic and Linguistic Minorities Over-Represented in Jobs with a High Level of Compensated Risk? Results from a Montréal, Canada Study Using Census and Workers' Compensation Data. *Am. J. Ind. Med.* **2010**, *53*, 875–885. [CrossRef] [PubMed]
5. Centers for Disease Control and Prevention. People at Increased Risk and Other People Who Need to Take Extra Precautions. Available online: https://www.cdc.gov/coronavirus/2019-ncov/need-extra-precautions/index.html (accessed on 28 April 2021).
6. Castañeda, E.; Smith, B.; Vetter, E. Hispanic Health Disparities and Housing: Comparing Measured and Self-Reported Health Metrics Among Housed and Homeless Latin Individuals. *J. Migr. Health* **2020**, *1–2*, 100008. [CrossRef] [PubMed]
7. Moya, E.M.; Zamore, C.; Perez, L.M.; Tellez, K.; Avila, A.; Aragones, A. COVID-19 Imperils Access to Health and Human Services in El Paso, Texas and New York City: Perspectives from Hispanic Parents. *J. Racial Ethn. Health Disparities* **2022**, *9*, 1024–1029. [CrossRef] [PubMed]

8. Castañeda, E. Latinos in El Paso at Risk from COVID-19. Available online: https://ernestoc.medium.com/latinos-in-el-paso-at-risk-from-covid-19-1c508c564d24 (accessed on 11 December 2022).
9. The High COVID-19 Death Toll in Texas-Mexico Border Towns. Available online: https://time.com/6074581/covid-19-deaths-texas-mexico-border/ (accessed on 11 December 2022).
10. Moore, R. A Year into the Pandemic, COVID-19 Has Ravaged El Paso. Available online: http://elpasomatters.org/2021/03/14/a-year-into-the-pandemic-covid-19-has-ravaged-el-paso/ (accessed on 11 December 2022).
11. Castañeda, E. Speaking about Health Disparities: A Teachable Moment about Structural Racism. Available online: https://ernestoc.medium.com/speaking-about-health-disparities-a-teachable-moment-about-structural-racism-2774dc5f44b (accessed on 11 December 2022).
12. Reuters Graphics. COVID-19 Global Tracker. Available online: https://graphics.reuters.com/world-coronavirus-tracker-and-maps/ (accessed on 28 April 2021).
13. Reuters Graphics. Tracking the Novel Coronavirus in the U.S. Available online: https://graphics.reuters.com/HEALTH-CORONAVIRUS-USA/0100B5K8423/index.html (accessed on 28 April 2021).
14. Bureau of Communicable Disease Surveillance System. Age-Adjusted Rates of Lab Confirmed COVID-19. Available online: https://www1.nyc.gov/assets/doh/downloads/pdf/imm/covid-19-deaths-race-ethnicity-04162020-1.pdf (accessed on 16 April 2020).
15. NYC Health. COVID-19: Data, Details on Deaths. Available online: https://github.com/nychealth/coronavirus-data/blob/master/by-race.csv (accessed on 16 April 2020).
16. U.S. Census Bureau. U.S. Census Bureau QuickFacts: El Paso County, Texas. Available online: https://www.census.gov/quickfacts/fact/table/elpasocountytexas/PST045219? (accessed on 28 April 2021).
17. Lachica, J.; Castañeda, E.; McDonald, Y. (Eds.) *Poverty, Place, and Health along the US-Mexico Border*; Poverty and Health: A Crisis among America's Most Vulnerable. Volume 2: Place and Health among the Vulnerable; ABC-CLIO: Goleta, CA, USA, 2013.
18. KTSM Staff. El Paso COVID-19 Cases Surpass 1,000 Mark. Available online: https://www.ktsm.com/local/el-paso-news/el-paso-covid-19-cases-surpass-1000-mark/ (accessed on 28 April 2021).
19. Willard, K. Public Health Director in El Paso Resigns as City Response to COVID-19 Continues. Available online: https://kfoxtv.com/news/coronavirus/public-health-director-in-el-paso-resigns-as-city-response-to-covid-19-continues (accessed on 28 April 2021).
20. Coyne, M. The U.S. May Be Heading to A Second (or Even Fourth) Wave of the Coronavirus Epidemic. Here's What That Means. Available online: https://www.forbes.com/sites/marleycoyne/2020/04/02/the-us-may-be-heading-to-a-second-or-even-fourth-wave-of-the-coronavirus-epidemic-heres-what-that-means/ (accessed on 28 April 2021).
21. Cervantes Holguín, E.; Gutiérrez Sandoval, P.R. Resistir la Covid-19. Intersecciones en la Educación de Ciudad Juárez, México. *RIEJS* **2020**, *9*, 7–23. [CrossRef]
22. Pane, L.M.; Coronado, A. Virus Pushes Twin Cities El Paso and Juarez to the Brink. Available online: https://apnews.com/article/business-virus-outbreak-family-gatherings-north-america-mexico-e066bb7aaf4ad1c2417254c24c0e835c (accessed on 28 April 2021).
23. Berumen, J.; Schmulson, M.; Alegre-Díaz, J.; Guerrero, G.; Larriva-Sahd, J.; Olaiz, G.; Wong-Chew, R.M.; Cantú, C.; Ochoa-Guzmán, A.; Garcilazo-Ávila, A.; et al. Risk of Infection and Hospitalization by Covid-19 in Mexico: A Case-Control Study. *medRxiv* **2020**. [CrossRef]
24. Navarrete, B.; Sanchez, G. Risks and Challenges to Migrants, Asylum Seekers and Refugees Living Under COVID-19 in Ciudad Juárez, Mexico. *Migr. Policy Pract.* **2020**, *10*, 48–53.
25. Kahn, C. "Remain in Mexico" Policy's End Brings Renewed Hope to Asylum Seekers. Available online: https://www.npr.org/2021/02/14/967807189/remain-in-mexico-policys-end-brings-renewed-hope-to-asylum-seekers (accessed on 28 April 2021).
26. Castañeda, E. Expulsión de Migrantes Como Oportunidad Perdida y Tarea Para Sísifo. *Rev. Mex. De Sociol.* **2023**, *85*, 229–238.
27. Martinez, V. "Every Day I See Death": Gravediggers in Juarez Perform Grim Labor as COVID-19 Death Toll Rises in Mexico. Available online: https://www.elpasotimes.com/in-depth/news/local/juarez/2020/11/19/coronavirus-juarez-mexico-death-toll-cemetery-workers-covid-19/6248165002/ (accessed on 28 April 2021).
28. Neuman, W.L. *Social Research Methods: Qualitative and Quantitative Approaches*; Allyn & Bacon: Boston, MA, USA, 2011.
29. O'Hare, W.P. *Differential Undercounts in the U.S. Census: Who Is Missed?* Springer Nature: Berlin/Heidelberg, Germany, 2019; ISBN 978-3-030-10973-8.
30. El Paso Strong. City of El Paso COVID-19 Cases. Available online: https://www.epstrong.org/results.php (accessed on 28 April 2021).
31. U.S. Bureau of Labor Statistics. *Labor Force Characteristics by Race and Ethnicity, 2018*; BLS Reports; U.S. Bureau of Labor Statistics: Washington, DC, USA, 2019; pp. 1–83.
32. Passel, J.; Cohn, D. Share of Unauthorized Immigrant Workers in Production, Construction Jobs Falls Since 2007. Available online: https://www.pewresearch.org/hispanic/2015/03/26/share-of-unauthorized-immigrant-workers-in-production-construction-jobs-falls-since-2007/ (accessed on 28 April 2021).
33. Centers for Disease Control and Prevention. Health Equity Considerations & Racial & Ethnic Minority Groups. Available online: https://www.cdc.gov/coronavirus/2019-ncov/community/health-equity/race-ethnicity.html (accessed on 28 April 2021).
34. Villa, L. Millions of Americans Have Been Laid off Amid the Coronavirus Outbreak. Here's What It's Like to Be One of Them. Available online: https://time.com/5812538/coronavirus-economic-damage-workers/ (accessed on 28 April 2021).

35. Smith, R. Fact Sheet: Immigrant Workers' Eligibility for Unemployment Insurance. Available online: https://www.nelp.org/publication/immigrant-workers-eligibility-unemployment-insurance/ (accessed on 28 April 2021).
36. District of Columbia Department of Human Resources. E-DPM Instruction No. 12-51. 2013. Available online: https://dchr.dc.gov/sites/default/files/dc/sites/dchr/publication/attachments/edpm_12_51_guidelines_essential_and_emergency_personnel.pdf (accessed on 28 April 2021).
37. Stewart, E. The Essential Worker Trap. Available online: https://www.vox.com/2020/5/5/21245713/unemployment-insurance-recalled-workers-voluntary-quit-state-reopening (accessed on 28 April 2021).
38. Park, K.; Meagher, T.; Li, W. Tracking the Spread of Coronavirus in Prisons. Available online: https://www.themarshallproject.org/2020/04/24/tracking-the-spread-of-coronavirus-in-prisons (accessed on 28 April 2021).
39. The Marshall Project. A State-by-State Look at Coronavirus in Prisons. Available online: https://www.themarshallproject.org/2020/05/01/a-state-by-state-look-at-coronavirus-in-prisons (accessed on 28 April 2021).
40. Federal Bureau of Prisons. BOP: COVID-19 Update. Available online: https://www.bop.gov/coronavirus/ (accessed on 28 April 2021).
41. Nellis, A. The Color of Justice: Racial and Ethnic Disparity in State Prisons. Available online: https://www.sentencingproject.org/publications/color-of-justice-racial-and-ethnic-disparity-in-state-prisons/ (accessed on 28 April 2021).
42. Data USA. New Mexico. Available online: https://datausa.io/profile/geo/new-mexico (accessed on 28 April 2021).
43. The Sentencing Project. Latinx Disparities in Youth Incarceration. Available online: https://www.sentencingproject.org/publications/latino-disparities-youth-incarceration/ (accessed on 28 April 2021).
44. National Immigration Law Center. Immigrants and the Affordable Care Act (ACA). Available online: https://www.nilc.org/issues/health-care/immigrantshcr/ (accessed on 28 April 2021).
45. The Council of Economic Advisers. The State of Homelessness in America. Available online: https://www.whitehouse.gov/wp-content/uploads/2019/09/The-State-of-Homelessness-in-America.pdf (accessed on 1 May 2021).
46. Tsai, J.; Wilson, M. COVID-19: A Potential Public Health Problem for Homeless Populations. *Lancet Public Health* **2020**, *5*, e186–e187. [CrossRef] [PubMed]
47. Lebrun-Harris, L.A.; Baggett, T.P.; Jenkins, D.M.; Sripipatana, A.; Sharma, R.; Hayashi, A.S.; Daly, C.A.; Ngo-Metzger, Q. Health Status and Health Care Experiences among Homeless Patients in Federally Supported Health Centers: Findings from the 2009 Patient Survey. *Health Serv. Res.* **2013**, *48*, 992–1017. [CrossRef] [PubMed]
48. Oppenheimer, S.C.; Nurius, P.S.; Green, S. Homelessness History Impacts on Health Outcomes and Economic and Risk Behavior Intermediaries: New Insights from Population Data. *Fam. Soc.* **2016**, *97*, 230–242. [CrossRef] [PubMed]
49. Castañeda, E.; Klassen, J.D.; Smith, C. Hispanic and Non-Hispanic Homeless Populations in El Paso, Texas. *Hisp. J. Behav. Sci.* **2014**, *36*, 488–505. [CrossRef]
50. Centers for Disease Control and Prevention. Medical Conditions. Available online: https://www.cdc.gov/coronavirus/2019-ncov/need-extra-precautions/people-with-medical-conditions.html (accessed on 28 April 2021).
51. Garg, S. Hospitalization Rates and Characteristics of Patients Hospitalized with Laboratory-Confirmed Coronavirus Disease 2019—COVID-NET, 14 States, March 1–30, 2020. *MMWR Morb. Mortal. Wkly. Rep.* **2020**, *69*, 458. [CrossRef] [PubMed]
52. Alegria, M.; Canino, G.; Shrout, P.E.; Woo, M.; Duan, N.; Vila, D.; Torres, M.; Chen, C.-N.; Meng, X.-L. Prevalence of Mental Illness in Immigrant and Non-Immigrant U.S. Latino Groups. *Am. J. Psychiatry* **2008**, *165*, 359–369. [CrossRef] [PubMed]
53. Palloni, A.; Arias, E. Paradox Lost: Explaining the Hispanic Adult Mortality Advantage. *Demography* **2004**, *41*, 385–415. [CrossRef] [PubMed]
54 Medina-Inojosa, J.; Jean, N.; Cortes-Bergoderi, M.; Lopez-Jimenez, F. The Hispanic Paradox in Cardiovascular Disease and Total Mortality. *Prog. Cardiovasc. Dis.* **2014**, *57*, 286–292. [CrossRef] [PubMed]
55 Crosnoe, R. Studying the Immigrant Paradox in the Mexican-Origin Population. In *The Immigrant Paradox in Children and Adolescents: Is Becoming American a Developmental Risk?* American Psychological Association: Washington, DC, USA, 2012; pp. 61–76. ISBN 978-1-4338-1053-4.
56. Centers for Disease Control and Prevention. High Blood Pressure Symptoms and Causes. Available online: https://www.cdc.gov/bloodpressure/about.htm (accessed on 28 April 2021).
57. Centers for Disease Control and Prevention. Know Your Risk for Heart Disease. Available online: https://www.cdc.gov/heartdisease/risk_factors.htm (accessed on 28 April 2021).
58. National Heart, Lung, and Blood Institute. Blood Cholesterol. Available online: https://www.nhlbi.nih.gov/health-topics/blood-cholesterol (accessed on 28 April 2021).
59. American College of Allergy, Asthma & Immunology. Asthma Attack. Available online: https://acaai.org/asthma/symptoms/asthma-attack (accessed on 28 April 2021).
60. Centers for Disease Control and Prevention. Coronavirus Disease 2019 (COVID-19)—Symptoms. Available online: https://www.cdc.gov/coronavirus/2019-ncov/symptoms-testing/symptoms.html (accessed on 28 April 2021).
61. Centers for Disease Control and Prevention. COVID-19 Provisional Counts—Weekly Updates by Select Demographic and Geographic Characteristics. Available online: https://www.cdc.gov/nchs/nvss/vsrr/covid_weekly/index.htm#AgeAndSex (accessed on 28 April 2021).
62. American Stroke Association. Effects of Stroke. Available online: https://www.stroke.org/en/about-stroke/effects-of-stroke (accessed on 28 April 2021).

63. American Lung Association. Emphysema | American Lung Association. Available online: https://www.lung.org/lung-health-diseases/lung-disease-lookup/emphysema (accessed on 28 April 2021).
64. Boyles, S. COPD Care Suffers With High Insurance Deductibles. Available online: https://www.medpagetoday.com/meetingcoverage/ats/79988 (accessed on 28 April 2021).
65. World Health Organization. Hepatitis. Available online: https://www.who.int/news-room/q-a-detail/hepatitis (accessed on 28 April 2021).
66. HIV.gov. U.S. Statistics. Available online: https://www.hiv.gov/hiv-basics/overview/data-and-trends/statistics (accessed on 28 April 2021).
67. National Institute of Diabetes and Digestive and Kidney Diseases. What Is Chronic Kidney Disease? Available online: https://www.niddk.nih.gov/health-information/kidney-disease/chronic-kidney-disease-ckd/what-is-chronic-kidney-disease (accessed on 28 April 2021).
68. U.S. Census Bureau. *Census Bureau Projects U.S. and World Populations on New Year's Day*. Available online: https://www.census.gov/newsroom/press-releases/2019/new-years-population.html (accessed on 28 April 2021).
69. Centers for Disease Control and Prevention. HIV in the United States by Region. Available online: https://www.cdc.gov/hiv/statistics/overview/geographicdistribution.html (accessed on 28 April 2021).
70. World Health Organization. Tuberculosis (TB). Available online: https://www.who.int/news-room/fact-sheets/detail/tuberculosis (accessed on 28 April 2021).
71. Kilbourne, A.M.; Reynolds, C.F.; Good, C.B.; Sereika, S.M.; Justice, A.C.; Fine, M.J. How Does Depression Influence Diabetes Medication Adherence in Older Patients? *Am. J. Geriatr. Psychiatry* **2005**, *13*, 202–210. [CrossRef] [PubMed]
72. Peyrot, M.; Barnett, A.H.; Meneghini, L.F.; Schumm-Draeger, P.-M. Insulin Adherence Behaviours and Barriers in the Multinational Global Attitudes of Patients and Physicians in Insulin Therapy Study. *Diabet. Med.* **2012**, *29*, 682–689. [CrossRef] [PubMed]
73. Ross, S.A.; Tildesley, H.D.; Ashkenas, J. Barriers to Effective Insulin Treatment: The Persistence of Poor Glycemic Control in Type 2 Diabetes. *Curr. Med. Res. Opin.* **2011**, *27* (Suppl. 3), 13–20. [CrossRef] [PubMed]
74. Hu, J.; Amirehsani, K.; Wallace, D.; Letvak, S. The Meaning of Insulin to Hispanic Immigrants with Type 2 Diabetes and Their Families. *Diabetes Educ.* **2012**, *38*, 263–270. [CrossRef] [PubMed]
75. Hales, C.M.; Carroll, M.; Fryar, C.; Ogden, C. Prevalence of Obesity and Severe Obesity Among Adults: United States, 2017–2018. NCHS Data Brief; 2020. Available online: https://www.cdc.gov/nchs/products/databriefs/db360.htm (accessed on 1 May 2021).
76. National Center for Health Statistics. *Health, United States 2018*; Health; National Center for Health Statistics: Hyattsville, MD, USA, 2018; pp. 1–56.
77. Systematic Evidence Review from the Obesity Expert Panel, 2013; *Managing Overweight and Obesity in Adults*; NIH: National Heart, Lung, and Blood Institue: Bethesda, MD, USA, 2013; pp. 1–501.
78. Bailey, Z.; Krieger, N.; Agenor, M.; Graves, J.; Linos, N. Structural Racism and Health Inequities in the USA: Evidence and Interventions. *Lancet* **2017**, *389*, 1453–1463. [CrossRef] [PubMed]

International Journal of
Environmental Research and Public Health

MDPI

Article

Movement Pandemic Adaptability: Health Inequity and Advocacy among Latinx Immigrant and Indigenous Peoples

Mario Alberto Viveros Espinoza-Kulick

Ethnic Studies, Cuesta College, San Luis Obispo, CA 93405, USA; mario_espinozakulick@cuesta.edu; Tel.: +1-(805)-904-9225

Abstract: The COVID-19 pandemic exacerbated longstanding inequities in resources and healthcare, stacked on top of historical systems that exploit immigrants and communities of color. The range of relief, mutual aid, and advocacy responses to the pandemic highlights the role of social movement organizations in addressing the ways that immigration status creates systemic barriers to adequate health and wellbeing. This paper conceptualizes what I call, "movement pandemic adaptability," drawing from a decolonial-inspired study including participant-observation (September 2018–September 2020), interviews (n = 31), and focus groups (n = 12) with community members and health advocates. Data collection began before the COVID-19 pandemic (September 2018–February 2019) and continued during its emergence and the initial shelter-in-place orders (March 2019–September 2020). Movement pandemic adaptability emerged as a strategy of drawing from pre-existing networks and solidarities to provide culturally relevant resources for resilience that addressed vulnerabilities created by restrictions against undocumented people and language barriers for communities that speak Spanish and a range of Indigenous languages. This paper presents how the relationship between immigration status and health is influenced by the local context, as well as the decisions of advocates, policymakers, and community members.

Keywords: COVID-19; health equity; Latinx health; Latinx indigeneity; language; health access

Citation: Espinoza-Kulick, M.A.V. Movement Pandemic Adaptability: Health Inequity and Advocacy among Latinx Immigrant and Indigenous Peoples. *Int. J. Environ. Res. Public Health* **2022**, *19*, 8981. https://doi.org/10.3390/ijerph19158981

Academic Editor: Maria De Jesus

Received: 6 May 2022
Accepted: 21 July 2022
Published: 23 July 2022

1. Introduction

Groups that advocate for immigrants and immigrant rights rely on creative direct action strategies to organize for change [1,2]. Similarly, collective efforts related to addressing health inequities often utilize social movement strategies to target healthcare providers, insurance companies, and other aspects of the medical industry directly [3–8]. Scholars have documented major inequities in healthcare access and health outcomes within immigrant communities [9–12]. However, there has been little research examining the connections between immigrant health and advocacy movements. This paper bridges these research areas to analyze how immigrant health advocacy responded to the shifting political, social, and environmental context brought about by the COVID-19 pandemic.

Like other large-scale social and environmental events, the onset of a global pandemic creates a cascade of social changes [13–18]. The emergency response creates openings within the broader political setting for groups to amplify efforts for change [19,20]. Advocates draw on existing networks and communities of support to mobilize effectively during times of renewed opportunity [21]. Immigrant health movements, in particular, are accustomed to operating in limited-resource environments with political hostilities, leading to a range of creative and efficacious strategies [15]. However, researchers have yet to identify a conceptual framework for analyzing how immigrant health movements can inform broader work for health equity and access to care.

Unequal access and discrimination have systematic effects on the wellbeing of communities most at risk for disease [22]. Vocal xenophobic political ideologies and anti-immigrant policies—such as family separation, the widespread use of militarized enforcement raids, deportation, and detention—contribute to a culture of fear and reproduce health disparities [16,23,24]. These inequities have widespread effects on immigrant and Latinx communities, including mental health and chronic disease at the individual-, family-, and community-level. Academic researchers have spent considerable resources to document these inequities. With this knowledge well in hand, scholars can move beyond observing racial/ethnic disparities to document tenable strategies for ending systemic racism and its adverse effects on healthcare systems and practices [25–27]. This paper contributes to those efforts by demonstrating the interlinkages between immigrant advocacy and health advocacy [1,2,4,5,7,8,20,24,28–35].

Immigrant advocates have long contended with the risks facing immigrants [23,24]. Deportation, detention, and other punitive policies make direct action inherently risky for undocumented individuals and mixed-status families. However, "undocumented and unafraid" young people have also leveraged that risk to effectively gain visibility for policy change [30,31,36–38]. These creative responses to high-risk environments have prepared immigrant health advocates to lead equitably during the pandemic by prioritizing those most affected and at risk.

The concept of "movement pandemic adaptability" developed in this paper highlights how groups and organizations can lead through and beyond the COVID-19 pandemic with a central focus on equity. This theory emerged from a decolonial-inspired study of Latinx immigrant health advocacy on California's Central Coast. Movement pandemic adaptability includes building culturally responsive and language-accessible resources for community support, understanding opportunities in a changing world, identifying policies that impact communities at multiple levels, and drawing from localized expertise.

2. Materials and Methods

This study uses a decolonial-inspired ethnographic framework, based on deconstructing western research methods, privileging Indigenous and place-based knowledge production, and holding research accountable for its utility for underserved groups [39–44]. To better understand movement processes, data collection focused on participant observation between September 2018 to September 2020, and interviews with community members and advocates (n = 31) and focus groups with respondents from throughout the Central Coast (n =12). Community advocates played a crucial role in shaping the research questions and informing the study's priorities and commitments. In combination with the broader project, this provides a unique insight into the contexts of Latinx immigrant and Indigenous health advocacy.

A mixed-methods ethnographic approach was used to organize multiple types of data collection. Community input was especially prioritized through participant observation, a survey of community health needs and assets, and focus groups. Participant observation included attending collective action and public advocacy efforts and developing relationships with key informants [45]. Because I designed this project to be responsive to community needs, participant observation continued during the pandemic in a primarily digital environment [42,46,47]. Members of the community hold diverse and sometimes competing views, and thus I practiced reflexivity to organize and evaluate the perspectives presented through various data collection procedures including organizational communications and online archives of group events or meetings.

My family and I have lived on California's Central Coast for decades. I utilized aspects of my insider knowledge to gain greater insight into my observations. This helped me build relationships with individuals who do not occupy organizational leadership positions but play a key role in maintaining community relations and mobilizing grassroots actions. I shopped in locally owned stores and grocery markets, attended family celebrations, frequented public parks, participated in cultural events and holidays, accessed healthcare, and interfaced with local government agencies as a resident, constituent, and advocate. My daily investment in these communities has helped me to continuously center the need for effective and equitable solutions to healthcare disparities.

Individuals were recruited for interviews if they identified as one or both categories: immigrant community member (i.e., "Undocumented, Dreamers, mixed-status family member, resident and/or a naturalized citizen") or advocate (i.e., "individuals that actively participate in social change efforts toward advancing immigrant health equity"). Both groups were asked questions about health needs in the community, language and cultural diversity, and perceptions of the policy environment. Participants were recruited by phone, email, flyers, and social media ads. These efforts focused on groups that provide healthcare and legal aid for immigrant communities, community-based advocacy groups, schools, and community gathering places. Snowball sampling was used to recruit participants from the networks of previous interviewees [48]. This procedure is especially useful for recruiting participants and building trust among groups that have been historically marginalized and/or exploited by government agencies. I conducted 31 interviews before reaching saturation: the scope of new information in additional interviews was exceeded by repeated information from one or more previous interviews.

Focus groups were structured to include knowledge sharing from earlier interviews and the survey of health needs and assets. The conversations were structured around major themes in the study: political climate, health needs/assets, and language. Within each section, relevant findings were shared, and then participants had the opportunity to respond, ask questions, and discuss. Open-ended conversations set a tone for sharing knowledge and held the research accountable to the lived experiences of diverse community members [49,50]. The discussions allowed their voices to inform the interpretation of findings and set the priorities for analysis and dissemination of findings [51]. To facilitate opportunities for free-flowing discussions over Zoom, each of the six focus groups had up to four participants each. Participants were recruited from all counties represented in the study (Monterey, San Luis Obispo, Santa Barbara and Ventura). Half of the focus groups were conducted in English and the other half were conducted in Spanish ("cafecitos") based on language of preference. Incentives were provided for each interview and focus group participant (USD 25) and key informants with both community members and advocates (USD 30) in the form of cash or a gift card.

Data were coded using a grounded theory approach [52,53] with the software, Dedoose (Dedoose Version 8.3.43, Los Angeles, CA, USA). From participant observations, data included field notes, audio memos, recorded events, public materials, organizational documents, emails, newsletters, and news media. Codes were developed by closely reading materials and capturing relevant themes in participants' own words. The codebook developed from this stage was used for the analysis of interviews and focus groups. In continuing with the grounded theory approach, new codes were added upon comparing the interviews with field work documents [54]. A team of six research assistants were trained in coding techniques and completed line-by-line coding of each transcript. We established inter-rater reliability by meeting to discuss themes and resolve any discrepancies in the assignment of codes or creation of new codes. All items were coded by at least two research team members. When discrepancies existed, the team first sought to create consensus between the two coders. Agreement was reached in all such situations. Themes from these coding processes were then used for focused coding to interrogate social movement dynamics that bring together aspects of immigrant and health advocacy and how they changed during the pandemic.

3. Results

The COVID-19 pandemic has had a disparate impact on Latinx immigrant and Indigenous communities, a national trend [55,56] that is also reflected on the Central Coast [57]. Interviewees shared a range of reactions to the pandemic itself, including personal experiences and family loss. They also reflected on acts of collective resilience, which was evident in advocates' quick response to spread information and resources to protect vulnerable community members. During the same time period, the threats to Latinx immigrant and

Indigenous communities also included the proposed changes to the public charge rule and a systematic exclusion from government relief and aid programs.

To combat this unstable environment, groups used accessible language and culturally responsive communication to promote heath literacy and share relevant COVID-19 information. Direct support efforts worked to address the legal exclusion of immigrants from federal safety net programs. The practice of mutual aid and collective responsibility enacted during the pandemic builds from traditions of solidarity and kinship within Latinx immigrant and Indigenous communities. Furthermore, advocates went beyond repairing immediate harm to preventing future risk and exploitation. Working towards changing policies influences future opportunities for mobilization and can change systems. Throughout these actions, local experts were successful in implementing change when they bridged new information with meaningful cultural frameworks shared by multiple stakeholders.

3.1. Multilingual Interpretation for Health Access

Access to multilingual translation and interpretation facilitates inclusion for Spanish and Indigenous language speakers. On the Central Coast, the Mixteco/Indígena Community Organizing Project (MICOP) centralizes language interpretation in their work and provides Indigenous language access within networks of immigrant and health advocates. The group launched *Radio Indígena* in 2014, a local FM station with over 40 h of weekly live programming, featuring at least seven Mixteco languages, Zapoteco, and Purépecha. This service provides information and entertainment relevant to Indigenous farm working communities, such as support for low-income individuals to receive rental assistance, energy payment programs, and family paid leave.

This platform served a crucial role in spreading vital public health information during the COVID-19 pandemic. They quickly expanded to include Facebook Live broadcasts to supplement radio programming and demonstrate visually how testing works and show images of how others have participated in testing. These events are interpreted in at least one Indigenous language, often through consecutive interpretation. In engaging the audience, the speakers use a conversational style. The interpreter does not just repeat the words translated from Spanish but is trained to share the message in a relevant way for heterogenous audiences. For further accessibility, the videos include visual aids and photographs to guide individuals through practical steps to access transportation and where to arrive for testing. This visual demonstration helps to work against stigma and decrease fear of health services. The group emphasized overall health and wellbeing to encourage maximum prevention and safety when information about transmission was limited.

Interpretation services must be culturally responsive to regional diversity. One advocate interviewee elaborated on this, saying "Mixteco, there's not only one variant, there's 20 to 23, if not more. It is a big barrier, but that's why there's organizations like 805 UndocuFund or MICOP [Mixteco/Indígena Community Organizing Project], and IMPORTA" (Advocate Interview). MICOP created materials for World Languages Day to demonstrate regional differences between dialects from San Juan, Mixtepec, Piedra Azul, San Martín Peras, and Tlahuapa, Guerrero. Herencia Indígena is an organization that specializes in medical interpretation and partners with service providers to increase access to healthcare directly. Sharing complex medical information had increased salience during the pandemic. A *Radio Indígena* broadcast from June 2020 notified the community about a COVID-19 outbreak in H2A housing for farmworkers in Ventura County. The advocates shared information about how people could protect themselves from COVID, acknowledging the reality that social distancing is practically impossible in crowded common family and work areas. This broadcast was interpreted in Spanish, Mixteco, and Purépecha.

3.2. Creating Direct Support Mechanisms: Immigrants and Mutual Aid

While the virus was a central concern during the pandemic, it joined several longstanding issues affecting the community. As identified by the key informants, the 45th U.S. Presidential administration sponsored a number of hostile and xenophobic policies.

This included continuing to deport and detain migrants during a pandemic, increasing construction of a Border Wall, excluding immigrants from emergency and pandemic aid programs, and seeking to expand the public charge rule. These political hostilities advance a culture of threat and fear, but advocates support an alternate vision. As MICOP put it in an informational session on the public charge rule, "¡El conocimiento es la mejor defensa contral el miedo!" ("Knowledge is the best defense against fear"). They directly helped immigrants understand how certain policies do and do not affect them. Although information sharing is vital, it cannot reverse the exclusions that do exist.

To provide a direct and clear response to these exclusions, advocates organized networks of solidarity. These were typically organized around region or county, allowing service providers and businesses to coordinate and share resources with community members. These efforts mirror how state agencies seek to create wrap-around services with multiple points of access to resources, although these groups are usually organized on a voluntary basis or subsidized by personnel from non-profit and community-based organizations. Advocates demonstrated their tenacity and resourcefulness in mobilizing under hostile conditions. One community member shared her perspective when she said, "Nuestra estrategia es más que nada seguir insistiendo, seguir tocando puertas por puertas, seguir insistiendo dándoles la información correcta. Hay muchos recursos de los que ellos se pueden beneficiar ... Eso nos hace más fuertes." ("Our strategy is more than anything to keep insisting, keep knocking door to door, keep insisting by giving them the correct information. There are many resources for their benefit ... This makes us all stronger").

The 805 UndocuFund is a resource for immigrant communities that has provided substantial benefits in the face of legal exclusions from federal programs. The program was first started in response to the 2017 Thomas Fire as a collaboration between Central Coast Alliance United for a Sustainable Economy (CAUSE), MICOP, Future Leaders of America (FLA), and Ventura County Community Foundation. They fundraised over USD 5 million for struggling workers and their families during the COVID-19 pandemic. These funds were distributed to workers in small grants of USD 1000 each, but they were not able to meet the full level of demand within the community. Similar groups such as the San Luis Obispo County UndocuSupport group distributed community-generated funding to undocumented communities throughout the Central Coast. These funds are distributed by community groups with trusting relationships in the communities, who ward against fraud and scams.

3.3. Mobilizing for Farmworker Dignity

Latinx Immigrant and Indigenous advocates are heavily involved in improving working conditions for farm working communities. For example, youth leaders from CAUSE provided a powerful testimony at the Santa Barbara and Ventura County Board of Supervisors in July of 2021. One young person spoke about her parents' experience who were fired from the farm on the argument that there was no fruit to be harvested. She said:

> We all know that's a lie. It's the right season to grow fruit. It's also the right season to give the farmworkers the help they need. They are expected to work in the sun and feed this nation, how can we turn our back on them when they have been doing so much for us? How many more lives needs to be at risk before you bat an eye at them? How many more mothers are you going to take from us? I urge you to do the right thing and help them by providing masks, gloves, clean water, anything they need. They help feed our families and we should help keep their families safe. What are you going to do? Give them a helping hand, or wait until my mother or her coworkers also get COVID?

Advocates embraced and deployed the framing of farmworkers as "essential workers" to hold policymakers and farm owners accountable. The pandemic brought into sharp relief those aspects of the global economy that society cannot do without, including agriculture. Moreover, it also showed that the government can mobilize resources, funds, and services to communities in need, especially when "crises" are declared.

Policy change for farm workers includes organizational policies by individual farms, especially those that set industry standards for practices, pay rates, and conditions. For example, targets for social movement organizing included County Boards of Supervisors, as well as worker housing sites, employers, and labor contractors. During the pandemic, housing became an important site of direct advocacy to increase health regulations for testing and screening of COVID-19, as well as making opportunities available for quarantine when farm workers tested positive. Through an initiative called Housing for the Harvest, hotel rooms were made available along with services in English, Spanish, and Mixteco [58]. Because immigrants are excluded from most formal relationships with the state, employers also play a more pronounced role in influencing community members' daily experiences.

During 2020, advocates in Santa Maria organized farm workers to obtain a pay raise and improve working conditions. The central victory at Rancho Laguna Farms included a raise of USD 2.10 per box of strawberries [59], in addition to increased access to shade for safe and socially distanced breaks as well as training for more effective communication by supervisors. After over a decade with no wage increases, this change was a historic win for organizers. Successful mobilization was a result of multiple strategies, including petitions, a work stoppage, and public demonstrations [60]. This action inspired resistance among the farm owners, who attempted to suppress organizing by contacting law enforcement officers. CAUSE was able to successfully win a settlement through the California Agricultural Labor Relations Board of USD 30,000 for 212 farmworkers in Santa Maria as compensation for damages caused by unlawful retaliation. The farm owners were additionally required to provide training on farmworkers' rights to supervisors under the Agricultural Labor Relations Act, including the right to organize. By exercising their collective power, farm workers inspire others to honor the dignity and value created by essential workforces, during and beyond the pandemic.

4. Discussion

Latinx Immigrant and Indigenous Health movements demonstrated adaptability in the pandemic environment by building from existing resources and networks of solidarity. These strategies were culturally responsive and language accessible and provided support resources to the community. These strategies are characteristic of both health access movements and constituency-based movements [5,6,61,62]. However, the efficacy of information is limited by structural constraints such as housing conditions, racism, and xenophobic policies [63–65]. Advocacy and direct action disrupted patterns of exploitation and mobilized supportive decision makers at the local and state levels [30–32,37,66,67]. The state of California polarized against the federal government's hostilities toward immigrants, creating political openings for policy change. For instance, advocates won Medi-Cal expansion to include income-eligible minors and young adults up to age 26.

This study's strengths are rooted in the decolonial-inspired framework, including the use of multiple forms of data, the level of rapport between the researcher and the community, and the deployment of locally-specific explanations of events and perspectives. However, there are also some study limitations, especially in terms of time and scope. Future researchers would benefit from examining these dynamics over time in other communities of Latinx immigrant and Indigenous people. While some basic aspects of temporal change were observed between 2018 to 2020, this study is limited to the COVID-19 pandemic and its early days in the United States. More research is needed to understand how these strategies evolved over time.

Immigrant health movements depended on grassroots mobilization to build trusting relationships between community leaders and those most in need. Due to historic systems of exploitation, Latinx communities mistrust government agencies and mainstream healthcare providers. The shared experiences of structural exclusion shape an embodied experience of health risk [68], so that being an "essential worker" becomes politicized as a condition of health risk. This demonstrates how health social movements mobilize collective identities beyond illness itself [5,27]. This mobilization was effective because of the expertise of community leaders who advocate for systems change at every level.

Legislative change, organizational policy, and local actions can further improve the health of Latinx Immigrant and Indigenous communities. These recommendations build from the movement pandemic adaptability of local organizers and state-level advocates. In California, state legislation can lead the way for national change that is more inclusive and equitable for Latinx Immigrant and Indigenous communities. State legislators have recently expanded state public health insurance (Medi-Cal) to undocumented elders aged 50 and up. Policymakers are poised to further expand Medi-Cal to include undocumented adults of all ages, with the Governor's draft budget for 2022–2023 funding coverage to start in 2024. If this moves forward as planned, California will be the first state to remove immigration status as a barrier to public health insurance. However, insurance and access only addresses part of the issue.

City, county, state, and federal governments can declare racism a public health crisis and take immediate action accordingly. Taking aggressive action against racism means immediately ending practices that reproduce health disparities. For instance, policymakers can disallow county sheriffs and city police from coordinating with federal immigration agencies such as Immigration and Customs Enforcement. Appropriate action also includes providing funding, resources, and capacity support for anti-racist and immigrant-serving organizations. Local groups can contribute to equity and access by regularly hiring multilingual interpreters. In a medical context, this action is necessary to ensure access to care for all individuals. In all contexts, translation and interpretation services need to be responsive to local audiences, including Indigenous language speakers.

5. Conclusions

Researchers have documented the widespread existence of health inequities for Latinx immigrant and Indigenous communities. Discrimination and systemic oppression are major drivers behind these realities. Scholars have also examined the successful advocacy strategies of immigrant rights groups, as well as constituencies invested in improving healthcare access and outcomes. This paper brought together research on these topics to examine the specific dynamics of immigrant health movements in the context of the COVID-19 pandemic. The concept of "movement pandemic adaptability" highlights the implementation of culturally responsive strategies for healthcare rooted in collaborations between diverse community leaders and healthcare experts. Future research is needed to extend this concept to examine other community pandemic responses, as well as to evaluate the role of responsive community-based strategies within public health systems in a range of crisis settings.

Funding: This research was funded by the Robert Wood Johnson Foundation (Dissertation Award, Dissemination Award, and Health Policy Research Scholars Fellowship), Scholars Strategy Network, Community Change Leadership, California Polytechnic State University, San Luis Obispo (Believe, Educate & Empower, Advocate, Collaborate and Nurture (BEACoN) Grant). The APC was funded by the University of California Santa Barbara Migration Initiative.

Institutional Review Board Statement: The study was conducted in accordance with the Declaration of Helsinki and approved by the Institutional Review Board of the University of California, Santa Barbara (Procotol Number: 22-19-0595).

Informed Consent Statement: Informed consent was obtained from all subjects involved in the study.

Data Availability Statement: Reports of the data presented in this study are available in English and Spanish online at https://lagenteunidacc.wixsite.com/recursosdesalud/reports-reportes, accessed on 21 July 2022.

Acknowledgments: Thank you to the participants in this study.

Conflicts of Interest: The author declares no conflict of interest.

References

1. Burciaga, E.M.; Martinez, L.M. How Do Political Contexts Shape Undocumented Youth Movements? Evidence from Three Immigration Destinations. *Mobilization Int. Q.* **2017**, *22*, 451–471. [CrossRef]
2. Mora, M.D.J.; Rodriguez, R.; Zermeño, A.; Almeida, P. Immigrant Rights and Social Movements. *Sociol. Compass* **2018**, *12*, e12599. [CrossRef]
3. Archibald, M.E.; Crabtree, C. Health Social Movements in the United States: An Overview: Health Social Movements in the United States. *Sociol. Compass* **2010**, *4*, 334–343. [CrossRef]
4. Banaszak-Holl, J.C.; Levitsky, S.R.; Zald, M.N. *Social Movements and the Transformation of American Health Care*; Oxford University Press: New York, NY, USA, 2010; ISBN 978-0-19-974214-1.
5. Brown, P.; Zavestoski, S.; McCormick, S.; Mayer, B.; Morello-Frosch, R.; Altman, R.G. Embodied Health Movements: New Approaches to Social Movements in Health. *Sociol. Health Illn.* **2004**, *26*, 50–80. [CrossRef]
6. Brown, T.M.; Fee, E. Social Movements in Health. *Annu. Rev. Public Health* **2014**, *35*, 385–398. [CrossRef]
7. Taylor, V.; Leitz, L. *From Infanticide to Activism: The Transformation of Emotions and Identity in Self-Help Movements. Peace Faculty Books and Book Chapters*; Oxford University Press: Oxford, UK, 2010.
8. Taylor, V.; Zald, M. Health Movements (United States). In *The Wiley-Blackwell Encyclopedia of Social and Political Movements*; American Cancer Society: Hoboken, NJ, USA, 2013; ISBN 978-0-470-67487-1.
9. Barcellos, S.H.; Goldman, D.P.; Smith, J.P. Undiagnosed Disease, Especially Diabetes, Casts Doubt On Some Of Reported Health 'Advantage' Of Recent Mexican Immigrants. *Health Aff.* **2012**, *31*, 2727–2737. [CrossRef]
10. Becerra, D.; Hernandez, G.; Porchas, F.; Castillo, J.; Nguyen, V.; Perez González, R. Immigration Policies and Mental Health: Examining the Relationship between Immigration Enforcement and Depression, Anxiety, and Stress among Latino Immigrants. *J. Ethn. Cult. Divers. Soc. Work Innov. Theory Res. Pract.* **2020**, *29*, 43–59. [CrossRef]
11. Cabrera-Nguyen, E.P. Estimating the Prevalence and Correlates of Psychiatric Disorders and Mental Health Problems among Undocumented Mexican Immigrants Using the National Latino and Asian American Study. Doctor's Dissertation, Washington University, St. Louis, MO, USA, 2015.
12. Garcini, L.M.; Renzaho, A.M.N.; Molina, M.; Ayala, G.X. Health-Related Quality of Life among Mexican-Origin Latinos: The Role of Immigration Legal Status. *Ethn. Health* **2018**, *23*, 566–581. [CrossRef]
13. Bloss, W. Escalating U.S. Police Surveillance after 9/11: An Examination of Causes and Effects. *Surveill. Soc.* **2007**, *4*, 208–228. [CrossRef]
14. Earl, J. Information Access and Protest Policing Post-9/11: Studying the Policing of the 2004 Republican National Convention. *Am. Behav. Sci.* **2009**, *53*, 44–60. [CrossRef]
15. Falicov, C.; Niño, A.; D'Urso, S. Expanding Possibilities: Flexibility and Solidarity with Under-Resourced Immigrant Families During the COVID-19 Pandemic. *Fam. Process* **2020**, *59*, 865–882. [CrossRef] [PubMed]
16. Golash-Boza, T.M. *Immigration Nation: Raids, Detentions, and Deportations in Post-9/11 America*, 1st ed.; Routledge: Boulder, CO, USA, 2012; ISBN 978-1-59451-838-6.
17. Maira, S.M. *The 9/11 Generation: Youth, Rights, and Solidarity in the War on Terror*; Reprint edition; NYU Press: New York, NY, USA, 2016; ISBN 978-1-4798-8051-5.
18. Rechitsky, R.; Hoekstra, E. *Humanitarianism and Mass Migration: Confronting the World Crisis*; SAGE Publications Sage CA: Los Angeles, CA, USA, 2020.
19. Griffin, R.W. Political Opportunity, Resource Mobilization, and Social Movements: The Case of the South Texas Farm Workers. *Soc. Sci. J.* **1992**, *29*, 129–152. [CrossRef]
20. Hoekstra, E. Bordered Resistance: Immigrant Health Justice, Biocitizenship, and the Racialized Criminalization of Health Care. Ph.D. Dissertation, University of Minnesota, Minneapolis, MN, USA, 2019.
21. Taylor, V. Social Movement Continuity: The Women's Movement in Abeyance. *Am. Sociol. Rev.* **1989**, *54*, 761–775. [CrossRef]
22. Molina, N. *Fit to Be Citizens?: Public Health and Race in Los Angeles, 1879–1939*; University of California Press: Berkeley, CA, USA, 2006; ISBN 978-0-520-24649-2.
23. Lopez, W.D. *Separated: Family and Community in the Aftermath of an Immigration Raid*; Johns Hopkins University Press: Baltimore, MD, USA, 2019; ISBN 978-1-4214-3331-8.
24. Prieto, G. *Immigrants Under Threat: Risk and Resistance in Deportation Nation*; New York University Press: New York, NY, USA, 2018.
25. Ford, C.L.; Griffith, D.M.; Bruce, M.A.; Gilbert, K.L. *Racism: Science & Tools for the Public Health Professional*; American Public Health Association: Washington, DC, USA, 2019; ISBN 978-0-87553-303-2.
26. Ford, C.L.; Airhihenbuwa, C.O. The Public Health Critical Race Methodology: Praxis for Antiracism Research. *Soc. Sci. Med.* **2010**, *71*, 1390–1398. [CrossRef]
27. Viruell-Fuentes, E.A.; Miranda, P.Y.; Abdulrahim, S. More than Culture: Structural Racism, Intersectionality Theory, and Immigrant Health. *Soc. Sci. Med.* **2012**, *75*, 2099–2106. [CrossRef]
28. Best, R.K. Disease Campaigns and the Decline of Treatment Advocacy. *J. Health Politics Policy Law* **2017**, *42*, 425–457. [CrossRef]
29. Costanza-Chock, S. Digital Popular Communication: Lessons on Information and Communication Technologies for Social Change from the Immigrant Rights Movement. *Natl. Civ. Rev.* **2011**, *100*, 29–35. [CrossRef]
30. Costanza-Chock, S. *Out of the Shadows, into the Streets! Transmedia Organizing and the Immigrant Rights Movement*; The MIT Press: Cambridge, CA, USA, 2014; ISBN 978-0-262-02820-2.

31. Enriquez, L.E.; Saguy, A.C. Coming out of the Shadows: Harnessing a Cultural Schema to Advance the Undocumented Immigrant Youth Movement. *Am. J. Cult. Sociol.* **2016**, *4*, 107–130. [CrossRef]
32. Mensink, S. Prefiguration, Strategic Interaction and Political Belonging in Undocumented Migrant and Solidarity Movements. *J. Ethn. Migr. Stud.* **2020**, *46*, 1223–1239. [CrossRef]
33. Rusch, D.; Walden, A.L.; DeCarlo Santiago, C. A Community-based Organization Model to Promote Latinx Immigrant Mental Health through Advocacy Skills and Universal Parenting Supports. *Am. J. Community Psychol.* **2020**, *66*, 337–346. [CrossRef]
34. Taylor, V. Self-Labeling and Women's Mental Health: Postpartum Illness and the Reconstruction of Motherhood. *Sociol. Focus* **1995**, *28*, 23–47. [CrossRef]
35. Taylor, V.; Van Willigen, M. Women's Self-Help and The Reconstruction of Gender: The Postpartum Support and Breast Cancer Movements. *Mobilization Int. Q.* **1996**, *1*, 123–142. [CrossRef]
36. Baker-Cristales, B. Mediated Resistance: The Construction of Neoliberal Citizenship in the Immigrant Rights Movement. *Lat. Stud.* **2009**, *7*, 60–82. [CrossRef]
37. FitzGerald, D.; Cook-Martín, D. *Culling the Masses: The Democratic Origins of Racist Immigration Policy in the Americas*; Harvard University Press: Cambridge, MA, USA, 2014; ISBN 978-0-674-72904-9.
38. FitzGerald, D.S.; Skrentny, J.D. (Eds.) *Immigrant California: Understanding the Past, Present, and Future of U.S. Policy*; Stanford University Press: Stanford, CA, USA, 2021; ISBN 978-1-5036-1439-0.
39. Wray-Lake, L.; Wells, R.; Alvis, L.; Delgado, S.; Syvertsen, A.K.; Metzger, A. Being a Latinx Adolescent under a Trump Presidency: Analysis of Latinx Youth's Reactions to Immigration Politics. *Child. Youth Serv. Rev.* **2018**, *87*, 192–204. [CrossRef]
40. Fortuna, L.R.; Noroña, C.R.; Porche, M.V.; Tillman, C.; Patil, P.A.; Wang, Y.; Markle, S.L.; Alegría, M. Trauma, Immigration, and Sexual Health among Latina Women: Implications for Maternal–Child Well-being and Reproductive Justice. *Infant Ment. Health J.* **2019**, *40*, 640–658. [CrossRef]
41. Fujiwara, L.H. Immigrant Rights Are Human Rights: The Reframing of Immigrant Entitlement and Welfare. *Soc. Probl.* **2005**, *52*, 79–101. [CrossRef]
42. Hing, B.O.; Johnson, K.R. *The Immigrant Rights Marches of 2006 and the Prospects for a New Civil Rights Movement*; Social Science Research Network: Rochester, NY, USA, 2006.
43. Hondagneu-Sotelo, P.; Salas, A.; Gutiérrez, R.A.; Almaguer, T. What Explains the Immigrant Rights Marches of 2006?: Xenophobia and Organizing with Democracy Technology. In *The New Latino Studies Reader, A Twenty-First-Century Perspective*; University of California Press: Berkeley, CA, USA, 2016; pp. 609–621. ISBN 978-0-520-28484-5.
44. Nicholls, W.J. *The DREAMers: How the Undocumented Youth Movement Transformed the Immigrant Rights Debate*; Stanford University Press: Stanford, CA, USA, 2013; ISBN 978-0-8047-8869-4.
45. Terriquez, V. Intersectional Mobilization, Social Movement Spillover, and Queer Youth Leadership in the Immigrant Rights Movement. *Soc. Probl.* **2015**, *62*, 343–362. [CrossRef]
46. Yukich, G. Constructing the Model Immigrant: Movement Strategy and Immigrant Deservingness in the New Sanctuary Movement. *Soc. Probl.* **2013**, *60*, 302–320. [CrossRef]
47. Blackwell, M.; Boj Lopez, F.; Urrieta, L. Special Issue: Critical Latinx Indigeneities. *Lat. Stud.* **2017**, *15*, 126–137. [CrossRef]
48. Fox, J.; Rivera-Salgado, G. *Indigenous Mexican Migrants in the United States*; Center for U.S.-Mexican Studies, Center for Comparative Immigration Studies, UCSD: San Diego, CA, USA, 2004; ISBN 978-1-878367-50-1.
49. Jacob, M.M. *Yakama Rising: Indigenous Cultural Revitalization, Activism, and Healing*; University of Arizona Press: Tucson, AZ, USA, 2013; ISBN 978-0-8165-9921-9.
50. Jolivette, A.J. *Indian Blood: HIV and Colonial Trauma in San Francisco's Two-Spirit Community*; University of Washington Press: Seattle, WA, USA, 2016; ISBN 978-0-295-99849-7.
51. Manzo, R.D.; Brazil-Cruz, L.; Flores, Y.G.; Rivera-Lopez, H. *Cultura y Corazón: A Decolonial Methodology for Community Engaged Research*; Illustrated edition; University of Arizona Press: Tucson, AZ, USA, 2020; ISBN 978-0-8165-3766-2.
52. McGuire, S.S. Agency, Initiative, and Obstacles to Health Among Indigenous Immigrant Women From Oaxaca, Mexico. *Home Health Care Manag. Pract.* **2006**, *18*, 370–377. [CrossRef]
53. McGuire, S. Borders, Centers, and Margins: Critical Landscapes for Migrant Health. *Adv. Nurs. Sci.* **2014**, *37*, 197–212. [CrossRef] [PubMed]
54. Rodriguez-Lonebear, D. Building a Data Revolution in Indian Country. In *Indigenous Data Sovereignty: Toward an Agenda*; Kukutai, T., Taylor, J., Eds.; Australian National University Press: Canberra, Australia, 2016; pp. 253–272.
55. Smith, L.T. *Decolonizing Methodologies: Research and Indigenous Peoples*, 2nd ed.; Zed Books: London, UK, 2012; ISBN 978-1-84813-950-3.
56. Brown, P.; Morello-Frosch, R.; Zavestoski, S.; Senier, L.; Altman, R.G.; Hoover, E.; McCormick, S.; Mayer, B.; Adams, C. Field Analysis and Policy Ethnography in the Study of Health Social Movements. In *Social Movements and the Transformation of American Health Care*; Banaszak-Holl, J.C., Levitsky, S.R., Zald, M.N., Eds.; Oxford University Press: New York, NY, USA, 2010; pp. 101–116. ISBN 978-0-19-974214-1.
57. Best, R.K. *Contested Illnesses: Citizens, Science, and Health Social Movements*; Brown, P., Morello-Frosch, R., Zavestoski, S., The Contested Illnesses Research Group, Eds.; University of California Press: Berkeley, CA, USA, 2012; p. 324. ISBN 9780520270213.
58. Hoffman, B. Health Care Reform and Social Movements in the United States. *Am. J. Public Health* **2003**, *93*, 75–85. [CrossRef] [PubMed]

59. Keefe, R.H.; Lane, S.D.; Swarts, H.J. From the Bottom Up: Tracing the Impact of Four Health-Based Social Movements on Health and Social Policies. *J. Health Soc. Policy* **2006**, *21*, 55–69. [CrossRef] [PubMed]
60. Epstein, S. The Politics of Health Mobilization in the United States: The Promise and Pitfalls of "Disease Constituencies". *Soc. Sci. Med.* **2016**, *165*, 246–254. [CrossRef]
61. Epstein, S. *Impure Science: AIDS, Activism, and the Politics of Knowledge*; University of California Press: Berkeley, CA, USA, 1996.
62. Rabeharisoa, V.; Moreira, T.; Akrich, M. Evidence-Based Activism: Patients', Users' and Activists' Groups in Knowledge Society. *BioSocieties Lond.* **2014**, *9*, 111–128. [CrossRef]
63. Armstrong, E.A.; Bernstein, M. Culture, Power, and Institutions: A Multi-Institutional Politics Approach to Social Movements. *Sociol. Theory* **2008**, *26*, 74–99. [CrossRef]
64. Kukutai, T.; Taylor, J. *Indigenous Data Sovereignty: Toward an Agenda*; ANU Press: Canberra, Australia, 2016; ISBN 978-1-76046-031-0.
65. Mendoza, F.S. Health Disparities and Children in Immigrant Families: A Research Agenda. *Pediatrics* **2009**, *124*, S187–S195. [CrossRef]
66. Vargas, E.D.; Ybarra, V.D. U.S. Citizen Children of Undocumented Parents: The Link Between State Immigration Policy and the Health of Latino Children. *J. Immigr. Minority Health* **2017**, *19*, 913–920. [CrossRef]
67. Telles, E. Race and Social Problems. *Race Soc. Probl.* **2012**, *4*, 1–4. [CrossRef]
68. Becot, F.; Inwood, S.; Bendixsen, C.; Henning-Smith, C. Health Care and Health Insurance Access for Farm Families in the United States during COVID-19: Essential Workers without Essential Resources? *J. Agromed.* **2020**, *25*, 374–377. [CrossRef]

International Journal of
Environmental Research and Public Health

MDPI

Concept Paper

The Most Vulnerable Hispanic Immigrants in New York City: Structural Racism and Gendered Differences in COVID-19 Deaths

Norma Fuentes-Mayorga [1,*] and Alfredo Cuecuecha Mendoza [2]

1 The Colin Powell School for Civic and Global Leadership, The City College New York (CCNY), New York, NY 10031, USA
2 Centro de Investigación e Inteligencia Económicas-UPAEP, Puebla 72410, Mexico; alfredo.cuecuecha@upaep.mx
* Correspondence: nfuentes@ccny.cuny.edu

Abstract: This paper explores the structural and group-specific factors explaining the excess death rates experienced by the Hispanic population in New York City during the peak years of the coronavirus pandemic. Neighborhood-level analysis of Census data allows an exploration of the relation between Hispanic COVID-19 deaths and spatial concentration, conceived in this study as a proxy for structural racism. This analysis also provides a more detailed exploration of the role of gender in understanding the effects of spatial segregation among different Hispanic subgroups, as gender has emerged as a significant variable in explaining the structural and social effects of COVID-19. Our results show a positive correlation between COVID-19 death rates and the share of Hispanic neighborhood residents. However, for men, this correlation cannot be explained by the characteristics of the neighborhood, as it is for women. In sum, we find: (a) differences in mortality risks between Hispanic men and women; (b) that weathering effects increase mortality risks the longer Hispanic immigrant groups reside in the U.S.; (c) that Hispanic males experience greater contagion and mortality risks associated with the workplace; and (d) we find evidence corroborating the importance of access to health insurance and citizenship status in reducing mortality risks. The findings propose revisiting the Hispanic health paradox with the use of structural racism and gendered frameworks.

Keywords: New York City; Hispanic population; COVID-19 death rates; Hispanic immigrants; structural racism; spatial concentration; gendered analysis; Hispanic health paradox

Citation: Fuentes-Mayorga, N.; Cuecuecha Mendoza, A. The Most Vulnerable Hispanic Immigrants in New York City: Structural Racism and Gendered Differences in COVID-19 Deaths. *Int. J. Environ. Res. Public Health* **2023**, *20*, 5838. https://doi.org/10.3390/ijerph20105838

Academic Editors: Maria De Jesus and Ernesto Castañeda

Received: 24 January 2023
Revised: 24 April 2023
Accepted: 6 May 2023
Published: 16 May 2023

1. Introduction

The U.S. COVID-19 pandemic unraveled an unprecedented health and economic crisis in which historically racialized and vulnerable minorities paid the highest price with their lives. Federal policy defines "Hispanic" not as a race but as an ethnicity. Additionally, it prescribes that Hispanics can, in fact, be of any race. However, some authors argue that standard U.S. racial categories might either be confusing or not provide relevant options for Hispanics to describe their racial identity. A good share of Hispanics considers their Hispanic background to be part of their racial background, while others think of it as their ethnic background. A good share considers the label both an ethnic and racial identity [1]. The disproportionally higher death rates decimated the Hispanic population of New York City which made it clear that legacies of structural and social inequalities combined to increase the higher risk of mortality for the group [2–60]. In 2020, for example, during the peak year of the pandemic, the Hispanic population experienced a decline in life expectancy at birth, shrinking the group's survival advantage over the white population from over three years to less than one year [3]. As of June 2022, in New York City, at the epicenter of the pandemic, Hispanics exhibited the highest cumulative COVID-19 infection rates (28,025 per 100,000 people) and death rates (871 per 100,000) and the second-highest hospitalization rates (2150 per 100,000 people) among all racial and ethnic groups for whom the city collects data [56]. This is the case even when both Hispanic adults and eligible children in New York City have higher vaccination rates compared to the white and black populations [57]. Currently, at 60.6 million, Hispanics are the largest minority group and the youngest of all racial and ethnic groups, with an average age of 30 in the U.S. These young adults compose disproportionately the largest share of voters, workers, and consumers among Latinos. During the first and peak year of the pandemic, they suffered the highest excess mortality rates of any other racial or ethnic group in the nation [58]. In California, for example, Hispanics ages 20 to 54 were 8.5 times more likely than white Americans to die of COVID-19 [45]. In New Jersey, young Latino men between the ages of 18–49 died at 4.5 times the rate of Latino women and 7 times the rate of white men in the same age category. However, to this date, we lack insights in New York City as to which Hispanic subgroups experienced the worst risks or mortality caused by the COVID-19 pandemic.

On-going qualitative research in New York City by the lead author [4] suggests that Hispanic families in households with mixed immigrant status experienced the worst forms of economic and health vulnerabilities due to COVID-19. Accordingly, living arrangements, family structures, education, and years of residence help explain the higher rates of infection, hospitalization, and deaths in these households. These preliminary insights also suggest that Hispanic women living with a spouse or male partner experienced higher risks of COVID-19 infections and hospitalizations than those who headed home on their own. In addition, emerging COVID-19 literature has argued that, nationally, while women experienced labor market shocks, losing jobs at much higher rates than men, the latter paid a higher price with their lives [41]. An established epidemiological scholarship also documents that while women tend to experience higher comorbidities and a lower quality of health, especially as they age, men tend to develop more chronic illnesses and die sooner. These findings contribute to what has been conceptualized as a gender health paradox [42]. The results have led these and other scholars to advocate for inter-disciplinary studies bridging public health and social sciences scholarships to distinguish the main factors affecting men's and women's health choices, resources, and outcomes. Beyond structural drivers of discrimination, implicit bias by health care providers based on gender, race, ethnicity, and other characteristics is now associated with the exclusion or misdiagnosis of women and those of other minority groups' health conditions [61].

Given the higher than usual COVID-19 death rates among different populations in specific spatial locations, researchers have also emphasized that we pay attention to geography in explaining the higher COVID-19 risks and death rates among the US Hispanic population [3]. This is particularly the case in specific regions where the Hispanic population has traditionally concentrated [5,6,60]. The higher-than-average death rates among Hispanic groups are surprising, as close to four decades of studies have consistently documented the health advantages of foreign-born Hispanics when compared to whites or their native-born counterparts. The phenomenon has been conceptualized as the Hispanic health paradox (HHP) [2,7–10,22]. However, researchers now argue that the COVID-19 pandemic has eroded the health advantage of Hispanics given the higher death rates experienced by the group since the pandemic.

Beyond geography, scholars have also examined the role of structural racism [11], one especially exacerbated by the nesting effects of intersectional inequalities the Hispanic population confronts in the US, such as concentration in low-wage service occupations with higher risk of COVID-19 exposures [6]; limited access to health care services [9] such as vaccinations [6] or preventive care; and the weathering effect of living in highly concentrated, poor, inner-city neighborhood areas [11].

Studies have also shown that the positive correlation observed between death rates and the concentration of Hispanics seems to vanish at the county level when socio-economic characteristics linked to structural racism are controlled [12]. Ample research has documented the role of geography on life expectancy [13,14], the rate of COVID-19 spread [15], and the relation of air pollution concentration to deaths because of COVID-19 [16]. Most significantly, these emerging insights reveal that COVID-19 deaths are linked to spatial location at the county level [17]. However, other studies [17] based on national data at the county level find no spatial correlation between COVID-19 deaths and the Hispanic population. Yet, our analysis of panel data at the level of the unit of metropolitan areas [PUMA] for New York City finds a positive spatial correlation between the Hispanic population's COVID-19 death rate during the peak year of the pandemic. This result is consistent with previous studies, also based in New York City, documenting the correlation between neighborhood characteristics and spatial distribution in determining the health needs of specific groups [18].

Informed by the above scholarship, this paper further examines how structural racism (measured by spatial segregation) and intersectional forms of gendered inequality (measured by family structure, employment, and citizenship status) combine to explain the disproportionally higher rates of COVID-19 deaths among Hispanic groups in New York City during the first and most devastating year of the pandemic. Beyond the analysis of spatial correlations, we document differences in gendered vulnerabilities associated with the risk of Hispanic men and women dying from COVID-19. An important caveat in our study is that once we control for neighborhood (PUMA) characteristics, the positive correlation between the death rate and the Hispanic population vanishes for women but not for men. This result is new and invites further research by gender, spatial stratification, and public health scholars, especially among proponents of the Hispanic health paradox. Our analysis of different subsamples reveals that Hispanic men with a shorter time of residence in the U.S., citizenship status, and health insurance have better health outcomes than those with a longer residence. We interpret the importance of the time spent in the US as proof that the weathering process matters [11] in decreasing the health advantage of Hispanic groups. We also interpret the importance of health insurance and citizenship status as class indicators increasing access to preventive health services, such as vaccination [6].

We perform further analysis focused on women to understand what characteristics of the PUMA data help eliminate the positive correlation between COVID-19 deaths and the Hispanic population share. A separate, ongoing qualitative study by the lead author [4] in New York City suggests that Hispanic immigrant women who import at least one year of higher education and who act as sole heads of household experience lower risks of COVID-19 infection and deaths. Our quantitative analysis reveals that for different subsamples of women, only the inequality variables of the Townsend index explain in all the subsamples the positive correlation between deaths and the Hispanic population. These variables include the share of the Hispanic population that lives in overcrowded households, uses public transportation, is unemployed, has children, and lives in poverty.

This paper is organized as follows: the first part discusses our theoretical considerations of the Hispanic health paradox, structural racism, gender inequality and its relation to health outcomes, and the applicability of this scholarship for framing our findings on the role of spatial segregation and social inequality on the disproportionate death rates observed for the Hispanic population in New York City; the second part of the paper introduces our empirical models used to calculate death differentials for the Hispanic population; the third part presents the data and results of findings; the fourth part presents our discussion and conclusion as well as recommendations for future research.

2. Theoretical Considerations

2.1. The Hispanic Health Paradox

Ample research has documented the health advantage of foreign-born Latinos when compared to the non-Hispanic, native-born population [7–10]. The Hispanic health paradox (HHP), for example, explains the observed higher-than-average life expectancy among the Hispanic population despite their lower-than-average socioeconomic characteristics. It is termed a "paradox" because, despite their lower socioeconomic position, Hispanics, when compared to whites, have better health outcomes on some measures such as mortality, cardiovascular disease, and premature births [19,20] than native-born white groups. The "paradox" is especially pronounced for first-generation immigrants and those from Mexico and parts of Central and South America [21–23].

However, even prior to the coronavirus pandemic, scholars had already noted several health trends challenging the HHP, especially among Mexican Americans. The U.S.'s Mexican American population exhibits higher obesity rates, higher Type 2 diabetes rates, higher absolute increases in the prevalence of diabetes, and much higher mortality rates due to diabetes compared to the white population [24–26]. A recent study [59] in El Paso, Texas, reveals that a high share, or 49.3%, of Hispanic respondents had been previously diagnosed with a high-risk co-morbidity and that this history increased their likelihood of hospitalization or dying from COVID-19-related illnesses. Additional forms of inequalities, such as poverty, homelessness, and the lack of citizenship status and medical insurance, increased these risks. Other research has evidenced that Hispanics in general also exhibit higher rates of disability, lower rates of health insurance, and lower access to quality health care [27,28]. Many of these studies also show that the health advantage of Hispanic immigrants declines significantly the longer they reside in the US, despite increases in socioeconomic status, with middle-class, native-born Hispanics reporting higher risks of non-communicable disorders, such as diabetes and stroke, even when compared to their lower-SES co-ethnics and the white population [14,29]. Beyond our findings' contribution to the revisiting of the Hispanic health paradox, we contribute a new analysis focused on spatial segregation], as a measure of structural racism, to understand the correlation between spatial concentration and health outcomes and explain the determinants of the higher death rates experienced by New York City Hispanics.

2.2. Structural Racism and Health Outcomes

A legacy of structural racism [30] (p. 1457) put in place with the US institutions of slavery and Jim Crow Laws, leading to the institutionalization of racist practices and ideologies, has benefited the life chances of majority white groups at the expense of African Americans, Hispanics, and other people of color in this nation [31]. There is also evidence that, beyond structural inequality resulting from overt racial discrimination, implicit racism, which is harder to measure, combines to negatively affect the quality of health services non-white individuals receive [32,34,61]. Implicit racism has been defined as ethnic or racial bias impacting the behavior of health care providers in the delivery of care. It is not "consciously acknowledged and operates through subtle ways" [33] (p. 44). Although focused mainly on measuring structural racism through spatial segregation, our findings also have implications for the added effect of implicit racism or discrimination in increasing the vulnerabilities of COVID-19 contagion, hospitalization, and deaths for Hispanic groups in specific neighborhood areas of New York City, as our findings will reveal.

2.3. Structural Inequality, Sexism and the Health Outcomes of Women and Men

An established literature has documented that gender discrimination, or sexism, is a significant determinant of lower health outcomes and higher rates of comorbidities for women than for men [49,50] However, most studies focused on explaining discrimination along gender lines are focused on individual effects or aggregates at the group level [50,51]. More recent scholarship has argued that the health discrimination women experience is multilayered and reinforced by institutions such as the labor market, the political system, and even the health care system [49,52]. For example, lower wages and limited access to insurance and gainful employment have proven to negatively impact women's access to quality and timely care delivery, increasing their risk of discrimination within the health care system. Emerging COVID-19-focused research now also documents that intersectional forms of gendered and race-based inequalities combine to impact health, which is defined as "the totality of ways in which societies foster racial discrimination through mutually reinforcing systems of housing, education, employment, earnings, benefits, credit, media, health care, and criminal justice [44,46]. These patterns and practices, in turn, reinforce discriminatory beliefs, values, and the distribution of outcomes of hospitalized COVID-19 patients, with white minority groups experiencing the higher adverse risks [53,58].

A recent U.S. study focused on structural inequality and gendered disparities in health care access and health outcomes [47,49] traces the impact of state sexism on the lower health outcomes of women. Drawing on the national consumer survey of health care access, the scholars find that in states with more widespread access to medical insurance, such as Medicaid, including resources from the Safety Net, women enjoy better health outcomes. Most importantly, structural sexism is a strong predictor of higher rates of morbidity and mortality for women, as in states with higher levels of economic inequality, women and children experience higher rates of mortality [48,50,51]. The opposite is also observed. In states where women experience lower institutional sexism, women have fewer barriers to care and access to more comprehensive health care than men. Drawing on this literature, our paper explores how structural and social intersectional forms of inequalities combine to affect the higher COVID-19 death rates among subgroups of Hispanic men and women in New York City.

2.4. Structural Racism and the Fates of Hispanic Groups during the COVID-19 Pandemic

The higher death rate due to COVID-19 reported among the Hispanic population [3,5,6] has led researchers [2] to conclude that the health advantages the group had enjoyed have been reduced by the ravages of the COVID-19 pandemic and ensuing decimation of the population. However, scholars disagree about the plausible causes. One scholar [11] attributes the higher death rate to structural racism, specifically to three characteristics observed among the Hispanic population: (a) a higher risk of COVID-19 exposure; (b) lower quality of health care and limited access to health insurance; and (c) the negative and cumulative impact of a weathering process with more years of residence and acculturation in the U.S. [8]. Another scholar [6] has argued that the occupations of the Hispanic population and the lower vaccination rates among the group also contribute to higher-than-average death rates. Yet, the qualitative insights of a longitudinal qualitative study by the lead author and her colleague [4] reveal that Hispanic immigrants in New York City have had the highest rate of COVID-19 vaccinations among other groups. Some other authors have shown that the positive correlation observed between COVID-19 death rates and the share of the Hispanic population at the county level vanishes when the socioeconomic characteristics of the county, which are linked to structural racism, are controlled [12]. We further explore this analysis in the paper.

2.5. Spatial Concentration and Death Rates

Studies have documented the existence of spatial concentration patterns in the spread of COVID-19 cases and deaths. One study [15] shows that over time, key nodes of regional concentration and expansion of the disease formed mostly within five metropolitan areas in the continental U.S.: New York, Chicago, Los Angeles, Miami, and Houston. These scholars argue that these five regional nodes formed due to different economic, social, and environmental factors. However, other scholars [16] have shown that deaths concentrated within metropolitan areas are due to the correlation between high pollution and the severity of the COVID-19 disease. Interestingly, among the top metropolitan areas identified as having the highest concentration of Hispanic populations, New York continues to rank among the top cities where Hispanics experience the highest indexes of spatial segregation and inequality [55].

Bronx County, for example, has the largest share of Latinos in New York State [17,55]. In explaining the impact of structural inequality on the higher death rates of U.S. minorities, scholars have analyzed spatial concentration at the Bronx County level. They find a significant correlation between spatial segregation and deaths for non-Hispanic black groups but not a significant correlation between spatial segregation and death rates for Hispanics. However, our more focused analysis of spatial concentration at the neighborhood level in New York City shows that spatial segregation increased the risk of death for Hispanics in the Bronx. We also explore how different forms of gender and class inequality, measured by education, employment, and citizenship, combine to further increase the vulnerability of COVID-19 infections, hospitalizations, and deaths among different Hispanic subgroups.

3. Methodology

As a complete data set that disaggregates deaths by PUMA (Public Use Microdata Areas (PUMAs) are non-overlapping, statistical geographic areas that partition each state or equivalent entity into geographic areas containing no fewer than 100,000 people each) by race and ethnicity is not available, researchers have looked at the correlation between specific population shares and the total number of deaths [12,35,36]. In this paper, we follow the approach of McLaren [12] to indirectly estimate the differential mortality ratio between Hispanics and the rest of the population. The estimation of this mortality differential is the first objective of this paper. The method consists of estimating the partial correlation between total deaths and the Hispanic population, as shown in Equation (1):

$$D_i = \beta_0 + \beta_1 hispanic_i + u_i \tag{1}$$

where D_i represents deaths at PUMA i; $hispanic_i$ represents the share of Hispanic population in PUMA i; u_i represents the usual error term; and β_1 represents the correlation between deaths at PUMA level and the Hispanic population share. Following [12], define the weighted average deaths in PUMA i by Equation (2):

$$D_i = hispanic_i d_{h,i} + (1 - hispanic_i) d_{-h,i} \tag{2}$$

where $d_{h,i}$ represents deaths among Hispanics in PUMA i, and $d_{-h,i}$ represents deaths among the rest of the population in PUMA i.

Differentiating Equations (1) and (2) with respect to $hispanic_i$

$$\frac{dD_i}{dhispanic_i} = \beta_1 \tag{3}$$

$$\frac{dD_i}{dhispanic_i} = d_{hispanic,i} - d_{-hispanic,i} \tag{4}$$

Which implies that:

$$\beta_1 = d_{h,i} - d_{-h,i} = \Delta_h^* \tag{5}$$

Δ_h^* is the death mortality differential for the Hispanic population. If $\beta_1 > 0$, the Hispanic population has a higher mortality ratio than the rest of the population. Studies usually introduce variables that can measure structural racism. If the mortality differential does not disappear, then the residual differential is not explained by structural racism [11,34]. If $\beta_1 < 0$, we would argue that the Hispanic population has a lower death prevalence, which is explained by the Hispanic health paradox [8–10].

Equation (1) suffers from biases generated by a model that is not well specified because of the nature of the data and the existence of more covariates. Consequently, we include more control variables that could explain the mortality differentials, taking into consideration the nature of the data. Given the panel data structure of our data for deaths and the cross-section nature of the data on the PUMA characteristics, we estimate a random effect estimation on the change in death rate by PUMA:

$$\Delta D_{it} = \beta_0 + \beta_1 hispanic_i + \sum_{k=1}^{K} \gamma_i X_{ik} + u_{it} \tag{6}$$

where X_{ik} represents control variable k. As control variables, we include the share of the population with some college or more education, the share of the population with high school completed, the share of the population working in 13 specified occupation categories, the median household income, the share of the insured population, the share of the population that drives to work, the share of the unemployed population, the share of the population that rents, the share of overcrowded households, and the fraction of households with child poverty. These variables are linked to structural racism [12] and the Townsend Index [36,43], a deprivation index that has been found to be correlated with geographic areas with high health problems [35]. This specification has the advantage of eliminating any potential time trend existing in the death rate.

Equation (7) shows a second specification where we exploit the spatial distribution of the data to consider the potential spatial distribution of deaths [15,16]. Specifically,

$$\Delta D_{it} = \beta_0 + X_i\beta + \overline{X}_i\gamma + \lambda W \Delta D_{it} + \rho M u_i + \epsilon_{it} \tag{7}$$

where X_i includes all control variables and the Hispanic population, $\overline{X}_i$ includes the spatial lags for control variables, W and M are spatial weighting matrices, and λ and ρ are scalar parameters. In this specification, each variable is said to have a direct and an indirect effect. Direct effects refer to impacts that are not linked to spatial correlation, while indirect effects are linked to the different sources of spatial correlation that are present in Equation (7).

Exploiting the spatial panel nature of the data has certain advantages over an OLS estimation. First, by considering the spatial correlation, we obtain a better estimation than the one offered by OLS. Second, the spatial specification allows us to obtain direct and indirect effects, which allows the determination of the importance of spatial correlations in determining the effects of each variable.

The second analytical objective of this paper is to obtain gendered estimations for Equations (1), (6), and (7). The data on deaths is aggregated; consequently, we cannot separate it by gender. The data at the PUMA level, however, comes from the American community survey (ACS) and allows for the calculation of characteristics by gender by aggregating the PUMA characteristics only for the population of adult men and women, respectively.

A third objective of the paper is to further analyze the origins of the results. We will do so by generating different subsamples at the PUMA level, which will allow us to do a comparison of the estimations of Equations (1), (6), and (7) for the different partitions of the data. The analysis is explained fully in Section 4.4.

4. Results

4.1. Data Sources

Zip code data on mortality comes from New York City health [NYCH], which provides COVID-19 cases and deaths by zip code [37]. The data was collected for the months of November 2020 through June 2021. Data was transformed to PUMA level using a cross walk available from Baruch College's Newman Library [38].

As Figure 1 shows, the average death rate by PUMA for the period of November 2020 to June 2021 shows a positive spatial correlation with the Hispanic population in New York City. The dark blue areas indicate a higher concentration of the Hispanic population, with the highest share concentrated in the Bronx and Queens, where death rates for the group have been highest. Our analysis shows that this correlation is statistically significant at the 1 percent level with a chi squared of 10.81 and with 1 degree of freedom.

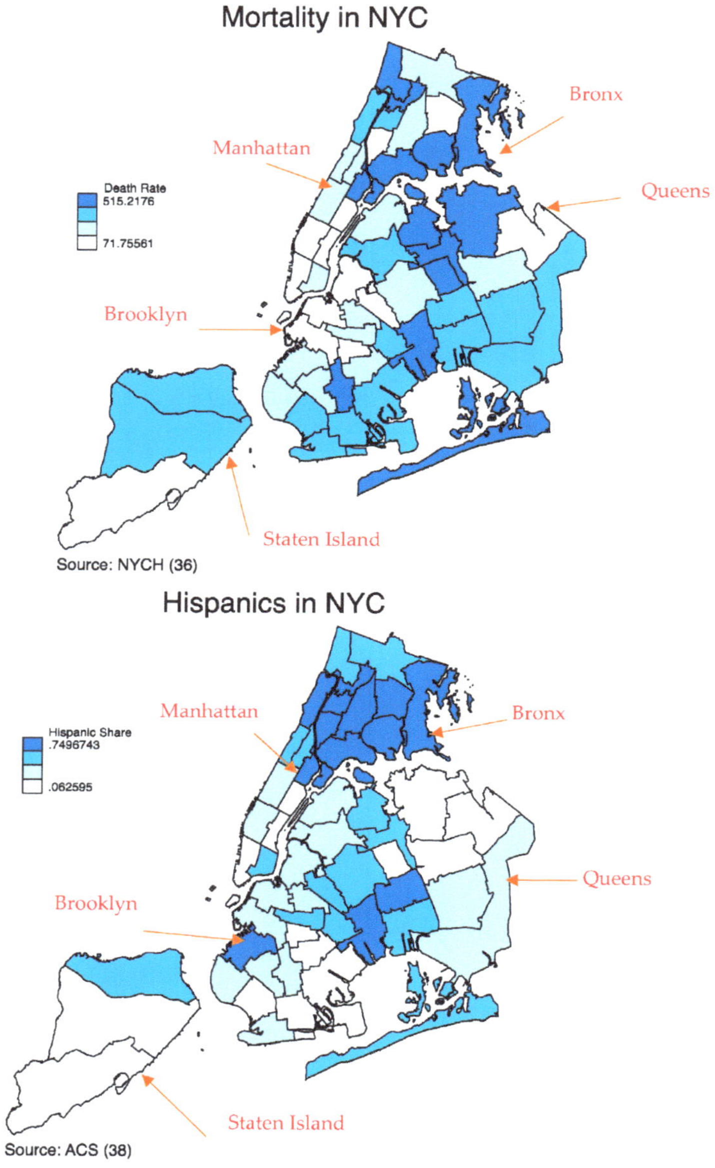

Figure 1. Source: Own calculations with data from NYCH [37] and ACS [39].

The significance of the spatial correlation contrasts with results reported by Saffary et al. [17] at the county level for the entire US, since they report that the spatial correlation between county COVID-19 death rate and Hispanic population is not significant.

Table 1 shows the average death rate per PUMA for the period beginning in November 2020 and ending in June 2021. It clearly shows a positive increase in the death rate during the specified time period.

Table 1. COVID-19 Death rate in 55 NYC PUMAs.

Period	Mean	S.E.
November 2020	186	78
December 2020	186	78
January 2021	195	79
February 2021	216	86
March 2021	236	92
April 2021	253	97
May 2021	263	100
June 2021	267	102

Source: own estimations based on [37].

The data for the Hispanic population was obtained from the 2019 American community survey (ACS) 5-year sample obtained from Public Use Microdata Areas (PUMAS) [39]. The data selected were men and women 18 years of age and older. Table 2 shows the average values for the different variables obtained from this source. In particular, the median income in 2019 was USD 29,000, the Hispanic population was 20% of the population, 56% of the population have high school or more education, 22% of the population have college or more education, 92% of the population have health insurance, 26% of the working-age population drive to work, 3.7% of the population are unemployed, 12% of the population have an occupation in management related activities, 3.9% have an occupation in computer-related activities, 11% of the population have activities related to education, 3.9% of the population have activities related to health services, 14.2% of the population work in other service occupations, 7% of the population work in sales, 8.7% work in offices, 0.1% in farming, 2.8% in construction, 1.4% in installation, 2.3% in production, 4.6% work in transportation, and 0.1% in the military. The table also shows that 45% of the population rents, 75% live in overcrowded conditions or have more than one individual per room, and 21% of households have children living below or at the poverty line.

Table 2. Mean values for selected variables.

	Mean	S.E.
Median income	29,746	14,486
	Shares	
Hispanic	20.4%	15.1%
High School completed	56.1%	12.8%
College or more	22.4%	7.3%
Health Insurance	92.5%	2.9%
Drive to work	26.6%	13.3%
Unemployed	3.7%	0.9%
Management	11.8%	5.7%
Computers	3.9%	1.6%
Education	11.0%	3.9%
Health	3.9%	1.2%
Services	14.2%	4.2%
Sales	7.0%	1.1%
Office	8.7%	1.4%
Farming	0.1%	0.1%
Construction	2.8%	1.2%
Installation	1.4%	0.6%
Production	2.3%	1.1%
Transportation	4.6%	1.7%
Military	0.1%	0.4%
Rent	45.3%	15.0%
Overcrowded	74.8%	8.1%
Child poverty	21.0%	9.3%

Source: 5-year public sample, 2019 American Community Survey (ACS) [39].

4.2. Random Panel Estimation for Monthly Death Rates

Table 3 presents the estimations for Equations (2), (6), and (7). In the three equations, we use the change in the logarithm of the death rate as the dependent variable. Column (1) in Table 3 shows a negative correlation between the change in the COVID-19 death rate and the Hispanic population. This result has the opposite sign from that explained in the previous section. This shows that the positive correlation between deaths and the Hispanic population exists at certain levels, but at the first difference, the correlation becomes negative, which is consistent with the predictions advanced by the Hispanic health paradox for the group. This result, however, is not robust to the inclusion of the characteristics of the PUMAs, or to the spatially correlated terms. These results imply that when we control for structural racism (based on the characteristics of the PUMAs), no correlation is found between deaths and the Hispanic population.

Table 3. Results for RE and spatial RE models. NYC PUMAs, November 2020–June 2021.

Model	RE Model	RE Model	Spatial RE Model		
			Direct Effect	Indirect Effect	Total Effect
Hispanic	−0.03 *	0.06	0.24	2.14	2.39
	[0.015]	[0.04]	[0.16]	[2.07]	[2.22]
Median income		-4.4×10^{-7}	2.4×10^{-7}	-3.3×10^{-6}	-3×10^{-6}
		[7.5×10^{-7}]	[3.8×10^{-6}]	[3.8×10^{-5}]	[4.2×10^{-5}]
High School completed		−0.15	−0.75 **	−5.68	−6.42
		[0.13]	[0.37]	[3.82]	[4.16]
College or more		0.13	1.04 *	9.80	10.84
		[0.19]	[0.58]	[6.46]	[7.01]
Health Insurance		−0.25	−1.09 ***	−5.20	−6.29 *
		[0.21]	[0.41]	[3.46]	[3.83]
Drive to work		−0.14 **	−0.45 **	−5.13 *	−5.58 *
		[0.07]	[0.20]	[3.16]	[3.34]
Unemployed		−0.09	1.27	11.52	12.79
		[0.52]	[2.56]	[19.04]	[21.49]
Management		−0.18	−0.84	−6.42	−7.26
		[0.30]	[1.12]	[10.48]	[11.54]
Computers		0.46	1.62	13.41	15.03
		[0.55]	[2.13]	[20.21]	[22.27]
Education		−0.26	−0.11	0.96	0.84
		[0.17]	[0.29]	[2.74]	[2.95]
Health		−0.79 *	0.01	22.57	22.57
		[0.47]	[1.68]	[20.64]	[22.26]
Services		−0.22	−0.13	−0.03	−0.17
		[0.20]	[0.47]	[3.99]	[4.44]
Sales		−0.42	−1.56	4.83	3.28
		[0.43]	[1.26]	[12.71]	[13.79]
Office		0.31	0.22	2.71	2.93
		[0.32]	[0.76]	[8.41]	[9.11]
Farming		0.23	16.62	201.52	218.14
		[4.41]	[15.21]	[157.51]	[171.83]
Construction		−1.09 *	−4.03 **	−23.12	−27.15
		[0.59]	[2.09]	[18.13]	[20.14]
Installation		−1.68	−4.87	−31.74	−36.62
		[1.20]	[4.32]	[41.02]	[45.11]

Table 3. *Cont.*

Model	RE Model	RE Model	Spatial RE Model		
			Direct Effect	Indirect Effect	Total Effect
Production		−0.05	0.40	4.94	5.34
		[0.85]	[2.90]	[27.34]	[30.00]
Transportation		−0.42	−0.27	4.56	4.29
		[0.51]	[1.54]	[13.94]	[15.20]
Military		0.97	1.09	3.94	5.03
		[0.64]	[1.59]	[14.91]	[16.33]
Rent		−0.10 *	−0.33 **	−3.06 *	−3.40 *
		[0.06]	[0.15]	[1.82]	[1.95]
Overcrowded		0.11	0.55 *	3.14	3.69
		[0.07]	[0.32]	[3.39]	[3.70]
Child poverty		−0.18 **	−0.40	−1.34	−1.74
		[0.09]	[0.41]	[3.31]	[3.71]
Constant	0.06 ***	0.54	Na	Na	Na
	[0.004]	[0.28]			
N	385	385		385	
Pseudo R2	1%	8.40%		12.64%	

*** Significant at 1%, ** Significant at 5%, * Significant at 10%. Source: own calculations with data from [37,39].

Table 3 also shows in Column (2) that in the random effect estimation, a negative correlation is found between the share of individuals that drive to work and deaths, which is expected given that people driving to work would maintain social distance. Table 3 also shows a negative correlation between the share of individuals that work in health services and death rates, which probably shows that individuals in the health industry were more aware of taking measures to avoid infections. Table 3 shows a negative correlation between the share of individuals working in construction and deaths, probably because individuals working in construction stop working and therefore avoid risks. Table 3 also shows a negative relationship between people who rent and deaths, probably showing that houses under rent had better conditions that avoided infection risks, such as lower levels of overcrowding. Finally, PUMAs with a larger share of children living in poverty show a negative correlation with the death rate, perhaps because in households with younger individuals, there were fewer deaths or because individuals in these households were forced to remain at home to take care of small or school-age children when schools closed or transitioned to online education, reducing the risk of COVID-19 contagion.

Columns (3), (4), and (5) in Table 3 show the results for the spatial random effect model. They show the direct, indirect, and total effects estimated for each variable. This model shows different results as compared to the random effect model. Now, the share of individuals with high school or more years of education has a direct negative effect on deaths. No indirect effect or total effect is found. This result probably shows that individuals with high school or higher education were less exposed to the disease, had access to resources, including vaccines, or had the education to obtain information about timely prevention.

Table 3 shows that having a college education or more has a positive direct effect on deaths, while no indirect or total effect is found to be significant. This result shows that, on average, Hispanics with a college education or more were more exposed to the disease, as these individuals' jobs probably required more social or direct interactions with the public or people they serve. This result is correlated with the qualitative findings from ongoing research conducted by the lead author and her colleague in New York City [4].

Table 3 shows that the share of the population with health insurance is negatively correlated with deaths in both direct and total effects. No indirect effect is found. This result is important and in line with Garcia et al. [11], who find that structural racism explains the disproportionate impact of the COVID-19 pandemic on black and Latinx people since the lower availability of health insurance among the Hispanic population is mentioned as a risk factor.

Table 3 also shows that the share of the population that drives to work has direct, indirect, and total negative effects, illustrating the importance of social distancing for avoiding infections and deaths. Table 3 also captures a negative direct effect for the share of the population that works in construction, but no indirect or total effect is found. The result indicates that individuals working in this sector probably were laid off or lost their jobs as the industry closed and consequently avoided risks of infections and deaths.

Table 3 shows that the share of individuals who rent has a negative direct, indirect, and total effect. This probably shows that the housing conditions for individuals in rented housing were more protective of infections and deaths. However, individuals living in overcrowded households showed a positive direct effect but not an indirect or total effect associated with deaths. This shows that individuals in overcrowded households had more difficulty avoiding infections or keeping social distance.

4.3. Estimations for Men and Women

Table 4 presents estimations for men and women. We first look at the positive correlation that exists between the level of COVID-19 deaths and Hispanic men, which indicates that they have 0.78 more deaths than the non-Hispanic male population. In the case of women, the excess death rate is 0.72. Once we introduce the spatial correlation, we can see that the positive direct effect of being Hispanic and male is 1.13, while the indirect effect is −1.08. The total effect is not very significant. These results imply evidence of both implicit and structural discrimination, while the effect of the spatial correlation is factually positive. This result is consistent with other findings showing that spatial concentration in New York City somehow mediated the ability of some Hispanic individuals to combat the pandemic [40]. For women, the direct effect of spatial concentration is 1.15, almost identical to the effect observed for men. The indirect effect of spatial concentration is −1.20, which is larger than the effect observed for men. The total effect of spatial concentration we find to be negative and insignificant in explaining COVID-19's higher death rates. In fact, our findings suggest that women benefit more from living in segregated or concentrated neighborhood areas than men, and this deserves further research by spatial stratification, poverty, and public health scholars.

Table 4. Excess deaths for Hispanics, spatial correlation, and gendered effects.

	Direct Effect	Indirect Effect	Total Effect
	No controls, no spatial correlation, levels		
Men	N/A	N/A	0.78 **
			[0.36]
Women	N/A	N/A	0.72 **
			[0.36]
	With no controls, only spatial correlation, levels		
Men	1.13 ***	−1.08 *	0.06
	[0.42]	[0.62]	[0.52]
Women	1.15 ***	−1.20 **	−0.04
	[0.42]	[0.61]	[0.50]
	With controls, spatial correlation, changes		
Men	0.26 **	1.44	1.70
	[0.11]	[1.29]	[1.39]
Women	−0.07	−0.13	−0.19
	[0.12]	[1.72]	[1.83]

Source: own calculations with data from [37,39]. *** Significant at 1%, ** Significant at 5%, * Significant at 10%.

Table 4 also shows that once we introduce the PUMA characteristics, for men, the direct effect of spatial concentration is 0.26, while the indirect effect and the total effect are not significant. This would imply that after controlling for spatial concentration or structural racism, Hispanic men still observe an excess death of 0.26, which evidences that the higher risk of dying for Hispanic males is also explained by implicit bias. In the case of women, after controlling for the characteristics of the PUMA, the direct, indirect, and total effects remain all non-significant in explaining COVID-19's higher death rates. This is consistent with an earlier study [12] that found that after controlling for characteristics, there was no evidence of implicit bias for Hispanics. However, our result finds that such a result holds only for Hispanic women but not for men.

4.4. Using Different Hispanic Subsamples: Time in the U.S., Citizenship, Employment Status, Health Insurance, Never Married, and Heads of Household

In this section, we show the results of generating further analysis among subsamples of Hispanic groups to identify potential explanations for the different levels of intersectional vulnerabilities that combined to differently increase the death rates of Hispanic men and women in New York City. The analysis uses years of residence as a proxy for nativity or for the correlation between the weathering effect or reduction of protective health factors associated with nativity or with acculturation to the US's culture [8].

Time in the U.S. and Citizenship: Table 5 looks at subsamples generated for individuals who arrived in the U.S. since the year 2000 and for individuals who are also U.S. citizens. The first variable measures if the time spent in the U.S. is linked to mortality results, given the importance of the weathering process [11]. The weathering hypothesis implies that health outcomes should deteriorate the longer Hispanics reside in the U.S. In the case of citizenship, the argument is that it should be positively related to better health outcomes. Table 5 shows that for the two subsamples, the positive correlation between deaths and the Hispanic population is observed at the same levels for men and women. When the spatial correlation is considered, the direct effect is positive for both men and women, and the indirect effect is negative. The total effect is non-significant. If we control for the characteristics of the PUMA, no significant correlation between deaths and the Hispanic population is observed for either men or women. This would imply that the characteristics of the PUMA, and consequently of spatial concentration or structural racism, explain the excess deaths of Hispanic men and women. Considering that for the entire sample of men, we did find a positive correlation between deaths and the Hispanic population, this result would imply that individuals that have less time in the U.S. and that are citizens have better health outcomes, which consequently shows that the weathering hypothesis applies [11] and that citizenship matters. This second aspect may indicate that a vulnerable immigrant status or lack of legal documentation also negatively impacts access to preventive care for individuals living in New York City, perhaps due to a fear of apprehension in the search for medical care.

Table 5. Excess deaths for Hispanics, spatial correlation, and gendered effects.

	Recently Arrived Immigrants			**Citizens**		
	Direct Effect	**Indirect Effect**	**Total Effect**	**Direct Effect**	**Indirect Effect**	**Total Effect**
	No controls, no spatial correlation, levels					
Men	N/A	N/A	0.61 **	N/A	N/A	0.79 **
			[0.30]			[0.39]
Women	N/A	N/A	0.54 *	N/A	N/A	0.73 **
			[0.30]			[0.38]
	With no controls, only spatial correlation, levels					
Men	0.80 **	−0.65	0.16	1.21 ***	−1.24 *	−0.04
	[0.35]	[0.51]	[0.42]	[0.46]	[0.67]	[0.56]
Women	1.10 ***	−1.15 **	−0.06	1.20 ***	−1.33 **	−0.13
	[0.42]	[0.59]	[0.44]	[0.44]	[0.64]	[0.53]
	With controls, spatial correlation, changes					
Men	−0.10	−0.28	−0.38	0.17	0.56	0.73
	[0.11]	[0.86]	[0.97]	[0.13]	[1.41]	[1.52]
Women	0.10	0.75	0.84	−0.03	−0.32	−0.36
	[0.08]	[0.79]	[0.86]	[0.11]	[1.32]	[1.42]

Source: own calculations with data from [37,39]. *** Significant at 1%, ** Significant at 5%, * Significant at 10%.

Employment and Health Insurance: Table 6 presents results for subsamples of individuals that are employed and also those with health insurance. In the case of employed individuals, the argument is that their higher exposure to the virus may deteriorate their health status [6,11]. In the case of individuals with health insurance, access to health services may explain better health outcomes [11]. Table 6 shows that there is a positive correlation between deaths and the Hispanic population for both men and women included in these subsamples. Controlling for spatial correlation renders a positive direct effect, while a negative indirect effect is found. If we control for the PUMA characteristics, in the case of the subsample individuals that are male and employed, we observe a positive correlation between deaths and the Hispanic population. The direct, indirect, and total effects are found to be significant and positive. This would imply that employment alone cannot explain the positive correlation between deaths and the Hispanic population.

Table 6. Excess deaths for Hispanics, spatial correlation, and gendered effects.

	Employed Individuals			Individuals with Health Insurance		
	Direct Effect	Indirect Effect	Total Effect	Direct Effect	Indirect Effect	Total Effect
	No controls, no spatial correlation, levels					
Men	na	na	0.78 **	Na	na	0.78 **
			[0.34]			[0.37]
Women	na	na	0.75 **	Na	na	0.73 **
			[0.34]			[0.36]
	With no controls, only spatial correlation, levels					
Men	1.03 ***	−0.81	0.22	1.46 **	−1.51 **	−0.06
	[0.40]	[0.57]	[0.47]	[0.48]	[0.69]	[0.55]
Women	1.13 ***	−1.00 *	0.13	1.49 **	−1.60 **	−0.12
	[0.44]	[0.60]	[0.47]	[0.48]	[0.67]	[0.53]
	With controls, spatial correlation, changes					
Men	0.28 ***	1.78 *	2.06 **	0.22	0.94	1.16
	[0.08]	[0.92]	[0.99]	[0.14]	[1.58]	[1.72]
Women	−0.03	−0.38	−0.41	−0.06	−0.70	−0.76
	[0.12]	[1.13]	[1.25]	[0.09]	[1.31]	[1.39]

Source: own calculations with data from [37,39]. *** Significant at 1%, ** Significant at 5%, * Significant at 10%.

In the case of individuals with health insurance, once we control for the PUMA characteristics, the correlation between deaths and the Hispanic population vanishes. This would imply that individuals with access to health insurance have better health outcomes. In the case of Hispanic women, once we control for PUMA characteristics, the positive correlation vanishes. These results corroborate emerging labor market research showing that the ravages of the pandemic led men to lose their lives, while women mostly lost their jobs, as many of these jobs concentrated in the 'care' or low-wage service industry, with higher levels of interaction with the public, leading to higher unemployment rates among women than men [41], and consequently, lower risks of COVID-19 infections and deaths.

Family Structure and Gendered Effects: Table 7 presents results for subsamples of individuals that have never married and that are single, as well as for individuals that are heads of households. Single individuals may have a higher risk of exposure, assuming they face more barriers to keeping social distance. Heads of households may have a lower risk of exposure, assuming they delegate who gets to carry out errands. Table 7 illustrates that for the two gender subsamples, there is a positive correlation between the level of deaths and the Hispanic population, both for men and women. If we control for spatial correlation, the direct effect is positive, while the indirect effect is negative. If we control for PUMA characteristics for the subsample of never-married men, we find that the direct and indirect effects are positive, as is the total effect. This would imply that marital status cannot explain the positive correlation observed between deaths and the Hispanic population. In the case of the sample of male heads of households, the direct effect is found to be statistically significant. This would imply that household headship alone would not explain the positive correlation observed between COVID-19 deaths and the Hispanic population. In the case of women, once we control for PUMA characteristics, the positive correlation vanishes.

Table 7. Excess deaths for Hispanics, spatial correlation, and gendered effects.

	Never Married/Single Individuals			Only Heads of Household		
	Direct Effect	Indirect Effect	Total Effect	Direct Effect	Indirect Effect	Total Effect
	No controls, no spatial correlation, levels					
Men	N/A	N/A	0.78 **	N/A	N/A	0.83 **
			[0.36]			[0.39]
Women	N/A	N/A	0.73 **	N/A	N/A	0.70 **
			[0.35]			[0.36]
	With no controls, only spatial correlation, levels					
Men	1.21 ***	−1.07 *	0.14	1.38 ***	−1.38 **	−0.005
	[0.45]	[0.63]	[0.49]	[0.48]	[0.70]	[0.59]
Women	1.21 ***	−1.08 *	0.13	1.52 ***	−1.75 ***	−0.24
	[0.47]	[0.63]	[0.47]	[0.47]	[0.67]	[0.53]
	With controls, spatial correlation, changes					
Men	0.34 ***	3.18 **	3.52 ***	0.16 *	0.69	0.85
	[0.10]	[1.29]	[1.38]	[0.10]	[0.96]	[1.04]
Women	0.09	1.36	1.45	−0.13	−0.97	−1.10
	[0.12]	[1.32]	[1.43]	[0.10]	[0.95]	[1.05]

Source: own calculations with data from [37,39]. *** Significant at 1%, ** Significant at 5%, * Significant at 10%.

Age and Weathering Effects: Table 8 presents estimations based on a comparison by age for two different Hispanic subsamples. The first subsample comprises younger individuals, between 18 and 35 years old, while the second includes older individuals, between 36 and 53 years old. According to the weathering process hypothesis [11], younger individuals should experience better health outcomes than individuals with more time in the US, which in principle should be observed among medium-aged individuals. On the other hand, if younger individuals are more likely to be undocumented, they may concentrate in jobs with higher risks of exposure [6,11] or have lower access to health insurance [11]. Table 8 shows that a positive correlation is found at levels between the Hispanic population and deaths, both for men and women. Once we control for spatial correlation, the direct effect is found to be significant, the indirect effect is negative, and the total effect is non-significant. This would imply that spatial concentration actually helps reduce the impact of the pandemic [40]. If we control for PUMA characteristics and differentiate the data, for young men, a positive total effect is found, while for young women, the correlation vanishes. In the case of middle-aged men, the correlation vanished, while for medium-aged women, the correlation became negative, confirming the prediction of the weathering effects, which are foundational for proponents of the Hispanic Health Paradox.

Table 8. Excess deaths for Hispanics by age, spatial correlation, and gendered effects.

	Young Adults (18 to 35 Years Old)			Medium Age Adults (36 to 53 Years Old)		
	Direct Effect	Indirect Effect	Total Effect	Direct Effect	Indirect Effect	Total Effect
	No controls, no spatial correlation, levels					
Men	N/A	N/A	0.75 **	N/A	N/A	0.81 **
			[0.33]			[0.35]
Women	N/A	N/A	0.72 **	N/A	N/A	0.71 **
			[0.33]			[0.33]
	With no controls, only spatial correlation, levels					
Men	1.11 ***	−0.92 *	0.19	1.11 ***	−0.92	0.18
	[0.41]	[0.55]	[0.43]	[0.41]	[0.57]	[0.48]
Women	1.18 ***	−1.03 *	0.14	1.11 ***	−1.08 **	.03
	[0.43]	[0.57]	[0.42]	[0.39]	[0.55]	[0.45]

Table 8. *Cont.*

	Young Adults (18 to 35 Years Old)			Medium Age Adults (36 to 53 Years Old)		
	Direct Effect	**Indirect Effect**	**Total Effect**	**Direct Effect**	**Indirect Effect**	**Total Effect**
	With controls, spatial correlation, changes					
Men	0.19 ***	1.36	1.55 *	0.03	0.19	0.23
	[0.07]	[0.87]	[0.94]	[0.05]	[0.51]	[0.56]
Women	0.002	−0.05	−0.05	−0.23 ***	−1.93 *	−2.17 **
	[0.06]	[0.55]	[0.60]	[0.09]	[1.05]	[1.13]

Source: own calculations with data from [37,39]. *** Significant at 1%, ** Significant at 5%, * Significant at 10%.

4.5. Using Less Control Variables for Women

Table 9 presents estimations for the different subsamples of women, using less control variables than those used in Tables 5–7.

Table 9. Excess deaths for Hispanic women, spatial correlation for different subsamples, and control variables.

	Direct Effect	Indirect Effect	Total Effect	Direct Effect	Indirect Effect	Total Effect	Direct Effect	Indirect Effect	Total Effect
	Full Sample				Employed			Citizens	
Occupations	0.003	0.64 **	0.65 **	0.01	0.44	0.45	−0.02	0.20 ***	0.18 ***
	[0.03]	[0.31]	[0.33]	[0.04]	[0.30]	[0.32]	[0.02]	[0.06]	[0.06]
Median income	−0.02	−0.02	−0.04	0.002	−0.17 *	−0.16	−0.01	−0.03	−0.04
	[0.02]	[0.03]	[0.03]	[0.02]	[0.10]	[0.10]	[0.02]	[0.03]	[0.03]
Education	−0.01	−0.07	−0.08	−0.004	−0.08	−0.08	−0.002	−0.05	−0.05
	[0.02]	[0.11]	[0.12]	[0.02]	[0.11]	[0.12]	[0.02]	[0.12]	[0.13]
Townsend index	0.03	0.02	0.05	0.03	−0.11	−0.08	0.03	−0.08	−0.05
	[0.03]	[0.22]	[0.24]	[0.03]	[0.19]	[0.21]	[0.03]	[0.17]	[0.19]
	Recently arrived migrants				Health Insurance			Never Married/Single	
Occupations	−0.03	0.24	0.21	0.01	0.45 *	0.46 *	0.04	0.07	0.11
	[0.03]	[0.25]	[0.27]	[0.03]	[0.25]	[0.27]	[0.03]	[0.16]	[0.18]
Median income	−0.05 ***	−0.01	−0.06 ***	−0.02	−0.02	−0.04	−0.02	−0.02	−0.04
	[0.02]	[0.02]	[0.02]	[0.02]	[0.03]	[0.03]	[0.02]	[0.03]	[0.03]
Education	−0.03 *	−0.09	−0.12	−0.01	−0.07	−0.08	−0.004	−0.03	−0.03
	[0.02]	[0.07]	[0.08]	[0.02]	[0.11]	[0.12]	[0.02]	[0.11]	[0.12]
Townsend index	−0.01	0.09	0.08	0.04	−0.04	0.002	0.02	−0.09	−0.07
	[0.02]	[0.13]	[0.14]	[0.03]	[0.17]	[0.18]	[0.02]	[0.14]	[0.15]
	Heads of household								
Occupations	−0.01	0.16	0.15						
	[0.03]	[0.20]	[0.22]						
Median income	0.01	−0.20 *	−0.19						
	[0.02]	[0.12]	[0.12]						
Education	−0.01	−0.09	−0.10						
	[0.02]	[0.10]	[0.11]						
Townsend index	0.03	0.03	0.06						
	[0.03]	[0.17]	[0.19]						

Source: own calculations with data from [37,39]. *** Significant at 1%. ** Significant at 5%. * Significant at 10%.

Additionally, for the full sample of women, Table 9 shows that controlling for occupations is not enough to explain the positive correlation between deaths and the Hispanic population. On the contrary, median income, education, and the variables of the Townsend index are enough to explain by themselves the positive correlation between COVID-19 deaths and the Hispanic population. Similar findings are observed for the subsample of women with health insurance and the subsample of citizens. For the subsample of recently arrived women, neither median income nor education can explain the positive correlation between deaths and the Hispanic population. Only occupations and the variables of the Townsend index can explain this positive correlation. For the subsample of heads of household that are women and employed, median income cannot explain the positive correlation between deaths and the Hispanic population. However, occupations, education, and the variables of the Townsend index can explain the effect of structural racism.

For the subsample of women who are never married and single, the occupations, the median income, the education, and the variables of the Townsend index can explain structural racism. These results imply that these women have better health outcomes and that structural racism can be explained by almost any of the PUMA characteristics.

5. Discussion

This paper studies the relationship between death rates at the PUMA level and the Hispanic population of New York City. Our census-based analysis confirms results by other scholars [3,60] documenting a positive correlation between COVID-19 death rates and the share of the New York City population that is Hispanic. Our analysis further shows that the death rate is spatially correlated with the Hispanic population, which offers a new and more varied understanding than is provided by earlier studies [12,17]. In addition, when we control for PUMA neighborhood characteristics on death rates, the positive correlation between Hispanic population and death rates vanishes for women but not for men. The first result confirms findings by McLaren [12], while the second gendered result for women is new. This implies that in neighborhoods with a high concentration of Hispanic population, women may experience higher protective factors that decrease the risks of dying from COVID-19, while we did not observe this for men. Some of these factors may be mediated by women's access to more diverse networks among people with longer tenure in the US or within local or mainstream institutions, such as schools and migrant-servicing agencies. This in turn increases access to health-preventive information or even access to the safety net.

Different subsamples of Hispanic individuals from different age groups confirm the results of our analysis for women. In fact, for medium-aged women, we find evidence of the Hispanic Health Paradox, since a negative correlation between deaths and the Hispanic population is found among individuals with longer tenure in the U.S. In the case of men, individuals with less time residing in the U.S., access to medical insurance, and U.S. citizenship tend to have better health outcomes than those with more years of residence in the U.S. These results substantiate earlier studies [4,11], except for our finding about the higher risk of death for young Hispanic men, which is a new finding in the literature. This may be due to younger men being more likely to live in neighborhood areas with higher population concentration, which exert greater traditional expectations on them as providers; or these men may be concentrated in jobs with higher exposure or less protective factors, such as access to health insurance. These risks translate to higher COVID-19 vulnerabilities for younger or immigrant males in more recent cohorts.

In the case of women, different specifications of the model are analyzed for the different subsamples. We find that in all subsamples, the variables of the Townsend index explain the positive correlation between deaths and the Hispanic population, which confirms results found by McLaren [12] and other scholars in other geographic areas where the Hispanic population concentrates [60]. In the case of the occupations, we find that they can explain the positive correlation between subsamples of women that are recent immigrants, heads of households, employed, and never married/single, which confirm results found by García et al. [11] and Riley et al. [6]. The median income can explain the positive correlation between deaths and the Hispanic population for those with citizenship status, for women with health insurance, and for those never married/single, confirming results by EDQ [40]. The variables for education can explain the positive correlation between deaths and the Hispanic population in the case of heads of household, women who are employed, have health insurance, are citizens, and those never married/single, confirming results by EDQ [40]. These results also imply that women who have never married and are single are over-represented among the subsample of Hispanic individuals with better health outcomes. These results confirm those by Fuentes and Kucheva [4].

6. Conclusions

The first objective of this paper was to estimate the correlation between deaths caused by COVID-19 and the Hispanic population. If the estimation is performed at neighborhood levels, our results show a positive correlation between deaths and the Hispanic population, revealing a larger death rate among the Hispanic population when compared with the rest of the population of New York City. If the estimation is performed among subgroups, we obtain a negative correlation between deaths and the Hispanic population, substantiating the predictions of the Hispanic Health Paradox. If we control for spatial correlation effects and variables related to structural racism, the correlation between deaths and the Hispanic population vanishes.

The second objective of the paper is to estimate the correlation between deaths and the Hispanic population separately for men and women, controlling for the gendered characteristics of the PUMA. The results show that the same results obtained for the entire sample are obtained for women, while for men, we find a positive direct effect that is offset by the indirect effects of spatial correlation, rendering a non-significant total effect. For men, four elements are found to negatively affect their health in the U.S.: (1) the time spent in the U.S.; (2) their employment status; (3) their civil status or never married/single, and (4) their young age. Three elements are found to positively affect health outcomes: (1) US citizenship, (2) access to health insurance, and (3) being of medium age. In the case of women, only the characteristic being of medium age is found to positively affect the health status of individuals. In all other cases, the control variables linked to structural racism explain the positive correlation observed at different levels.

These findings reveal that women, despite suffering infections from COVID-19, had lower death rates, as has been found for all women nationally [50]. We argue that these results highlight the need for additional studies to better understand why Hispanic women seem to derive a more protective effect from living in areas with a higher concentration of the population. Women appear to be more resilient to COVID-19, particularly when the results are linked to the occupations they perform, their access to better health services, or other biomedical reasons for these results. The results also highlight the need for improving the health services for the immigrant young men population of New York City, since they seem to perform riskier and essential jobs for the city and to experience higher limitations or vulnerability when accessing health insurance, and as research shows, they died at higher rates during the pandemic. Our results also suggest the need for further research on the needs of older immigrant adults, such as women, since we find evidence that the weathering hypothesis continues to matter or to shorten their presumed immigrant health advantages. Our results also emphasize that it is imperative that federal, state, and local governments collect and release comprehensive data on the number of confirmed COVID-19 cases and deaths by race/ethnicity and immigrant status, as well as age, to better gauge the impact of the outbreak across non-white Hispanic groups in mixed-status immigrant households. Finally, we claim that our results also highlight the need for a discussion among academics and policymakers of the different incremental steps to be taken to reduce the disproportionate burden of other potential future pandemics among minorities, given the decimation that the pandemic has caused among older black and vulnerable Hispanic populations in the U.S. Our results mainly emphasize the need for transformative actions that address structural racism to achieve greater health equity among historically racialized U.S. minorities. Finally, as Hispanics and Latinos make up a disproportional share of the young U.S. population, projected by 2030 to compose 22 percent of the U.S.'s labor force [1], the size and composition of the population and its contribution to the U.S. economy make it more imperative to design policy solutions to reduce structural racism and other forms of social inequalities that threaten the recovery of the group from the ravages of the pandemic and its future members contributions to our society.

Funding: This research received no external funding.

Institutional Review Board Statement: Not applicable.

Informed Consent Statement: Not applicable.

Data Availability Statement: We will provide datasets analyzed or generated during the study only upon request.

Conflicts of Interest: The authors declare no conflict of interest.

References

1. Gonzalez-Barrera, A.; Lopez, H. Is being Hispanic a Matter of Race, Ethnicity or Both? Pew Research Center. 2015. Available online: https://www.pewresearch.org/fact-tank/2015/06/15/is-being-hispanic-a-matter-of-race-ethnicity-or-both/) (accessed on 7 November 2019).
2. Saenz, R.; García, M. The disproportionate impact of COVID-19 on older Latino mortality: The rapidly diminishing Latino paradox. *J. Gerontol. B Psycol. Sci. Soc. Sci.* **2021**, *76*, e81–e87. [CrossRef] [PubMed]
3. Andrasfay, T.; Goldman, N. Reductions in 2020 US life expectancy due to COVID-19 and the disproportionate impact on the Black and Latino populations. *Proc. Natl. Acad. Sci. USA* **2021**, *118*, e2014746118. [CrossRef] [PubMed]
4. Fuentes, N.; Kucheva, Y. Revisiting the Hispanic Health Paradox: The Housing and Work Experiences of Immigrants in NYC during the COVID-19 Pandemic. 2021. Available online: https://covid19research.ssrc.org/grantee/revisiting-the-hispanic-health-paradox-the-housing-and-work-experiences-of-immigrants-in-nyc-during-the-covid-19-pandemic/ (accessed on 17 September 2020).
5. Laurencin, C.T.; Wu, Z.H.; McClinton, A.; Grady, J.J.; Walker, J.M. Excess Deaths among Blacks and Latinx Compared to Whites during COVID-19. *J. Racial Ethn. Health Disparities* **2021**, *8*, 783–789. [CrossRef] [PubMed]
6. Riley, A.R.; Chen, Y.-H.; Matthay, E.C.; Glymour, M.M.; Torres, J.M.; Fernandez, A.; Bibins-Domingo, K. Excess death among Latino people in California during the COVID-19 pandemic. *medRxiv* **2021**. *preprint*. [CrossRef]
7. Markides, K.S.; Coreil, J. The Health of Hispanics in the Southwestern United States: An Epidemiologic Paradox. *Public Health Rep.* **1986**, *101*, 253–265. [PubMed]
8. Vega, W.A.; Rodriguez, M.A.; Gruskin, E. Health disparities in the Latino population. *Epidemiol. Rev.* **2009**, *31*, 99–112. [CrossRef] [PubMed]
9. Dominguez, K.; Penman-Aguilar, A.; Chang, M.H.; Moonesinghe, R.; Castellanos, T.; Rodriguez-Lainz, A.; Schieber, R. Vital signs: Leading causes of death, prevalence of diseases and risk factors, and use of health services among Hispanics in the United States—2009–2013. *Morb. Mortal. Wkly. Rep.* **2015**, *64*, 469.
10. Ruiz, J.M.; Steffen, P.; Smith, T.B. Hispanic Mortality Paradox: A systematic review and meta-analysis of the longitudinal literature. *Am. J. Public Health* **2013**, *103*, e52–e60. [CrossRef]
11. Garcia, M.; Homan, P.; García, C.; Brown, T.H. The Color of COVID-19: Structural Racism and the Disproportionate Impact of the Pandemic on Older Black and Latinx Adults. *J. Gerontol. B Psychol. Sci. Soc. Sci.* **2021**, *76*, e75–e80. [CrossRef]
12. McLaren, J. Racial Disparity in COVID-19 Deaths: Seeking economic roots with Census data. *B.E. J. Econ. Anal. Policy* **2020**, *21*, 897–919. [CrossRef]
13. Hochschild, A.R. *Strangers in Their Own Land*; The New Press: New York, NY, USA, 2016.
14. Fuentes-Mayorga, N.; Burgos, G. Generation X and the Future Health of Latinos. *Generations* **2017**, *41*, 58–67.
15. Zhu, D.; Ye, X.; Manson, S. Revealing the spatial shifting pattern of COVID-19 pandemic in the United States. *Sci. Rep.* **2021**, *11*, 8396. [CrossRef]
16. Bossak, B.H.; Andritsch, S. COVID-19 and Air Pollution: A Spatial Analysis of Particulate Matter Concentration and Pandemic-Associated Mortality in the US. *Int. J. Environ. Res. Public Health* **2022**, *19*, 592. [CrossRef] [PubMed]
17. Saffary, T.; Adegboye, O.A.; Gayawan, E.; Elfaki, F.; Kuddus, M.A.; Saffary, R. Analysis of COVID-19 Cases' Spatial Dependence in US counties Reveals Health Inequalities. *Front. Public Health* **2020**, *8*, 579190. [CrossRef] [PubMed]
18. Kahn, J.X.; Seligson, A.L.; Dragan, K.L. Identifying New York City neighborhoods at risk of being overlooked at interventions. *Prev. Chronic Dis.* **2020**, *17*, 190325. [CrossRef]
19. Fenelon, A.; Blue, L. Widening Life Expectancy Advantage of Hispanics in the United States: 1990–2010. *J. Immigr. Minor. Health* **2014**, *17*, 1130–1137. [CrossRef] [PubMed]
20. Markides, K.S.; Eschbach, K. Aging, Migration, and Mortality: Current status of research on the hispanic paradox. *J. Gerontol.* **2005**, *60*, S68–S75. [CrossRef] [PubMed]
21. Lara, M.; Gamboa, C.; Kahramanian, M.I.; Morales, L.S.; Hayes Bautista, D.E. Acculturation and Latino Health in the United States: A review of the literature and its sociopolitical context. *Annu. Rev. Public Health* **2005**, *26*, 367–397. [CrossRef]
22. Palloni, A.; Arias, E. Paradox Lost: Explaining the Hispanic adult mortality advantage. *Demography* **2004**, *41*, 385–415. [CrossRef]
23. Riosmena, F.; Wong, R.; Palloni, A. Migration Selection, Protection, and Acculturation in Health: A Binational Perspective on Older Adults. *Demography* **2012**, *50*, 1039–1064. [CrossRef]
24. Goldman, N. Will the Latino Mortality Advantage Endure? *Res. Aging* **2016**, *38*, 263–282. [CrossRef] [PubMed]
25. Kposowa, A.J. Mortality from Diabetes by Hispanic Groups: Evidence from the US National Longitudinal Mortality Study. *Int. J. Popul. Res.* **2013**, *2013*, 571306. [CrossRef]
26. O'Bryant, S.E.; Johnson, L.; Reisch, J.; Edwards, M.; Hall, J.; Barber, R.; Devous, M.D.; Royall, D.; Singh, M. Risk factors for mild cognitive impairment among Mexican Americans. *Alzheimer's Dement.* **2013**, *9*, 622–631. [CrossRef] [PubMed]
27. Hayward, M.D.; Hummer, R.A.; Chiu, C.-T.; Gonzalez-Gonzalez, C.; Wong, R. Does the Hispanic paradox in U.S. adult mortality extend to disability? *Popul. Res. Policy Rev.* **2014**, *33*, 81–96. [CrossRef] [PubMed]
28. Hummer, R.A.; Hayward, M.D. Hispanic older adult health & longevity in the United States: Current patterns & concerns for the future. *Daedalus* **2015**, *144*, 20–30. [CrossRef] [PubMed]
29. Goldman, N.; Pebley, A.R.; Creighton, M.; Teruel, G.M.; Rubalcava, L.; Chung, C. The consequences of migration to the United States for short term changes in the health of Mexican immigrants. *Demography* **2014**, *51*, 1159–1173. [CrossRef]

30. Bailey, Z.; Krieger, N.; Agenor, M.; Graves, J.; Linos, N.; Basset, M.T. Structural Racism and Health Inequities in the USA: Evidence and interventions. *Lancet* **2017**, *389*, 1453–1463. [CrossRef]
31. Leong, N. Racial Capitalism. *Harv. Law Rev.* **2013**, *126*, 2151–2225. [CrossRef]
32. Jost, J.T.; Rudman, L.A.; Blair, I.V.; Carney, D.R.; Dasgupta, N.; Glaser, J.; Hardin, C.D. The existence of implicit bias is beyond reasonable doubt: A refutation of ideological and methodological objections and executive summary of ten studies that no manager should ignore. *Res. Organ. Behav.* **2009**, *29*, 39–69.
33. Blair, I.V.; Steiner, J.F.; Fairclough, D.L.; Hanratty, R.; Price, D.W.; Hirsh, H.K.; Wright, L.A.; Bronsert, M.; Karimkhani, E.; Magid, D.J.; et al. Clinicians' Implicit Ethnic/Racial Bias and Perceptions of Care among Black and Latino Patients. *Ann. Fam. Med.* **2013**, *11*, 43–52. [CrossRef]
34. Millet, G.; Jones, A.; Benkeser, D.; Baral, S.; Mercer, L.; Beyrer, C.; Honerman, B.; Lankiewicz, E.; Mena, L.; Crowley, J.; et al. Assesing differential impacts of COVID-19 on black communities. *Ann. Epidemiol.* **2020**, *47*, 37–44. [CrossRef] [PubMed]
35. Brown, C.S.; Ravallion, M. *Inequality and the Coronavirus: Socioeconomic Covariates of Behavioral Responses and Viral Outcomes across US Counties*; NBER Working Paper No. w27549; National Bureau of Economic Research: Cambridge, MA, USA, 2020.
36. Nagaraja, C.H. *Deprivation Indices for Census Tracts in Bronx and New York Counties*; Global Healthcare Innovation Management Center: New York, NY, USA, 2015.
37. New York City Health. Neighborhood Data Profiles. Consulted between November 2020 and June 2021. 2022. Available online: https://www1.nyc.gov/site/doh/covid/covid-19-data-neighborhoods.page (accessed on 22 January 2023).
38. Newman Lybrary. New York City Data on Neighborhoods. Consulted on February 2022. 2022. Available online: https://guides.newman.baruch.cuny.edu/nyc_data/nbhoods (accessed on 10 February 2022).
39. Ruggles, S.; Flood, S.; Goeken, R.; Schouweiler, M.; Sobek, M. *IPUMS USA: Version 12.0*; IPUMS: Minneapolis, MN, USA, 2022. [CrossRef]
40. Economic Development Quartely (EDQ). COVID-19 and the New York City Economy. 2021. Available online: https://edc.nyc/sites/default/files/2021-03/NYCEDC-ERP-EDQ3-COVID-19-New-York-City-Economy.pdf (accessed on 3 October 2022).
41. Albanesi, S. *Changing Business Cycles: The Role of Women's Employment*; NBER Working Paper: New York, NY, USA, 2020.
42. Bird, C.E.; Rieker, P.P. *Gender and Health*; Cambridge University Press: New York, NY, USA, 2008; p. 256.
43. Townsend, P.; Phillimore, P.; Beatie, A. *Health and Deprivation: Inequalities and the North*; Croom Helm: London, UK, 1988.
44. NYC. COVID-19: Data. Available online: https://www1.nyc.gov/site/doh/covid/covid-19-data-totals.page (accessed on 16 August 2022).
45. Martínez, L.E.; Bustamante, A.; Balderas-Medina Anaya, Y.M.D.; Domínguez-Villegas, R.; Santizo-Greendwood, S.; Diaz, S.F.M.; Hayes-Bautista, D. COVID-19 in Vulnerable Communities: An Examination by Race/Ethnicity in Los Angeles and New York City. *Res. Rep.* 2020. Available online: https://latino.ucla.edu/wp-content/uploads/2021/08/LPPI-LA-v-NY-Report.pdf (accessed on 10 February 2022).
46. Krieger, N. Measures of Racism, Sexism, Heterosexism, and Gender Binarism for Health Equity Research: From Structural Injustice to Embodied Harm—An Ecosocial Analysis. *Annu. Rev. Public Health* **2020**, *41*, 37–62. [CrossRef] [PubMed]
47. Rapp, K.S.; Volpe, V.V.; Hale, T.L.; Quartararo, D.F. State-level sexism and gender disparities in health care access and quality in the United States. *J. Health Soc. Behav.* **2022**, *63*, 2–18. [CrossRef] [PubMed]
48. Pabayo, R.; Cook, D.M.; Harling, G.; Gunawan, A.; Rosenquist, N.A.; Muennig, P. State-Level Income Inequality and Mortality among Infants Born in the United States 2007–2010: A Cohort Study. *BMC Public Health* **2019**, *19*, 1333. [CrossRef]
49. Homan, P. Structural Sexism and Health in the United States: A New Perspective on Health Inequality and the Gender System. *Am. Sociol. Rev.* **2019**, *84*, 486–516. [CrossRef]
50. Moss, N.E. Gender Equity and Socioeconomic Inequality: A Framework for the Patterning of Women's Health. *Soc. Sci. Med.* **2002**, *54*, 649–661. [CrossRef]
51. Harnois, C.E.; Bastos, J.L. Discrimination, Harassment, and Gendered Health Inequalities: Do Perceptions of Workplace Mistreatment Contribute to the Gender Gap in SelfReported Health? *J. Health Soc. Behav.* **2018**, *59*, 283–299. [CrossRef]
52. Krieger, N. Theories for Social Epidemiology in the 21st Century: An Ecosocial Perspective. *Int. J. Epidemiol.* **2001**, *30*, 668–677. [CrossRef]
53. Pal, S.; Gangu, K.; Garg, I.; Shuja, H.; Bobba, A.; Chourasia, P.; Shekhar, R.; Sheikh, A.B. Gender and Race-Based Health Disparities in COVID-19 Outcomes among Hospitalized Patients in the United States: A Retrospective Analysis of a National Sample. *Vaccines* **2022**, *10*, 2036. [CrossRef]
54. Frey, W.H. Neighborhood Segregation Persists for Black, Latino or Hispanic, and Asian Americans. 2021. Available online: https://www.brookings.edu/research/neighborhood-segregation-persists-for-black-latino-or-hispanic-and-asian-americans/ (accessed on 10 February 2022).
55. Wikkipedia. List of Majority-Hispanic or Latino counties in the United States. Available online: https://en.wikipedia.org/wiki/List_of_majority-Hispanic_or_Latino_counties_in_the_United_States (accessed on 10 February 2022).
56. NYC. COVID-19: Data—Trends and Totals. Available online: https://www1.nyc.gov/site/doh/covid/covid-19-data-totals.page (accessed on 16 August 2022).
57. NYC. COVID-19: Data—Vaccines. Available online: https://www1.nyc.gov/site/doh/covid/covid-19-data-vaccines.page#nyc (accessed on 16 August 2022).

58. Izzy, S.; Tahir, Z.; Cote, D.J.; Al Jarrah, A.; Roberts, M.B.; Turbett, S.; Kadar, A.; Smirnakis, S.M.; Feske, S.K.; Zafonte, R.; et al. Characteristics and Outcomes of Latinx Patients with COVID-19 in Comparison with Other Ethnic and Racial Groups. *Open Forum Infect. Dis.* **2020**, *7*, ofaa401. [CrossRef]
59. Cione, C.; Vetter, E.; Jackson, D.; McCarthy, S.; Castañeda, E. The Implications of Health Disparities: A COVID-19 Risk Assessment of the Hispanic Community in El Paso. *Int. J. Environ. Res. Public Health* **2023**, *20*, 975. [CrossRef] [PubMed]
60. Sabin, J.A. Tackling implicit bias in health care. *New Engl. J. Med.* **2022**, *387*, 105–107. [CrossRef] [PubMed]
61. Millán, I.; Noel, N.; Pérez, L.; Pulido, A. US Hispanic and Latino lives and livelihoods in the recovery from COVID-19 | McKinsey. *McKinsey Co.* **2020**, *17*, 2021.

International Journal of
Environmental Research and Public Health

MDPI

Article

COVID-19 and Policy-Induced Inequalities: Exploring How Social and Economic Exclusions Impact 'Temporary' Migrant Men's Health and Wellbeing in Australia

Daile Lynn Rung

Freemasons Centre for Male Health and Wellbeing, Faculty of Health, Charles Darwin University, Casuarina 0810, Australia; daile.rung@cdu.edu.au

Abstract: The Australian government swiftly put in place a number of economic relief measures and policies to support people during the COVID-19 crisis. However, the government's COVID-19 response policies excluded people with 'temporary' migrant status living in the country and encouraged people holding temporary visas who lost jobs and could no longer afford to support themselves to 'go home'. This paper draws upon sub-citizenship theory to explore how Australia's immigration and COVID-19 response policies are likely to impact the health and wellbeing of 'temporary' migrant men and their families. Through focusing on Australia's policy approach towards 'temporary' migrants and the social, health, and human rights implications among men with temporary migrant status during the pandemic, this paper contributes to emerging literature that considers the intersectional implications of immigration and COVID-19 response policies as they pertain to people with precarious migration status. Applying sub-citizenship theory to analyse how Australia's COVID-19 response policies intersect with 'temporary' migration schemes offers a useful way to think about and unearth how structural, and often legislated, exclusions can affect the health and wellbeing of marginalised groups.

Keywords: temporary migrants; migrant men; men's health; wellbeing; social exclusion; economic insecurity; COVID-19; Australia; policy; welfare; work rights

Citation: Rung, D.L. COVID-19 and Policy-Induced Inequalities: Exploring How Social and Economic Exclusions Impact 'Temporary' Migrant Men's Health and Wellbeing in Australia. *Int. J. Environ. Res. Public Health* **2023**, *20*, 6193. https://doi.org/10.3390/ijerph20136193

Academic Editors: Maria De Jesus and Ernesto Castañeda

Received: 9 April 2023
Revised: 21 May 2023
Accepted: 1 June 2023
Published: 21 June 2023

1. Introduction

Since the COVID-19 pandemic emerged in December 2019, communities around the world have faced immense stressors upon their health and wellbeing. The pandemic has brought to the forefront structural vulnerabilities faced by marginalised groups and individuals [1]. Globally and in Australia, people with temporary migrant status have emerged as one of the most vulnerable groups to experience health and wellbeing inequalities associated with COVID-19 [2–5].

As the coronavirus infection spread, public health directives in most countries began to call for social distancing along with various policies and measures, including border lockdowns aimed at slowing down the spread of the virus. In its bid to pursue a zero-COVID suppression policy aimed to minimize community transmission of COVID-19, Australia closed its borders to all non-residents on 20 March 2020 and only fully opened its borders to international visitors in February 2022. Throughout 2020 and 2021, different states and territories within Australia were implementing lockdowns and social restrictions to various degrees to try to curb community transmission [6]. In Australia, this strategy, known as 'flattening the curve', was supported by the government through physical distancing policies and economic support packages, known as Jobkeeper and Jobseeker [7]. However, the government's economic support policies in response to COVID-19 did not make support available to all people living in Australia. From the outset of the COVID-19 pandemic, 'citizens' and 'permanent residents' were prioritised, while 'temporary' migrants were explicitly excluded [2–4,8–11]. The Australian government rationalised this exclusion as needing to 'draw a line somewhere' [12] and encouraged people holding temporary visas to 'go home' if they cannot economically support themselves [13].

There are an estimated 1.9 million temporary visa holders in Australia as of June 2022 [14]. Temporary migrants are a diverse group of people who hold temporary visas for work, education, and family purposes in Australia. Temporary migrants include international students, New Zealanders on Special Category visas, working holiday makers, skilled and low-skill workers, post-study graduate visa holders, and partner and family visa holders. In 2022, the top three nationalities of all temporary visa holders in Australia included nationals from New Zealand (34.6 per cent), India (14.7 per cent), and China (7.3 per cent) [14]. Although not officially counted as 'temporary' migrants, another substantial group of people who may hold temporary visas include refugees and asylum seekers on temporary protection and bridging visas.

Unfortunately, as people with temporary migrant status are without voting rights, there is little political will to explore and understand how their social and economic conditions impact their health and wellbeing. Scholarship is needed to explore how exclusionary social policies might affect the health and social and emotional wellbeing among different sub-sets of temporary migrants as they comprise a large and diverse group. To contribute to this work, this paper explores how COVID-19 policy exclusions have compounded pre-existing social and economic exclusions faced by men living in Australia with temporary migrant status.

Drawing upon sub-citizenship theory [15,16], I aim to explore how 'temporary' migrant men's health and wellbeing may be affected by an array of pre-existing social and economic exclusions, which were compounded by exclusionary social and economic policies in response to the pandemic. Concentrating on the role of exclusionary policies and social practices in the context of COVID-19, I intend to analyse the health and wellbeing implications of men living in Australia with temporary migrant status and, by extension, those of their families and children. To accomplish this, I consider how pre-existing vulnerabilities and exclusions from work, welfare supports, and free public services, including healthcare and education, are likely to affect the health and wellbeing of 'temporary' migrant men and their families.

People with temporary migrant status in Australia have been excluded from accessing public services and welfare safety nets for many years, long before the global pandemic. However, as people holding temporary visas in Australia were uniformly excluded from accessing the government's roll out of COVID-19 support measures, it is important to ascertain how the compounding of exclusionary immigration, public health, and pandemic response policies pre- and post-COVID may affect the health and wellbeing of temporary migrant men and their families in the country.

There is increasing consensus among researchers investigating the impact of the virus from medical, public health, and sociological perspectives that intersectional analyses are urgently needed to create more equitable pandemic policies and interventions [17–19]. Intersectional approaches that analyse how biological sex, sociological aspects of gender, and diverse social inequalities affect people's health and wellbeing are helpful to build understandings of how COVID-19 affects diverse groups of people in different ways.

Addressing the nexus between COVID-19, equity, and men's health from a public health perspective, Smith et al. [17] note: the vulnerability of certain groups are rarely acknowledged in popular and social media in comparison to broader population-wide discussions about COVID-19; and seldom have these recognised the inequalities faced by men (p. 51).

Through focusing upon men with temporary migrant status in Australia, this paper contributes to emerging scholarship that explores "how future public health pandemic approaches could better respond to the needs of the most vulnerable and marginalised groups of boys and men in a timely way" [17] (p. 49). The economic and social impact of COVID-19 policies upon migrant men, who are often the breadwinners in migrant households, will undoubtedly have health and wellbeing implications for migrant fathers and their families.

Many of the issues raised in this paper focused on men with temporary migrant status also apply to women, children, LGBT communities, and undocumented migrants, albeit in complex and varied ways. This paper's focus on men holding temporary visas should not be taken as a statement that they face more structural inequalities than women and LGBT communities who hold temporary visas or other groups of migrants, including undocumented migrants.

While this paper's intersectional approach focuses on men with temporary migrant status, it acknowledges that certain sub-groups of temporary migrant men, including LGBT migrants, experience compounded forms of social, economic, and health inequalities [20]. It must also be acknowledged that certain groups of migrants, including undocumented migrants, are more at risk of experiencing social, economic, and health inequalities. For example, Australia's punitive immigration detention regime confines undocumented migrants in close quarters in detention centres where they faced extremely high risks of COVID-19 infection and possibly death [21]. Viewing this issue through a sub-citizenship lens, undocumented migrants are institutionally positioned at lower levels of the sub-citizenship hierarchy, making them more vulnerable to state-led violence and subordination.

This critical social policy analysis paper has two interrelated aims. First, it explores how Australia's neoliberal approach to immigration creates social and economic exclusions and barriers for all people who hold temporary visas in the country. Second, building upon this key insight, it considers how Australia's COVID-19 response policies have deepened pre-existing social and economic exclusions that are likely to present certain health and wellbeing challenges for men with temporary migrant status and, by extension, their families.

Two broad threads of literature are drawn upon to provide the necessary contextual background to explore 'temporary' migrant men's health and wellbeing in the context of COVID-19 in Australia. First, literature pertaining to COVID-19 and men's health suggests that men are a highly vulnerable group with respect to COVID-19. Second, I draw upon literature and public policies in Australia focused on temporary migrants' health and wellbeing pre- and post-COVID. The paper sheds clarity around the notion of 'temporary' migrants through discussing how it has come to be that millions of people hold this precarious migration status in Australia and elsewhere.

To operationalise the critical social policy approach, I apply an intersectional sub-citizen lens to explore how Australia's COVID-19 policy responses multiplied and compounded pre-existing economic and social exclusions faced by people with temporary migration status. Sub-citizenship theory [16] enables a deep consideration of how the predominance of neoliberal dynamics underpinning immigration and public policies works to sort and categorise people to experience different levels of subordination and inequalities largely based upon the allocation of migration and citizenship status. Through a sub-citizenship approach, the focus is on how it has come to be that pre-existing exclusions and vulnerabilities with respect to work and access to welfare supports and public services have become compounded for those with temporary migrant status and how such exclusions are likely to result in adverse health and wellbeing among temporary migrant men.

The premise underlying this paper is that COVID-19 public health and pandemic response policies should have the end goal of improving the health and wellbeing of all people in society regardless of their gender, race, age, migration/citizenship status, socioeconomic status, sexual orientation, or any other attribute. The United Nations' Sustainable Development Goals (SDG) can be advanced through inclusive public health, immigration, and social policies that promote good health and wellbeing (SDG 3) and reduce inequality (SDG 10) [22]. With these goals in mind, this paper aligns with scholarship advocating for a gendered and human rights lens in public health and pandemic research and policy responses.

2. COVID-19 and Men's Health

The available evidence suggests that being male is a key factor determining the health and wellbeing outcomes of people who contract COVID-19. Sex-disaggregated epidemiological analyses across different parts of the world reveal a gender gap associated with the virus [23].

Globally, epidemiological findings indicate that men are more vulnerable to COVID-19 than women, with men experiencing higher morbidity and mortality rates [23,24]. Indeed, most countries with available data indicate a higher male-to-female case fatality ratio [25]. Data from China indicate that the majority (66.7%) of COVID-19 patients have been male. In Italy, men accounted for 58% of infected patients and 70% of COVID-19-related deaths. In the United States, 53.5% of reported COVID-19 deaths have been in men [26].

At the present time, it is too early to tell what accounts for this gender gap in COVID-19-related deaths, although some have speculated it may be related to sex-based immunological differences between males and females; gendered lifestyle behaviours, such as higher rates of smoking and drinking; and less adherence to preventative measures, such as handwashing and mask-wearing, that may put men more at risk [23]. Most of the available literature exploring the COVID-19 gender health gap has been bio-medically focussed on the possible role that biological sex differences, such as hormones and chromosomes, may play with health and wellbeing differences between men and women.

There has been less attention focused on the underlying social and contextual factors that may shape men and women's health outcomes with respect to COVID-19 [26,27]. Focusing exclusively on decontextualised statistics about sex differences is dangerous because it obscures other factors that may be equally—as or perhaps more—relevant than biological sex in shaping people's vulnerability to the virus itself and the knock-on social and economic consequences associated with the global pandemic. Sociological studies offer the benefit of adding much-needed contextual analyses through critically analysing the factors that connect individuals to their social landscape. Thus, there is a great need for sociological approaches, as they allow us to better understand the underlying factors that may be accounting for the gender gap observed in the rich epidemiological data already available. Investigating how different groups of people were and continue to be affected in a post-COVID world would benefit from intersectional approaches that take account of how gender, sex, age, race, socio-economic status, and other markers of difference make some groups more vulnerable to certain health and wellbeing challenges.

While we know that COVID-19 has negatively impacted men's health and wellbeing in a general sense, little information is available about how the health and wellbeing of migrant and refugee men's has been impacted. Borgkvist [28], Adamson and Smith [29], and Rung and Adamson [30] note there is limited research on groups of marginalised fathers, including migrants and refugees. Internationally and in Australia, there is a critical gap in knowledge about 'temporary' migrant men's mental health and wellbeing in general and in the context of COVID-19. To address this gap, this paper contributes to sociologically oriented literature to understand how complex social and economic factors may impact the health and wellbeing of 'temporary' migrant men and, by extension, their families living in Australia in the aftermath of COVID-19.

Most of the available data that pertain to migrant men's health and wellbeing in the Australian context draws upon the Longitudinal Study of Australian Children (LSAC), which excludes people with temporary migrant status. However, as the LSAC includes people from migrant and refugee backgrounds who have Australian citizenship or permanent residency status, it provides some indication of the health and wellbeing challenges faced by migrant men who have more secure migration and citizenship statuses. Men with less secure migration and citizenship statuses may have similar (and likely more complex) health and wellbeing challenges as migrant men who hold permanent residency visas or are citizens. However, to date, no studies have focused upon the health and wellbeing of men with temporary migrant status pre or post pandemic.

Overall, a small number of studies that draw upon LSAC data suggest that migrant and refugee men with more secure residency and citizenship status are at risk of poorer mental and general health, particularly when they face employment challenges. Whilst these studies draw upon LSAC data that pre-dates the emergence of COVID-19, these findings show that migrant and refugee men in Australia are more vulnerable to health and wellbeing challenges and job conditions have a strong impact upon the health and wellbeing of migrant men.

Considering that the social and emotional wellbeing of fathers from migrant and refugee backgrounds is strongly linked to fulfilling what they view as their cultural role as financial and figurative providers [30], there is a need to explore how certain employment and financial challenges associated with COVID-19 may affect the health and wellbeing of 'temporary' migrant men and their families in Australia.

However, to shed some clarity around the highly misleading term, 'temporary' migrant, it is useful to first understand how it has come to be that millions of people with temporary migrant status live in Australia and why they are institutionally positioned as a highly vulnerable group of people.

3. 'Temporary' Migrants in Australia

In Australia, people are lawfully classified into three general categories: citizens, permanent residents, and short-term visitors. Australia's immigration system divides migrants into two main categories: permanent migrants, who hold visas to live in Australia indefinitely, and temporary migrants, whose visas have time limitations.

There are three important points to keep in mind about people living in Australia with temporary migrant status. First, temporary migrants represent a significant population in Australia, with nearly 2 million temporary migrant visa holders in the country [31]. Second, temporary migrants can—and increasingly do—live long-term in Australia [16,32–35]. Third, temporary migrants are highly diverse in terms of gender, race, socio-economic status, age, and sexuality.

While 'temporary' implies that this group lives in a country on a short-term basis, 'temporary' migrants can—and increasingly do—live long term in Australia [16,32–35]. Mares's (2016) [33] notion of 'long-term temporary migrants' is useful as it denotes that people often hold this precarious migration status for many years. It is most useful and accurate to view the term 'temporary' migrant a *status* rather than an indicator of how long a person has actually lived in and contributed to society [15,16,33]. Australian immigration policy changes over the past thirty years have resulted in millions of long-term temporary migrants [16,33].

Hugo (2014) [35] notes that the growth of temporary migration is one of the most significant developments to the dynamics of Australian immigration policy. In many countries, including Australia and Canada, there has been a sharp increase in temporary migrant schemes at the expense of both permanent immigration and humanitarian resettlement programs [36]. Over the past few decades, policy changes to the composition of immigration pathways have fundamentally changed Australia from the settler society model of the 20th century into what is now arguably best characterised as a temporary migrant society [15,33,35]. In fact, since 2000, temporary migrants have far outnumbered permanent ones [37].

Millions of migrants holding temporary visas live in Australia long term, work, study, pay taxes, obey laws, form social attachments, develop feelings of home and belonging, and contribute to the social, economic, and cultural life of the nation. However, due to their status, this group of people lacks access to a range of public services and benefits—including healthcare, education, and social safety nets—and are denied voting rights [33]. However, it should be noted that 'temporary' migrants in Australia are considered residents for tax purposes only [38]. This means that all public services, welfare supports, Medicare, and other social and economic safety nets are funded through the tax contributions of a group of people who are deemed ineligible to access free public services, supports, and safety nets in times of need. People holding temporary visas in Australia usually must pay for all services, such as healthcare and education for their children, until they acquire permanent resident and/or citizenship status. In recent years, immigration policy changes have required permanent residents to serve a 'waiting period' before they can access Australia's income support system [39]. As of July 2021, the government announced that permanent residents would have to wait four years to access most welfare support services. In the previous policy, the waiting period was two years. It should be noted that time spent in the country as a 'temporary' migrant does not count towards the waiting period.

While most people with temporary migration status in Australia have some degree of working rights and pay taxes, they are more at risk of experiencing exploitation and other forms of mistreatment in the workplace [40]. As 'temporary migrants do not stand on the same firm legal ground as citizens and permanent residents' [33] (p. 6) they run a far greater risk of experiencing exploitation and abuse in the workplace.

Welfare restrictions contribute to economic insecurities among temporary migrants, particularly if they lose their employment. Being excluded from welfare and other supports puts temporary migrants in a highly precarious economic position, which in turn makes them more willing to do the 'dirty, difficult and dangerous jobs that nationals will not' [40] (p. xiii). Without access to freely available public services and safety nets, temporary migrants are more vulnerable to underpayment, wage theft, superannuation theft, and other forms of mistreatment as they have limited supports and alternatives to leave unscrupulous employers and abusive workplace conditions.

This paper acknowledges that the barriers to social, political, and economic participation currently confronting 'temporary' migrants is not an accidental or unlucky occurrence, but rather should be viewed as "a direct consequence of dramatic and deliberate changes in immigration policy since the 1990s" [3] (p. 62). The expansion in both the number of 'temporary' migrants and the elongation of time that many people occupy this status has come about through deliberate changes to Australian immigration and citizenship policies. This begs the question, "What accounts for the policy changes that have increased the number 'temporary' migrant and the length of time they hold this precarious status in Australia?".

4. Temporary Migration Schemes and Neoliberal Citizenship

Neoliberal economic doctrines that first emerged in the 1970s and came into prominence in the 1980s have had an immense influence upon how nation-states retool immigration and citizenship policies [41]. Under neoliberal economic theory, everything has a 'market value', including social belonging vis à vis access to immigration and citizenship pathways. Australia is not the only country whose approach to immigration and citizenship policy has been retooled in neoliberal terms, as this global trend towards commodifying immigration and citizenship policies has become particularly apparent in affluent, western countries. Australia's immigration system and its militarised, securitised approach to border enforcement is arguably one of the most extreme manifestations of neoliberal citizenship in the world [15,16,42].

Neoliberal citizenship is characterised by "a contractual view that sees citizenship no longer primarily as a prima facie right but as a prized possession that is to be earned and can be lost if not properly cultivated" (p. 408) [43]. Through reframing citizenship in an increasingly contractual and contingent manner, the nation-state provides the institutional machinery necessary to redraw and reengineer the boundaries and tenor of citizenship though the creation of market-driven policies [41]. Under neoliberal terms, citizenship and the rights associated with it are no longer regarded as human rights connected to dwelling in a territorial space and being a member of a particular society, but as commodified, contractual rights [41,43].

Neoliberal citizenship is marked by progressively tightening people's access to even the most basic services, safety nets, and human rights [16,44–47]. A marker of the advance of neoliberal citizenship is found in reframing access to 'public' services, welfare, and social safety nets as only being available people who the nation-state deems as 'belonging', based upon migrant and/or citizenship status. Neoliberal approaches to citizenship and immigration pathways tend to work against the mobility, security, and human rights of people who have less-than-full status in their county of residence (i.e., 'non-citizens') [16]. Those whom the nation-state construes as not belonging to its imagined community [48] face compounded, and often legislated, exclusions. Increasingly, access to welfare support in many countries is only available to those deemed 'deserving', often based their demonstrated ability to work in the formal economy.

One of the main ways that neoliberal citizenship is being realised in Australia is through the expansion of temporary migration schemes. As the nation-state shifts the rules, pathways, requirements, and monetary commitments required for immigrants to attain more secure migration and citizenship statuses, the result has been more long-term temporary migrants. Castles (1995) [49] warns that immigration policy models that bar people from attaining permanent settlement creates 'differential exclusion' among migrants and stands in direct opposition to the democratic principle of including all members of society. Temporary migrant schemes are neoliberal policy models par excellence due to their ability to incorporate immigrants into certain areas of society, above all the labour market, whilst excluding millions of people from accessing welfare and social safety nets, permanent residency, and citizenship rights, including political participation.

Australian immigration intakes are increasingly displaying a preference for 'staggered' or 'two-step' pathways towards permanent residence [33,50]. In 2012–2013, less than half (40.2%) of permanent visas were obtained onshore i.e., people who lived in the country as 'temporary' migrants [51]. By comparison, in 2019–2020, nearly two-thirds (64.5%) of permanent residence visas in Australia were granted to people through the onshore program [52].) As people who obtain permanent residency status are predominately former temporary migrants, this trend suggests that the regulatory processes governing Australia's immigration system have been retooled to allow for a more drawn-out immigration process. Extending temporary migration pathways is highly lucrative for nation-states and immigration intermediaries, yet highly precarious for people with temporary migrant status [16,36,50,53].

Immigration pathways leading from temporary residency to permanent residency to citizenship are far from certain. The longer people are construed as 'temporary' migrants, the more precarious their lives become as they do not have access to the same social protections and legal footing as permanent residents and citizens. Not having access to welfare supports and services can be detrimental to people who experience normal life events such as sickness, separation, domestic violence, pregnancy, raising children, or losing a job. When the global pandemic emerged in Australia in early 2020, temporary migrants were among the most vulnerable due to their precarious social status in the country.

In recent years, it has become increasingly common for temporary visa holders to go through numerous temporary visas, where they run the risk of becoming long-term and potentially indefinite temporary residents [33]. As Mares [33] explains, temporary visa holders are in danger of "moving around in circles, jumping repeatedly from one temporary visa to another. If they cannot leap to a safe landing before their temporary visa options are exhausted, then they are out" (p. 32). Elongated and staggered immigration policy approaches ensure that 'temporary' migrants contribute to the economy, yet most will not find a pathway towards permanent residence and the social, economic, and political rights associated with that status.

5. Viewing 'Temporary' Migrants through a Sub-Citizen Lens

Sub-citizenship theory provides an open-ended and relational approach to explore how people's experiences with social, political, and economic exclusions and access to human rights are connected to institutionalised processes governing migration and citizenship. In earlier work, I defined sub-citizenship as "translocal processes of subordination that create various hierarchal conditions of precarity and dehumanization for different groups of people primarily based upon, but not wholly determined by, migration and citizenship status" [16]. Sub-citizenship is structurally produced and enacted though immigration policies and processes that sort, classify, and assign people into a hierarchical array of migration and citizenship statuses. This process is underpinned by nation-states' monopoly on classifying people as belonging to one of two constructed binaries: 'citizens' and 'non-citizens' [16].

This paper's use of sub-citizenship theory focusing on the health and wellbeing implications among temporary migrant men in the context of COVID-19 policy exclusions expands upon previous approaches to sub-citizenship that have analysed how policies and practices led to the subordination and dehumanisation of other groups of migrants including children with illegalised migrant status in Australia and America [16], the UK's 'Windrush scandal' [54], migrant workers and Australia's COVID-19 governmental responses [4], the conflation of globalisation and migration [55], integration and transnational practices of New Zealand migrants in Australia [56], and alternatives to immigration detention in Indonesia [57].

Structurally linked to the neoliberal market paradigm, sub-citizenship is a process that creates and draws upon disempowered migrant labour to expand markets and prop up the empowered labour, wages, and social protections enjoyed by people with more secure migration and citizenship status, i.e., citizens and permanent residents [16]. Nation-states create and sustain the legal frameworks, policies, and practices that perpetuate and expand sub-citizenship though crafting boundaries that differentially exclude [48] certain groups of people socially, politically, and economically.

While primarily aimed at expanding the global capitalist economy, sub-citizenship subjects all people to various forms of social, political, economic, and territorial expulsion [16]. Those positioned at lower levels of the sub-citizenship hierarchy are more vulnerable to social and economic exclusion, exploitation, state-led violence, and human rights abuses. The imposition of torture and indefinite detention without the right to habeas corpus is increasingly deployed against those positioned at the bottom of the sub-citizen hierarchy, i.e., people with illegalised migration statuses [16,58].

Within sub-citizenship's hierarchical structure, 'temporary' migrants are institutionally positioned as a highly vulnerable group of 'non-citizens' due to their precarious, or insecure, migration status. Living in countries, often long-term, with less than full status puts temporary visa holders at risk of numerous and overlapping social, political, economic, and human rights exclusions [36].

Under Australia's current immigration policies, 'temporary' migrants:

- lack the right to permanently reside in the country;
- have partial work rights, which are temporary in nature;
- are often dependent on a third party (such as an employer who acts as their 'sponsor') to secure their employment and residency rights;
- do not have access to free public services, such as healthcare and education
- lack access to welfare and social protections, including COVID-19-related pandemic responses (Jobseeker and Jobkeeper);
- lack voting rights; and
- are at risk of being deported or detained if they breach their visa conditions [4,9,16,33,36].

As nation-states retool their immigration and citizenship policies, temporary migrant status often becomes a mechanism that bars certain people from accessing welfare and public services, such as healthcare and education, while at the same time ensuring that this differentially excluded group serves as a net contributor to the public purse.

6. Australia's COVID-19 Policy Impacts upon 'Temporary' Migrants

In Western countries, the most vulnerable populations tend to be people without permanent legal status, such as asylum seekers and temporary visa holders, and other poor, marginalised citizens with limited or no access to healthcare. People with temporary migrant status have long been among the most marginalised populations around the world, as they have limited (and often no) access to public health care, social protection, work rights, public education, permanent residency, and voting rights [3,9,16,36,59].

Through an intersectional, sub-citizen lens, we can develop better understandings of how Australia's immigration and COVID-19 response policies sorted, classified, and excluded certain groups of people based on the citizen/non-citizen construct. The sections below explore how ordering people into migration classifications and legal statuses exacerbated pre-existing social and economic inequalities among temporary migrants who were excluded from Australia's pandemic assistance schemes based on their low positioning within the sub-citizenship hierarchy.

7. Heightened Job Insecurities

Predating the emergence of COVID-19, people with temporary migrant status in Australia faced multiple and overlapping vulnerabilities and exclusions from accessing fair work, including exploitative and unsafe working conditions [40,60] with wage theft and underpayment endemic in occupations and industries that employ temporary migrant workers [61–63]. In 2018, a survey of 1433 international student visa holders found that 100% of those working in the restaurant and retail sectors were underpaid [62]. Clibborn (2018) [62] speculated that the international students in the study tolerated the underpayment because it was viewed as a widespread and normalised behaviour among this disenfranchised group of workers.

The pandemic undoubtedly intensified pre-existing economic insecurities and workplace vulnerabilities among people with temporary migration status in Australia. In early 2020, Australia began to enforce social distancing and lockdowns to contain the spread of COVID-19. As a result of these policies, certain sectors, such as tourism, retail, and restaurants, and the informal economy were among the first to shed jobs. Temporary migrants, who are concentrated in heavily casualised and informal sectors of the economy, were among the first to lose their jobs during the government's COVID-19 lockdowns. As many temporary visa holders, most notably international students, often do not have full work rights, they are more economically vulnerable if they experience job loss or reduction of work hours. While the 40 h per fortnight limitation placed on work hours was relaxed for international student visa holders working in essential services such as supermarkets and aged care [64], this move was not enough to combat wide-spread job losses and economic insecurities experienced by this marginalised group of workers.

To date, one large-scale study has focused on how Australia's COVID-19 response policies impacted temporary visa holders living in the country. In July 2020, over 6100 temporary migrants in Australia were surveyed, including over 5000 international students and further thousand temporary migrant visa holders including Working Holiday Makers, Temporary Graduate visa holders, Temporary Skill Shortage visa holders, refugees, and people seeking asylum [2]. Key findings from the study include temporary migrants reporting:

- a critical loss of income from job loss and/or diminished family support;
- an inability to meet basic living needs;
- a belief their financial crisis will substantially worsen;
- financial supports being inadequate to meet need;
- a diminished sense of wellbeing at work and home; and
- widespread experiences of racism [2].

During the pandemic, many temporary visa holders lost their jobs and incomes, and many reported experiencing more exploitative working conditions and abuse [2]. More than 70% of temporary migrants reported either job loss or substantially reduced work hours. Many also reported reduced hourly wages (21%), doing unpaid work (11%), being forced to do tasks they were uncomfortable with (13%), and performing work in exchange of food and/or housing rather than wages (13%) [2].

8. Exclusion from Welfare, Public Services, and COVID-19 Supports

Prior to the pandemic, people with temporary migrant status in Australia were excluded from all welfare supports and, in most instances, were not entitled to free public services such as healthcare and public education for their children. As this group cannot access welfare and usually must pay for public services, they are at risk of poverty, homelessness, and food insecurity, particularly if they lose their job.

In keeping with the above trend of excluding temporary visa holders from welfare support, Australia explicitly excluded 'temporary' migrants from accessing the government's emergency COVID-19 economic assistance measures. In April 2020, then Prime Minister Scott Morison delivered a 'go home' message to people holding temporary visas who experienced job losses and could no longer afford to sustain themselves in Australia. However, it is important to note that Australia's response towards temporary visa holders was at odds with other countries. The United Kingdom, Canada, New Zealand, Ireland, and other countries recognised temporary migrants as valuable members of society and responded through extending wage subsidies and other forms of support, including unemployment payments and housing support, to temporary migrants residing in these countries [2].

Excluding members of society with temporary migrant status from essential economic aid and support during a global pandemic can be viewed as part of the institutional machinery producing sub-citizenship through drawing sharp divisions between people based on migration and citizenship status [4,16]. Symington (2021) [4] notes that "despite being taxpayers that contribute a crucial sector to the Australian workforce, migrants holding temporary visas were forced in much of Australia to rely on their savings and superannuation and, where those were exhausted or non-existent, charity" (p. 10).

Framing temporary visa holders as undeserving of pandemic response measures compounded pre-existing economic and social inequalities faced by this group. As the government's Jobkeeper and Jobseeker payments were not made accessible to workers with temporary migrant status, some employers responded through laying off temporary migrant employees en masse whilst retaining people with permanent residency and citizenship status [65,66]. Given that Australia's COVID-19 response policies penalised businesses that employ temporary migrant workers [10], it is hardly surprising that some employers responded through standing down employees with temporary migrant status in favour of those who were eligible for the government's COVID-19 economic response payments.

9. COVID-19 Response Policy's Implications for 'Temporary' Migrant Men and Families

Having reviewed how Australia's COVID-19 policies exacerbated pre-existing social and economic insecurities among temporary migrants, we can now consider how widespread job losses and financial hardship alongside exclusions from COVID-19 supports and free public services may impact the health and wellbeing of temporary migrant men and their families.

Prior to the emergence of the COVID-19 pandemic, Wickramage et al. (2018) [59] observed that people residing in nation-states with 'non-citizen' status 'may be disproportionately affected in the event of health emergencies' due to of a combination of political, sociocultural, economic, and legal barriers that results in their 'limited access to and awareness of health and welfare services' (p. 251). As previously discussed, before COVID-19, temporary migrants in Australia were far more vulnerable to experience job, housing, and food insecurity than those who held more secure migration and citizenship statuses. Australia's pandemic response policies exacerbated the already precarious economic and social situation faced by temporary migrants living in the country, as they were among the first to lose their jobs; were ineligible to access any form of welfare support or free public services, including healthcare and public education; and often have little or no social support networks to rely upon [10,67].

As discussed earlier, there is a dearth of information available on temporary migrant men's health and wellbeing in general in the context of COVID-19. Through piecing together the available information on migrant men's work and fathering practices, migrant men's health and wellbeing, and Berg and Farbenblum's (2020) [2] recent survey findings of temporary migrants in Australia during COVID-19, we can infer some of the likely post-COVID health and wellbeing implications for men and their families with temporary migration status.

It is widely known that fathers, both migrant and non-migrant, are more likely to be the breadwinners in the family [68–71], with emerging evidence indicating that many migrant and refugee families heavily rely on the male partner's income to survive [30]. Migrant and refugee fathers in Australia strongly identify as being providers for their families [30,72–74]. Moreover, their sense of wellbeing and capacity for engaged fathering often hinges on fulfilling the breadwinner role [30].

The available data in the Australian context focus specifically on the mental health and wellbeing of migrant and refugee-background fathers with more secure migration and citizenship statuses, (i.e., permanent residents and citizens). The key learnings from a small number of studies that draw upon LSAC data prior to the pandemic suggest that migrant and refugee men's mental health and wellbeing is strongly influenced by their employment and job conditions [75] and that migrant and refugee fathers, particularly those from non-English speaking countries, are more likely to experience poorer mental and physical health than Australian-born fathers [76].

While, presently, there is no empirical data focused on the health and wellbeing of temporary migrant men in Australia in the context of COVID-19, we can deduce with some degree of confidence from the available evidence that men holding temporary visas are at least as likely to experience similar general health and mental health challenges as those with more secure residency and citizenship statuses. Taking this line of reasoning a step farther, it is likely that 'temporary' migrant men are at risk of experiencing more pronounced mental health and general health challenges than those with permanent residency and citizenship status, as migrant men's employment conditions strongly influence their health and wellbeing.

Alongside the findings above pertaining to the intersections between employment, fathering, and health and wellbeing among migrant and refugee men, one large-scale study focusing on people with temporary migrant status in Australia found that widespread job losses in the context of exclusionary COVID-19 response policies had devastating financial and social impacts upon this group [2]. The findings of this large-scale study demonstrate that temporary migrants in Australia faced increased economic, job, and housing insecurity; unfair and exploitative working conditions; and increased experiences of racism and abuse during the pandemic.

As migrant families often rely upon fathers to survive economically, if a migrant father faces employment challenges or a reduced income, the family falls into a very difficult financial position. The situation is more economically precarious for temporary migrants in Australia as they are ineligible for welfare, COVID-19 supports, and access to free public services, such as healthcare and public education for their children. Being excluded from social safety nets and supports puts additional pressure on 'temporary' migrant men to economically support their families.

When migrant men are unable to fulfill the breadwinner role, they often undergo emotional and mental stress and suffer a crisis of masculinity [74,77]. As migrant men on temporary visas are more vulnerable to exploitative work conditions and are ineligible for COVID-19 schemes or other forms of economic and social supports, they have fewer options available to leave unscrupulous employers. Under such conditions, 'temporary' migrant men may continue working in jobs where they experience abuse and exploitation as they as they feel compelled to fulfill what they regard as their cultural duty of being financial providers to their families.

10. Summary and Conclusions

This paper applied an intersectional sub-citizen lens to explore how Australia's COVID-19 policy responses multiplied and compounded pre-existing economic and social exclusions faced by temporary migrant men. Migrant men are often the breadwinners who feel a cultural obligation to be financial providers for their families. As temporary visa holders in Australia were more likely to experience employment-related stresses, including job loss, reduced work hours, exploitation, and racism, and were ineligible for COVID-19 welfare and income safety nets, it is likely that temporary migrant men were less able to fulfill the role of being financial providers for their families. Being excluded from welfare safety nets and services, including access to COVID-19 economic supports, is likely to adversely impact the health and wellbeing of 'temporary' migrant men and their families.

People holding temporary visas are positioned low in the sub-citizen hierarchy. Due to their classification as 'non-citizens', temporary migrants have highly precarious and limited work and residency rights within the nation-state. Through applying a sub-citizenship lens to men with temporary migrant status, this paper explored how construing temporary visa holders as non-citizen outsiders rendered millions of men, women, and children as ineligible for social and economic support in Australia during the global pandemic.

COVID-19 undoubtedly heightened health, wellbeing, and economic insecurities for people around the world. People with temporary migration status have long been a highly vulnerable group, especially in times of crises. The global pandemic brought to the surface and deepened long-standing structural and legislated inequalities among temporary migrants. These exclusions hinge upon nation-states construing people who hold temporary visas as 'non-citizen' outsiders regardless of how long they have lived, worked, and contributed to the country.

Temporary visa holders face numerous intersecting inequalities that are likely to undermine their health and wellbeing at the best of times. During Australia's COVID-19 recession, temporary migrants experienced disproportionate health, wellbeing, and economic disadvantages, which were compounded as the country opted not to recognise this group as belonging to society and deserving of access to welfare supports, public services, and safety nets.

In the absence of studies focused on temporary migrant men's health and wellbeing in the context of COVID-19, this paper has pieced together the available global literature on men's health and COVID-19, migrant men's health and wellbeing, and the social and economic conditions of temporary migrants in Australia during the pandemic. Viewing these threads of literature though a sub-citizen lens, it contends that exclusionary social and economic policies faced by temporary migrants have been compounded during the pandemic. The combination of Australian immigration and COVID-19 response policies likely undermined the health and wellbeing of temporary migrant men and their families.

Certainly, there is a great need for future empirical research to explore how the health and wellbeing of temporary migrant men and their families have been impacted post-COVID. Comparative studies drawing upon the voices of diverse groups of temporary migrants living in Australia and different countries would be a welcome advancement in this space. Such scholarship would build an evidence base to understand how policy responses impact the health and wellbeing of diverse groups of temporary migrants in different countries and contexts around the world.

Through reinforcing the social boundaries and hierarches between 'citizens' and 'non-citizens', Australia's COVID-19 policy responses have deepened pre-existing social and economic exclusions among a highly vulnerable group of people living, often long-term, with precarious residency status in the country. In failing to extend new and existing welfare supports and COVID-19 response measures to temporary migrants and communicating a 'go home' message to those who experienced job loss, the country refused to accept responsibility for millions of people who live, pay taxes, contribute to social and economic life, and call Australia their home. We have yet to see what the long-term impact of exclusionary COVID-19 response policies will be on temporary migrant men and families and on the willingness of future immigrants to make Australia their home.

Funding: This research received support from the Freemasons Centre for Male Health and Wellbeing, Northern Territory.

Institutional Review Board Statement: Not applicable.

Informed Consent Statement: Not applicable.

Conflicts of Interest: The author declares no conflict of interest.

References

1. Team, V.; Mandrson, L. How COVID-19 reveals structures of vulnerability. *Med. Anthropol.* **2020**, *39*, 671–674. [CrossRef] [PubMed]
2. Berg, L.; Farbenblum, B. As if We Weren't Humans: The Abandonment of Temporary Migrants in Australia during COVID-19. 2020. Available online: https://www.migrantjustice.org/publications-list/report-as-if-we-werent-humans (accessed on 3 February 2021).
3. Clibborn, S.; Wright, C.F. COVID-19 and the policy-induced vulnerabilities of temporary migrant workers in Australia. *J. Aust. Political Econ.* **2020**, *85*, 62–70.
4. Symington, A. Migrant workers and the COVID-19 crisis in Australia: An overview of governmental responses. *Aust. J. Hum. Rights* **2020**, *26*, 507–519. [CrossRef]
5. Ullah, A.A.; Nawaz, F.; Chattoraj, D. Locked up under lockdown: The COVID-19 pandemic and the migrant population. *Soc. Sci. Humanit. Open* **2021**, *3*, 100126. [CrossRef] [PubMed]
6. Bennett, C. COVID-19 in Australia: How did a country that fought so hard for extra time end up so ill prepared? *BMJ* **2023**, *380*, 469. [CrossRef] [PubMed]
7. Australian Government. Jobkeeper Payment. 2020. Available online: https://www.ato.gov.au/general/jobkeeper-payment/ (accessed on 18 February 2021).
8. Phillips, M. Responding to migrant workers: The case of Australia. In *State Responses to COVID-19: A Global Snapshot at 1 June 2020*; Georgeou, N., Hawksley, C., Eds.; Western Sydney University: Penrith, Australia, 2020; pp. 12–13.
9. Tham, J.C. COVID-19, labour rights and the role of the state. *J. Aust. Political Econ.* **2020**, *85*, 71–83.
10. Tham, J.C. Why Temporary Migrants Need Jobkeeper. The Conversation. 2020. Available online: https://theconversation.com/why-temporary-migrants-need-jobkeeper-135688 (accessed on 25 April 2021).
11. Shakespeare-Finch, J.; Bowen, H.; Cashin, M.; Badawi, A.; Wells, R.; Rosenbaum, S.; Steel, Z. COVID-19: An Australian Perspective. *J. Loss Trauma* **2020**, *25*, 662–672. [CrossRef]
12. Ministers Treasury Portfolio. 'Interview with Ali Moore, ABC Melbourne Mornings', Job-Keeper Package and Legislation; Economic Response to Coronavirus Transcript. Available online: ministers.treasury.gov.au/ministers/josh-frydenberg-2018/transcripts/interview-ali-moore-abc-melbourne-mornings (accessed on 8 April 2020).
13. Van Kooy, J. COVID-19 and Humanitarian Migrants on Temporary Visas: Assessing the Public Costs. 2020. Available online: https://www.refugeecouncil.org.au/covid-19-assessing-the-public-costs/ (accessed on 16 May 2021).
14. Australian Government. Australia's Migration Trends 2021–2022 Highlights. 2023. Available online: https://www.homeaffairs.gov.au/research-and-stats/files/migration-trends-2021-22.pdf (accessed on 31 May 2023).
15. Rung, D.L. To Move and to Resettle: The Elusive Goals of Precarious 'Non-Citizens': An Institutional Ethnography of Human (Im)mobility within Transnational Regimes of Social Motion. Ph.D. Thesis, Charles Darwin University, Darwin, Australia, 2018. Available online: https://ris.cdu.edu.au/ws/portalfiles/portal/23670929/Thesis_23670895_Rung_D.pdf (accessed on 1 November 2018).
16. Rung, D.L. Processes of Sub-Citizenship: Neoliberal Statecrafting 'Citizens,' 'Non-Citizens,' and Detainable 'Others'. *Soc. Sci.* **2020**, *9*, 5. [CrossRef]
17. Smith, J.; Griffith, D.M.; White, A.; Baker, P.; Watkins, D.C.; Drummond, M.; Semlow, A. COVID-19, equity and men's health: Using evidence to inform future public health policy, practice and research responses to pandemics. *Int. J. Men's Soc. Community Health* **2020**, *3*, e48–e64. [CrossRef]
18. Walter, L.A.; McGregor, A.J. Sex- and Gender-specific Observations and Implications for COVID-19. *West. J. Emerg. Med.* **2020**, *21*, 507–509. [CrossRef]
19. Wenham, C.; Smith, J.; Morgan, R.; Gender and COVID-19 Working Group. COVID-19: The gendered impacts of the outbreak. *Lancet* **2020**, *395*, 846–848. [CrossRef]
20. Kline, N.S. Rethinking COVID-19 Vulnerability: A Call for LGBTQ+ Im/migrant Health Equity in the United States During and After a Pandemic. *Health Equity* **2020**, *4*, 239–242. [CrossRef] [PubMed]
21. Vogl, A.; Fleay, C.; Loughnan, C.; Murray, P.; Dehm, S. COVID-19 and the relentless harms of Australia's punitive immigration detention regime. *Crime, Media, Cult. Int. J.* **2020**, *17*, 43–51. [CrossRef]
22. United Nations. Making the SDGS a Reality. Available online: https://sdgs.un.org/#goal_section (accessed on 13 March 2023).
23. Bwire, G.M. Coronavirus: Why men are more vulnerable to COVID-19 than women? *SN Compr. Clin. Med.* **2020**, *2*, 874–876. [CrossRef] [PubMed]
24. Dehingia, N. Sex differences in COVID-19 case fatality: Do we know enough? *Lancet* **2020**, *9*, e14–e15. [CrossRef]
25. Griffith, D.M.; Sharma, G.; Holliday, C.S.; Enyia, O.K.; Valliere, M.; Semlow, A.R.; Stewart, E.C.; Blumenthal, R.S. Men and COVID-19: A Biopsychosocial Approach to Understanding Sex Differences in Mortality and Recommendations for Practice and Policy Interventions. *Prev. Chronic Dis.* **2020**, *17*, E63. [CrossRef]

26. Danielsen, A.C.; Noll, N. Communicating about COVID-19 and Sex Disparities: A Guide for Media, Scientists, Public Health Officials, and Educators. 2020. Available online: https://www.genderscilab.org/blog/covid-communication (accessed on 3 September 2021).
27. Berkeley Media Studies Group. Communicating about Racial Equity and COVID-19: Connecting Data to Context. 2020. Available online: http://www.bmsg.org/resources/publications/communicating-about-racial-equity-and-covid-19-connecting-data-to-context/ (accessed on 15 January 2021).
28. Borgkvist, A.; Moore, V.; Eliott, J.; Crabb, S. 'I might be a bit of a front runner': An analysis of men's uptake of flexible work arrangements and masculine identity. *Gender Work. Organ.* **2018**, *25*, 703–717. [CrossRef]
29. Smith, J.A.; Adamson, E. Exploring the Links between Fathering, Masculinities and Health and Well-Being for Migrant Fathers: Implications for Policy and Practice. *Int. J. Mens Soc. Community Health* **2020**, *3*, e58–e65. [CrossRef]
30. Rung, D.L.; Adamson, E. Renegotiating roles as fathers and workers: Exploring the experiences of migrant and refugee men in Australia. *Int. J. Men's Soc. Community Health* **2022**, *5*, e1–e14. [CrossRef]
31. Australian Government. Coronavirus and Temporary Visa Holders. 2020. Available online: https://minister.homeaffairs.gov.au/davidcoleman/Pages/Coronavirus-and-Temporary-Visa-holders.aspx (accessed on 12 January 2021).
32. Mares, P. Temporary Migration and Its Implications for Australia. Presented at the Australian Senate Occasional Lecture Series, Canberra, Australia, 23 September 2011.
33. Mares, P. *Not Quite Australian: How Temporary Migration is Changing the Nation*; Text Publishing: Melbourne, Australia, 2016.
34. Robertson, S. The temporalities of international migration: Implications for ethnographic research. *Inst. Cult. Soc. Occas. Pap.* **2014**, *5*, 1–16. [CrossRef]
35. Hugo, G. Change and Continuity in Australian International Migration Policy. *Int. Migr. Rev.* **2014**, *48*, 868–890. [CrossRef]
36. Goldring, L.; Landolt, P. Caught in the Work–Citizenship Matrix: The Lasting Effects of Precarious Legal Status on Work for Toronto Immigrants. *Globalizations* **2011**, *8*, 325–341. [CrossRef]
37. Phillips, J.; Simon-Davies, J. Migration to Australia: A Quick Guide to the Statistics. 2017. Available online: http://parlinfo.aph.gov.au/parlInfo/download/library/prspub/3165114/upload_binary/3165114.pdf (accessed on 9 April 2020).
38. Australian Government. (n.d.). Residency for Tax Purposes. Available online: https://www.ato.gov.au/uploadedFiles/Content/IND/Downloads/Occupation_guides/n75127-DE-5543_Residency-for-tax-purposes-factsheet_W.pdf (accessed on 12 March 2022).
39. Australian Government. Social Security Payments–Residence Criteria. 2020. Available online: https://www.dss.gov.au/about-the-department/international/policy/social-security-payments-residence-criteria#:~:text=Those%20granted%20a%20permanent%20visa,immediately%2C%20if%20they%20are%20eligible (accessed on 14 May 2021).
40. Berg, L. *Migrant Rights at Work: Law's Precariousness at the Intersection of Immigration and Labour*; Routledge: London, UK, 2016.
41. Wacquant, L. Three steps to a historical anthropology of actually existing neoliberalism. *Soc. Anthr.* **2012**, *20*, 66–79. [CrossRef]
42. Bowling, M. Academic Robert Manne: Why Australia Has a 'Uniquely Harsh' Border Control System. 2016. Available online: http://catholicleader.com.au/analysis/academic-robert-manne-why-australia-has-a-uniquely-harsh-border-control-system (accessed on 11 August 2017).
43. Van Houdt, F.; Suvarierol, S.; Schinkel, W. Neoliberal communitarian citizenship: Current trends towards 'earned citizenship' in the United Kingdom, France and the Netherlands. *Int. Sociol.* **2011**, *26*, 408–432. [CrossRef]
44. Brodie, J. Meso-discourses, state forms and the gendering of liberal-democratic citizenship. *Citizsh. Stud.* **1997**, *1*, 223–242. [CrossRef]
45. Grace, B.L.; Nawyn, S.J.; Okwako, B. The Right to Belong (If You Can Afford It): Market-based Restrictions on Social Citizenship in Refugee Resettlement. *J. Refug. Stud.* **2017**, *31*, 42–62. [CrossRef]
46. Sagy, T. Do Human Rights Transcend Citizenship? Lessons from the Buduburam Refugee Camp. *Soc. Leg. Stud.* **2013**, *23*, 215–236. [CrossRef]
47. Somers, M. *Genealogies of Citizenship: Markets, Statelessness, and the Right to Have Rights*; Cambridge University Press: Cambridge, UK, 2008.
48. Anderson, B. *Imagined Communities*; Verso: London, UK, 1983.
49. Castles, S. How nation-states respond to immigration and ethnic diversity. *J. Ethn. Migr. Stud.* **1995**, *21*, 293–308. [CrossRef]
50. Robertson, S.; Runganaikaloo, A. Lives in limbo: Migration experiences in Australia's education–migration nexus. *Ethnicities* **2013**, *14*, 208–226. [CrossRef]
51. Australian Government. 2013–2014 Migration Programme Report. Department of Immigration and Border Protection. 2014. Available online: http://www.border.gov.au/ReportsandPublications/Documents/statistics/report-migration-programme-2013-14.pdf (accessed on 20 May 2018).
52. Australian Government. Australia's Migration Trends 2019–2020 Highlights. 2020. Available online: https://www.homeaffairs.gov.au/research-and-stats/files/migration-trends-highlights-2019-20.pdf (accessed on 10 June 2022).
53. Goldring, L.; Landolt, P. *Immigrants and Precarious Employment in the New Economy Project, Brief 2: Immigrants and Precarious Work*; York University: Toronto, ON, Canada, 2009.
54. Lee-Browne, K. 'In the Cruel Shadow of Empire': A Case Study on the Illegalisation, Migrantisation and Sub-Citizenship of the Windrush. Bachelor's Thesis, Malmo University, Malmo, Sweden, 2020.

55. Castañeda, E.; Shemesh, A. Overselling Globalization: The Misleading Conflation of Economic Globalization and Immigration, and the Subsequent Backlash. *Soc. Sci.* **2020**, *9*, 61. [CrossRef]
56. Morey, M.R. Policy, Occupation and Transnationalism: New Zealanders Living in Australia. Ph.D. Thesis, University of Adelaide, Adelaide, Australia, 2020.
57. Missbach, A. Substituting immigration detention centres with 'open prisons' in Indonesia: Alternatives to detention as the continuum of unfreedom. *Citizsh. Stud.* **2020**, *25*, 224–237. [CrossRef]
58. Amnesty International. Australia: Island of Despair: Australia's "Processing" of Refugees on Nauru. 2016. Available online: https://www.amnesty.org (accessed on 20 May 2018).
59. Wickramage, K.; Gostin, L.O.; Friedman, E.; Prakongsai, P.; Suphanchaimat, R.; Hui, C.; Harper, D.R. Missing: Where are the migrants in pandemic influenza preparedness plans? *Health Hum. Rights J.* **2018**, *20*, 251–258.
60. Berg, L. At the border and between the cracks: The precarious position of irregular migrant workers under international human rights law. *Melb. J. Int. Law* **2007**, *8*, 1–34.
61. Berg, L.; Farbenblum, B. Wage Theft in Australia: Findings of the National Temporary Migrant Work Survey. 2018. Available online: https://static1.squarespace.com/static/593f6d9fe4fcb5c458624206/t/5bd26f620d9297e70989b27a/1540517748798/Wage+theft+in+Silence+Report.pdf (accessed on 5 March 2019).
62. Clibborn, S. Multiple frames of reference: Why international student workers in Australia tolerate underpayment. *Econ. Ind. Democr.* **2018**, *42*, 336–354. [CrossRef]
63. Howe, J.; Clibborn, S.; Reilly, A.; van der Broek, D.; Wright, C.F. *Towards a Durable Future: Tackling Labour Challenges in the Australian Horticulture Industry*; The University of Sydney: Sydney, Australia, 2019.
64. Australian Government. Boosting Health and Disability Worker Numbers during the Coronavirus [Press Release]. Available online: https://formerministers.dss.gov.au/18988/boosting-health-and-disability-worker-numbers-during-the-coronavirus/ (accessed on 23 April 2020).
65. Karp, P. Sydney Laundry Condemned for Standing Down Migrant Workers Ineligible for Jobkeeper. *The Guardian*. Available online: https://www.theguardian.com/australia-news/2020/apr/30/sydney-laundry-condemned-for-standing-down-migrant-workers-ineligible-for-jobkeeper (accessed on 30 April 2020).
66. Rajish, A. Stood Down en Masse, More Than 100 Nepali Workers at a Sydney Laundry Still Awaiting Support. SBS Nepali. Available online: https://www.sbs.com.au/language/english/stood-down-en-masse-more-than-100-nepali-workers-from-a-sydney-laundry-still-awaiting-support (accessed on 27 May 2020).
67. Boucher, A. COVID-19 Is Not Only a Health Crisis, It's a Migration Crisis. 2020. Available online: https://www.lowyinstitute.org/the-interpreter/covid-19-not-only-health-crisis-it-s-migration-crisis (accessed on 1 March 2021).
68. Baxter, J. Fathers and Work. 2018. Available online: https://aifs.gov.au/sites/default/files/4_fathers_and_work_1909_0.pdf (accessed on 19 May 2021).
69. Baxter, J.; Gray, A.M.; Alexander, M.; Strazdins, L.; Bittman, M. *Mothers and Fathers with Young Children: Paid Employment, Caring and Wellbeing*; Department of Families, Community Services and Indigenous Affairs, Commonwealth of Australia: Canberra, Australia, 2007.
70. Coles, L.; Hewitt, B.; Martin, B. Contemporary fatherhood: Social, demographic and attitudinal factors associated with involved fathering and long work hours. *J. Sociol.* **2018**, *54*, 591–608. [CrossRef]
71. Craig, L.; Mullan, K. Australian fathers' work and family time in comparative and temporal perspective. *J. Fam. Stud.* **2012**, *18*, 165–174. [CrossRef]
72. Forget, G.; Correa-Velez, I.; Dee, M. Being a Father in My New Society: A Qualitative Study of the Fathering Experiences of Men from Refugee Backgrounds Resettled in Australia. *J. Refug. Stud.* **2019**, *32*, 322–339. [CrossRef]
73. Pease, B. Immigrant men and domestic life: Renegotiating the patriarchal bargain? In *Migrant Men: Critical Studies of Masculinities and the Migration Experience*; Donaldson, M., Hibbins, R., Howson, R., Pease, B., Eds.; Routledge: New York, NY, USA, 2009; pp. 79–95.
74. Tan, G.; Rung, D.L.; Golebiowska, K. (Forthcoming). Coordinating Settlement (Im)mobilities: Exploring the Social Organisation of Secondary Migration Patterns and Resettlement Geographies among Humanitarian Migrants in Regional Australia. *Aust. Geographer*.
75. Cooklin, A.R.; Giallo, R.; Strazdins, L.; Martin, A.; Leach, L.S.; Nicholson, J.M. What matters for working fathers? Job characteristics, work-family conflict and enrichment, and fathers' postpartum mental health in an Australian cohort. *Soc. Sci. Med.* **2015**, *146*, 214–222. [CrossRef]
76. Giallo, R.; Riggs, E.; Lynch, C.; Vanpraag, D.; Yelland, J.; Szwarc, J.; Duell-Piening, P.; Tyrell, L.; Casey, S.; Brown, S.J. The physical and mental health problems of refugee and migrant fathers: Findings from an Australian population-based study of children and their families. *BMJ Open* **2017**, *7*, e015603. [CrossRef]
77. Rung, D.L.; Hetz, H.; Radford, D. 'I came to Australia with very big hope, big wishes, big goals': Applying 'mobility work' and 'resettlement work' to explore the emotional labour and subaltern masculinities of refugee-background men. In *Migratory Men: Place, Transnationalism and Masculinities*; Stahl, G., Zaho, Y., Eds.; Routledge: London, UK, 2023.

International Journal of
Environmental Research and Public Health

MDPI

Article

"Es Muy Tranquilo Aquí": Perceptions of Safety and Calm among Binationally Mobile Mexican Immigrants in a Rural Border Community

Rebecca M. Crocker [1,*], Karina Duenas [1], Luis Vázquez [2], Maia Ingram [3], Felina M. Cordova-Marks [1], Emma Torres [2] and Scott Carvajal [3]

1 Department of Health Promotion Sciences, Zuckerman College of Public Health, University of Arizona, Tucson, AZ 85724, USA; krduenas@arizona.edu (K.D.); felina@arizona.edu (F.M.C.-M.)
2 Campesinos Sin Fronteras, Somerton, AZ 85350, USA; lvazquez@campesinossinfronteras.org (L.V.); etorres@campesinossinfronteras.org (E.T.)
3 Arizona Prevention Research Center, Department of Health Promotion Sciences, Zuckerman College of Public Health, University of Arizona, Tucson, AZ 85724, USA; maiai@arizona.edu (M.I.); carvajal@arizona.edu (S.C.)
* Correspondence: rcrocker@arizona.edu

Abstract: Perceptions of community can play an important role in determining health and well-being. We know little, however, about residents' perceptions of community safety in the Southwestern borderlands, an area frequently portrayed as plagued by disorder. The qualitative aim of this community-based participatory research study was to explore the perceptions of Mexican-origin border residents about their communities in southern Yuma County, Arizona. Our team of University of Arizona researchers and staff from Campesinos Sin Fronteras, a grassroots farmworker support agency in Yuma County, Arizona, developed a bilingual interview guide and recruited participants through radio adds, flyers, and cold calls among existing agency clientele. Thirty individual interviews with participants of Mexican origin who live in and/or work in rural Yuma County were conducted remotely in 2021. Participants overwhelmingly perceived their communities as both calm and safe. While some participants mentioned safety concerns, the vast majority described high levels of personal security and credited both neighbors and police for ensuring local safety. These perceptions were stated in direct contrast to those across the border, where participants had positive familial and cultural ties but negative perceptions regarding widespread violence. In conclusion, we argue that to understand environmental factors affecting health and well-being in Mexican immigrant populations, it is critical to examine the role of binational external referents that color community perceptions.

Keywords: Mexican immigrants; U.S.-Mexico borderlands; community perceptions; safety; violence; well-being; binational; external referents

Citation: Crocker, R.M.; Duenas, K.; Vázquez, L.; Ingram, M.; Cordova-Marks, F.M.; Torres, E.; Carvajal, S. "Es Muy Tranquilo Aquí": Perceptions of Safety and Calm among Binationally Mobile Mexican Immigrants in a Rural Border Community. *Int. J. Environ. Res. Public Health* **2022**, *19*, 8399. https://doi.org/10.3390/ijerph19148399

Academic Editors: Maria De Jesus and Ernesto Castañeda

Received: 20 April 2022
Accepted: 7 July 2022
Published: 9 July 2022

1. Introduction

The extent to which individuals hold positive perceptions of their neighborhoods and communities may have important implications for their health and wellbeing [1]. Growing awareness of the importance of upstream influences has led to increased interest in "place effects", or the impact of our social and physical environments on human health [2]. Such ties have been explored in the literature about geographies of health and well-being, where the material and socioeconomic conditions of one's lived environment have been assigned a seat at the table next to individual and family factors as determinants of variation and inequities in individual wellbeing [3,4]. While much of this research has addressed negative contributing factors such as violence, lack of infrastructure, and unsightly surroundings, the theory of "therapeutic landscapes" has been widely employed to identify the places or milieus (both physical and psychological) that can, by contrast, promote healing and wellness [5].

Perceptions of a community may be influenced by a broad variety of factors attendant to individual and community level priorities and needs for wellbeing [6]. These include aesthetic and safety features such as lighting and sidewalks, housing style and affordability [7] and the availability of local resources like parks and schools [8]. It also incorporates less tangible socio-cultural aspects founded in community history, ethnic identity and social networks, with social cohesion acting as a major contributor to wellbeing [9]. In addition, perceived personal safety has been associated with enhanced wellbeing and health promoting physical activity [10], whereas fear and experiences of crime have a negative influence on how individuals assess their neighborhoods and can carry long-term health consequences [11,12].

While the U.S.–Mexico border region has been a locus of media attention characterizing the region as unfavorably affected by uncontrolled migration, "spillover" drug related violence from Mexico, and poor public safety, we know little about how border inhabitants themselves perceive and experience their lived environments. This scarcity of data on border residents limits our access to what Castañeda and Chiappetta (2020) term an "authentic interpretation of border security," independent from sensationalized media portrayals [13] (p. 11). Crime statistics, however, indicate that the region has been mischaracterized. They demonstrate that cities and settlements on the U.S. side of the international border have lower than average crime rates as compared to other regions of the U.S. [14,15]. Moreover, crime rates in U.S. border cities are decreasing faster than in the rest of the country, even at a time when drug war related violence has spiked in many Mexican towns and cities right across the border [16,17].

Moreover, the limited available data indicates that most border residents have positive perceptions of their communities and local safety, reflecting these official low crime rates [13]. Communities in the U.S. borderlands are populated largely by Mexican origin residents, and their shared sociocultural identity alone may confer a health advantage [18]. Evidence from El Paso, Texas indicates that the primarily Mexican origin residents positively described their city as "safe", "calm", and "good" and did not perceive that community safety was dependent on the border wall [13,19]. This is somewhat surprising given that Mexican immigrants are often disproportionately vulnerable to attacks and robberies and are less likely to report crimes to the police due to concerns over immigration status [20,21].

It has been suggested that when interpreting place-based perceptions of safety and other community attributes, it may be important to consider changes in referents due to residential mobility [3]. This is particularly relevant in studies along the U.S.–Mexico border, where a significant portion of residents were born in Mexico and have regular and constant cross-border exposures. A binational lens has been incorporated elsewhere to better understand immigrants' perceptions of other critical health-related issues, including blocked access to medical care post-migration, the relevance of preventive dental care, and ties between trauma and mental health [22–24]. Moreover, for Mexicans living in the United States, the change in place of residence often entails a significant loss of civic and human rights due to the dearth of legalized immigration pathways for them. The realities of living as long-term "undocumented" residents of a foreign country experiencing a wave of anti-immigrant public sentiment and exclusionary legislation likely color all nature of community perceptions.

Further exploration of how border residents perceive their communities within this binational context is warranted, particularly given the link between perceptions of social and physical environments and human health. In this article, we present the qualitative results of a study that aimed to explore the perceptions of Mexican-origin border residents about their communities in southern Yuma County, Arizona.

2. Materials and Methods

2.1. Study Aims

This article presents data from the first data collection phase of a community-based participatory research (CBPR) project, taking an ecological approach to identifying sources of stress and resilience among Mexican-origin persons in Yuma County, Arizona [25,26].

2.2. Study Design

This multi-year, mixed-methods study employed a CBPR approach bringing together researchers from the University of Arizona (UA) and a workforce of community health workers (known in Spanish as *promotoras*) and behavioral health technicians from Campesinos Sin Fronteras (CSF). CSF is a grassroots community organization in Yuma County, Arizona founded by farmworkers to address unmet health and social needs they identified in their community. The 6th author is CSF's current Executive Director and one of its founders. The study's CBPR approach was based on over 20 years of partnership addressing the health and safety of agricultural workers in the region. This study's focus on stress and resilience among Latino/a adults grew out of the team's previous work on farmworker experiences of stress and discrimination, and ongoing concern from CSF regarding poor access to mental health services and support [27]. In addition to increasing the quality of the research, this strong academic–community collaboration ensures that the research is responsive to community priorities and provides community benefit [28,29].

The development of aim 1 of this study began in August 2020 with weekly meetings between the UA research team and the CSF team. These meetings were guided by reviewing the study's stated aims but were held in an open format that encouraged all members of the study team to discuss key areas of interest relating to sources of stress and potential areas of resilience in southern Yuma County. These meetings were held remotely via zoom and participants were encouraged to speak in their preferred language and a bilingual member of the team provided translation in the Zoom chat feature. This design was aimed to ensure that all team members felt comfortable expressing their ideas, opinions and expertise to the entire group. Team building and team collaboration was also enhanced by an immersion tour of Somerton and San Luis, Arizona hosted by CSF in September 2021, aimed to build cultural and community specific familiarity.

Based on a careful review of notes summarizing the priority areas and themes identified during team discussions, the lead author developed a draft qualitative interview guide in English and Spanish. This draft was reviewed by the entire team for representation of salient themes and cultural and community congruence, and the Spanish version was edited by native speakers for regional appropriateness. The resulting semi-structured interview guide (see Supplementary File S1: Interview Guide English/Spanish) focused on five domain areas in the context of living on the border and in a binational environment: 1. health concepts, 2. personal health and wellbeing, 3. sources of resilience, 4. sources of stress, and 5. community. We also included a short demographic questionnaire aimed to capture individual characteristics including gender, birth year, marital status, household members, family size, binational connection, and employment.

2.3. Sample Participants

Participants for the study (N = 30) were recruited by the CSF promotora workforce through existing CSF client networks, phone calls, flyers placed in the CSF waiting room, radio advertisements on the CSF radio station, a feature run in a local Spanish newspaper, and word of mouth. Inclusion criteria included that the person: (1) be of Latino/a origin, (2) live in the border region of either southern Yuma County, Arizona, or northern Sonora, Mexico, (3) be between the ages of 18–70, and (4) have access to a telephone or computer for Zoom-based calls. After describing the study to potential participants, the promotoras screened them for eligibility. Those who were interested and eligible were then consented verbally, provided with a copy of the consent disclosure for their records, and scheduled for an interview as soon as possible.

2.4. Data Collection

While data collection was originally planned to be in person, the team switched to password protected Zoom audio calls due to the onset of the COVID-19 pandemic. In order to assist participants with Zoom technology, CSF promotoras sent interview reminders, provided instructions on connecting to the Zoom platform, and completed a follow-up call after the interview was completed. Three members of the UA team and two CSF behavioral health technicians led the qualitative interviews. All five were bilingual and experienced at conducting culturally congruent interviews with Latino/a populations. In preparation for data gathering, the two behavioral health technicians received training on protection of human subjects, ethics, and providing informed consent. In addition, the lead author conducted a bilingual interview training for the interview team.

The promotoras piloted the semi-structured interview questions with Spanish speaking CSF staff. Once participant recruitment began, we implemented the interview guide with three participants and then reviewed the interview guide implementation to ensure fluidity and the tailoring of questions to cover all areas of study aims. Interviews were conducted in the participants' preferred language (29 in Spanish and one in English) and lasted between 40–80 min. Participants were given a $40 Walmart gift card incentive for their time.

2.5. Data Analysis

Audio files of the interviews were transcribed in the language spoken by a bilingual, bicultural graduate student and a professional transcription company (GMR Transcription). Interviewers then conducted quality assurance checks of transcriptions. After reviewing transcripts, the research team agreed that data saturation had been reached and salient themes were evident. At this point, transcripts were uploaded to Dedoose data management software (www.dedoose.com, accessed on 19 April 2022) and two UA members of the research team independently coded 15 interview transcripts each (see Supplementary Materials Table S1: Code Tree). Notations of the rationale for additional codes and revised codes were discussed for consensus, and following completion of coding, the research team discussed the most prominent findings, surprises in the data, and weighed the relative impact of the findings to prioritize dissemination in the framework of the team's research priorities and CSF's areas of interest.

2.6. Ethical Considerations

This study's CBPR approach facilitated our recruitment process and ensured open and culturally consonant communication with research participants. Given the sensitive nature of questions surrounding immigration, we encouraged participants to verbalize any discomfort throughout the interview process and assured them that they could refrain from answering any question or stop the interview at any time. At the time of receiving their incentive, the promotoras inquired with each participant about their experience in the interview and accepted any feedback that was provided. This study was approved by the UA human subjects' protections review board (2003462440). To protect participant privacy, pseudonyms are used throughout this article.

3. Results

This study sample of Mexican origin participants included 17 women and 13 men, with an average age of 35. Half of participants were married, while the remaining 15 were primarily single or in domestic partnerships, and most (23/30) had at least one child. Most participants (23/30) were born in the Mexican border states of Sonora or Baja California Norte, three were from other states in Mexico (Guanajuato, Michoacán and Sinaloa), and four were born in the U.S. border states of Arizona and California. Most participants lived in Yuma County, Arizona (17 in San Luis, Arizona, six in Somerton, and three in Yuma), while four lived in the Mexican border city of San Luis Río Colorado, Sonora. Occupations in the sample varied and included retail positions, maintenance, and clerical work, but the most common were in agriculture (8/30) and teacher or teacher's aide (5/30). Five participants were either unemployed or stay-at-home mothers. For a full presentation of sample demographic characteristics, see Table 1.

Table 1. Characteristics of Mexican Origin Study Participants.

Characteristics	Median/n	%/Range
Age (years)	35	21, 60
Females (% yes)	17	56.6
Married (% yes)	15	50.0
Have Children (% yes)	23	76.6
Place of Origin		
From Mexican Border States	23	76.6
From other Mexican States	3	10.0
From U.S. Border States	4	13.3
Place of Current Residence		
San Luis, Arizona	17	56.6
Somerton, Arizona	6	20.0
Yuma, Arizona	3	10.0
San Luis Río Colorado, Mexico	4	13.3
Employment		
Employed (% yes)	25	83.3
Teaching or Aide (% yes)	5	16.6
Agriculture (% yes)	8	26.6

Study participants overwhelmingly reported that the small towns of Somerton and San Luis, Arizona provided safe and calm environments in which to live and raise families. They frequently described their communities as "tranquilo" (meaning calm, tranquil, peaceful, or quiet) and safety and calm were identified as major advantages to living in southern Yuma County (For original quotes in Spanish, see Supplementary Materials Table S2: Original Quotes in Spanish). Three primary themes emerged in relationship to these findings: (1) Perception of Calm, with a sub-theme of how calm environments reduce stress; (2) Comparing Safety in Yuma County and Mexico, with sub-themes on safety concerns in Yuma County, comparisons to higher levels of violence in Mexico, and the roles of neighbors and police in promoting safety; and (3) Appreciation of Safety in Southern Yuma County, with a sub-theme on the compromises made for gaining safety.

3.1. Perceptions of Calm

Most participants living on the U.S. side of the border described the places where they lived as calm and peaceful, perceptions that were often related to these places being relatively small towns in a predominantly rural region. This notion of "small town" was tied to several specific benefits, including the absence of excessive noise, crowded environments, and dangerous or frustrating transportation issues. Luis, a resident of San Luis, Arizona expressed: "I think that, first and foremost, what I like is that it's a quiet city, right? There isn't—it's not a very big city, it's not noisy."

The region's sense of calm was often compared positively to other larger cities in both Mexico and the US. Most participants had had prior experience living in larger cities, most commonly San Luis Rio Colorado, Sonora, the fourth largest city in state of Sonora, and the large urban center of Mexicali, Baja California Norte. Others had been exposed to other large cities in Mexico or had traveled to work in urban areas in the U.S. southwest and west, such as Los Angeles or Salinas, California, and Tucson or Phoenix, Arizona. Manuela explained that while San Luis, Arizona was larger than Somerton, "It is quieter than, I don't know, I have been to California and places like that, Phoenix, and it seems to me like there is a lot of traffic. Here I can go out in the street without being scared of, well of driving, because I'm a really nervous driver." While some acknowledged that the size of their towns limited opportunities for entertainment and recreation, many participants felt there were enough stores, restaurants, and parks to serve their basic needs.

In addition to appreciating the small size of the communities where they lived, participants also attributed the region's calm environment to the fact that their neighbors were either older or lived in family units, were work-focused ("gente de trabajo"), and generally kept to themselves. Anita, a married woman living in Somerton said: "In terms of tranquility, here where I am living, I live around many elderly people, so it is a very quiet community. I used to live in Yuma and it was like a trailer park where I lived, and there was a lot of disorder, a lot of problems. Not here, here everything is really quiet." Many participants specifically acknowledged the lack of altercations with their neighbors and the fact that no one appeared interested in starting problems. For example, Francisca, a widow who had lived in the region for over 30 years, commented that: "Well it's very peaceful, very calm, because my neighbors are not rowdy. I have never had a fight with anyone there. Very peaceful, very calm."

A Calm Environment Reduces Stress

Participants frequently commented that the small and calm nature of their communities created ease in their daily lives and made it less stressful than living in a large city or other places where one had more daily concerns. Many mentioned specific practical advantages of living in a quiet place that reduced stress, including ready access to stores, restaurants and other facilities. Adán, who moved to Somerton from Yuma 22 years ago stated: "But what can I tell you? The market is just a three-minute walk away, I have stores here. I live right along the main street and we have everything close by. You don't get stressed out about the traffic. Here when you go to the store, you walk."

Other participants commented more generally that living in a small town afforded a slower pace of life. When asked if the stressors in her community were similar to those experienced elsewhere, Somerton resident Monica replied: "No I don't think they are the same because I feel that both the community and the city are a bit calmer and there are other places where everything is faster paced. So, I don't think they are the same." Some participants noted that this slower pace both reduced stress and enabled them to enjoy their daily lives more fully. Evaristo, who had lived in the United States for 20 years commented that in general life north of the border felt very rushed and focused around work, but that in San Luis: "Here I feel that, yes, you enjoy it a little bit more. But I don't know exactly how to explain it but I feel calmer in this area than in a city."

For Somerton resident Olger, a married father of three originally from the Sonoran capital of Hermosillo, this calm translated as his "comfort zone." He explained:

"It's not very stressful here, because it is basically a small town. I would say this place is not very stressful ... Sometimes we have talked about buying a house and we ask ourselves: 'where? Where would we go?' And I have always said: 'well not Yuma, not Yuma.' Because it could be really pretty in some parts, in some parts quiet. But you do feel the stress of living in the city a bit more because of all the traffic, perhaps lots of malicious people, etc. And here it is really a little calmer. Yes, it's basically, it's like my space, my comfort zone, and it's even like—I live in apartments, I mean, I don't have a house still, right? And in fact, I live where I work. And I feel comfortable and safe here. Why? Because I am familiar with my surroundings, I know all the people here, the neighbors, I know how the facilities are. So, I don't have much to worry about."

For most participants, limiting stress was understood to be an important component to mental and physical health. For example, Manuela, an agricultural field-worker who lived in Yuma, explained: "I think that living a life with lots of stress deteriorates you, it wears you down." Because of this, many participants believed that finding calm was a critical element of health maintenance.

3.2. Comparing Safety in Southern Yuma County and Mexico

3.2.1. Safety Concerns in Southern Yuma County

A few participants raised safety concerns about their communities in Yuma County, some of which were common to the broader region, such as car accidents and gang activity, while others were closely tied to the region's proximity of the US–Mexico border, such as recruitment of youth into the drug trade, undocumented migration, and border surveillance. For example, Rosie, whose home was very close to the border wall and had an unfenced yard, described:

"Immigration officials go there, behind my house. Helicopters are out starting early in the morning ... and you can't know if there might be, if someone might be running or have a gun. That has never happened because I don't think they come to do those things. They cross because they want to get ahead. But still, there have been many cases in which they don't come armed but the police themselves can shoot off their guns just because they want to catch someone."

Others mentioned concerns about "spillover violence" from Mexico, noting the disappearance and subsequent murders of two young women from the area in 2021, a crime that participants felt was reminiscent of violence in Mexico. Chucho, a young man originally from Los Angeles, said that he was starting to hear about "the violence, like cartels doing like killings and gun shootings across the border ... like that type of like news has been increasing and that like the only worry is like, when will it spill over to this side?"

3.2.2. Comparison to Higher Violence Levels in Mexico

Participants named far more safety concerns, however, when speaking about Mexico and particularly the northern border region. Most participants (23/30) were originally from the border states of Sonora and Baja California Norte, and had witnessed dramatic increases in drug-related violence over the past decades. While the majority of participants (26/30) now lived on the US side of the border, they had frequent exposure to Mexico through regular border crossings to visit with family, friends, and significant others, attend celebrations and family events, doctors' appointments, and shopping. Those who lived in San Luis, Arizona described living "right on the border", and being able to see Mexico and the busy crossing lines from their homes. The four participants who lived in Mexico crossed the border daily or weekly.

These binational cultural and community ties afforded participants first-hand experiences with issues around compromised public safety in Mexico. For example, Ana, originally from San Luis Río Colorado, explained: "Right now there is a lot of crime, and they say this is because everyone wants to take control of the borders. Right now in San Luis Río Colorado there has been a lot of, well something that we had never seen here: murders, kidnappings in broad daylight."

Many participants described a declining arc of public safety in Mexico due to the drug trade that made living there and even visiting potentially risky. They mentioned threats to security including vandalism, robbery, violent attacks, gun fights, accidents, killings, and kidnappings. Diego, who moved to San Luis four years ago from Mexicali, explained: "Oh yes, it's really different by comparison to where I lived in Mexico, because there it was, well where I lived it was a really dangerous block. There were many people doing drugs ... and just leaving my house you could get assaulted. That happened many times, not to us, but to other people."

3.2.3. Perceptions of Relative Safety in Southern Yuma County

Participants' binational frame of reference had a direct impact on the way they perceived security in the cities and towns on the U.S. side of the border, with the vast majority reporting that the communities in southern Yuma County felt very safe by comparison. Monica, originally from Mexicali, Baja California Norte, said: "Look, the community where we are now is actually calm. But if you're talking about Mexico, Mexico is really hectic. In Mexicali everything is go, go, go. But everything in Yuma County is peaceful. Here there are more older people so it's quieter, all things considered." Often participants living in the U.S. could not think of anything that made them feel unsafe in their communities and described a deep level of personal security both in terms of protection from acts of violence as well as the security of their possessions.

Elia, lamented that the Sonoran ejido of her childhood had been a safe place but that public safety had declined dramatically since then. She stated: "Here in San Luis, Arizona, I feel very safe. There's not, how can I say, like in Mexico, so many gangs, so many addictions, so much alcohol, so many bad people in the street. I feel very safe, very safe here, more peaceful. I can, yes, I can leave my girls outside while I go in for a drink of water or something. I have my fence and everything, but I can leave them outside briefly."

Participants' conceptualization of regional safety was often defined by the absence of major violent events such as shoot-outs, kidnappings, and murders. Angeles, a young woman originally from the city of Mexicali, Baja California Norte, explained that what she liked about San Luis, Arizona was that: "You almost never hear about there being problems. Lately there are a lot of car accidents, but I mean, you don't hear about gunshots, horrible things like that, they're unheard of."

Francisca indicated that the lack of such violent outbursts gave her a sense of freedom with her children. She explained: "Here, one can comfortably take the kids to the park or get them out on a walk. Yes, it's very rare that you hear about anything bad here in San Luis, Arizona, like that someone was killed or run over or something. There [in Mexico] no. There no. There you look at someone the wrong way and you don't make it."

3.2.4. The Role of Neighbors in Promoting Safety

In reflecting on why their communities in Yuma County felt safe to them, participants frequently commented on the helpful roles played by their neighbors. While many participants reported not knowing their neighbors well, most described generally positive relationships and appreciation of the fact that their neighbors did not start verbal or physical altercations with each other. Tomás explained: "the families all keep to themselves."

Moreover, participants remarked that their neighbors supported community safety by taking good care of their own properties, alerting each other to any issues, and watching out for each other's personal safety and belongings. For example, Sabina noted that her neighbors were always willing to lend a hand. She explained: "I truly feel that this is a safe community. I feel so safe here where I live, so safe that—and this is my fault—that sometimes I say: 'I left the bicycle outside without putting the outside light on. And the bicycle is still there in the morning!' (laughter) ... so I feel that, ay, yes, my neighbors will watch it for me."

A few participants expressed that the fact that most local residents were of Mexican origin and Spanish speaking greatly eased their ability to communicate and support each other in keeping the area safe. For example, one thing that Tomás appreciated about his home in San Luis, Arizona was the constant influx of new immigrants from Mexico. He explained: "What makes it different is that new young people from Mexico are always arriving. So, there is a little more Mexican culture here. And they settle here, and you could say that that is why we make a good match, because we basically have the same roots and the same behaviors."

Diego, who had moved to San Luis four years prior described a neighborhood Facebook group that added an additional layer of cooperation around basic safety and caretaking. He said that through that group: "We also make sure that, like if they see something strange, then they let us know on there, or if a pet got loose and they find it somewhere else, you know, they also notify us, things like that. We are, like, in close communication."

3.2.5. The Role of Police in Promoting Safety

Participants also noted that local police forces played a critical role in making them feel safe and protected. Given that our team had previously documented stress deriving from the multiple overlapping jurisdictions of police and border authorities in Yuma County [30], our study team included the following question to directly assess the presence of and impact of such stress: "Do you feel that the presence of border patrol and police is a cause of stress for you or members of your family or community?"

Contrary to what we expected based on this prior research, the majority of participants replied that the police played a positive role in regional security. Francisca, a woman in her mid-40s who lived in San Luis responded: "Well, not really. I think they are a means of security for the community and for those around us on both sides of the border." Malena, who was originally from central Mexico, felt similarly. She said: "The police control makes me feel safer. Yes, I think that, as far as I can see, they do their job well. And, what can I say? Well, I don't know, I am very at ease here."

Several participants expressed appreciation for the constant presence and proximity of the police forces in the region, with a few mentioning being glad to have members of the police force as their close neighbors. Ivis, a mother of three who lived in Somerton stated: "Yes, it is calm here, I feel safe. And then I also have neighbors who are police here. I have neighbors who are police, I have five neighbors who are police." Another Somerton resident, Adán, remarked that: "It makes me feel safer here because, just 30 seconds away, we have the police and fire department. That makes me feel very safe, because it's not as if just because we live here nothing more will ever happen, right? But that gives us a lot of peace of mind."

Others commented on how regularly the police passed through the areas where they lived. Pancho, originally from Culiacán, Sinaloa expressed: "It makes me feel safe that here there is always, always really constant surveillance. Even though I live on Main Street, on the main drag, every day at the same time a patrol car passes by ... always doing their rounds."

Several participants remarked specifically on appreciating the responsiveness of the police forces, an observation that was linked both to the towns being small and to the professional training of the local forces. Sabina, a preschool teacher who had lived in San Luis for 20 years, said: "I feel protected in this community. I think the police department does its job well. I think that when people need to call them, they are there to assist them, because it's not a very big community." Ernesto, a young man born in U.S. but with significant cross-border family and cultural ties stated: "I feel like it makes me feel safe that here in San Luis, Arizona you can call 911 for an emergency and they respond very quickly. The officials here are, yes, they are very well-equipped, very well-trained professionals."

While most participants referred to the local police agencies of their towns in their responses, a few mentioned also welcoming the presence of other police jurisdictions, including those from the nearby Cocopah Indian Tribe as well as federal forces. For example, Luis, a young man employed in the lettuce fields, explained how more soldiers and National Guards had recently been sent to the border near his home in San Luis, Arizona. He said: "They say there is more mobilization around public safety, right? Or of the armed forces. And the truth is that you start to feel a little more at ease, because, I mean, like when they started to arrive, the level of insecurity declined, isn't that right?"

3.3. *Appreciation of Safety in Southern Yuma County*

When asked what they liked about where they lived, participants living in southern Yuma County overwhelmingly expressed great appreciation for how safe they felt in their small communities. Many participants offered specific examples of how they had reduced their levels of precaution and vigilance since moving to the area due to their perceived low risk of personal attacks and robbery. For example, Ami a married mother of three children stated: "I feel—let me give you an example—I feel free to have my car windows down without having to look all around me. I feel calm here, at ease."

Participants recognized that the lack of violence, vandalism, and traffic danger positively affected many areas of their daily lives, allowing them to feel at ease while going outside to walk, shop, and eat, and being on the street. For example, Tomás stated that: "In terms of tranquility, before the pandemic one could go to the parks without any problem at all. There is no uncontrolled vandalism." Likewise, Mario, a married father living in San Luis, commented that the lack of traffic dangers facilitated walking in public places. He said: "The good thing is that [San Luis] has, that one can walk at ease in the streets. The cars don't go fast, they respect the traffic signals, they respect you. It's very good."

This sense of calm also extended to participants' homes and personal belongings. They described being surprised upon realizing that their belongings were safe when left unsecured, and enjoying the ease of not always having to lock homes and cars. Evaristo, a fieldworker with two children stated: "It's simply the fact that I have felt so comfortable when I go out. I come home and sometimes I say to myself 'ay, the door was left open, and ay look, what happened?' And how peaceful it feels to go out and know that you can even not lock up, because you know that everything will be okay."

Some also described novel feelings around their own personal safety in their homes, including the freedom to come home alone and unaccompanied, even at night. Sabina, a single mother of five children explained: "I feel safe, so safe that sometimes I have to go to a training or something, and sometimes I forget to turn on the light. And I don't feel scared coming home, I don't come home like 'oh no, my house is dark. Let me call someone to see if they can accompany me home.' No, with all the trust in the world, I open the door to my house and I turn on the light."

Making Compromises for Safety

In several instances, participants indicated that their appreciation of the region's safety and calm had influenced their decision to move to or remain in the area, despite noting its disadvantages in other areas. Some participants indicated, for example, that they were willing to forego better economic opportunity and more developed infrastructure and services potentially available in other areas of the United States in exchange for a safe local environment. Belem noted: "Here the community is very peaceful, where we live you rarely hear much about, like in other places that they stole something or there are lots of gangs, almost nothing like that. It's like, even though the situation here in terms of work and pay is not very good, you feel like it's a good place to raise your kids, all considering."

Several participants recognized that moving to the quiet communities of southern Yuma County led to a loss of social cohesion or "convivencia" (shared living experiences) they had enjoyed in Mexico. For example, Linda explained that to her what was missing from her community was: "a little more life, more of that Mexican part—or maybe another kind of culture— but it's almost, almost like you come here to Somerton and, it's as if, like everyone is shut away, everyone is closed off. Even before COVID, everyone was shut away in their houses." Likewise, Vanessa noted of her home in Somerton that: "The other place I lived before was like a million times better. But the truth is, the environment around there was a little more [dangerous]. And so, I think that is the most important factor that makes me—even though I know that it's like better there—that I still prefer to be here."

Sabina concluded that the calm and safe environment of San Luis, Arizona was a deciding factor for her family. She stated: "It's a quiet town. If one wants to live peacefully, I think it is a peaceful town. I compare it to San Luis Río Colorado, and I can say that for the calm and safety, I'll stay in Arizona."

4. Discussion

Over the past decades, there has been growing recognition that place and people's perceptions of it are woven into the fabric of what creates health-inducing environments. Moreover, individuals' experiences of the communities and neighborhoods in which they live are contributing factors to the widespread variation and inequities observed in individual wellbeing [3,4]. Latino/a-origin populations in the United States are documented to face a disproportionate burden of both incidence of and complications from many diseases, including diabetes and liver disease [31,32]. From the lens of social determinants of health, they face some of the largest disparities among U.S.-based ethnic groups in areas including inequities in health care access, education, and occupational protections [33]. However,

Latino/as also exhibit lower overall mortality rates as compared to non-Hispanic Whites, a phenomenon known as the "immigrant epidemiological paradox" [34]. The potential for place-based factors to act as sources of both added stress and mitigating resilience among U.S.-based Latino/as is a topic that warrants further exploration [1,35,36].

In this article we explore community perceptions of Mexican origin residents who live in rural Yuma County, Arizona. This locale merits study due to both the under-reporting of border residents' (and especially foreign-born residents') community perceptions and because of the common media portrayals of this region as plagued by violence and disorder [13]. The fact that a majority of residents of this region are foreign born and have regular cross-border contact facilitates a binational study framework that brings to the forefront the important role of external referents as influencers of individuals' community perceptions and health promoting practices [3].

Findings reported here reveal that participants overwhelmingly perceived their rural communities in southern Yuma County, Arizona as both calm and safe. While these results contradict popular media characterizations of the borderlands, they are consistent with crime statistics demonstrating an inverse relationship between crime and both border proximity and high immigrant density [37,38]. In addition, our results mirror findings from Castañeda and Chiappetta's (2020) quantitative study in the border city of El Paso, Texas, in which 42.3% of survey participants used the word "calm" to describe the area and 97% reported feeling safe or very safe [13].

Study participants' descriptions of calm were primarily tied to their homes being in small towns that had a slow pace of life, were walkable for basic needs, and promoted a low stress environment that encouraged participation and ease in their communities. These findings reflect prior research showing that walkability enhances opportunities for recreation and community engagement [10]. Participants also linked feelings of calm to easeful relationships with their primarily Mexican origin neighbors and familiarity with the region. The multiple benefits of the "ethnic enclave effect" have been previously documented, including increased social control and decreased all-cause mortality and morbidity related to stroke, cancer, and hypertension [18,39]. The fact that participants' communities in Yuma County boasted both a largely Mexican population and proximity to Mexico meant that they provided a positive balance of physical safety and cultural familiarity. This resulted in participants being able to appreciate perceived safety and calm in Yuma County while also taking advantage of the opportunities for sustained cultural and familial ties and maintenance of cultural practices.

Participants' perceptions of calm in rural Yuma County were partially formed in relationship to external referents developed in large metropolises in both Mexico and U.S. border states where they had previously worked or lived. Study staff from Campesinos Sin Fronteras noted with interest participants' common perception of regional calm given that San Luis is second busiest port of entry in the state of Arizona and the primary gateway for Mexican agricultural workers heading north, meaning that significant cross border traffic is a constant presence.

The salience of external referents was even more noticeable in the realm of participants' perceived safety. Despite substantial and positive cross border ties to family, culture, and hometowns, participants made repeated references to murders, extortion, kidnappings, and drug trafficking in Mexico. Over the past several decades, drug-related violence has escalated in many Mexican communities, fueled by U.S. demand for illegal substances, official crackdown by the Mexican government, and U.S. exports of firearms and military training [40]. This phenomenon has unfolded with particular brutality along Mexico's northern border, and Mexicali, Baja California Norte and San Luis Río Colorado, Sonora have experienced a dramatic uptick in drug related homicides in recent years [16,17]. Study staff from Campesinos Sin Fronteras reinforced these findings, noting that some residents of San Luis and Somerton, Arizona had been victims of the wave of kidnappings and murders across the border, plunging several families into unspeakable pain and anxiety.

Thus, despite mentioning important safety concerns in Yuma County including drug trafficking and potential spillover violence from Mexico, participants overwhelmingly perceived the area as safe, based on the absence of extreme acts of violence and threats to material belongings. Castañeda and Chiappetta (2020) likewise found that people born outside of El Paso (many of whom were from Mexico) were more likely to describe the El Paso area as safe, concluding that: "This may be because many of those not raised in El Paso are immigrants, and their referents for safety are more unsafe than El Paso" [13] (p. 9).

Luna-Arocas and Tang (2015) argue that the significance of external referents is not uniform but rather enhanced by cultural and other factors that determine the weight assigned to the object of comparison [41]. The regularity with which participants mentioned safety and their willingness to forego the potential advantages of other places in exchange for regional safety indicate that safety and security are of prime importance to Mexican origin border residents. As such, we argue that the comparison between safety levels in the United States and Mexico acted as a central determinant to individuals' perceptions of their communities in Yuma County. This finding parallels the 1996 World Health Organization's declaration of violence as a growing global public health crisis that undermines individual and community level health and wellbeing [12,42]. Violence and fear of violence have been linked to decreased physical activity in the neighborhood setting and declines in overall physical and mental well-being [11,43,44].

Lastly, our findings indicated that participants credited both neighbors and local police forces as key collaborators in the promotion of safety in southern Yuma County. Many participants indicated that their neighbors—who were overwhelmingly of Mexican origin—promoted safety by avoiding conflicts among each other and safeguarding each other's belongings. The social control mechanisms sometimes present in ethnic enclaves have been shown to promote mutual trust and reliance and carry positive implications for health and wellness [13,39]. More specifically, a sense of "collective efficacy"—shared norms around taking action to ensure community wellness—has been linked to lower actual crime rates and perceptions of crime, as well as more distally to decreases in obesity and enhanced opportunities for physical activity [11,45,46].

The fact that the Mexican origin participants of this study widely heralded the active police presence and vigilance in their communities warrants close examination. Mexican immigrants' negative interactions with police and immigration patrol in the form of daily encounters and immigration raids have been repeatedly shown to generate widespread fear and carry negative health implications [47,48]. Moreover, in a representative sample of residents surveyed in this same region over a decade prior, members of this study team found that residents frequently complained of the overbearing presence of law enforcement in the region, a presence that was characterized by structural racism [30].

Several factors may help explain positive police perceptions in this sample. First, the fact that most study participants had legal residency status in the United States (as evidenced by regular border crossings at official ports of entry) meant they had the ability to engage with police forces without significant fear of deportation or immigration-related detainment. This may explain the contrast between our results and other studies which found that immigrants are frequent targets of theft and other crimes and that they report those crimes less frequently to the police [21,49]. Our respondents were also well-established in their communities and the majority had long-term employment.

Study partners from CSF noted several possible explanations for this finding. They commented that few undocumented people remain in rural Yuma County given the regular border surveillance. In addition, they noted that participants' lack of complaints related to immigration enforcement authorities may be related to the closures of check-points in the region and a decline in community-level immigration vigilance due to the increasing impermeability of the international border wall as well as a shift in focus toward the surge of Central American refugees. Lastly, they posited that residents' trust in local police agencies may have been boosted by the fact that most members of the police forces in the region were of Mexican descent and lived locally in the communities they police. Community partners identified many local outreach and support efforts undertaken by the local police forces and identified by name many police officers who were highly appreciated for their community-based efforts. As evidenced by prior work on community policing, improved trust in local police forces is an important predictor of their perceived efficacy [50].

And finally, the role of external referents was again highly relevant in determining participants' positive perceptions of the local police agencies and the credit they ascribed to them for keeping the region safe and orderly. Community partners described the role of binational referents as a mirror effect, in which the negative reference point of the police forces in San Luis Rio Colorado and other border regions in Sonora improved the way participants viewed U.S. based police forces. They maintain that police forces in San Luis Río Colorado are known as corrupt for accepting bribes and that they are ineffective in fulfilling the duties of public security, sending a message to the public that nothing can stop or punish criminals who act with impunity in broad daylight. Corruption of Mexican armed forces more broadly has been previously shown to undermine popular trust and support [51]. Due to this juxtaposition, the regular surveillance, professionalism, and responsiveness of police forces in Yuma County provided a welcome contrast to experiences pre-migration and/or during cross border visits.

Study Limitations

There are limitations to this study. Our sample was dominated by people with legal residency status in the United States and thus does not adequately reflect the experiences of undocumented people who would likely feel significantly less safe in this region especially in regards to police and border patrol surveillance. Additionally, we conducted the interviews during a wave of COVID-19 infections that hit the border area disproportionately, reducing opportunities for contact with extended networks in the community. The experiences related to the pandemic thus tended to dominate our conversations regarding sources of stress and resilience.

5. Conclusions

Given demonstrated inequities in morbidity and mortality amongst U.S.-based Latino/as, it is imperative to identify environmental factors that may exacerbate health stressors or alternately promote resilience, wellbeing, and positive health practices among Latino/a sub-groups. This article has demonstrated the potential for perceived safety and calm to serve as important contributors to health supporting environments among Mexican origin people living in the U.S. borderlands. Furthermore, threats of violence in Mexico may act to accentuate perceived safety among people of Mexican origin in the U.S. borderlands, indicating an important role for external—and specifically binational—referents in driving community perceptions in this region. However, the undermining of public safety in northern Mexico has the potential to erode the benefits of safe and calm borderland environments by minimizing immigrants' ability to sustain contacts with family and culture that serve to reduce social isolation and promote cultural continuity. In addition, Mexican immigrants' opportunities to benefit from secure local environments in the U.S. borderlands are highly contingent on their legal status and their ability to become integrated members of their communities with the full range of civil rights.

Supplementary Materials: The following supporting information can be downloaded at: https://www.mdpi.com/article/10.3390/ijerph19148399/s1, File S1: Interview Guide English/Spanish, Table S1: Code Tree, Table S2: Original Quotes in Spanish.

Author Contributions: Conceptualization, S.C., R.M.C., L.V., E.T. and M.I.; methodology, R.M.C., L.V., S.C., E.T. and M.I.; formal analysis, R.M.C. and M.I.; investigation, R.M.C., K.D., L.V. and M.I.; writing—original draft preparation, R.M.C., M.I., K.D.; writing—review and editing, S.C., R.M.C., M.I., F.M.C.-M.; project administration, K.D.; funding acquisition, S.C. All authors have read and agreed to the published version of the manuscript.

Funding: This research was funded by the National Institute on Minority Health & Health Disparities (NIH), grant #1R01MD014150-01A1.

Institutional Review Board Statement: The study was conducted in accordance with the Declaration of Helsinki, and approved by the Institutional Review Board of the University of Arizona on 24 March 2020 (Protocol #2003462440).

Informed Consent Statement: Informed consent was obtained from all subjects involved in the study.

Data Availability Statement: Not applicable.

Acknowledgments: The authors thank Campesinos Sin Fronteras staff members Rosa Guerra, Idolina Castro, Rogelio Torres, Laura Ramirez, Betsabe Ruiz, Laura del Villar, and Maria Figueroa for the essential role they played in study design, recruitment, scheduling, and interpretation of results. In addition, we thank UA team members Jill de Zapien, Carlos Figueroa, Thaddeus Pace, John Ruiz, and Melissa Flores for their roles in study design and reflections on findings. Lastly, we thank Josselyne Sanchez for her assistance with transcriptions.

Conflicts of Interest: The authors declare no conflict of interest. The funders had no role in the design of the study; in the collection, analyses, or interpretation of data; in the writing of the manuscript, or in the decision to publish the results.

References

1. Stroope, S.; Cohen, I.F.; Tom, J.C.; Franzen, A.; Valasik, M.A.; Markides, K.S. Neighborhood perception and self-rated health among Mexican American older adults. *Geriatr. Gerontol. Int.* **2017**, *17*, 2559–2564. [CrossRef]
2. Macintyre, S.; Ellaway, A.; Cummins, S. Place effects on health: How can we conceptualise, operationalise and measure them? *Soc. Sci. Med.* **2002**, *55*, 125–139. [CrossRef]
3. Curtis, S.; Congdon, P.; Atkinson, S.; Corcoran, R.; MaGuire, R.; Peasgood, T. Adverse conditions for wellbeing at the neighbourhood scale in England: Potential and challenges for operationalising indicators relevant to wellbeing in and of places. *Wellbeing Space Soc.* **2020**, *1*, 100009. [CrossRef]
4. Tunstall, H.V.; Shaw, M.; Dorling, D. Places and health. *J. Epidemiol. Community Health* **2004**, *58*, 6–10. [CrossRef] [PubMed]
5. Williams, A. Therapeutic landscapes in holistic medicine. *Soc. Sci. Med.* **1998**, *46*, 1193–1203. [CrossRef]
6. Diez Roux, A.V.; Mair, C. Neighborhoods and health. *Ann. N. Y. Acad. Sci.* **2010**, *1186*, 125–145. [CrossRef]
7. Smetcoren, A.S.; De Donder, L.; De Witte, N.; Buffel, T.; Dury, S.; Kardol, M.J.M.; Verte, D. Influence of Housing Quality on Feelings of Wellbeing and Neighborhood Integration. In Proceedings of the 67th Annual Scientific Meeting of the Gerontological Society of America, Washington, DC, USA, 5–9 November 2014.
8. Van Den Berg, A.E.; Maas, J.; Verheij, R.A.; Groenewegen, P.P. Green space as a buffer between stressful life events and health. *Soc. Sci. Med.* **2010**, *70*, 1203–1210. [CrossRef]
9. Osborne, C.; Baldwin, C.; Thomsen, D. Contributions of Social Capital to Best Practice Urban Planning Outcomes. *Urban Policy Res.* **2016**, *34*, 212–224. [CrossRef]
10. Iroz-Elardo, N.; Adkins, A.; Ingram, M. Measuring perceptions of social environments for walking: A scoping review of walkability surveys. *Health Place* **2020**, *67*, 102468. [CrossRef]
11. Roman, C.G.; Chalfin, A. Fear of Walking Outdoors: A Multilevel Ecologic Analysis of Crime and Disorder. *Am. J. Prev. Med.* **2008**, *34*, 306–312. [CrossRef]
12. Tan, S.-Y.; Haining, R. Crime victimization and the implications for individual health and wellbeing: A Sheffield case study. *Soc. Sci. Med.* **2016**, *167*, 128–139. [CrossRef] [PubMed]
13. Castañeda, E.; Chiappetta, C. Border residents' perceptions of crime and security in El Paso, Texas. *Soc. Sci.* **2020**, *9*, 24. [CrossRef]
14. Castañeda, E.; Heyman, J.M. Is the Southwestern Border Really Unsafe. Cambridge: Scholars Strategy Network. 2012. Available online: https://scholars.org/contribution/southwestern-border-really-unsafe (accessed on 29 February 2020).
15. Miller, H.V.; Peguero, A. *Routledge Handbook on Immigration and Crime*; Routledge: London, UK, 2018.
16. Correa-Cabrera, G. Security, Migration, and the Economy in the T exas–T amaulipas Border Region: The "Real" Effects of M exico's Drug War. *Politics Policy* **2013**, *41*, 65–82. [CrossRef]
17. Rramos. Rising Violence Along Baja California-Sonora Border Tied to Larger Organized Crime Disputes. 2021. Available online: https://justiceinmexico.org/violence-border-larger-organized-crime (accessed on 7 April 2022).
18. Eschbach, K.; Ostir, G.V.; Patel, K.V.; Markides, K.S.; Goodwin, J.S. Neighborhood context and mortality among older Mexican Americans: Is there a barrio advantage? *Am. J. Public Health* **2004**, *94*, 1807–1812. [CrossRef] [PubMed]
19. Landler, M.; Romero, S. Trump Takes Border Wall Fight to El Paso; Beto O'rourke Fires Back. *The New York Times*, 11 February 2019.
20. Barranco, R.E.; Shihadeh, E.S. Walking ATMs and the immigration spillover effect: The link between Latino immigration and robbery victimization. *Soc. Sci. Res.* **2015**, *52*, 440–450. [CrossRef] [PubMed]

21. Nuño, L.F. Mexicans in New York City. *Soc. Bord.* **2013**, *8*, 80–101.
22. Horton, S.B.; Barker, J.C. A latino oral health paradox? using ethnography to specify the biocultural factors behind epidemiological models. *NAPA Bull.* **2010**, *34*, 68–83. [CrossRef]
23. Li, M. Pre-migration Trauma and Post-migration Stressors for Asian and Latino American Immigrants: Transnational Stress Proliferation. *Soc. Indic. Res.* **2015**, *129*, 47–59. [CrossRef]
24. Crocker, R.M. The Impact of Binational Barriers to Medical Care on the Care-Seeking Practices of Mexican Immigrants. *Qual. Health Res.* **2021**, *31*, 1043–1055. [CrossRef]
25. Stokols, D.; Misra, S.; Runnerstrom, M.; Hipp, J.A. Psychology in an age of ecological crisis: From personal angst to collective action. *Am. Psychol.* **2009**, *64*, 181–193. [CrossRef]
26. Roura, M. The Social Ecology of Power in Participatory Health Research. *Qual. Health Res.* **2020**, *31*, 778–788. [CrossRef] [PubMed]
27. Carvajal, S.C.; Rosales, C.; Rubio-Goldsmith, R.; Sabo, S.; Ingram, M.; McClelland, D.J.; Redondo, F.; Torres, E.; Romero, A.J.; O'Leary, A.O.; et al. The border community and immigration stress scale: A preliminary examination of a community responsive measure in two Southwest samples. *J. Immigr. Minor. Health* **2012**, *15*, 427–436.
28. Brush, B.L.; Mentz, G.; Jensen, M.; Jacobs, B.; Saylor, K.M.; Rowe, Z.; Israel, B.A.; Lachance, L. Success in Long-Standing Community-Based Participatory Research (CBPR) Partnerships: A Scoping Literature Review. *Health Educ. Behav.* **2019**, *47*, 556–568. [CrossRef]
29. Wallerstein, N.; Duran, B. Community-Based Participatory Research Contributions to Intervention Research: The Intersection of Science and Practice to Improve Health Equity. *Am. J. Public Health* **2010**, *100*, S40–S46. [CrossRef]
30. Sabo, S.; Shaw, S.; Ingram, M.; Teufel-Shone, N.; Carvajal, S.; De Zapien, J.G.; Cecilia, R.; Flor, R.; Gina, G.; Rubio-Goldsmith, R. Everyday violence, structural racism and mistreatment at the US–Mexico border. *Soc. Sci. Med.* **2014**, *109*, 66–74. [CrossRef]
31. Kposowa, A.J. Mortality from Diabetes by Hispanic Groups: Evidence from the US National Longitudinal Mortality Study. *Int. J. Popul. Res.* **2013**, *2013*, 1–12. [CrossRef]
32. Rich, N.E.; Oji, S.; Mufti, A.R.; Browning, J.D.; Parikh, N.D.; Odewole, M.; Mayo, H.; Singal, A.G. Racial and Ethnic Disparities in Nonalcoholic Fatty Liver Disease Prevalence, Severity, and Outcomes in the United States: A Systematic Review and Meta-analysis. *Clin. Gastroenterol. Hepatol.* **2017**, *16*, 198–210.e2. [CrossRef]
33. Velasco-Mondragon, E.; Jimenez, A.; Palladino-Davis, A.G.; Davis, D.; Escamilla-Cejudo, J.A. Hispanic health in the USA: A scoping review of the literature. *Public Health Rev.* **2016**, *37*, 1–27. [CrossRef]
34. Markides, K.S.; Coreil, J. The health of Hispanics in the southwestern United States: An epidemiologic paradox. *Public Health Rep.* **1986**, *101*, 253–265.
35. Escobar, K.M.; Sivaram, M.; Gorey, K.M. Multiplicative Advantages of Hispanic Men Living in Hispanic Enclaves: Intersectionality in Colon Cancer Care. *Soc. Welf.* **2018**, *46*, 4.
36. Ruiz, J.M.; Steffen, P.; Smith, T.B. Hispanic Mortality Paradox: A Systematic Review and Meta-Analysis of the Longitudinal Literature. *Am. J. Public Health* **2013**, *103*, e52–e60. [CrossRef] [PubMed]
37. Martinez Jr, R.; Stowell, J.I.; Lee, M.T. Immigration and crime in an era of transformation: A longitudinal analysis of homicides in San Diego neighborhoods, 1980–2000. *Criminology* **2010**, *48*, 797–829. [CrossRef]
38. Martinez, R.; Stowell, J.I.; Iwama, J.A. The Role of Immigration: Race/Ethnicity and San Diego Homicides Since 1970. *J. Quant. Criminol.* **2016**, *32*, 471–488. [CrossRef]
39. Zhou, M.; Bankston, C. *Growing up American: How Vietnamese Children Adapt to Life in the United States*; Russell Sage Foundation: New York, NY, USA, 1998.
40. Hunt, E. Staying the course in Mexico: The role of the US in the drug war, 2006–present. *Third World Q.* **2019**, *40*, 1184–1205. [CrossRef]
41. Luna-Arocas, R.; Tang, T.L.-P. Are You Satisfied with Your Pay When You Compare? It Depends on Your Love of Money, Pay Comparison Standards, and Culture. *J. Bus. Ethic* **2014**, *128*, 279–289. [CrossRef]
42. Olofsson, N. A life course model of self-reported violence exposure and ill-health with a public health problem perspective. *AIMS Public Health* **2014**, *1*, 9. [CrossRef]
43. Danielsson, I.; Olofsson, N.; Gådin, K.G. Consequences of violence—A public health issue. Strong connection between violence/threat and illness in both women and men. *Lakartidningen* **2005**, *102*, 938–940.e942.
44. Garcia-Moreno, C.; Jansen, H.A.; Ellsberg, M.; Heise, L.; Watts, C.H. Prevalence of intimate partner violence: Findings from the WHO multi-country study on women's health and domestic violence. *Lancet* **2006**, *368*, 1260–1269. [CrossRef]
45. Browning, C.R.; Cagney, K.A. Neighborhood Structural Disadvantage, Collective Efficacy, and Self-Rated Physical Health in an Urban Setting. *J. Health Soc. Behav.* **2002**, *43*, 383–399. [CrossRef]
46. Sampson, R.J.; Raudenbush, S.W.; Earls, F. Neighborhoods and Violent Crime: A Multilevel Study of Collective Efficacy. *Science* **1997**, *277*, 918–924. [CrossRef]
47. LeBrón, A.M.W.; Schulz, A.J.; Gamboa, C.; Reyes, A.; Viruell-Fuentes, E.A.; Israel, B.A. "They Are Clipping Our Wings": Health Implications of Restrictive Immigrant Policies for Mexican-Origin Women in a Northern Border Community. *Race Soc. Probl.* **2018**, *10*, 174–192. [CrossRef]

48. Lopez, W.D.; Kruger, D.J.; Delva, J.; Llanes, M.; Ledón, C.; Waller, A.; Harner, M.; Martinez, R.; Sanders, L.; Harner, M.; et al. Health Implications of an Immigration Raid: Findings from a Latino Community in the Midwestern United States. *J. Immigr. Minor. Health* **2016**, *19*, 702–708. [CrossRef] [PubMed]
49. Golash-Boza, T.M. *Immigration Nation: Raids, Detentions, and Deportations in Post-9/11 America*; Routledge: London, UK, 2015.
50. Torres, J.A. Predicting perceived police effectiveness in public housing: Police contact, police trust, and police responsiveness. *Polic. Soc.* **2015**, *27*, 1–21. [CrossRef]
51. Ugues, A., Jr.; Esparza, D. The relationship between crime victimization, corruption, and public attitudes of Mexico's armed forces. *Democr. Secur.* **2018**, *14*, 211–237. [CrossRef]

International Journal of
Environmental Research and Public Health

MDPI

Article

Indigenous Border Migrants and (Im)Mobility Policies in Chile in Times of COVID-19

Carlos Piñones-Rivera [1,*], Nanette Liberona [2], Rodrigo Arancibia [3] and Verónica Jiménez [4]

1 Escuela de Psicología y Filosofía, Universidad de Tarapacá, Arica 1000000, Chile
2 Departamento de Antropología, Universidad de Tarapacá, Arica 1000000, Chile
3 Cooperativa Apacheta, Iquique 1100000, Chile
4 Programa de Doctorado en Psicología, Escuela de Psicología y Filosofía, Universidad de Tarapacá, Arica 1000000, Chile
* Correspondence: carlospinonesrivera@gmail.com

Abstract: The commodification of healthcare and the structural violence towards the migrant population in the Chilean system materialize in a series of structural barriers to accessing healthcare. In the face of this structural vulnerability, cross-border health mobility is one of the primary resources of indigenous border migrants living in the Tarapacá region (Chile). This involves crossing the border of both people (specialists/patients) and objects (such as ritual supplies or biomedicines), which play a crucial role as, in many cases, it is the only way to satisfy their healthcare needs. The security-orientated geopolitics of border closure (Plan Frontera Segura) has been reinforced by immobility policies linked to the COVID-19 pandemic. While doing so leaves people without the fundamental resource of healthcare mobility or obliges them to cross the border via unauthorized crossings, exposing them to criminalization and abuse by different agents of violence (the military, people smugglers, etc.). In this paper, we will offer a description of these processes of (im)mobility, analyzing their conformation both by the current policies of the Chilean State and by the notorious deficiency in indigenous and migrant rights, denouncing the material impact they have on the health/illness/care process of indigenous migrants.

Keywords: healthcare mobility; borders; immigrant health; indigenous health; structural violence; structural vulnerability; social determinants of health; health inequality

Citation: Piñones-Rivera, C.; Liberona, N.; Arancibia, R.; Jiménez, V. Indigenous Border Migrants and (Im)Mobility Policies in Chile in Times of COVID-19. *Int. J. Environ. Res. Public Health* **2022**, *19*, 9728. https://doi.org/10.3390/ijerph19159728

Academic Editors: Ernesto Castañeda and Maria De Jesus

Received: 20 June 2022
Accepted: 4 August 2022
Published: 7 August 2022

Publisher's Note: MDPI stays neutral with regard to jurisdictional claims in published maps and institutional affiliations.

1. Introduction

Neoliberal reforms to the healthcare system are linked to a worsening of collective health [1,2]. The commodification of all vital arrangements that is typical of neoliberalism in Chile has not only turned it into one of the countries with the highest out-of-pocket spending among the member nations of the Organization for Economic Co-operation and Development (OECD) [3,4] but also to have one of the highest costs for medications in Latin America [5]. The latter is due to the structure of a strongly monopolized pharmaceutical market focused on sectorial decisions rather than on people's rights and needs [6]. Additionally, waiting lists for hospital treatment present serious problems: just between January and June 2018, there were 9724 deaths of people on such waiting lists [7]. In general, the system systematically pushes people into debt for basic subsistence, shaping a subjectivity that, in addition to suffering structural inequity, is held responsible for such suffering [8].

One phenomenon studied on the northern border of Chile is related to the journeys people make to neighboring countries to seek healthcare attention [9]. The literature indicates that this form of mobility is not carried out due to nomadic customs, nor for the pleasure of traveling. Instead, it is often motivated by the system's inequity, based on a neoliberal model that strengthens the healthcare market and leads to a population segmentation according to income and risks [10], thus hindering most people's access to quality care [1–5]. This problem becomes more acute when it affects migrant populations, who also suffer the compounded effect of phenomena such as cyclic irregularity [11], racism in healthcare [12], as well as other aspects included in the category of "Social Determinants" [13–17].

Although the studies of healthcare mobility have contributed new perspectives in understanding health/disease/care processes, we can observe two main limitations. The first has consisted of focusing restrictively on biomedical care while ignoring the contribution of other forms of knowledge that contribute to the medical pluralism of the current regions of Arica and Parinacota, and Tarapacá in northern Chile. Such is the case of Andean traditional medical knowledge, which plays a vital role for the Chilean and migrant population. The second is that although these works consider the relationship between mobility and territory along the lines proposed by Tarrius [18], they have not analyzed the role of medical knowledge in specifying how it actually circulates. Thus, circular knowledge appears as an abstract and unspecific term in these studies.

Our research questions are: what are the processes of (im)mobility that affected the health mobility in the Tarapacá region (Chile) in COVID-19 times? How does this (im)mobility process impact the health/illness/care process of indigenous migrants? How do the current policies of the Chilean State and its deficiency in indigenous and migrant rights give form to that (im)mobility process?

Our main argument is that the security-focused geopolitics of the border closure (Secure Border Plan) [19] has been reinforced by COVID-19 immobility policies. Those policies leave people without the fundamental resource of healthcare mobility or oblige them to use unauthorized border crossings, thus exposing themselves to criminalization and abuse from different agents of violence (such as people smugglers or the military) [20]. For this purpose, we will focus on what happens on the Chile-Bolivia border (Colchane) (see Figure 1). We wish to offer a description of these processes of (im)mobility, analyzing their conformation both for the current policies of the Chilean State and for the notorious absences in the area of indigenous and migrant law, revealing the material impact they have on the health/disease/care process of indigenous migrants.

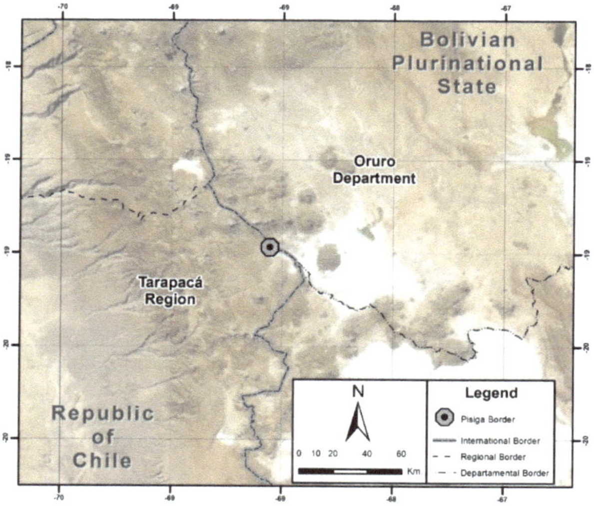

Figure 1. The Chile–Bolivia cross border region.

1.1. *(Im)Mobility Policies in Border Studies*

1.1.1. Thoughts on (Im)Mobility

Border studies are increasingly interested in the interaction and links that occur through them and that people deploy in their constant crossings [21,22], which is how mobility takes a prominent place in the analysis. These studies question the generalized use of the notion of migration because it prevented the capture of some population movements. Heyman [23] posits that mobility makes "fewer judgments about the nature of the movement (duration, purpose, social position)" (p. 427). Tarrius, for his part, developed a paradigm of mobility based on the space-time-identity triad within the framework of the anthropology of movement, which allows "understanding how crossings of space are always also crossings of social hierarchies" [18] (p. 45). He thus posed that any "social, cultural and economic mobility leaves a mark in space and time" [18] (p. 45). Based on an analysis of migratory circulations (a notion derived from French social geography), as evidenced in his studies on the trade between Marseille, Algeria, and Morocco [24], this author identified the convenience of the notion of circulatory territory, which "confirms the socialization of spaces according to logics of mobility" [18] (p. 55). From these perspectives, border regions are understood as the right place to capture the variety of movements and to observe them from a territorial perspective [25].

Due to the discussion regarding spatial mobility and territory, an interest arose concerning its counterpart, as immobility allows mobility to be visualized. Following this argument, we refer through processes of (im)mobility to the mobility/immobility continuum as a dialectical relationship in the production of space, as well as a relational experience, differentiated and located in geographical and historical terms, which is a consequence of the unequal exercise of power [26]. The authors point out that mobility cannot be understood without immobility because they are dialectically related and determine each other. We adopt this concept from critical human geography, as it allows us to realize that the movement of people is an embodied experience that produces and reproduces space.

Nevertheless, contemporary border studies consider both the mobility of people and that of goods, capital, and information [27], while the border, for its part, functions as a filter or system of differentiated flows [28]. In this sense, Heyman's theoretical contribution is relevant, given that by stating that there is unequal mobility [27], he introduces the analysis of border control policies as mobility control policies. Heyman explains that unequal mobility is understood from two fundamental points: firstly, it occurs in contemporary capitalism (with a connection between unequal mobility, borders, labor, and capital); and, secondly, it is the result of a complex relationship between policies and the functional needs of capitalism.

Thus, the cross-border space that we observe in this work results from the (im)mobility produced in this case by people subject to forced displacement, border migration, and objects that circulate in relation to Andean medical knowledge. However, the (im)mobility processes are determined by border and migratory control policies that we will present below.

1.1.2. Securitization and (Im)Mobility Policies

As we have mentioned, the processes of (im)mobility are the focus of policies that seek to control the borders and the various movements across them. These include migration, interpreted as a security problem for states. The international literature has identified securitization as one of the main trends pertinent to these policies. As such, it is associated with the political establishment's fear of losing symbolic control over their territorial limits and has been structured by the habitus of security professionals and by the globalization of surveillance technologies. Ultimately, however, securitization is based on the discomfort of citizens who feel they cannot deal with the uncertainties of everyday life in a neoliberal society [29]. Other theoretical approaches define securitization as a response to migration perceived as a political-identitarian threat [30,31] or a socioeconomic thread [32,33].

Such security-focused policies view migrants as dangerous subjects, and one of their manifestations is the criminalization of such people [34]. The Chilean approach to migration adopted the figure of the migrant as the enemy within the State during Pinochet's dictatorship [35]. However, securitization is far from just a Chilean phenomenon and responds to a global trend [36,37]. Eduardo Domenech [38] proposed that South American immigration policies have turned towards a "punitive approach" in recent years, intensifying state violence towards migrants in a context of essential changes in migratory patterns. Examples of these changes are the militarization of the Peru-Ecuador and Chile-Bolivia borders in 2020 to control and limit mobility. Likewise, the imposition of visas to Venezuela from 2019 by Ecuador, Argentina, and Chile. These trends are adapted to the creation of a regime of global migration control, characterized by "the emergence of new ways of thinking and acting on migrations such as migration management" [38] (p. 22), the purpose of which is the regulation of international migrations in a neoliberal global framework. These policies focus on preventing, eliminating, and regulating "migratory pressures". One of the culminating instances of this global regime is the Global Compact for Migration (2018), which assumes migration as "safe, orderly and regular". After analyzing the narratives of international agencies, Pécoud affirmed that the use of the term migration management is reassuring; "a managed phenomenon is a phenomenon under control, which will probably not escape the regulatory capacity of States". [39] (p. 22). In this context, migrations are conceived as a positive phenomenon that can benefit multiple stakeholders if adequately administered. This positive image conceals the structural vulnerability that directly affects people in movement.

2. Materials and Methods

The data analyzed for this research has resulted from collaborative ethnographic work, focused on socio-legal and health support for migrants who reside in or transit through the Tarapacá region (Chile) and who have encountered the leading organization dedicated to the defense of the human rights of migrants in the said region: the Open Assembly of Migrants and Pro-Migrants (Spanish acronym, AMPRO). Such support in their migratory procedures and access to social rights represent the main instances in which observation of participants is carried out and field notes collated. Collaborative work was fundamental for establishing a connection with the people and for the team's conformation, including a migrant facilitator and leader.

In our current research project, the main stakeholders are people requesting refugee status, who are residents or are in transit through the cities of Arica, Iquique, and Alto Hospicio, and who entered Chile via border crossings in the regions of Arica and Parinacota, and Tarapacá (Table 1).

To compare the information gathered from participants with that of local and national institutional actors, we conducted semi-structured interviews with key informants, such as local authorities and technical personnel, to understand how migration and border policies are interpreted and applied. Other key informants were members of NGOs (such as the Red Cross, Jesuit Migrant Service, and UNHCR), along with social organizations that provide legal and social assistance to this population segment (Table 2). We also made observations at the frontier crossings in the regions of Arica and Parinacota, and Tarapacá.

In addition, we conducted a documentary analysis of various related national and international regulatory bodies and reviewed requests for official documents through the Chilean government's Transparency website, which provides access to public information. We also monitored the local, national, and international media regarding the border closure due to public health concerns.

The study was conducted in accordance with the Declaration of Helsinki and approved by the Institutional Review Board (or Ethics Committee) of Universidad de Tarapacá for studies involving humans. Informed consent was obtained from all subjects involved in the study.

Table 1. List of immigrants interviewed.

Actor	Gender	Nationality	Age	Residence	Date	Interview Modality
Immigrant	Female	Bolivian	Adult	Iquique (Chile)	apr-21	Virtual
Immigrant	Male	Bolivian	Adult	Iquique (Chile)	apr-21	In person
Immigrant	Female	Bolivian	Adult	Iquique (Chile)	may-21	In person
Immigrant	Female	Bolivian	Adult	Iquique (Chile)	apr-21	In person
Immigrant	Female	Bolivian	Adult	Iquique (Chile)	mar-21	In person
Immigrant	Female	Bolivian	Adult	Iquique (Chile)	apr-21	In person
Immigrant	Male	Bolivian	Adult	Iquique (Chile)	may-21	Virtual
Immigrant	Female	Bolivian	Adult	Iquique (Chile)	may-21	In person
Immigrant	Male	Bolivian	Adult	Iquique (Chile)	may-21	In person
Immigrant	Female	Colombian	Adult	In transit	nov-21	In person
Immigrant	Male	Colombian	Elderly	In transit	nov-21	In person
Immigrant	Male	Colombian	Elderly	In transit	nov-21	In person
Immigrant	Male	Colombian	Young	In transit	nov-21	In person
Immigrant	Female	Colombian	Elderly	In transit	nov-21	In person
Immigrant	LGBTQ+	Cuban	Adult	In transit	nov-21	In person
Immigrant	Female	Ecuadorian	Adult	In transit	nov-21	In person
Immigrant	Female	Venezuelan	Young	In transit	nov-21	In person
Immigrant	Female	Venezuelan	Young	In transit	nov-21	In person
Immigrant	Male	Venezuelan	Young	In transit	nov-21	In person
Immigrant	Female	Venezuelan	Young	In transit	nov-21	In person
Immigrant	Female	Venezuelan	Young	In transit	nov-21	In person
Immigrant	Male	Venezuelan	Adult	In transit	nov-21	In person
Immigrant	Male	Venezuelan	Young	In transit	nov-21	In person
Immigrant	Female	Venezuelan	Young	In transit	nov-21	In person
Immigrant	Male	Venezuelan	Young	In transit	nov-21	In person
Immigrant	Male	Venezuelan	Adult	In transit	nov-21	In person
Immigrant	Female	Venezuelan	Adult	In transit	nov-21	In person
Immigrant	Female	Venezuelan	Adult	In transit	nov-21	In person
Immigrant	Female	Venezuelan	Adult	In transit	nov-21	In person
Immigrant	Female	Venezuelan	Adult	In transit	nov-21	In person
Immigrant	Female	Venezuelan	Young	In transit	nov-21	In person
Immigrant	Female	Venezuelan	Young	In transit	nov-21	In person
Immigrant	Male	Venezuelan	Adult	In transit	nov-21	In person
Immigrant	Male	Venezuelan	Adult	In transit	nov-21	In person
Immigrant	Female	Venezuelan	Adult	In transit	nov-21	In person
Immigrant	Male	Venezuelan	Adult	In transit	nov-21	In person
Immigrant	Female	Venezuelan	Young	In transit	nov-21	In person
Immigrant	Male	Venezuelan	Adult	In transit	nov-21	In person
Immigrant	Male	Venezuelan	Young	In transit	nov-21	In person
Immigrant	LGBTQ+	Venezuelan	Young	In transit	nov-21	In person
Immigrant	Female	Venezuelan	Young	In transit	nov-21	In person
Immigrant	Female	Venezuelan	Young	In transit	nov-21	In person

Table 2. Key informants interviewed.

Actor	Gender	Nationality	Age	Residence	Date	Interview Modality
Yatiri	Male	Peruvian	Elderly	Tacna (Perú)	feb-21	In person
Yatiri	Male	Peruvian	Elderly	Tacna (Perú)	feb-21	In person
Yatiri	Male	Bolivian	Elderly	Alto Hospicio (Chile)	feb-21	In person
Yatiri	Male	Bolivian	Elderly	Oruro (Bolivia)	feb-21	In person
Human Rights Lawyer	Male	Chilean	Adult	Iquique (Chile)	dic-21	In person
Church Volunteer	Male	Chilean	Adult	Iquique (Chile)	mar-22	In person
Immigrant leader	Female	Bolivian	Adult	Iquique (Chile)	apr-21	In person
Psychologist	Female	Chilean	Adult	Iquique (Chile)	feb-22	In person
Lawyer NGO	Female	Chilean	Adult	Iquique (Chile)	may-22	In person

3. Results and Discussion

3.1. Cross-Border (Im)Mobility Processes in Times of COVID-19

The COVID-19 pandemic led to a state of exception in Chile, which included border closures (Supreme Decree 104 of 18 March 2020). However, it is possible to describe a continuity between said closures and other border policies related to migratory control and the control of illegal activities. Just as a political and media link was developed internationally between migration, organized crime, and terrorism [40,41], in Chile, migration was consistently associated with drug trafficking and smuggling [42–44].

The link-up between these three aspects clearly manifests the securitizing tendency that has permeated Chile's immigration and border policies. This focus on security has impacted the process of (im)mobility, strengthening the restriction of people's movements. A clear example of this is the package of measures announced by former President Sebastián Piñera on 23 April 2018, which included a migration bill, an anomalous migration regularization process, increased entry restrictions for Haitians through the imposition of a consular tourist visa, the creation of a Democratic Responsibility visa, exclusively for Venezuelans, the elimination of the temporary work visa, the strengthening of mechanisms to carry out expulsions and the implementation of the Secure Border Plan in the five regions of northern Chile. It is essential to highlight that the focus on certain national groups (especially Haitians and Venezuelans) shows that these are racist-influenced policies, as we have analyzed in other works [45].

A speech introducing this law, made by former President Piñera, clearly shows its criminalizing characteristics:

> The main objective of this new law is to Put our House in Order through an orderly, safe, and regular migration policy, which allows legal migration and combats illegal migration [...] those who enter or try to enter our country clandestinely by unauthorized means, not only commit a crime, they also risk being subject to expulsion. [46]

As Dufraix et al. [19] have shown, the result of these policies, adhering to the concept of "ordering the house", have not led to orderly, safe, and regular migration; instead, they have increased migratory irregularity. For example, the Democratic Responsibility Visa (DRV) presented by the government of Sebastián Piñera in Cúcuta only granted 27% of all applications up to January 2021. Moreover, the Consular Tourism Visa (CTV), which came into force in 2019, has only been issued for 21% of all applications up to January 2021 [47].

The same is also true of the asylum law. Celebrated as a law drafted to the level of international standards, it has been neutralized by the political decision to make it inapplicable [48]. Proof of this is that in 2019, having registered 16,748 requests for asylum before the Chilean border authority by Venezuelan nationals, the Chilean State recognized the refugee condition of only five such citizens. In 2020, only seven Venezuelans were recognized as refugees after 1629 applications were officially processed [47]. In 2021, the processing of asylum applications decreased considerably due to a policy of disincentives and access barriers, as revealed by the Comptroller's Report on the closure of this process by the country's border authorities for the year 2021. Through Decree 7.196 of 2021, the government instructs to suspend, in certain provincial governorates, the reception of applications for recognition of refugee status under Law 20.430. Likewise, "State agents have hindered the possibilities of persons seeking international protection to claim the right to request asylum" [48] (p. 408).

Lastly, and shortly before the Piñera government left office, the Ministry of Interior and Public Security ordered a modification to the Regulation of the Law of Asylum (Decree 125), imposing a pre-admissibility measure, which was previously used arbitrarily, to limit the processing of asylum requests, thus institutionalizing this practice.

One interesting aspect is that these securitizing measures have adopted the language of migrant protection, concerning the dangers inherent to people trafficking networks and "the risks derived from such people's irregular situation in the country" (paragraph 3 of decree 776 of the Ministry of Interior and Public Security). However, as Huysmans and

Squire [49] have analyzed, such a humanitarian discourse is part of the securitizing strategy, hence its dual nature.

In the case of the border with Bolivia, which we analyze in this article, the principal measures established have been restrictions on mobility. However, as we will analyze further, such measures then acquired a new characteristic and legitimacy concerning the processes of (im)mobility propitiated by the COVID-19 pandemic.

3.1.1. (Im)Mobility Policies Linked to the Pandemic

Immobility acquires its meaning in a broader political context when promulgating a state of exception. It confers special powers to the State, placing limits on the exercise of rights, for example, those of mobility. However, the fact that rights are limited is not a problematic issue in itself. The basis of rights' limitation is the need to reconcile the exercise of each right with the protection of certain valuable assets for the greater good or with the exercise of the rights of third parties. What is problematic is the identification of these limits and the scope of the restrictions allowed by the legal system. In the case of pandemics such as COVID-19, states can limit the exercise of rights to protect public health. Moreover, unlike what happens with other protected interests by which rights are limited, such as national security, public order, or public morals, in the case of public health, criteria and technical reasons customize more defined and objective profiles applied in the context of migration control [50]. Thus, the closure of borders generates an unquestioned consensus in the context of a pandemic, overshadowing political processes such as the securitization or criminalization of migration, actions that then experience a previously controversial legitimacy.

On 17 March 2020, through Decree 102, the Chilean government ordered the temporary closure of borders due to the presence of cases of COVID-19. The argument was the "health alert for a period of one year [...] due to a public health emergency of international importance, caused by the outbreak of the new coronavirus". According to article 57 of the health code, "adequate measures must be established to prevent international transmission". All of the above occurred because "the State must protect the population, as it is responsible for coordinating and controlling actions related to the population's health".

However, borders are never an absolute barrier but rather an exercise that transforms the mobility of people into politics to decide how and who can effectively cross them [51]. The regulations segmented entry into the country based on specific criteria: the entrance route (land or air); nationality (Chilean/foreign); immigration status (foreigner with permanent residence/undocumented foreigner/foreigner with exceptional credentials, such as diplomatic visas); family links (with children or parents resident in Chile/or without them). Thus, the border policy excluded people who entered by land routes, did not have special documents, and had no resident parent or children in Chile. This control was strictly applied in the terrestrial border crossings and much more flexible in the aerial entry points, which indicates a class bias in its implementation.

In this scenario, it is essential to clarify that the conditions for traveling to the country with a resolved migration situation were restricted. Thus, the publicized Democratic Responsibility Visas (in force since 2018) were suspended in November 2020. According to the information given to applicants, this was attributed to the sanitary closure of Chilean borders, "due to which the completion period of the administrative process has been surpassed", referring to the Democratic Responsibility Visa [52]. This was how the massive rejection of such visa applications was justified. The possibilities of formalizing their migratory status once inside the country were also tricky. Indeed, eliminating the work visa meant that many people who had entered as tourists could no longer formalize their situation.

However, the most shocking occurrence in terms of media exposure was the illegal group expulsions that heralded the so-called "Colchane Plan". Almost a year after the border closure, inter-institutional coordination was established to implement the said plan, the purpose of which was to counter the increase in the number of illegal crossings through the Colchane Pass on the Chile-Bolivia border. Within this context, and between 3 and 8 of February 2021, four expulsion orders were issued that led to the deportation of 138 foreign nationals (Figure 2). The expulsions consisted of authentic cases of media staging that, through criminalizing migration, increased the hostility of the Chilean population towards migrants while justifying the illegality of the actions carried out by the Chilean State, given that the expulsions were massive and did not adhere to legal standards of due process.

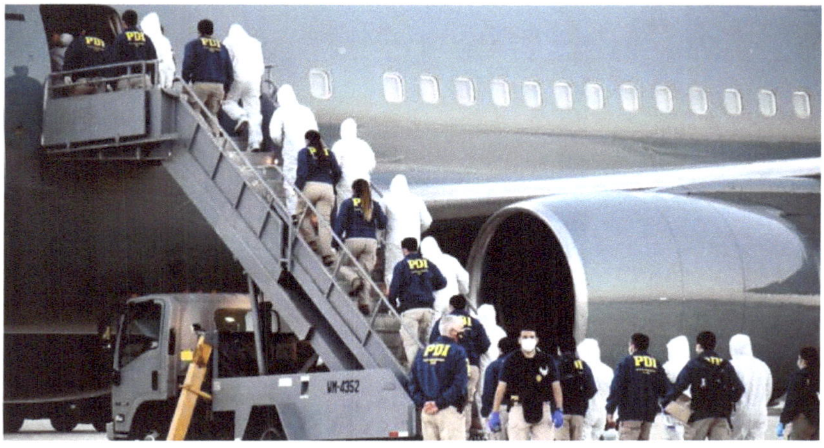

Figure 2. Expulsion of 138 foreign nationals under the Colchane Plan.

According to the analysis carried out by Jiménez [53], in none of these resolutions was there an individual, objective and rational evaluation of the circumstances of each person (criminal records, their previous background in their countries of origin, or any analysis related to the family or working roots of the people, or any deliberation of people's welfare related to the above). This violates the principle of non-refoulment, which corresponded in most cases to Venezuelans expelled from Chile, the vast majority of whom represented cases of forced migration, thus meeting the conditions to receive refuge according to the Convention relating to the Status of Refugees of 1951. Furthermore, there was no guarantee of access to an appeal against the expulsion order, as the period to lodge such a plea was 24 h, which made it completely unviable, given that the court specified for the procedure was the Supreme Court of Chile, located in the country's capital almost 2000 km away.

Conceptually, all these measures were intended to prevent the international transmission of the coronavirus. However, the securitization criterion absorbed the health criterion, as we can conclude from some specific situations related to health. One of the most significant in this regard was the requirement of voluntarily reporting to the Investigations Police (PDI) to access preventive quarantine for all people who entered the country using an unauthorized route. Consequently, a registry of those who entered by irregular means was established, while it was unclear what the purpose of this procedure was.

While some people were told that this would serve them in any subsequent regularization process, the authorities also announced expulsing those who had entered by such irregular routes. Consequently, many people avoided going to the healthcare-quarantine residences for fear of being exposed to expulsion. Moreover, this was carried out according to a rationale of minimally sufficient healthcare provision. That is to say, once people received minimal care, the next step was their expulsion.

Another example in which the security objective became paramount to the health objective can be observed in the initial approach regarding the vaccination of undocumented foreigners. Indeed, the first instruction was that migrants with tourist visas and those that were undocumented would not be vaccinated. This instruction provoked strong criticism from migrant and pro-migrant organizations, which finally reversed said directive.

Finally, the policy to close the border led directly to an increase in irregular crossings, thus encouraging the criminal activity of the so-called "coyotes" or people smugglers, who profit by aiding people to cross the border. This policy leaves migrants in a highly vulnerable situation, and many have suffered abuse from smugglers or even lost their lives [20].

As can be seen in these examples, although the State of exception was based on sanitary reasons, the political decisions often subordinated health reasons to securitization.

3.1.2. Militarization for Public Health

Another aspect worthy of analysis of the Colchane Plan is related to the process of militarization that accompanied it. On 4 February 2021, the Chilean government, through a modification of decree 265, authorized the Armed Forces to assist the police in matters of migration to protect the borders through technology and patrols.

In addition to the media staging of the expulsions analyzed above, the militarization of the borderlands generated impacts on local indigenous communities. They, in turn, denounced the discriminatory treatment they were receiving, as stated in the application for protection corresponding to Court Inscription No. 21-2021, presented by Adimelia Moscoso, Elías Mamani, and Bárbara Montecino:

> [The army] frequently confuses Chilean Aymaras with Bolivian Aymaras, treating them with discrimination related to identity control and the native language of the Aymara people. In this sense, there is no equality of rights regarding movements between Chilean and Bolivian Aymaras, concerning the hundreds of migrants who cross the border, in which it can be observed that they are not subject to any control. [54] (s/p)

Furthermore, it also hampered cross-border mobility between Chile and Bolivia, typically undertaken by members of indigenous communities:

> Aymara communities, in this sense, have been prevented from accessing a series of products they exchange or get a reasonable price for in surrounding communities. This has increased the cost of living of Aymara families and led to a shortage of specific products such as gas, non-perishable food, and coca leaves, among others, which are vital for our people. In addition, they have prevented members of the community from going to the aid of family members, including the elderly, who in the communities have a fundamental role as they are custodians of the knowledge and wisdom of ancestral uses and customs. The high level of administrative surveillance of 'official border crossings' has caused a greater flow through 'unauthorized' crossings. Our communities have seen an increase in the frequency and quantity of vehicles (including caravans of up to 40 vehicles), sometimes related to drug trafficking, smuggling, and other crimes". [54] (s/p)

This was reflected in comments made by the Mayor of Colchane, who stated as follows:

> The militarization and placement of two armored vehicles on the border, along with military personnel, has only controlled our people, not the immigrants, as the army provides humanitarian assistance to migrants [...]. I believe that what is needed here is some self-criticism and to sit down and get to work, as it is not just this issue of the humanitarian point of view of the rights that migrants have to migrate, but also the rights that we have, for example, the indigenous peoples, as we deal with this migratory phenomenon, which is not our responsibility, and that is clearly detrimental to our cultural identity.

One clear example is the issue of coca leaves. These leaves play an integral role in the life of the Aymara as food as well as medicine (in its ritual aspects and chemical properties); this is a sacred plant used in the offering rituals made to the Pachamama and protective beings. However, it is not grown in Chile, so it enters the country mainly from Bolivia and

Peru. Although it crosses into Chile via unauthorized routes, thus avoiding border controls, officials of the Agricultural and Livestock Service (Servicio Agrícola y Ganadero-SAG) and customs officials, who understand its importance, allow the entry of small amounts of leaves for personal consumption.

In the context of the closure and militarization of Chile's borders, this criterion has been suspended, as those bringing in coca leaves are obliged to use unauthorized routes, thus exposing people to having to explain themselves to the military, who do not possess such an understanding of the customs specific to the territory. Moreover, neither have soldiers been trained to use flexible criteria when dealing with a heavily criminalized plant. Such criminalization has a long history, led by the United States, which, based on the Geneva Convention (1936), obliged other states to pursue drug trafficking and any actions involving "harmful drugs". Furthermore, an essential step in the criminalization of coca leaves was their inclusion in the Single Convention on Narcotic Drugs of 1961 of the United Nations (1961 Convention), modified by the Geneva Protocol in 1972, signed by 74 countries [55].

Thus, the movement of vital elements for the region's indigenous communities, such as the entry of coca leaves, was affected not only by the closure of borders but also by their consequent militarization, generating an inadvertent impact on health. To understand this impact, we must consider the existing medical pluralism, specifically the role of so-called "traditional" knowledge. Of course, the value of such knowledge is not restricted to the native people's or neighboring countries' populations. As we have shown [56], it also constitutes one of the primary resources for the undocumented migrant population.

Paradoxically, this impact on health was implemented based on legal arguments regarding health. What happened is that, in the context of COVID-19, the health domain was reduced to the coronavirus domain. Thus, the monocultural, biomedical approach of the State once again shows its limitations. However, to get a broader idea of the impact on health caused by such immobility policies, it is necessary to leave aside the monocultural rationale and observe the impact they had from the point of view of Andean medical knowledge.

3.2. Impact on the Health/Disease/Care Process

> I traveled first ... the first year I was making the journey every three months, because as I did not have a visa, so I had to leave no matter what, because they told me: you have to have your papers in order to be able to get the visa, so you cannot have anything out of order, things like that. Then, I went every three months, and I saw them and came back again. I entered [...] I was almost a month, and then I returned. [...] The last time I left was just before the pandemic ... and then a month went by, and just when the pandemic was beginning, I returned. That month that we came, the pandemic had started, we had already entered, and I could not leave ... (N., Bolivian woman, interviewed in May 2021, Iquique.)

The mobility of people was affected, including healthcare mobility. As we have shown in previous works [56,57], cross-border healthcare mobility is a frequent and essential socio-spatial practice in Tarapacá. This mobility does not consist only of searching for patented drugs or biomedical attention. It also includes the search for supplies such as medicinal plants, naturist preparations, and products made by the respective domestic producers based on local herbal remedies. Furthermore, an essential part of health mobility is to provide elements related to the healing practices of Andean medical knowledge [57].

Since time immemorial, Andean medical knowledge has drawn on the different ecological foundations. For this reason, it has been and is transnational and cross-border in nature. The origin of its inputs shows a complex interrelation of legal spaces and regimes. Thus, the elements sold for ritual 'mesas' or sacred offerings in the territory of Tarapacá come from Oruro, while many of the naturist products are sourced from the national industries of Peru and Bolivia. Medicinal plants come from the different ecological floors present in these three countries.

Moreover, the ways that they enter the country also vary. According to a Chilean customs officer, most likely, the bulk of these products enter the country thanks to small-scale smuggling. They use the so-called "traveler franchise" that allows a person to enter the country with everything in their luggage. Thus, when someone wants to introduce a more considerable volume of products, they are distributed among people paid to carry them as part of their luggage [58,59]. Another modality is the payment of bribes to officials to let contraband trucks pass through the border checkpoints. Some Bolivian informants said they pay about US$5000 for this purpose, making a collection among all those interested in the truck coming across the border.

These strategies of transporting therapeutic goods pass through various regulatory spaces [60], of which the dominant one is that of the State. Within the framework we are analyzing, this means that the assets of Andean medical knowledge are, in general, criminalized objects. And this occurs either in their origin (when their production is prohibited), in one of the intermediate links by which they circulate (when the prohibition falls on the transfer from one country to another), or in their sale. The criminalization, illegalization, and State delegitimation of Andean medical knowledge is also applied to health and knowledge agents [61,62]. However, this does not prevent such agents from enjoying an important level of appreciation in the popular sectors, occupying a place characterized by the coexistence of legal rejection with the appraisal offered by social actors [60].

And while these networks are part of globalized processes, they take place within a context of strong historical roots in the Andean economic space [63], where indigenous people produce most of the goods sold. In addition, their flow through the commodity chain until they reach the consumers passes through various regulatory spaces where ethnic and kinship networks are indispensable for evading state control [64–66].

Thus, a significant impact is related to the difficulty of legally crossing the border to acquire supplies for treating health problems in adherence to an Andean rationale.

> Z.A.: So, whenever I travel to Bolivia, people in Chile ask me to bring back medicines, all from there. [. . .] I brought ovules for body pain, oil, and natural medicine. What they have confiscated are the maticos, the dry leaves. I've brought a lot of that, and they have confiscated it [. . .] I had about seven herbs, including chamomile, fresh chamomile, and here there is not any . . . the same with muña, and cola de caballo. There are two types of cola de caballo, one that's yellow and the other green. I brought the yellow one. I also brought boldo.
>
> C.P.: Ah, and you brought them from Cochabamba?
>
> Z.A.: From Cochabamba, without the stems. Just like they sell parsley, all tied together, just like that. (Z.A., Bolivian woman, interviewed in September 2020, Iquique.)

However, just as these anecdotes show the direct impact of the processes of (im)mobility in the practice of self-attention, a more significant impact can be observed in the obstacles imposed on the movements of traditional healthcare practitioners such as Yatiris (spiritual healers), Qulliris (bone setter and herbalists), and Usuyiris (traditional midwives).

These processes of outlawing such movements have been exacerbated in the context of (im)mobility caused by COVID-19. To illustrate this point, we find it appropriate to present the story of E.C., a Bolivian healer from the outskirts of La Paz (Bolivia) who now lives and works in Alto Hospicio (Chile). He reminds us that the specific nature of Andean medical knowledge requires that certain ingredients must be brought from beyond the borders: "Misa de rayo con tata Santiago [specific type of 'mesas' ritual offering] has to be carried out . . . and it does not exist here. Well, it exists, it is not that it is not here, but it is not my way of doing it, another way", as he well exemplified for us. Such practices are not taken into account by border control agents who, by preventing the open transit of such medicinal elements, force them to be transferred by illegal means. This situation has worsened since the implementation of the Secure Border Plan.

> E.C.: They wanted to confiscate that from me . . . in an apple box, you can fit 25 units of large 'mesas' offerings and about 40 little ones. When I was inspected by the SAG official [he said]: 'I am letting you go now, but sign this other form, do it for me. And if you carry this stuff again, I'm going to arrest you' [. . .] Last year it was not so bad . . . then I would bring about 2 or 3 crates of apple boxes, [. . .] brought them on the bus without any hassle. But now [since the border closure], it is just not on. You have to break the law and bring it all in illegally. (E.C., Bolivian yatiri healer, interviewed in July 2020, Alto Hospicio).

Despite what the case of E.C. shows, such flows continue from Chile to Bolivia. In general, control surveillance has focused on the dynamics of entry into Chile and mainly on the Venezuelan population due to their country's humanitarian "crisis". However, other permanent flows of people are associated with seeking attention for health problems and seeking options other than biomedical treatments, which have been systematically neglected.

One example of these flows and the validity of Andean medical knowledge was the seizure made by the Agricultural and Livestock Service (Servicio Agrícola y Ganadero-SAG) on 2 September 2020, of a truck from Bolivia passing through the Chungará border control post: the truck's load consisted of 200 kg of "forestry and agricultural products" that included "sacks of coca leaves [. . .], 74 L of alcohol for consumption purposes, and ten alpaca fetuses, the latter being quite unprecedented in the region and representing a high risk to public health" [67]. The confiscation also included black 'mesas' offerings (Figure 3), omitted in the official statement and newspaper reports. The director of SAG, Jorge Hernández, made the following remark:

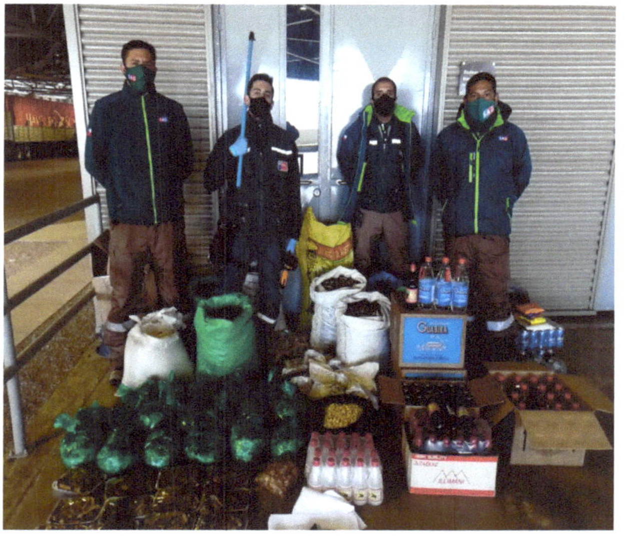

Figure 3. Confiscation of Bolivian truck cargo, including coca leaves, *'mesas'* offerings, and *'purito'* (90% proof alcohol), among other goods. Source: Agricultural and Livestock Service-SAG, September 2020.

> . . . This type of cargo, specifically the alpaca fetuses, which are domestic South American camelids, represent an extreme risk to domestic (animal) health, as they can carry exotic diseases not present in the country, which could have a considerable impact on domestic production and affect the export of Chilean products to critical foreign markets.

Curiously, the presence of alpaca fetuses in a region where these animals are widespread is described as "unprecedented". Also, curious seems to claim a high risk to animal health in a border zone where livestock transport from one side of the border occurs regularly. Moreover, when the cross-border networks of the popular economy make these elements available daily for the ritual and health needs of the population. Nevertheless, this is how the border control practices of the Chilean State have fostered the "criminal life" [60] of essential objects of Andean medical knowledge.

3.3. Deficits in Indigenous and Migrant Law

Chile has signed and ratified numerous human rights instruments. The so-called constitutionalization of the different branches of law enables the direct application of such treaties under the provisions of the second paragraph of article 5 of the Political Constitution of the Republic, either as self-executing norms or as norms that serve for the systematic or organic interpretation of Chilean laws. However, in many cases, the implementation and exercise of these rights are subject to the adaptation of internal regulations, which in monocultural structural contexts is challenging to implement. Thus, the immobility processes reported in this article are supported by significant deficiencies in the domestic law for migrant and indigenous populations.

Human rights represent the backbone of international law; thus, the need to prevent discrimination and abuses suffered by migrants is a long-standing concern that has been led by international bodies, with the right to freedom of movement and to choose a place of residence expressly recognized in the Universal Declaration of Human Rights (1948) and the International Covenant on Civil and Political Rights (1966).

At the regional level, regional integration initiatives, such as the Southern Common Market (MERCOSUR), have established free movement agreements, particularly regarding border areas. Bolivia and Chile are associate members of MERCOSUR, through their respective Economic Complementation Agreements, and must therefore respect the Agreement on Residence for Nationals of the MERCOSUR States Parties, Bolivia, and Chile. The latter involves facilities for the movement of workers in border areas. In the field of health and border, an important step was taken with the signing of the 2019 Agreement on Linked Border Localities [68]. However, the assessment of access to biomedical health in MERCOSUR border areas in pandemic contexts is rather negative. Considering all States opted to prevent the spread of the virus contagion by closing borders, a rebordering effect was produced [69], limiting interaction at the borders, mainly affecting local communities. The PAHO has expressed concern because these areas are home to vulnerable populations, including indigenous people, communities living in remote areas, and immigrants [70]. Regarding indigenous rights, given the institutional structure of MERCOSUR, the contribution of this instrument depends on the recognition that each State party or associated State gives to its indigenous peoples; and Chile still has not recognized indigenous peoples' existence in its constitution [71].

Considering all the above, the main effects on migrants relate to the right to admission to Chile, the right to legalize their residency status, the right to receive refuge, the right to non-return to their country of origin, the right to due process concerning their humanitarian situation and the right to receive healthcare without discrimination. In this case, the adverse effects and the dramatic impacts on health arise from the primacy of a security-orientated form of being treated, particularly regarding the medical treatment associated with COVID-19. Thus, appropriate measures have not been witnessed that would allow migrants to avoid the risk associated with their vulnerability, especially in the case of children, or to avoid being exposed to acts of xenophobia, discrimination, and stigmatization.

In the case of native peoples, it must be taken into account that specific rights enshrined in international law refer to cross-border mobility. Ultimately, these rights are based on the right to cultural integrity, the right to culture, and cultural heritage. The first thing to point out is that Supreme Decree 104, which declares a state of constitutional exception of catastrophe and allows the restriction of certain rights, has ignored the right to participate in measures that directly affect peoples and communities. Consequently, the measures implemented to protect the security and life of citizens lack any sense of interculturality, given that regulations emanating from the central level are established, with total ignorance of the regional territorial dynamics of native peoples and cross-border existence.

Regarding healthcare, this has led to a setback in the dialogue held with the State. Just to give an example, during the process of participation and subsequent indigenous consultation of article 7 of Law 20,584 (a process that lasted for more than five years), the representatives of native peoples of the whole country informed the Chilean State of the necessary conditions to guarantee the right to healthcare with cultural relevance, pointing to problems such as being obliged to use practices of the biomedical model, among many others. For each problem identified, proposals were drawn up by consensus between the State and the different native peoples in a detailed document submitted to the Office of the Comptroller General of the Republic. Today, this entire process of dialogue has not only been ignored but has been made entirely imperceptible, as if the government had to provide solutions to the pandemic without any previous guidance in this regard.

In terms more directly related to cross-border mobility, international regulations have made progress in establishing, as stated in the American Declaration on the Rights of Indigenous Peoples, the right to association, assembly, organization, and expression and to exercise them without interference. Furthermore, it explicitly guarantees the right to "travel and to maintain and develop contacts, relations, and direct co-operation, including activities for spiritual, cultural, political, economic and social purposes, with their members and other peoples" (Article XX). Although Chilean legislation has not been aligned with the American Declaration (ADRIP, 2016), the ILO Convention 169 of 1989 has been ratified, which, being a more limited instrument in terms of standards, establishes that governments must "take appropriate measures, including by means of international agreements, to facilitate contacts and co-operation between indigenous and tribal peoples across borders, including activities in the economic, social, cultural and environmental fields".

Mobility for healthcare purposes represents a process directly associated with what is established by law, as it consists of economic activities (exchange, sale, consumption), as well as those of a social and cultural nature, due to the symbolic and ritual activity that is inherent to them. Likewise, it comprehends environmental activities, as reciprocal relationships with the territory are cultivated, taken care of, and reproduced in the environment and communities.

Furthermore, Andean medical knowledge constitutes an essential part of the cultural integrity of the indigenous peoples of this territory. In this regard, Convention 169 established that "Governments shall have the responsibility of developing, with the participation of the peoples concerned, coordinated and systematic action to protect the rights of these peoples and to guarantee respect for their integrity". The aforementioned right is specified and expanded in more advanced formulations such as the United Nations Declaration on the Rights of Indigenous Peoples or the American Declaration, which establishes the right to "their own cultural identity and integrity and to their cultural heritage", whether this is tangible or intangible, and not limited to the present, as it includes historical and ancestral heritage (Article XIII).

In the case of Andean medical knowledge, we are in the presence of an institution that is key to maintaining cultural integrity [72], as it maintains an essential part of the cosmovision, spirituality, and the relationship with the territory. This knowledge is embodied in institutions, practices, beliefs, and values. Likewise, agents with this knowledge represent carriers of a tangible and intangible cultural heritage. Thus, neither they nor their activities should be persecuted or criminalized but protected.

In this sense, the American Declaration states: "Indigenous peoples have the right to recognition and respect for all their ways of life, cosmovisions, spirituality, uses, customs, norms, traditions, forms of social, economic and political organization; forms of transmission of knowledge, institutions, practices, beliefs, values, dress, and languages, recognizing their interrelationship as established in this Declaration" (Article XIII). This right does not concern only to "protection, preservation, maintenance", but rather the "development of that cultural heritage for their collective continuity and that of their members and so as to transmit that knowledge to future generations" (Article XIII). Therefore, protecting and developing indigenous culture is fundamental, as cultural continuity correlates with good mental health, lower suicide levels, and lower school dropouts in indigenous communities [73].

Although the limitation of rights is inherent to the legal system, the problem can be redirected to the fundamental aspects on which the rights are limited. Referring to the limitation of mobility in the COVID pandemic, one of the main problems is that the State operates according to a monocultural rationale. This rationale is rooted in the structure of the State and hindered the implementation and adaptation of internal regulatory frameworks to comply with international standards fully. Consequently, the rights of native peoples related to cultural integrity and cross-border mobility were not included in the design of the proposals implemented. As a result, a paradox was conformed in which measures taken in the name of health end up producing negative impacts on the population's health.

4. Conclusions

Three questions guided our research: What processes of (im)mobility affected the health mobility in the Tarapacá region (Chile) in COVID-19 times? How did this (im)mobility process impact the health/illness/care process of indigenous migrants? How do the current policies of the Chilean and its deficiency in indigenous and migrant rights give form to that (im)mobility process? Regarding these questions, we want to highlight some ideas that have emerged from our work.

The immobility processes reviewed can be summarized in two groups, depending on whether they respond to processes determined by the immigrant condition or whether they operate independently of this condition. For the first set, we show how the (im)mobility processes were forged in continuity with racist immigration policies oriented towards security. In this framework, the apparent rationality of the health measures served as a legitimizing element of security policies, several of which were directly discriminatory and contrary to law, such as collective expulsions, the denial of the right to refuge, and violation of the right of non-refoulment.

In the second set, we found the (in)mobility processes related to the border closure. Border closure policies linked to COVID-19, created in terms of a monocultural rationale, impacted the health of indigenous people and communities. Those policies affected the socio-cultural, economic, and political exchange necessary for social reproduction and protecting life and health. One concealed aspect is the impact these had on the necessary mobility of Andean medical knowledge in terms of elements used and patients and agents of health (such as *Yatiris*, *Qulliris*, and *Usuyiris*). Border closure affected the dynamics of Andean medical knowledge, impacted its cultural integrity, and strengthened its criminalization, contrary to the recognition, protection, and development enshrined by international law.

In the intersection of both processes, militarization also impacted the health of immigrants and indigenous communities, reflected in racism and abuses perpetrated by members of the armed forces, not prepared to deal with this complexity, much less in cross-border and intercultural contexts.

These aspects combined allow us to understand why measures that are supposed to protect public health end up producing negative impacts on the health of certain groups and peoples, for they lead us to verify once again that policies have a differential impact on the population, according to the structural vulnerability involved. Furthermore, they also invite us to think about who pays the price for the defense of public health when health-related arguments give space and legitimacy to the securitizing and racist tendencies still present in the state structure of a country such as Chile.

Our research poses specific challenges: further study of health (im)mobility is needed. Previous work has focused chiefly on health mobility, neglecting the dialectical processes of immobility that the pandemic brought to the forefront. As we do here, those studies may embrace medical pluralism to analyze the effects on health from the point of view of the different medical knowledge present in the territories, surpassing the medical monism that assumes biomedicine is the only worthy knowledge. Finally, more research is needed to show the gap between what the legislation establishes and what the States do. This research will help us shed more light on the permanent contradiction of States that consider themselves democratic, but based on their neoliberal matrix, permanently and selectively reproduce structural violence against populations such as indigenous and immigrants.

Author Contributions: Conceptualization, C.P.-R.; methodology, C.P.-R. and N.L.; formal analysis, C.P.-R.; investigation, C.P.-R.; resources, C.P.-R.; data curation, C.P.-R.; writing—original draft preparation, C.P.-R.; writing—review and editing, C.P.-R., N.L., R.A. and V.J.; project administration, N.L.; funding acquisition, N.L. All authors have read and agreed to the published version of the manuscript.

Funding: This research and the APC was funded by Agencia Nacional de Investigación y Desarrollo (ANID) Chile, Fondecyt Regular 1210602.

Institutional Review Board Statement: The study was conducted in accordance with the Declaration of Helsinki and approved by the Institutional Review Board (or Ethics Committee) of Universidad de Tarapacá for studies involving humans.

Informed Consent Statement: Informed consent was obtained from all subjects involved in the study.

Conflicts of Interest: The authors declare no conflict of interest.

References

1. Cid, C. Causas Estructurales de Los Problemas de Inequidad En El Acceso a La Salud En Chile. *Rev. Chil. Salud Pública* **2008**, *12*, 57–96. [CrossRef]
2. Homedes, N.; Ugalde, A. Privatización de los servicios de salud: Las experiencias de Chile y Costa Rica. *Gac. Sanit.* **2002**, *16*, 54–62. [CrossRef]
3. Oyarte, M.; Espinoza, M.; Balmaceda, C.; Villegas, R.; Cabieses, B.; Díaz, J. Gasto de Bolsillo en Salud y Medicamentos en Chile. Out-of-Pocket Expenditures in Health and Medications in Chile: Comparative Analysis Between 1997, 2007, and 2012. *Value Health Reg. Issues* **2018**, *17*, 202–209. [CrossRef] [PubMed]
4. Villalobos Dintrans, P. Out-of-Pocket Health Expenditure Differences in Chile: Insurance Performance or Selection? *Health Policy* **2018**, *122*, 184–191. [CrossRef]
5. Álvarez, R.; González, A. *Análisis Comparativo de Precios de Medicamentos en América Latina*; Series Documentos de Trabajo; Repositorio Académico de la Universidad de Chile: Santiago, Chile, 2018.
6. Fiscalía Nacional Económica. *Estudio de Mercado Sobre Medicamentos*; Fiscalía Nacional Económica: Santiago, Chile, 2019.
7. CNN. 9.724 Pacientes Murieron Mientras Estaban en Lista de Espera en el Primer Semestre de 2018. Available online: https://www.cnnchile.com/pais/pacientes-fallecidos-lista-de-espera-en-2018-minsal_20190213/ (accessed on 19 July 2022).
8. Marambio-Tapia, A. Endeudamiento "saludable", empoderamiento y control social. *Polis. Rev. Latinoam.* **2018**, *17*, 11.
9. Liberona, N.; Tapia, M.A.; Contreras Gatica, Y. Movilidad Por Salud Entre Arica y Tacna: Análisis de Una Demanda No Satisfecha y de Una Oferta Atractiva Del Otro Lado de La Frontera. *Geopolítica* **2017**, *8*, 253–278. [CrossRef]
10. Cid, C.; Uthoff, A. La reforma a la salud pendiente en Chile: Reflexiones en torno a una propuesta de transformación del sistema. *Rev. Panam. Salud Pública* **2017**, *41*, 170–179. [CrossRef]
11. Cortez, A. Migración internacional: Un desafío para las políticas públicas de Chile. In *Niños y Niñas Migrantes: Políticas Públicas, Integración e Interculturalidad*; Quimantú: Santiago, Chile, 2007; pp. 105–118. ISBN 978-956-8656-00-3.
12. Liberona, N.; Mansilla, M.A. Pacientes ilegítimos: Acceso a la salud de los inmigrantes indocumentados en Chile. *Salud Colect.* **2017**, *13*, 507–520. [CrossRef]
13. Cabieses, B.; Bernales, M.; McIntyre, A.M. *La Migración Internacional Como Determinante Social de la Salud en CHILE: Evidencia y Propuestas Para Políticas Públicas*; Facultad de Medicina, Clínica Alemana-Universidad del Desarrollo: Concepción, Chile, 2017; ISBN 978-956-374-000-4.
14. Castañeda, H.; Holmes, S.M.; Madrigal, D.S.; Young, M.-E.D.; Beyeler, N.; Quesada, J. Immigration as a Social Determinant of Health. *Annu. Rev. Public Health* **2015**, *36*, 375–392. [CrossRef]
15. Liberona, N. De La Alterisación a La Discriminación En Un Sistema Público De Salud En Crisis: Conflictos Interétnicos a Propósito De La Inmigración Sudamericana En Chile. *Rev. Cienc. Soc.* **2012**, *28*, 19–38.
16. Liberona, N.; Piñones-Rivera, C. *Informe Técnico Encuesta Vida de Inmigrantes*; UNAP: Iquique, Chile, 2019.
17. Morey, B.N. Mechanisms by Which Anti-Immigrant Stigma Exacerbates Racial/Ethnic Health Disparities. *Am. J. Public Health* **2018**, *108*, 460–463. [CrossRef] [PubMed]

18. Tarrius, A. Leer, Describir, Interpretar Las Circulaciones Migratorias: Conveniencia de La Noción de Territorio Circulatorio. Los Nuevos Hábitos de La Identidad. *Relac. Estud. Hist. Y Soc.* **2000**, *21*, 38–56.
19. Dufraix, R.; Ramos, R.; Quinteros, D. "Ordenar La Casa": Securitización y Producción de Irregularidad En El Norte de Chile. *Sociologias* **2020**, *22*, 172–196. [CrossRef]
20. Liberona, N.P.; Piñones Rivera, C.D.; Dilla, H. De la migración forzada al tráfico de migrantes: La migración clandestina en tránsito de Cuba hacia Chile. *Migr. Int.* **2021**, *12*, 1–23. [CrossRef]
21. Morales, A. Desentrañando Fronteras y Sus Movimientos Transnacionales Entre Pequeños Estados. Una Aproximación Desde La Frontera Nicaragua-Costa Rica. In *Migraciones y Fronteras: Nuevos Contornos Para la Movilidad Internacional*; Anguiano, M., López, A., Eds.; Icaria: Barcelona, Spain, 2010; pp. 185–224.
22. Parella, S. Una exploración de las prácticas transfronterizas en la zona urbana Caléxico (Estados Unidos)-Mexicali (México). In *Regiones Fronterizas, Migración y Los Desafíos Para Los Estados Nacionales Latinoamericanos*; Tapia, M., González, A., Eds.; RIL Editores: Santiago, Chile, 2014; pp. 41–69. ISBN 978-956-01-0048-1.
23 Heyman, J. Construcción y Uso de Tipologías: Movilidad Geográfica Desigual En La Frontera México-Estados Unidos. In *Métodos Cualitativos y Su Aplicación Empírica: Por Los Caminos de la Investigación Sobre Migración Internacional*; Ariza, M., Velasco, L., Eds.; National Autonomous University of Mexico, Institute of Social Research: Mexico City, Mexico, 2012; pp. 419–454.
24. Tarrius, A. La mundialización por abajo. In *El Capitalismo Nómada en el Arco Mediterráneo*; Editorial Hacer: Barcelona, Spain, 2007; ISBN 978-84-96913-02-8.
25. Tapia, M.; González, A. *Regiones Fronterizas: Migración y Los Desafíos Para Los Estados Nacionales Latinoamericanos*; RIL Editores: Santiago, Chile, 2014.
26. Glockner, V.; Álvarez-Velasco, S. Espacios de vida cotidiana y el continuum movilidad/inmovilidad: El protagonismo de niñxs y adolescentes migrantes en el continente americano. Un proyecto etnográfico multimedia. *An. Antropol.* **2021**, *55*, 59–72. [CrossRef]
27. Heyman, J. Capitalismo, Movilidad Desigual y La Gobernanza de La Frontera México-Estados Unidos. In *Desafiando Fronteras Control de la Movilidad y Experiencias Migratorias en el Contexto Capitalista*; Aquino, A., Varela, A., Décasse, F., Eds.; Frontera Press: Mexico City, Mexico, 2012; pp. 25–40.
28. Heyman, J. Cuatro Temas En Los Estudios de La Frontera Contemporánea. In *El Río Bravo Mediterráneo: Las Regiones Fronterizas en la Época de la Globalización*; Ribas, N., Ed.; Bellaterra: Barcelona, Spain, 2011; pp. 81–97.
29. Bigo, D. Security and Immigration: Toward a Critique of the Governmentality of Unease. *Alternatives* **2002**, *27*, 63–92. [CrossRef]
30. Sayad, A. L'immigration et La Pensée d'Etat, Réflexions Sur La Double Peine. *Sci. Sociales. EUR17472 Coast A* **1996**, *2*, 11–29.
31. Balibar, É. *Le Frontiere Della Democrazia, Manifestolibri*; Manifestolibri: Rome, Italy, 1993.
32. Castel, R.; Beland, D. L'insécurité Sociale: Qu'est-Ce Qu'être Protégé? *Can. Rev. Sociol.* **2004**, *41*, 88.
33. Huysmans, J. The European Union and the Securitization of Migration. *JCMS J. Common Mark. Stud.* **2000**, *38*, 751–777. [CrossRef]
34. Quinteros, D. Nueva 'Crimigración' o La Vieja Economía Política Del Castigo? Dos Aproximaciones Criminológicas Para Entender El Control Punitivo de La Migración En Chile. *Astrolabio* **2016**, *17*, 81–113.
35. Stang, M.F. De la Doctrina de la Seguridad Nacional a la gobernabilidad migratoria: La idea de seguridad en la normativa migratoria chilena, 1975–2014. *Polis. Rev. Latinoam.* **2016**, *44*, 1–21. [CrossRef]
36. Mezzadra, S. Capitalismo, Migraciones y Luchas Sociales: La Mirada de La Autonomía. *Nueva Soc.* **2012**, *237*, 159–178.
37. Godenau, D.; López Sala, A.M. *Estados de Contención, Estados de Detención: El Control de La Inmigración Irregular En España*; TRAFICANTES: Barcelona, Spain, 2017; pp. 1–255.
38. Domenech, E. Las Políticas de Migración En Sudamérica: Elementos Para El Análisis Crítico Del Control Migratorio y Fronterizo. *Terc. Milênio Rev. Crítica Sociol. E Política* **2017**, *8*, 19–48.
39. Pécoud, A. Una Nueva «gobernanza» de La Migración? Lo Que Dicen Las Organizaciones Internacionales. *Migr. Desarro.* **2018**, *16*, 31–43. [CrossRef]
40. Mansur-Dias, G. Trata de Personas, Tráfico de Migrantes y La Gobernabilidad de La Migración a Través Del Crimen. *Etnografica* **2017**, *21*, 541–554. [CrossRef]
41. Ruiz, M.; Alvarez, S. Excluir Para Proteger: La "Guerra" Contra La Trata y El Tráfico de Migrantes y Las Nuevas Lógicas de Control Migratorio En Ecuador. *Estud. Sociológicos XXXVII* **2019**, *111*, 698–725.
42. García-Pinzón, V. Estado y frontera en el norte de Chile. *Estud. Front.* **2015**, *16*, 117–148. [CrossRef]
43. Iturra, L. El Cuerpo Otro y Los Otros Espacios. In *El Afán de Cruzar Las Fronteras: Enfoques Transdisciplinarios Sobre Migraciones y Movilidad en Sudamérica y Chile*; Tapia, M., Liberona, N., Eds.; RIL Editores: Santiago, Chile, 2018; ISBN 978-956-01-0528-8.
44. Liberona, N. De las fronteras geopolíticas a las fronteras sociales: La migración boliviana a través de la prensa de Tarapacá (1990–2007). *Estud. Front.* **2015**, *16*, 41–74. [CrossRef]
45. Liberona, N. Fronteras y Movilidad Humana En América Latina. *Nueva Soc.* **2020**, *289*, 49–58.
46. Gobierno de Chile Presidente Piñera Promulga Nueva Ley de Migraciones Para Chile. Available online: http://prensa.presidencia.cl/discurso.aspx?id=173742 (accessed on 19 July 2022).
47. Servicio Jesuita a Migrantes Migración En Chile. In *Anuario 2020 Medidas Migratorias, Vulnerabilidad y Oportunidades En Un Año de Pandemia (N°2)*; SJM: Santiago, Chile, 2021.
48. Pascual-Ricke, T. La [Des]Protección de Los Derechos Humanos En Contextos de Movilidad Humana En Chile: Expulsiones Administrativas y Soli-Citudes de Protección Internacional. *Anu. Derechos Hum.* **2020**, *16*, 381–410. [CrossRef]

49. Huysmans, J.; Squire, V. Migration and Security. In *Handbook of Security Studies*; Dunn, M., Mauer, V., Eds.; Routledge: London, UK, 2009; ISBN 978-0-415-46361-4.
50. Mayorga, R. Control Migratorio y Salud Pública: Restricciones a La Movilidad Humana Por Razones Médicas o Sanitarias En Tiempos Del Covid-19. *Rev. Derecho* **2021**, *34*, 203–223. [CrossRef]
51. De Genova, N. Extremities and Regularities: Regulatory Regimes and the Spectacle of Immigration Enforcement. In *The Irregularization of Migration in Contemporary Europe: Detention, Deportation, Drowning*; Jansen, Y., Celikates, R., Bloois, J., Eds.; Rowman Littlefield: Lanham, MD, USA, 2014; pp. 3–14. ISBN 978-1-78348-171-2.
52. El Mostrador Cancillería Suspendió Trámite de Visa de Responsabilidad Democrática Para Venezolanos, Pero Aclara Que Se Trata de Un Reinicio. Available online: https://www.elmostrador.cl/dia/2020/11/13/cancilleria-suspendio-tramite-de-visa-de-responsabilidad-democratica-para-venezolanos-pero-aclara-que-se-trata-de-un-reinicio/ (accessed on 19 July 2022).
53. Jiménez, V.T. Expulsiones Colectivas En El "Plan Colchane": La Necesidad y Propuesta de Un Concepto de Expulsión Colectiva. *Anu. DDHH* **2021**, *17*, 405. [CrossRef]
54. Moscoso, A.; Mamani, E.; Montecino, B. *Recurso de Protección Rol Corte 21-2021*; Iquique, Chile, 2021.
55. Muro, A.; Aguirre, P.; Parra, D.; Piza, M. *Usos, Impactos y Derechos: Posibilidades, Políticas y Jurídicas Para La Investigación de La Hoja de Coca En Colombia*; Elementa: Bogotá, Colombia, 2018.
56. Piñones-Rivera, C.; Liberona Concha, N.; Mansilla, M.Á. Itinerarios Terapéuticos Transfronterizos: Hacia El Estudio Del Pluralismo Médico y La Movilidad Humana Transfronteriza. *Si Somos Am.* **2020**, *20*, 9–37. [CrossRef]
57. Piñones-Rivera, C.; Muñoz, W.; Liberona, N. Te Mueves o Te Mueres: La Movilidad Del Saber Médico Andino En La Triple Frontera Bolívia, Chile y Perú. In *Fronteira, Território e Ambiente: Diálogos Entre América Latina e Europa*; Ferrari, M., Gusman, I., Aparecido da costa, E., Lois González, R., Eds.; Edunioeste: Paraná, Brazil, 2020; ISBN 978-65-87438-16-0.
58. Chavarría, C.; Casquero, C.; Martínez, D. Contrabando: Importancia en la región trinacional frente a la estructura espacial. *Espac. Desarro.* **2012**, *24*, 75–88.
59. Dilla, H.; Álvarez, C. Arica/Tacna: Los Circuitos Económicos de Un Complejo Urbano Transfronterizo. *Diálogo Andin.* **2018**, *57*, 99–109. [CrossRef]
60. Van Schendel, W.; Abraham, I. *Illicit Flows and Criminal Things: States, Borders, and The Other Side of Globalization*; Tracking globalization; Indiana University Press: Bloomington, IN, USA, 2005; ISBN 978-0-253-34669-8.
61. Piñones-Rivera, C.D.; Liberona, N.P.; Montecino Quenaya, B. La Subordinación Ideológica Del Saber Médico Andino En La Salud Intercultural Chilena. *Polis (Santiago)* **2019**, *18*, 224–244. [CrossRef]
62. Piñones-Rivera, C.; Mansilla-Agüero, M.; Arancibia-Campos, R. El Imaginario de La Horizontalidad Como Instrumento de Subordinación: La Política de Salud Pueblos Indígenas En El Multiculturalismo Neoliberal Chileno. *Saude Soc.* **2017**, *26*, 751–763. [CrossRef]
63. Glave, L. *Trajinantes: Caminos Indígenas En La Sociedad Colonial Siglos XVI/XVII*; Instituto de apoyo agrario: Lima, Perú, 1989.
64. Albó, X. Aymaras Entre Bolivia, Perú y Chile. *Estud Atacameños* **2000**, *1*, 43–74. [CrossRef]
65. Benedetti, A.; Salizzi, E. Llegar, pasar, regresar a la frontera. Aproximación al sistema de movilidad argentino-boliviano. *Rev. Transp. Y Territ.* **2011**, *4*, 148–179. [CrossRef]
66. Tassi, N. *The Native World-System: An Ethnography of Bolivian Aymara Traders in the Global Economy*; Issues of globalization: Case studies in contemporary anthropology; Oxford University Press: Oxford, UK, 2017; ISBN 978-0-19-025522-0.
67. SAG. SAG Intercepta Más de 200 Kilos de Productos de Origen Animal y Vegetal En Chungará | SAG. Available online: https://www.sag.gob.cl/noticias/sag-intercepta-mas-de-200-kilos-de-productos-de-origen-animal-y-vegetal-en-chungara (accessed on 19 July 2022).
68. MERCOSUR. Acuerdo Localidades Fronterizas Vinculadas 2019. Available online: https://www.mercosur.int/documento/acuerdo-localidades-fronterizas-vinculadas/ (accessed on 25 July 2022).
69. Berzi, M.; Lemões, M.A.M.; Oddone, N. Obstáculos a La Movilidad de Pacientes En Zonas de Frontera Del Mercosur: Una Propuesta de Tipología. *Estud. Front.* **2021**, *22*, e072. [CrossRef]
70. Bravin, M.C.S.; Collado, A.P.; Covolo, M.L. Fronteras Amenazadas. Potencialidades y Desafíos Del MERCOSUR Para Responder a La Pandemia. *Rev. MERCOSUR Políticas Soc.* **2020**, *4*, 104–118. [CrossRef]
71. Observatorio Ciudadano. *El Convenio 169 de La OIT Sobre Pueblos Indígenas y Tribales a 10 Años de Su Ratificación Por El Estado de Chile: Análisis Crítico de Su Cumplimiento*; Central Unitaria de Trabajadores: Bogotá, Colombia, 2018.
72. Gundermann-Kröll, H.; González-Cortez, H. Sociedades Indígenas y Conocimiento Antropológico: Aymaras y Atacameños de Los Siglos XIX y XX. *Chungará* **2009**, *41*, 113–164. [CrossRef]
73. Kirmayer, L.J.; Sehdev, M.; Whitley, R.; Dandeneau, S.F.; Isaac, C. Community Resilience: Models, Metaphors and Measures. *Int. J. Indig. Health* **2009**, *5*, 62–117.

International Journal of
Environmental Research and Public Health

MDPI

Article

"Mi Corazón se Partió en Dos": Transnational Motherhood at the Intersection of Migration and Violence

Laurie Cook Heffron [1,*], Karin Wachter [2] and Esmeralda J. Rubalcava Hernandez [3]

1 School of Behavioral and Social Sciences, St. Edward's University, Austin, TX 78704, USA
2 School of Social Work, Watts College of Public Services and Community Solutions, Arizona State University, Phoenix, AZ 85004, USA
3 School of Social Work, University of Texas at Arlington, Arlington, TX 76019, USA
* Correspondence: lheffron@stedwards.edu

Abstract: In the recent Central American migrations spurred by violence, political instability, and economic insecurity, women grapple with whether and when to bring their children with them in pursuit of safety in another country, and with fulfilling their roles as mothers from afar. Drawing from the transnational motherhood literature and critical feminist theories, this interpretive qualitative study examined transnational motherhood grounded in the lived experiences of Central American women (n = 19) over the course of their migrations to the US. Informed by the principles of grounded theory, the inductive analysis identified five processes in which migration and violence shaped meanings of motherhood: risking everything, embodying separation, braving reunification, mothering others, and experiencing motherhood due to sexual violence. The findings contribute knowledge of how violence shapes and informs women's migrations and decision-making, and the consequences women endure in taking action to mitigate threats of violence in their own and their children's lives. The analysis furthermore highlights the specific and profound effects of family separation on mothers. The voices, perspectives, and experiences of migrating mothers and the ways in which migration and violence shapes notions and lived experiences of motherhood are imperative to research, practice, and advocacy to change oppressive immigration policies.

Keywords: migration; transnational motherhood; violence against women; intimate partner violence

Citation: Cook Heffron, L.; Wachter, K.; Rubalcava Hernandez, E.J. "Mi Corazón se Partió en Dos": Transnational Motherhood at the Intersection of Migration and Violence. *Int. J. Environ. Res. Public Health* **2022**, *19*, 13404. https://doi.org/10.3390/ijerph192013404

Academic Editors: Ernesto Castañeda and Maria De Jesus

Received: 1 August 2022
Accepted: 12 October 2022
Published: 17 October 2022

Publisher's Note: MDPI stays neutral with regard to jurisdictional claims in published maps and institutional affiliations.

1. Introduction

Against the backdrop of contemporary Central American migrations spurred by violence, political instability, and economic insecurity, mothers contend with leaving children behind in pursuit of safety in another country. Mothers migrate expecting to settle in the United States (US) and send for their children in hopes of securing their collective safety over the long-term. Immigration policies, including those that separate families and limit avenues for asylum, influence and restrict decisions, actions, and opportunities available to migrating mothers. In the midst of complex structural and interpersonal dynamics, lived experiences of family and motherhood are altered and reshaped. This study offers a nuanced examination of transnational motherhood, grounded in the lived experiences of Central American women in the shadows of violence and migration to the US.

1.1. Transnational Motherhood

Transnational motherhood acknowledges the ways in which people are anchored to multiple spaces and processes of mothering span geopolitical boundaries. Mothering across borders involves ongoing emotional care of, provision of financial support to, and communication with children from afar [1]. The identities and roles of women evolve, span across, and transcend national borders, as do socio-emotional and economic dimensions of parenting. Hondagneu-Sotelo and Ávila's seminal piece explored the meaning of motherhood in the context of immigration-related family separation [2]. Recent literature has resisted a binary conceptualization of transnational motherhood as either a sacrificial act or an abdication of responsibilities [3]. Contemporary scholarship suggests that mothering from afar is a prime example of how transnational identities function across social and physical spaces [4], expanding notions of gender and caretaking arrangements. Women who parent across borders face the basic question of "how to be socially and emotionally present while physically absent" [5] (p. 203). Rachel Hershberg uses the phrase "being present when forced to be absent" to describe how parents maintain and make meaning of transnational parenting [6]. Hershberg highlights consejos, the passing of conventional wisdom and advice from older to younger family members, as an example of adaptive communication between transnational parents and their children as a means of bridging distance and maintaining an emotional presence [6]. Horton describes transnational mothers feeling "physically absent but recognized and remembered in their home countries", while also "physically present yet invisible and disavowed in the United States" [7] (p. 17).

Recent studies have investigated how family is reorganized through separation, fears of separation, and upon reunification [8,9]. Transnational motherhood research also explores the role of those who take on caretaking responsibilities when mothers migrate and cross-border communication about parenting decisions, discipline, and child-rearing expenses [3,5,10,11]. Parent–child relationships are not fixed; multiple variables, such as children's age and developmental stage, communication, remittances, and the health and well-being of children, shape the experiences and outcomes of transnational motherhood [3,12]. Parents' migration can positively affect their children's economic well-being [11]. However, negative outcomes associated with migration-related separation include academic decline, 'acting out' behaviors, and poor self-esteem among children; and sadness, guilt, and loneliness among parents and caregivers [11,13–15]. Separation can also be associated with increased depression, anxiety, substance use, economic instability, and ambiguous loss for both children and parents [16]. Berger Cardoso and colleagues found that even when with their children, many parents feel a pervasive fear of separation and report that the risk of deportation, in addition to previous prolonged separations, alter family processes and family units [8].

1.2. Intersection of Migration and Violence

Women and girls in Central America are exposed to a constellation of violence, including from gendered impacts of criminal gang activity, to intimate partner violence (IPV), sexual violence, exploitation, and high rates of femicide [17,18]. Poverty, economic insecurity, underemployment, gender and age inequality, and patriarchal power structures intersect with risk of gender-based violence, placing women and girls at risk of experiencing abuse and violence and shrouding these experiences in silence with few outlets for support and protection [18]. Scholars describe migration as a strategy women employ to interrupt violence and ensure survival for themselves and their children [19–22]. Various forms of interpersonal, systemic, and structural violence intersect with the experience of migrating mothers. Non-partner sexual violence, IPV, and threats of violence, coercion, and abuse, for example, can make staying untenable [20]. Under these circumstances, women may migrate as an escape tactic or act of resistance [23,24]. The journey from Central America to the US, however, poses additional risks, during which women are exposed to verbal and physical abuse, sexual violence, exploitation, and other forms of violence [18,20,25]. Although studies describe the violence women face and their roles as mothers as embedded in the migration process from the beginning and playing critical roles in their decisions to migrate [20,21], motherhood is not widely addressed at the intersection of violence against women and migration.

1.3. The Current Analysis

The sensitive interplay between violence, migration, and motherhood represents an emerging and needed area of continued inquiry. This study draws from transnational feminisms, which recognize migration as a process involving complex, unsettled, and fluid senses of place, belonging, identity, and responsibility [10,26,27]. Feminist perspectives examine the many ways in which women assert power and resistance throughout migration, affirm women's decisions, and address the multiple contexts, identities, and experiences shaping migration [23,28–31]. These perspectives amplify the experiences and effects of migration as extending beyond migrating individuals to children, families and extended networks, recognizing how economic responsibilities, parenting roles, and communication evolve across geographic boundaries [8]. Rooted in the critical transnational literature, this qualitative analysis examined processes of transnational motherhood at the intersection of migration and violence, grounded in the perspectives of Central American women over the course of their migrations to the US.

2. Materials and Methods

Themes of motherhood presented in this articled emerged inductively from a study conducted in 2014, which examined violence against women and processes of migration among Central American women in the US [20]. The study was approved by the University of Texas at Austin Institutional Review Board and adhered to ethical guidelines in researching violence against women and migration to ensure the self-determination, safety, and wellbeing of participants [32,33].

2.1. Recruitment

Based on a purposive sampling approach, researchers recruited women based on inclusion criteria: (1) 18 years of age and over; (2) migration to the US within the past 15 years; and (3) Central American country of origin: El Salvador, Guatemala, or Honduras. These criteria reflect the original study's focus on contemporary patterns of migration from Central America to the US among adult women and women with children [20]. In recruiting potential participants, the first author drew on professional relationships with four organizations that provide shelter, social services, and/or legal services to immigrant communities in two cities in Texas. Staff presented the study to clients who matched the inclusion criteria and shared researchers' contact information with women who expressed interest in participating.

2.2. Participants

Nineteen (n = 19) women participated in the study, eight of whom originated from Honduras, six from El Salvador, and five from Guatemala. The average age of participants was 35 years (range: 25 to 53 years). Their average length of time in the US was 5.4 years (range: 2 months to 15 years). All participants identified as mothers, and on average women had 3.26 children (range: 1 to 7). Seventeen participants experienced one or more forms of intimate partner violence, sexual violence, and/or human trafficking.

2.3. Data Collection

The lead researcher conducted in-person interviews, using an iterative approach to adapt questions and probes as data collection progressed. The semi-structured interview guide, which evolved over time, queried women's motivations to migrate to the US and risks of violence prior to and during migration. Participants scheduled interviews at their preferred times and locations (e.g., the researcher's office, participants' homes, and service providers' offices). In an effort to build rapport and develop trust, the lead researcher reminded potential participants that their legal immigration status was not a topic of inquiry and that researchers would not report immigration status to any governmental or other entity [32]. All participants gave verbal informed consent and received written information about the study in both Spanish and English. All participants received $25 cash at the beginning of the interview, along with clear reminders that interviews could be suspended or stopped at any time. At the conclusion of each interview, the researcher (a licensed social worker) shared resources related to any unmet social service needs shared during the interview. Interviews lasted between one to two hours. All interviews were conducted in

Spanish and were digitally recorded and transcribed by a professional transcription service in Spanish. Data were stored in password-protected files accessible only to research staff.

2.4. Data Analysis

Informed by grounded theory analytical approaches [34], data analysis involved an ongoing examination of digital recordings, interview transcripts, field notes, and memos. The lead researcher first used line-by-line process coding to identify actions and processes across the first eight interview Spanish-language transcripts [34,35]. Next, she grouped these initial codes based on fit, frequency, or significance [34] and used these categories to code the full set of Spanish-language transcripts in NVivo. Participants' reflections on motherhood vis à vis migration and violence emerged inductively from this analytical process. Iterative comparisons within and across participants resulted in the five processes described below. Researchers utilized several strategies to enhance rigor and trustworthiness: memo-writing, reflexive practice, maintaining an audit trail, peer debriefing, and thick description [36]. The primary researcher regularly debriefed and consulted with practitioners and researchers with relevant expertise.

3. Results

Motherhood was a salient and ever-present factor throughout women's migrations from Central America to the US. The analysis identified five processes related to transnational motherhood at the intersection of migration and violence: risking everything, embodying separation, navigating reunification, mothering others, and experiencing motherhood due to sexual violence. All names are pseudonyms.

3.1. Risking Everything

Women's efforts and risk-taking to protect and provide their children a life free from violence directly influenced their meaning making of motherhood. While some women migrated with one or more children, most women left their children in their home country when they migrated to the US. Women talked about fearing for their children's safety back home and feeling guilt for having left them. María stated her hopes for her children: "tienen derecho a vivir un futuro sin violencia, sin problemas, sin amenazas de muerte". (*"They have a right to live a future without violence, without problems, without death threats."*) Isabel also described her efforts to break the cycle of violence she had experienced, "no quería que mi historia se repitiera en mis hijos y por eso yo he sido bien luchadora". (*"I didn't my kids to repeat my history and that's why I've been a fighter."*) Sierra was in an untenable position as a mother trying secure safety for herself and her two young children in the context of regional gang violence in Honduras. She had only enough money to pay for herself and one child to travel to the US. On the one hand, she was concerned about the gangs that controlled her community targeting her son; on the other hand, she had to consider the likelihood that her daughter would be at risk of sexual assault and exploitation if she remained in Honduras. Sierra weighed the risks and ultimately decided to bring her daughter to protect her from sexual violence, leaving her son in Honduras. María first migrated from Guatemala to the US without her children. She then returned to Guatemala, hoping to remain there with her family. However, her life was again threatened and she decided to make the journey again, this time with her children, which she and her mother both perceived as a decision to risk everything. With great emotion María shared,

> Agarré una mochila y metí la ropa que pude de mis niños, y otra bolsa la llené con comida. Y [mi mamá me dijo], No. Estás loca, vas a ir a matar a tus hijos, eres una asesina. Le dije no, no lo voy a hacer, pues si así pasa prefiero que muramos todos. (llorando) Le dije, no me importa, lo único que me importa es tratar de hacer algo por ellos, que no un día me voy a arrepentir y dije lo pude hacer y no lo hice. Y quería escapar, de ese infierno.
>
> *I grabbed a backpack and filled it as much as I could with my children's clothes and another bag I filled with food. [My mother told me], "No, you're crazy, you're going to*

> *get your children killed. You're a murderer." I said, "No, I'm not going to do that, and if that does happen I would rather we all die." (crying) I said, "I don't care, the only thing that matters is that I try to do something for them, I don't want to one day regret being able to do something and not doing anything. I want to escape from that hell.*

For María, taking leave from her mother in Guatemala also included a desire for her mother's permission and blessing, and she told her mother, "yo solo quiero su bendición es todo lo que le pido." (*"I just want your blessing, that's all I'm asking of you."*) Part of "risking everything" included the possibility that the decision to migrate could damage relationships with family at a time when they needed their loved one's blessings and emotional support to undertake a dangerous trip. The decision to migrate put the support and trust from their families and their most important relationships at risk.

3.2. Embodying Separation

When separated, mothers constantly thought about their children and worried about their safety, well-being, and schooling. Mothers spoke at length about the stress and sense of guilt related to arranging care across borders. They expressed concerns about how to send money, and whether it would arrive and adequately cover their children's needs. Despite feeling some satisfaction with being able to provide for their children's education or health needs, women felt distress at not being physically present to keep their kids safe from gang violence. Women experienced the separation from their children in terms of acute suffering and fear. Sierra recalled leaving her son in Honduras, "mi corazón se partió en dos, dejar la mitad allá y traerme mi otra mitad para aquí." (*"My heart broke in half, leaving one piece over there and bringing the other with me here."*) After talking with her children during her travels through Mexico, Clara said, "ponía a llorar después de oír a mi hijo. Y decía, ojalá que esto valga la pena." ("I would start crying after hearing my son. I would say, 'I hope this is worth it.'") Beatriz referred to these worries as, "las madres rompen la cabeza pensando." (*"mothers worry themselves sick."*) In addition to fear and concern, women felt a tremendous sense of guilt in having migrated and the resulting separation from their children. Beatriz, for example, returned to Guatemala after four years in the US, fulfilling a promise she had made to her children. When she arrived back in Guatemala, they passed by her in the airport without recognizing her. She said,

> Me sentía tan culpable haberlos abandonados cuatro años. El pequeño ya no me reconocía. Tuve que pegarme mucho a él para que me volviera a reconocer. Tuve que ganarme el cariño de los tres nuevamente, y pedirles perdón.
>
> *I felt so guilty after leaving them abandoned for four years. The smallest didn't recognize me. I had to stay close to him a lot so that he would remember me again. I had to win the affection of the three all over again and ask them for forgiveness.*

Women shared painful examples of how motherhood plays out in separation from home and children throughout migratory processes. While Celia migrated to the US with one child at great emotional and physical cost, she continued to grieve the death of her son, who had died before she left Honduras. Her physical distance from Honduras played a significant role in her grief. She was plagued with not being in Honduras to provide him a proper burial. She was no longer in contact with anyone who had known him and felt that she, alone, carried his memory. Furthermore, she carried the burden of her abusive husband blaming her for the boy's death. Hortensia shared another painful example of embodying separation during migration. While being held against her will in a drop house and having been sexually assaulted by smugglers, Hortensia learned that gang members had murdered her oldest daughter on the street in Guatemala. Hortensia was later able to bring two of her four surviving children to the US, though she remained physically separated from her two children in Guatemala and permanently separated from her deceased daughter. In spite of the separation, however, women described their children and motherhood as a source of strength. María, for example, shared "por mis hijos, no me da miedo nada." (*"because of my children, I'm not scared of anything."*) Women drew strength from having migrated for their children and felt supported by their children's love and encouragement from afar. Facing inconsistency of support systems over time and space, women described ongoing processes of losing support, building support, and re-building supportive relationships with their children and others.

3.3. Braving Reunification

All women in the study eventually brought some or all of their children to the US or were in the process of navigating reunifications with their children. Despite having survived harrowing journeys themselves, several women relied on unofficial means of bringing their children to live with them in the US. This involved paying a smuggler to bring them through Mexico and across the border, and exposing children to similar risks they endured while migrating, including exposure to the elements, lack of food and shelter, and vulnerability to robbery, violence, and exploitation. Isabel, for example, described sending for her children, losing track of them for an anxiety-ridden week, and being extorted by the criminal gang network that controlled border crossings. She shared,

> Yo puse en riesgo la vida de mis hijos, me los tuvieron ahí una semana exacta, ocho días sin saber nada, yo me estaba muriendo porque sentía que ¿dónde los iba a hallar? México también es grande, ¿dónde los iba a encontrar? Yo decía que si yo no sabía de ellos, yo me iba a ir a buscarlos de lugar en lugar, que yo los tenía que encontrar.
>
> *I put my children's lives in danger. [The smugglers] had them there for exactly one week, eight days without knowing anything. I was dying because I felt like Mexico is so big. Where was I going to find them? I said that if I didn't hear anything about them I would go place by place looking for them, I had to find them.*

The smugglers demanded Isabel send more money, ultimately totaling almost $20,000, which she did in desperation to secure the safety of her children, pleading to see them again. The smuggler said to her, "sí te los voy a entregar, cierto que eres una buena persona, una buena mamá, porque a pesar de que no sabes nada de ellos, sigues insistiendo" (*"Yes, I will give them to you. You are a good mother because despite not knowing anything about them, you kept insisting."*) The US border patrol finally located them and sent them to the hielera [*"freezer"* or *"ice box"* in reference to the temporary detention facility] where they spent three days. From there, US immigration officials sent them to a center for minors where Isabel went to get them. Karla had two children in Honduras and gave birth to a third child in the US. She and her husband worked hard to save money to bring the older children to the US. They twice collected the required money, only to have it stolen. The third time they paid $20,000, with the intention of bringing both boys safely, avoiding the danger and suffering they had experienced. Yet, despite promises of better conditions, the boys ultimately travelled for one month by train, slept outside, and went without food. After six years of separation, Karla described their reunification: "Estaban enojados con nosotros, porque dijeron cómo era posible que nosotros habíamos mandado traerles así. (*"They were angry. They said how was it possible that we would send for them to be brought like that?"*) Some women reported that they would never bring their children to the US unless they could do it by legal means. Natalia, for example, was determined not to subject her other children to the abuse she and her daughter had endured during the journey. She reflected,

> Es algo que a mi me llena de tristeza, y por eso es que yo ya no me animé a traer a mis hijos así, a mis otros dos hijos. Yo dije no, ya no más. Porque si mi niño no camina, o si a mi niña le pasa algo, y lo van a dejar botado, yo digo que no ya no.
>
> *It's something that fills me with sadness, and that's why I couldn't convince myself to bring my other children. I said no, because if my boy couldn't keep up with the walking, they would abandon him, or if something happened to my girl. I say no, no more.*

In two cases, women described how IPV complicated the process of reuniting with children. Once in the US, Karla's husband, became jealous, controlling, and abusive, which ultimately affected her ability to work and hindered their ability to save for their sons' travel to the US. Alma shared similar difficulties even though with a T Visa she had a legal avenue through which to bring her children. Her abusive ex-partner managed to thwart Alma's efforts to get the children's documentation and at the time of the interview, she had not yet been able to bring any of her four children to the US.

3.4. Mothering Others

Women's experiences with transnational motherhood also involved taking care of unaccompanied children they encountered along their journeys, particularly through Mexico. In the midst of missing their own children and maternal roles, women sometimes found themselves mothering others in transit. María, for example, helped care for eight-year-old twins during the entire journey through Mexico. Lorena spent several days taking care of a ten-year-old girl who had traveled alone from Guatemala, whom she encountered at a hotel. She shared,

> Nunca le pregunté cómo se llamaba, porque la niña estaba callada y no hablaba. La encontramos ahí en el hotel y yo la agarré como que era mi hija, como que traía acá. La bañé y la peiné. La regañe porque no se quería poner sweater. Lavé sus calzones, 'vete a cepillar los dientes' y así pasamos la noche. Nos subimos a otro bus y fuimos a otro pueblo. Y como la niña se pegó un poquito conmigo, entonces se quedó conmigo.
>
> *I never asked what her name was because the girl was quiet and didn't talk. We found her there in the hotel and I grabbed her like she was my daughter, as if I had brought her there. I bathed her and combed her hair. I scolded her because she didn't want to put on a sweater. I washed her underwear, [told her to] brush her teeth, and that's how we spent the night. We got another bus and went to another town. The girl got a little attached to me, so she stayed with me.*

Sierra travelled with her own child and took care of two other children who were travelling alone and hoping to reunite with their respective mothers in the US. To protect them from harm, she told people that they were her own children and her travel group did not realize they were not her children until after they had crossed the Rio Grande. While women cared for unaccompanied children as if they were their own, these relationships were temporary. During or shortly after crossing into the US, they separated. Lorena continued to worry about what happened to the child she took care of in Mexico, who was passed to other smugglers. She questioned, "¿Y porque va a estar mejor que contigo si a ti no te conoce? A mi tampoco pero ya tiene dos o tres días de estar conmigo, pero a ti ni una vez te ha visto." ("*Why is she going to be better off with you if she doesn't know you? She doesn't know me either but she's spent two or three days with me and she's never even seen you.*") Women took advantage of opportunities to care for other women's children, putting their strengths and skills to use while separated from their own children and in the absence of unaccompanied children's mothers.

3.5. Experiencing Motherhood due to Sexual Violence

Complicating the meanings women made of motherhood were experiences of sexual violence and resulting pregnancies. Three women in the sample disclosed (unprompted) that they had experienced or witnessed pregnancies following rape prior to, during, or post migration. Beatriz, for example, became pregnant resulting from sexual abuse by the man ("coyote" or smuggler) helping her cross through Mexico and into the United States. Lorena described immigration officials making women take a pregnancy test after they were apprehended while crossing the border into the US. She went on to say,

> Casi la mayoría de muchachas que vienen llegando y tienen sus hijos aquí fueron violadas en el camino y el bebé es consecuencia del camino. Es traumante. Porque aparte de que pasa esas penas en el camino todavía te queda un recuerdo para toda tu vida. (llorando)

Almost all the women who arrive and have their kids here were raped on the way, and the baby is a consequence of the trip. It is traumatic, because in addition to experiencing these challenges on the journey, you are left with a memory of it for your entire life. (crying)

Gloria, a mother of seven children, described what became a lengthy period of commercial sexual exploitation upon her arrival in the US after fleeing IPV in Honduras,

Cuando llegamos aquí nos amarraban de las manos y de los pies y un pañuelo en la boca y nos tiraban a una camioneta como una pelota. Cuando llegamos a una casa, nos compraban una ropa y nos obligaban a que nos vistieramos y traían una señora que los peinara y los pintara. Y nos obligaban a cosas que no queríamos. Y eso fue duro para mi. Pues mis hijos son de todo eso. Los tres hijos de aquí fueron del abuso.

When we got here they tied our hands and feet up, a handkerchief in our mouths and they threw us in a truck like a ball. When we got to a house, they bought us clothes and they made us put it on and there was a woman who brushed our hair and did our make-up. And they made us do things we didn't want to do. That was difficult for me. My children are from all of that, the three children here are from the abuse.

The spontaneous disclosures of these three women about the ways that violence forever marked motherhood in complex ways provide an additional and significant facet of transnational motherhood, deserving of further attention.

4. Discussion

The findings revealed the ways in which women who had migrated from Central America to the U.S. made meaning of their identities and roles as mothers, highlighting the centrality, power, and fluidity of motherhood at the intersection of migration and violence. Their roles as mothers and the imperative to risk everything to secure safety for themselves and their families served as constants in shaping their internal motivations and decisions to act. Women endured multiple separations from their children to secure safety, and braved the implications of reunifying with children who did not accompany them in their original journeys. In transit, they stepped in to mother children who were making the journey without a parent, fulfilling their roles as mothers even if only in passing. Some women would not make it to the U.S. without being sexually assaulted and experiencing motherhood as a direct result of violence. Together, the themes provide insights into complex processes shaping notions of motherhood and inform next steps for research, policy, and community practice.

Motherhood intricately intertwined with the violence-migration nexus, as women sought to protect their children from harm and create a violence-free future for their children and themselves. Experiences and possibilities of violence and migration rendered transnational mothering fraught and heavy with impossible decisions. In fleeing violence both at home from an intimate partner and in the public sphere (e.g., gangs), they confronted additional threats and assaults, as well as continued structural violence. A dominant factor in a mother's migration is often to ensure the economic survival of the family, which is largely interconnected with gendered poverty and structural oppression as well as the interpersonal economic coercion and control common in IPV [20]. Thus, any positive migration-related economic opportunities were still constrained by financial obligations back home and by IPV-related economic coercion persisting across borders and experienced anew in the US.

The findings from the current study add to the growing migration-related literature by highlighting the effects of family separation on mothers. The effects of temporary and enduring separations have profound and varied effects on parents, children, and caregivers [8,13–15,37]. What may be considered a temporary separation from children may become lengthy or even permanent, and women may be unprepared for the length of separation and the toll it takes on parent–child relationships [10]. Mothers interviewed for this study spoke at length about the stress and sense of guilt related to arranging care across borders and the social and emotional isolation and loss of support and trust from family members. Communication between mothers and children, as well as communication between mothers and their children's caregivers, is crucial to exchanging information, making parenting decisions, and maintaining emotional connections [5]. Women recognize the role of caretakers (primarily their children's maternal grandmothers) as critical in supporting their migration to the U.S. [11]. While some argue that leaving children behind is traumatic to children and contributes to family disintegration, others contend that parent substitutes are fully capable of taking on caretaking responsibilities [3]. Perhaps most impactful were the stress and trauma associated with the knowledge that their children continued to face danger back home, and the enduring and ambiguous losses associated with the death of a child or children. At the same time, women shared the positive impact of transnational mothering in the sense of agency and action incurred by doing what they had to do in the face of untenable circumstances and by taking advantage of opportunities to care for unaccompanied children in solidarity with other mothers facing similar circumstances.

The findings must be considered in the context of US immigration, detention, and deportation policies and practices, which directly influence and often manufacture family separation and exacerbate experiences of IPV. Contemporary policies, for example, have extended the duration of and uncertainty around family separation, restricted cross-border travel for transnational caretaking, and generally have made family reunification more difficult [5,16,20,38]. Menjívar argues that US immigration law exacerbates long and indefinite separations [39]. Family separation came to the foreground with the zero tolerance policy announced in May 2018, during which US officials tragically and haphazardly separated thousands of children from their parents [40]. Other recent policies, such as the Remain in Mexico Program (officially titled Migrant Protection Protocols), further restrict and hinder migrating parents' parenting decisions and actions. Under this practice, more than tens of thousands of asylum-seekers were detained along the US-Mexico border and forced back into Mexico to apply for asylum [41]. Waiting in makeshift camps, exposed to the elements and a host of other gendered dangers, many waited for months for their claims to be processed. Those travelling with children parented under these conditions and amidst great uncertainty, often unable to move neither north or south, and with few opportunities to create stability or safety for their children. While media coverage and public outrage over the zero tolerance policy and Remain in Mexico were merited, they overshadowed manifestations of family separation that occurred and continue to occur both as a common component of forced migration and as long-standing US government practice. The US system of immigration detention further strains mothering and mother-child relationships, particularly among those who have experienced IPV [42].

It is important that conceptualizations of transnational mothering acknowledge the power women exert as mothers. As this study illuminates, migrating with children and migration-related separation from children involves fluid and interconnected forms of coercion and/or force but also encompasses choice, autonomy, and self-determination. Even in the midst of the aforementioned policies and practices that restrict and criminalize the human experience of parenting, this study highlights the multiple ways in which women resist and challenge conditions and strategies that threaten to limit and constrict their roles as mothers. In warning of the dangers of maternal narratives that so easily blame mothers, rob women of agency, and promote one-dimensional and damaging narratives, Geraldine Pratt suggests that scholars instead aim to present "responses that affirm the testifier's capacity to respond and hence their agency and subjectivity" [43] (p. 10). These findings support Pratt's cautionary reminder about the responsibilities for scholars and researchers and extend to the ethical obligations of social workers, community organizers, and mental health practitioners. Efforts to respond in practice must identify, support, and expand women's agency and power as transnational mothers. Social workers, community organizers, and mental health providers working with immigrant communities must also work to address internalized guilt and shame and the larger social mechanisms that promote harmful narratives.

It is important to note certain limitations associated with this study, as it explored the process of migration in the context of violence for a narrow snapshot of migrating women and cannot represent all Central American women. Any research that focuses on migrating women runs a risk of essentializing migrant women and mothers, in particular, and it remains crucial to recognize the heterogeneity of migrating women and of migrants in general. In addition, researchers faced common impediments with recruiting, which were likely due to the social isolation and climate of fear experienced by undocumented and precariously documented immigrants, in addition to participant and resource constraints that did not allow for multiple interviews with each participant nor member-checking. There also exists potential bias related to participants' prior engagement with legal immigration systems and having already told, constructed, or re-constructed their stories for a different audience [44–46]. Sampling and recruitment procedures may have also resulted in bias towards those who had sought services, which could have included those who had faced more intense experiences of violence or hardship. Furthermore, while this study explored motherhood at the intersection of migration and violence, other elements of migrating parents' identities and experiences are missing. Not all migrant women share the same identities in terms of gender and sexual orientation, roles as mothers, or socioeconomic status, and this study only interviewed those identifying as women, excluding girls, men, and the transgender community. Further analysis and research should explore the ways in which racial, ethnic and indigenous social positions shape motherhood in the context of violence and migration, and investigate the parenting experiences of fathers and gender non-binary parents as well. Finally, this study did not directly or systematically investigate the critical issue of violence-related pregnancies, an aspect of transnational motherhood meriting further attention.

5. Conclusions

The findings from this analysis highlighted facets of transnational motherhood at the intersection of violence and migration, amplifying the perspectives and experiences of mothers as they "risked everything" to secure a safe future for themselves and their children. Transnational motherhood encompasses a multitude of parenting configurations, as mothers continue to parent from afar and to reconfigure their caretaking pre-migration, during migration, and after reunification. Centering the voices, perspectives, and experiences of women who embark on the migration journey to fight for themselves and their children is imperative to research, practice, and advocacy to address structural violence spurring migrations and to change oppressive immigration policies. The study reiterates the importance of understanding how violence shapes and informs women's migrations and decision-making, and the consequences women endure in taking action to change the inevitability of violence in their own and their children's lives.

Author Contributions: Conceptualization, L.C.H.; methodology, L.C.H.; software, L.C.H.; validation, L.C.H.; formal analysis, L.C.H.; investigation, L.C.H.; resources, L.C.H.; data curation, L.C.H.; writing—original draft preparation, L.C.H.; writing—review and editing, L.C.H., K.W. and E.J.R.H. visualization, L.C.H.; supervision, L.C.H.; project administration, L.C.H.; funding acquisition, L.C.H. All authors have read and agreed to the published version of the manuscript.

Funding: The study was made possible by following fellowships awarded to the first author: the Harrington Fellowship, Charles W. Laughton Endowed Presidential Scholarship, and Louis E. DeMoll Endowed Presidential Scholarship at The University of Texas at Austin, in addition to the P.E.O. Scholar Award.

Institutional Review Board Statement: The study was conducted in accordance with the Declaration of Helsinki, and approved by the Institutional Review Board of the University of Texas at Austin (#2013-04-0143 20 January 2015).

Informed Consent Statement: Informed consent was obtained from all subjects involved in the study.

Data Availability Statement: Not applicable.

Conflicts of Interest: The authors declare no conflict of interest.

References

1. Parreñas, R. Long distance intimacy: Class, gender and intergenerational relations between mothers and children in Filipino transnational families. *Glob. Netw.* **2005**, *5*, 317–336. [CrossRef]
2. Hondagneu-Sotelo, P.; Avila, E. "I'm here, but I'm there" the meanings of Latina transnational motherhood. *Gend. Soc.* **1997**, *11*, 548–571. [CrossRef]
3. Zentgraf, K.M.; Chinchilla, N.S. Transnational family separation: A framework for analysis. *J. Ethn. Migr. Stud.* **2012**, *38*, 345–366. [CrossRef]
4. Soerens, M.J. Violence in the borderlands: A dialogical approach to intimate partner violence among migrant women. *Psychol. Soc.* **2015**, *7*, 64–82.
5. Carling, J.; Menjívar, C.; Schmalzbauer, L. Central themes in the study of transnational parenthood. *J. Ethn. Migr. Stud.* **2012**, *38*, 191–217. [CrossRef]
6. Hershberg, R. Consejos as a family process in transnational and mixed-status Mayan families. *J. Marriage Fam.* **2018**, *80*, 334–348. [CrossRef]
7. Horton, S. A mother's heart is weighed down with stones: A phenomenological approach to the experience of transnational motherhood. *Cult. Med. Psychiatry* **2009**, *33*, 21–40. [CrossRef] [PubMed]
8. Cardoso, J.B.; Scott, J.L.; Faulkner, M.; Lane, L.B. Parenting in the context of deportation risk. *J. Marriage Fam.* **2018**, *80*, 301–316. [CrossRef]
9. Van Hook, J.; Glick, J. Spanning borders, cultures, and generations: A decade of research on immigrant families. *J. Marriage Fam.* **2020**, *82*, 229–235. [CrossRef]
10. Bernhard, J.K.; Landolt, P.; Goldring, L. Transnationalizing families: Canadian immigration policy and the spatial fragmentation of care-giving among Latin American newcomers 1. *Int. Migr.* **2009**, *47*, 3–31. [CrossRef]
11. Moran-Taylor, M.J. When mothers and fathers migrate north: Caretakers, children, and child rearing in Guatemala. *Lat. Am. Perspect.* **2008**, *35*, 79–95. [CrossRef]
12. Yeoh, B.S.; Lam, T. The costs of (im) mobility: Children left behind and children who migrate with a parent. *Perspect. Gend. Migr.* **2007**, *38*, 120–149.
13. Brabeck, K.; Lykes, M.B.; Hershberg, R. Framing immigration to and deportation from the United States: Central American immigrants make meaning of their experiences. *Community Work. Fam.* **2011**, *13*, 275–296. [CrossRef]
14. Davis, J. ¿Educación o desintegración? Parental migration, remittances and left-behind children's education in Western Guatemala. *J. Lat. Am. Stud.* **2016**, *48*, 565–590. [CrossRef]
15. Zayas, L.H.; Brabeck, K.M.; Cook Heffron, L.; Dreby, J.; Calzada, E.J.; Parra-Cardona, J.R.; Dettlaff, A.; Heidbrink, L.; Perreira, K.; Yoshikawa, H. Charting directions for research on immigrant children affected by undocumented status. *Hisp. J. Behav. Sci.* **2017**, *39*, 412–435. [CrossRef]
16. Capps, R.; Koball, H.; Campetella, A.; Perreira, K.; Hooker, S.; Pedroza, J.M. *Implications of Immigration Enforcement Activities for the Well-Being of Children in Immigrant Families*; Urban Institute: Washington, DC, USA; Migration Policy Institute: Washington, DC, USA, 2015.
17. Menjívar, C. *Enduring Violence*; University of California Press: Berkeley, CA, USA, 2011.
18. Obinna, D.N. Seeking sanctuary: Violence against women in El Salvador, Honduras, and Guatemala. *Violence Against Women* **2021**, *27*, 806–827. [CrossRef]
19. Amanor-Boadu, Y.; Messing, J.T.; Stith, S.M.; Anderson, J.R.; O'Sullivan, C.S.; Campbell, J.C. Immigrant and nonimmigrant women: Factors that predict leaving an abusive relationship. *Violence Against Women* **2012**, *18*, 611–633. [CrossRef]
20. Cook Heffron, L. "Salía de uno y me metí en otro": Exploring the migration-violence nexus among Central American women. *Violence Against Women* **2019**, *25*, 677–702. [CrossRef] [PubMed]
21. Ricoy, A.L.; Andrews, A.; Medina, A. Exit as care: How motherhood mediates women's exodus from violence in Mexico and Central America. *Violence Against Women* **2021**, *28*, 211–231. [CrossRef]
22. Schmidt, S. Endangered mothers or 'anchor babies'? Migration motivators for pregnant unaccompanied Central American teens. *Vulnerable Child. Youth Stud.* **2018**, *13*, 376–377. [CrossRef]
23. Nawyn, S.J.; Reosti, A.; Gjokaj, L. Gender in motion: How gender precipitates international migration. In *Perceiving Gender Locally, Globally, and Intersectionally*; Emerald Group Publishing Limited: Bingley, UK, 2009.
24. Wachter, K.; Cook Heffron, L. Intimate partner violence against women in forced migration. In *The Routledge Handbook of Domestic Violence and Abuse*; Devaney, J., Bradbury-Jones, C., Macy, R., Øverlien, C., Holt, S., Eds.; Routledge: London, UK, 2021.
25. United Nations High Commissioner for Refugees (UNHCR). Women on the Run. 2015. Available online: https://www.unhcr.org/en-us/publications/operations/5630f24c6/women-run.html (accessed on 31 July 2022).
26. McIlwaine, C. Migrant machismos: Exploring gender ideologies and practices among Latin American migrants in London from a multi-scalar perspective. *Gend. Place Cult.* **2010**, *17*, 281–300. [CrossRef]
27. Parrado, E.A.; Flippen, C.A. Migration and gender among Mexican women. *Am. Sociol. Rev.* **2005**, *70*, 606–632. [CrossRef]
28. Cook Heffron, L.; Snyder, S.; Wachter, K.; Nsonwu, M.; Busch-Armendariz, N. "Something is missing here:" Weaving feminist theories into social work practice with refugees. In *Contemporary Feminisms in Social Work Practice*; Wendt, S., Moulding, N., Eds.; Routledge: London, UK, 2016.

29. Fiddian-Qasmiyeh, E. Gender and forced migration. In *The Oxford Handbook of Refugee and Forced Migration Studies*; Fiddian-Qasmiyeh, E., Loescher, G., Long, K., Sigona, N., Eds.; Oxford University Press: Oxford, UK, 2014; pp. 176–197.
30. Johnson, C. Responsibility, affective solidarity and transnational maternal feminism. *Fem. Theory* **2020**, *21*, 175–198. [CrossRef]
31. Mohanty, C.T. *Feminism without Borders: Decolonizing Theory, Practicing Solidarity*; Duke University Press: Durham, NC, USA, 2003.
32. Baumann, A.N.A.; Rodríguez, M.D.; Parra-Cardona, J.R. Community-based applied research with Latino immigrant families: Informing practice and research according to ethical and social justice principles. *Fam. Process* **2011**, *50*, 132–148. [CrossRef] [PubMed]
33. Ellsberg, M.; Heise, L. Bearing witness: Ethics in domestic violence research. *Lancet* **2002**, *359*, 1599–1604. [CrossRef]
34. Charmaz, K. *Constructing Grounded Theory: A Practical Guide through Qualitative Analysis*; Sage: Thousand Oaks, CA, USA, 2006.
35. Miles, M.B.; Huberman, A.M.; Saldana, J. *Qualitative Data Analysis: A Methods Sourcebook*; Sage: Thousand Oaks, CA, USA, 2014.
36. Creswell, J.W.; Poth, C.N. *Qualitative Inquiry and Research Design*, 4th ed.; Sage Publications: Thousand Oaks, CA, USA, 2018.
37. Castañeda, E.; Jenks, D.; Chaikof, J.; Cione, C.; Felton, S.; Goris, I.; Buck, L.; Hershberg, E. Symptoms of PTSD and depression among Central American immigrant youth. *Trauma Care* **2021**, *1*, 99–118. [CrossRef]
38. Dreby, J. US immigration policy and family separation: The consequences for children's well-being. *Soc. Sci. Med.* **2015**, *132*, 245–251. [CrossRef]
39. Menjívar, C. Transnational parenting and immigration law: Central Americans in the United States. *J. Ethn. Migr. Stud.* **2012**, *38*, 301–322. [CrossRef]
40. Southern Poverty Law Center. Family Separation: A Timeline. 2022. Available online: https://www.splcenter.org/news/2022/03/23/family-separation-timeline (accessed on 31 July 2022).
41. American Civil Liberties Union [ACLU] Asylum Seekers Stranded in MEXICO Face Homelessness, Kidnapping and Sexual Violence. 2019. Available online: https://www.aclu.org/issues/immigrants-rights/immigrants-rights-and-detention/asylum-seekers-stranded-mexico-face (accessed on 31 July 2022).
42. Cook Heffron, L.; Serrata, J.V.; Hurtado, G. Latina Immigrant Women & Children's Well-Being & Access to Services after Detention. Casa de Esperanza's National Latino Network. 2019. Available online: https://www.nationallatinonetwork.org/images/Family_Detention_Report_English.pdf (accessed on 31 July 2022).
43. Pratt, G. Circulating sadness: Witnessing Filipina mothers' stories of family separation. *Gend. Place Cult.* **2009**, *16*, 3–22. [CrossRef]
44. Gubrium, J.F.; Holstein, J.A. Narrative practice and the transformation of interview subjectivity. In *The SAGE Handbook of Interview Research: The Complexity of the Craft*; Gubrium, J.F., Holstein, J.A., Marvasti, A.B., McKinney, K.D., Eds.; Sage: Thousand Oaks, CA, USA, 2012; pp. 27–44.
45. Riessman, C.K. *Narrative Methods for the Human Sciences*; Sage: Thousand Oaks, CA, USA, 2008.
46. Saltsman, A.; Majidi, N. Storytelling in research with refugees: On the promise and politics of audibility and visibility in participatory research in contexts of forced migration. *J. Refug. Stud.* **2021**, *34*, 2522–2538. [CrossRef]

International Journal of
Environmental Research and Public Health

MDPI

Article

The Influence of Media Coverage on the Negative Perception of Migrants in Chile

Andrés Scherman [1,2,3,*], Nicolle Etchegaray [3,4], Isabel Pavez [3,5] and Daniela Grassau [3,6]

1 Department of Communication, Universitat Pompeu Fabra, Roc Boronat 138, 08002 Barcelona, Spain
2 School of Communications and Journalism, Universidad Adolfo Ibáñez, Diagonal Las Torres 2640, Peñalolén, Santiago 7941169, Chile
3 Millennium Nucleus Center for the Study of Politics, Public Opinion and Media in Chile (MEPOP, NCS2021_063), Vergara 323, Santiago 8370139, Chile; nicole.etchegaray@udp.cl (N.E.); mipavez@uandes.cl (I.P.); dgrassau@uc.cl (D.G.)
4 School of Communication, Universidad Diego Portales, Vergara 240, Santiago 8370067, Chile
5 School of Communication, Universidad de los Andes, Mons. Álvaro del Portillo 12455, Las Condes, Santiago 7550000, Chile
6 School of Communications, Pontificia Universidad Católica de Chile, Avda. Libertador Bernardo O'Higgins 340, Santiago 8331150, Chile
* Correspondence: andres.scherman@uai.cl

Abstract: How mass media frame information about migrants is vital to further their well-being and social inclusion in the host society. However, it can also encourage forms of discrimination and xenophobia. In Chile, migration is a theme of great relevance due to a substantial increase in the flow of migrants over the last ten years, as well as the acts of extreme violence toward this group. Thus, this research analyzes how mass media coverage of migrants influences Chileans' perception of migrants. Adopting an experimental design, we implemented a large-scale, representative online survey with citizens over 18 years of age (N = 2227) and an experiment with combined access to positive and negative news about migrants in different news outlets. The regression analysis showed differences between citizens regarding the type of daily relationships they are willing to maintain with the migrant population. Furthermore, exposure to news about migration was the primary variable that explains why people consider this phenomenon one of the main problems affecting the country, confirming the agenda-setting theory. The experiment also indicated a causal relationship between the exposure to negative content and negative judgment about this group and their presence in the country.

Keywords: migration; well-being; mass media; Chile; framing

Citation: Scherman, A.; Etchegaray, N.; Pavez, I.; Grassau, D. The Influence of Media Coverage on the Negative Perception of Migrants in Chile. *Int. J. Environ. Res. Public Health* **2022**, *19*, 8219. https://doi.org/10.3390/ijerph19138219

Academic Editors: Maria De Jesus and Ernesto Castañeda

Received: 5 May 2022
Accepted: 29 June 2022
Published: 5 July 2022

1. Introduction

The migratory context in Chile is of high interest. There has been an increase in international immigrants in the last decade [1–3], mainly from the rest of Latin America [4–6]. Migration is especially relevant in Chile because foreign nationals increased from 2% to 7.6% of the total population of the country between 2002 and 2021, mainly due to the arrival of Venezuelan, Colombian, and Haitian immigrants [7]. Recently, a sharp increase in illegal crossings in the northern part of the country has increased conflict and negative attitudes toward immigrants. There have been attacks by the Chilean population on immigrants who are in precarious situations and are living on public roads [8], which has a negative impact not only on foreigners' lives but on social cohesion as well [9,10]. Thus, there is a complex scenario in part because migration is a recent cultural phenomenon where non-Chilean nationals are signified as outsiders regardless of their legal status or nationality [11,12]. Furthermore, it has fueled situations where migrants' rights are neglected and they are not treated as equals by the Chilean society [13]. For the purposes of the paper, we operationalize the term migrant by referring to the definition upheld by the

United Nations, which is "any person who is moving or has moved across an international border or within a State away from his/her habitual place of residence, regardless of (1) the person's legal status; (2) whether the movement is voluntary or involuntary; (3) what the causes for the movement are; or (4) what the length of the stay is" [14]. Although this new generation of migrants has triggered public policies to advance their welfare and social integration [6,15], they tend to have failed to successfully integrate due to prejudice, vulnerability, exclusion [16,17], and deliberate acts of violence towards this group [18]. The evidence also reveals media messages linked to negative stereotypes of migrants [19–21]. Consequently, evidence of migrants' experiences points to a sense of exclusion and alienation [22], depression, anxiety, and stress for those who legitimately seek to be part of Chilean society [20].

From a cultural perspective, the mass media as a social institution has a role in community formation, reaffirming ties, and sharing common values [23–25]. These practices could increase migrants' sense of belonging [26–28], providing a common language and references, as well as patterns, social orientations, and beliefs that allow coexistence in society [25,29–31]. However, it can also encourage the contrary, such as discrimination, xenophobia, and exclusion. The first set of practices contribute to facilitating social integration, whereas the latter set of practices undermine the process of social integration [32]. Social integration is defined as a process whereby newcomers have a degree of connection with the host society that allows them to claim that they belong in it [33]. In this regard, the mass media has a crucial role to play as they influence the beliefs and values of the population (see, e.g., [34,35]). Therefore, the main goal of this study is to explore the effect of the mass media on Chileans' perceptions of migrants, in a context where migration is still a relatively recent phenomenon in the country. We hypothesize that the mass media has a strong influence on migrants' social integration.

1.1. Framing and Agenda Setting: The Influence of Mass Media on Perceptions and Attitudes

Since the 1980s, the concept of framing has been one of the most used constructs to study the sociology of communications [36]. Consensus in the literature has shown that frames in informative stories can refer to (1) the particular way in which a story is composed to optimize the accessibility of the audience at a given time/limited space [34]; (2) the selection and emphasis of certain elements and the marginalization and minimization of others [37–39]; (3) a central organizing idea that defines the problem and the context [40]; and (4) deep value and ideological frameworks [41] that are inserted in a network of discourses with which they dialogue [42]. One of the most cited definitions of the concept of framing is the one proposed by Entman, who states that "framing essentially involves selection and salience. To frame is to select some aspects of a perceived reality and make them more salient in a communicating text, in such a way as to promote a particular problem definition, causal interpretation, moral evaluation, and/or treatment recommendation for the item described" [38].

There is a growing consensus that the mass media portrayal of migrants disseminates and reinforces prejudices and negative attitudes towards this group (see, e.g., [43,44]). This is because of the effect of a range of negative framings on audience perceptions, knowledge, attitudes, or even emotions [36,37,45]. Early findings indicated that audiences could not process the realities in all their complexity [46,47]; thus, they attempt to infer causal relationships from sensory information [36]. These frames of interpretation incorporate rules for processing reality and provide guidelines for future decoding and behavior [46]. They also provide a structure of interpretation that, once learned, reduces the complexity of the comprehension processes and can be applied in the elaboration of messages shared in social interaction [36].

On the one hand, the effects of frames on audiences would be conditioned, among other things, by their prominence or salience (position and repetition), by their cultural resonance (adjustment with existing schemes) [38], their accessibility in memory, and their applicability in the processing of immediate knowledge [48]. On the other hand, the effect of frames can also be conditioned by personal characteristics such as experience with the topic covered, levels of exposure to the media, and previous attitudes about the topic. This is demonstrated, for example, by the work of Druckman and Chong [49], which shows that the repetition of certain frames would have a greater impact on people with less knowledge and who are also more attentive to peripheral signals, while individuals with more knowledge would be more likely to engage in systematic information processing by comparing the relative strength of alternative frames in competitive situations.

Despite more studies on the effects of frames, several questions remain. Firstly, there is debate regarding the independence between the notion of framing and that of agenda setting [50]. Agenda setting, in very general terms, predicts a high degree of convergence between the agendas of the different news media and the public agenda, specifically regarding the importance of specific issues, political figures, and other objects of attention and the presence of attributes that are assigned to said objects [51]. In other words, from the perspective of the agenda-setting theory [50,52], media help public opinion to learn about an issue and determine the importance that it will assign to it: the elements frequently highlighted by the media become the elements on which public debate focus [51]. While the media agenda is measured based on the salience that they give to certain issues in their news, the public agenda has been defined as those issues of public interest that people evaluate as the most important and is usually operationalized based on the following question: "What do you think is the most important issue facing our country today?" [51,53]. Although the view of dependency between both theories (framing and agenda setting) is strongly resisted by the authors dedicated to the subject, who propose the existence of an autonomous theoretical conceptualization [41,54,55], this paper proposes that both perspectives are complementary and can help explain the role of the media in the perception of migrants in Chile.

1.2. Negative Media Portrayal of Migrants

The frames given by mass media news on migration have been extensively studied in developed countries through content analysis, confirming the tendency to link migration with delinquency, crime, terrorism, and other social problems, while the information on its positive contributions is delivered to a lesser extent [43,56–61]. Conflict is a prevalent frame, comprising news where migrants are typically portrayed as victims or criminals [22,60–62], as a challenge for border security [63], or as a major economic and social cost for the state [55,59,64,65]. Likewise, studies examining news on Hispanic immigration in the United States reveal that foreigners are shown as lazy, ambitious, and/or as a threat to national stability and Americans' job security (see, e.g., [53,62,66–68]). Similarly, Lakoff and Ferguson [54] analyze the framing of issues related to migration in the speech of former President George Bush as it was presented in the media. Among its conclusions, the focus on migration was as a problem that requires a solution, and as a detriment to the nation-state by utilizing frameworks such as globalization, humanitarian, civil rights, cheap labor, or economic refugees. The authors also highlight the superficial frameworks applied: equating migrants with illegality (for example, undocumented aliens), where "others" invade the country and threaten national security.

Similarly, in Chile, news framing has shown that migrants from Latin American countries tend to be linked to violence, crime, or negative portrayals, in contrast to those from Europe who are associated with positive news such as progress [19]. Scherman and Etchegaray [21] offer a deeper insight. They analyzed different media platforms covering print press, television, radio, and the Internet, finding that not all Latino migrants have the same press treatment and a new trend where migration is linked to conflict and political discussion. Latter research on mass media effects shows that the frames given to immigration have a significant influence on citizens' attitudes, opinions, and emotions [45,49,67,69]. Igartua and colleagues [45,49] consider that the effects of frames may be governed by what they call heuristic processing, assuming that when media consumers are not mainly motivated to process information, the presence of peripheral cues in the journalistic message may condition cognitive responses. In the case of migration coverage, they confirm that group cues, that is, references to the national, ethnic, or geographic origin of migrants, moderate the effects of framing. In their study, the reference to Moroccan migrants increased the perception of migration as a problem and a negative attitude towards immigration [49]. The opposite was confirmed when the news referred to Latin American migrants.

The current study builds on the previous research on the effects of frames on citizens' perceptions. We examine the following three questions:

RQ1: Are there differences between citizens regarding the type of relationships they are willing to maintain on a daily basis with the migrant population (living in a neighborhood with many immigrants, renting out their house or apartment to immigrants, working with immigrants, accepting their child marrying an immigrant, having their child in a school with many immigrant children, among other situations)?

RQ2: Is there a relationship between exposure to news about the situation of immigrants and the presence of this group of people in Chile as one of the issues that most affect Chileans (agenda-setting effect)?

RQ3: Is there a relationship between exposure to news with negative frames about immigrants and having a negative judgment about this group and their presence in the country (framing effect)?

2. Materials and Methods

2.1. Sample

In this study, we used a methodology that combined a survey with a large sample size (N = 2227 cases) and an experimental design. An online survey was used to do an experiment where researchers manipulated the independent variables of interest—journalistic texts with positive and negative thematic framing about immigrants on different information platforms—which were built considering the results of an earlier content analysis stage in which 400 news reports were reviewed. This content analysis has already been validated and its results have been published [21]. In this way, this research incorporates "experimental realism", which has been developed in other research with the goal that the experiments have greater external validity and can be generalized due to the combination of public opinion studies and the use of media content as experimental stimuli [68–71]

This type of experiment using surveys allowed us to approach our two following research questions: RQ2, the existence of an agenda-setting effect, and RQ3, the presence of a framing effect.

To conduct this experiment, we surveyed a total of 1800 people online (79.1%) and 477 in person (20.9%). The same experimental conditions and stimuli were used for both groups (news stories that dealt positively or negatively with migrants, coming from print media, websites, and radio; a control group that received no stimulus was also included); for more information, see Appendices A and B. The study included people living in all regions of the country.

The data were gathered between December 2020 and January 2021. This was a period with a low number of legal entries by foreigners, due to the pandemic, but during which there was a rise in illegal entries according to testimonies from border zone residents.

2.2. Experimental Design

Study participants were exposed to the experimental condition at the start of the questionnaire and were subsequently asked questions about the news story they read or heard to verify proper comprehension. People who did not correctly answer basic questions about the initial stimuli they received were not considered in the final analysis. The experiment considered seven conditions (see Table 1). In three of these, the respondents were exposed to a positive story (from radio, newspapers, or websites) while in another three they were exposed to negative stories from the same platforms. The seventh group received no stimulus and served as a control group. After exposing the respondents to their respective stimuli, they were asked different questions about foreigners' situation in Chile, ranging from the importance of this matter in public affairs to their level of favorability or negativity towards immigrants. The stimuli used can be seen in Appendix A. Prior to the experiment, we pre-tested that the positive and negative stimuli about immigrants were perceived in that way by people who were part of the survey target audience.

Table 1. Experimental conditions (platforms, framing) and number of cases.

Condition	Platform (a)	Predominant Framing (b)	Treatment	N
1	Print media (1)	Positive (1)	a_1b_1	300
2	Print media (1)	Negative (2)	a_1b_2	348
3	Web (2)	Positive (1)	a_2b_1	335
4	Web (2)	Negative (2)	a_2b_2	313
5	Radio (3)	Positive (1)	a_3b_1	377
6	Radio (3)	Negative (2)	a_2b_2	265
7 (Control)	Neither (0)	None (0)	a_0b_0	338

As part of the empirical analysis, we first carried out a cluster analysis using a battery of questions in which the interviewees were asked if they would accept or not maintain seven different types of relationships with immigrants. This analysis allowed a first descriptive approach with the aim of answering RQ1 and showing the types of relationships that respondents are willing to have with migrants.

2.3. Dependent and Independent Variables

In the regression analyses we used two dependent variables:

Agenda setting and migration. To measure the agenda-setting effect, we applied a variable where respondents were asked, "What is the principal problem currently affecting Chileans? What is the second biggest problem?" With these two answers, we created a dichotomous variable where value 1 was assigned to all respondents who mentioned immigration as the principal problem in their first or second choice, and value 0 was assigned to the rest of the sample (1 = 19.5%; 2 = 80.5%).

Frames and migration. The framing effect is measured by observing whether the impact of news with negative framing about migrants generates negative perceptions about this group. To construct this variable, we considered 10 ordinal variables asking about the level of agreement, on a scale of 1 to 5, with various affirmations about immigrants. These 10 affirmations were recodified and converted into binary variables (answers considering that immigrants' presence is not generating difficulties in Chile were coded with 1, and the other responses were coded with 0 in each variable; a counter was subsequently built to add up the responses from each respondent with a 1 value, that is, those which considered that migrants were not generating difficulties). Theoretically, the counter had a minimum value of 0, equivalent to having no positive opinion about migrants and a maximum value of 10, which would mean having positive opinions about migrants in each dimension surveyed (M = 3.3; SD = 2.9). This counter was subsequently used as a dependent variable in a Poisson regression presented in the Results section. Appendix B presents the details of the 10 variables used to build this dependent variable and its descriptive statistics.

The two principal independent variables related to the experiment performed were as follows:

Exposure to information. We used this variable to measure the existence of an agenda-setting effect, and separated the sample between people exposed to information about immigrants (positive and negative) and the control group which received no information about the topic (exposed to information = 81.8%; not exposed to information = 18.2%).

Exposure to different frames. This variable was used to measure the framing effect and was separated into three categories: exposed to positive framing about migrants (36.8%), exposed to negative framing about migrants (45%), and not exposed to any framing about migrants (18.2%).

Considering prior research, we decided to incorporate four additional control variables:

Evaluation of the economic situation. To measure perceptions of the economic situation, we asked, "In your judgment, currently, is the Chilean economy progressing, stagnant or declining?

Ideological position. This variable position was measured on a scale of 1 to 10, where 1 was the left and 10 was the right.

Degree of closeness with immigrants living in the country. To establish closeness level with immigrants in the country, we asked the respondents if they had any current contact with foreigners in five different situations, and built a counter with a minimum value of 0 and a maximum of 5. We asked whether the respondents had current contact with immigrants in the following five situations: (a) within their families; (b) among their friends; (c) in their workplaces; (d) in their places of study; and (e) in their neighborhoods.

Fear of crime. To measure the different levels of fear of crime we used the following question: "Currently, how afraid are you of being a victim of a crime?" The responses were on a Likert scale with 1 being "no afraid" to 4 being "very afraid".

Finally, we added three sociodemographic variables to the models: *gender*, *age*, and *social class*.

3. Results

To answer our first research question and evaluate the differences between citizens regarding the type of everyday relations they would be willing to have with the migrant population, we conducted a cluster analysis based on a battery of questions evaluating respondents' disposition to voluntarily relate with immigrants in seven different areas (1. living in the same neighborhood where many immigrants live; 2. renting a house or apartment to immigrants; 3. working or studying with immigrants; 4. having an immigrant be your boss at work; 5. letting your child bring immigrant friends home; 6. having a son or daughter marry an immigrant; and 7. having your child in a school where there are many children of immigrants). Response options were 1 = I would accept; 2 = I would try to avoid it; and 3 = I would reject it.

Using the two-stage method of cluster identification, we first conducted an inductive inspection of the segmentation using the two-step method. This allowed us to identify the number of segments to define, according to the criterion of an increase in the BIC index based on the possible models' fit. As a result, we defined the modeling of four clusters, whose description is detailed in the Results section. The segments' creation was developed based on the K-medians clustering method.

The clusters suggest an affirmative answer to RQ1 and indicate that attitudes towards migrants in Chile are segmented into four groups, with different levels of openness towards interaction with foreigners depending on the situations described in the battery of seven variables detailed in the previous section (see Table 2).

The first cluster (N = 1306) includes the largest number of individuals and is characterized by accepting relations with immigrants in all the social spaces mentioned. The second cluster (N = 572) is only different from the first in two variables: members of this group would try to avoid living in a neighborhood with a high number of immigrants and would also avoid renting out a home to any members of this group. The third cluster (N = 279) is characterized by avoiding contact with immigrants in all situations mentioned, as well as rejecting the idea of renting a home to foreigners. The final cluster (N = 96) concentrates the individuals with the least inclination to relate with immigrants, as they reject every form of interaction with foreigners that was polled.

To complement the clusters' descriptive analysis, we conducted bivariate analyses (ANOVA and Spearman's rho and Somers' d tests) to establish whether differences existed between the clusters according to the different control variables included in the regression analysis (see Tables 3 and 4).

Table 2. Cluster analysis.

In Each Case, Would You Accept This Type of Relation (1), Try to Avoid It (2), or Reject It (3)?	Cluster			
	1	2	3	4
P15.1 Live in a neighborhood with many immigrants	2	1	2	3
P15.2 Rent out a house or apartment you owned to immigrants	3	1	2	3
P15.3 Work/study with immigrants	2	1	1	3
P15.4 Have an immigrant be your boss at work	2	1	1	3
P15.5 Have your child bring immigrant friends home	2	1	1	3
P15.6 Have your child marry an immigrant	2	1	1	3
P15.7 Have your child in a school with many immigrant children	2	1	1	3

Table 3. ANOVA of association between clusters and numeric variables.

	Age (Years)		Political Position (Left = 1; Right = 10)	
	Median	SD	Median	SD
Cluster 1	44.60	15.353	4.70	2.185
Cluster 2	47.24	15.171	5.72	2.055
Cluster 3	50.61	15.408	6.06	2.651
Cluster 4	50.41	16.600	6.59	2.108
Total	46.23	15.513	5.19	2.298
F statistic	15.295		50.535	
Sig. (bilateral)	$p = 0.000$		$p = 0.000$	
N	2222		1984	

Table 4. Association between clusters and SES.

	Low	Middle	Upper	Total
Cluster 1	19.4%	37.6%	43.0%	100%
Cluster 2	24.0%	42.4%	33.6%	100%
Cluster 3	22.0%	41.2%	36.9%	100%
Cluster 4	40.9%	37.5%	21.6%	100%
Total	21.8%	39.2%	39.0%	100%
	Value	Sig. (bilateral)	N	
Spearman's rho	−0.076	0.000		
Somers' d (symmetric)	−0.073	0.000	2471	2160

This analysis shows that in all the statistical tests, the relation with immigrants was linearly ordered (from lowest to highest) for the majority of the variables analyzed. The average for the political positioning variables (1 = left; 10 = right) was significantly different between groups (F = 50.535; $p = 0.000$), with cluster 1, on average, being more towards the left (M = 44.60; SD = 2.18), while the highest average was found among individuals in cluster 4 (M = 6.59; SD = 2.10). A similar pattern is observed with age: people in cluster 1 had an average age of 44.6 years (SD = 15.3), while the median in cluster 4 was 50.4 years (SD = 16.6).

The socioeconomic level variable followed the pattern indicated. Cluster 1 had the largest proportion of people with greater purchasing power (upper class = 43%; lower class = 19.4%) while cluster 4 had the largest proportion of people with fewer resources (upper class = 21.6%; lower class = 40.9%), with an equally significant association between variables (Spearman's rho = −0.073, p = 0.000; Somers' d = −0.076, p = 0.000).

The results of Table 5 allow us to answer the second research question of this study. Exposure to news related to immigrants influences whether individuals view immigration as one of the most relevant issues in the country. Exposure to both positive and negative framings about migrants increases the chance of people considering immigration to be one of the two most important issues for the country to handle (The dependent variable for this analysis is categorical and has only two values: 1 (immigration is considered one of the most relevant issues on the country's public agenda) and 0 (immigration is not considered one of the most relevant issues on the public agenda). The negative and significant coefficients express a decrease in the chance of the presence of the dependent variable when the independent variable is modified; in the same way, negative and significant coefficients express an increase in the chance of the presence of the dependent variable in the same condition).

Table 5. Logistic regression of the determinants of agenda.

	B Unstandardized Coefficients
Men [Ref: Women]	−0.226 (0.129)
Age: 35–49 [Ref: 18–34]	0.044 (0.162)
Age: 50–64	−0.159 (0.171)
Age: 65+	−0.718 *** (0.212)
SES Middle [Ref: Low]	−0.022 (0.166)
SES Upper	−0.760 *** (0.182)
Political position [1 = Left; 10 = Right]	0.283 *** (0.030)
Economic situation: Stagnant [Ref: Making progress]	0.478 *** (0.183)
Economic situation: Declining	0.682 *** (0.218)
Low fear of crime [Ref: No afraid]	0.381 (0.481)
Somewhat afraid of crime	0.824 (0.468)
Very afraid of crime	1.519 *** (0.469)
Immigrant relations	0.095 ** (0.045)
Exposure positive frame (Ref: Not exposed to news)	0.891 *** (0.218)
Exposure negative frame	0.799 *** (0.222)
Intercept	−4.911 *** (0.582)
Observations	1897
Log likelihood	−905.210
Akaike Inf. Crit.	1842.419

** $p < 0.01$; *** $p < 0.001$.

Additionally, the results show that there is a positive relationship between having more personally intense or close relations with immigrants and whether this subject should have a more relevant spot on the media agenda. Similarly, those who were more afraid of becoming crime victims, those who consider that the economy is stagnant or declining, and those who have right-wing political positions were more likely to view migration as a highly relevant media agenda topic. By contrast, being male, being in a high socioeconomic level, and being 65 or older decreases the probability of someone considering that immigration is a priority subject for the public agenda.

Descriptive statistics of the independent variables are: *evaluation of the economic situation* (progressing = 12.5%, stagnant = 58.2%, declining = 29.2%), *ideological position* (M = 5.18, SD = 2.3), *degree of closeness with immigrants living in the country* (M = 1.31, SD = 1.18), *fear of crime* (no afraid = 4.1%, low fear = 28.7%, somewhat of afraid = 40%, and very afraid = 27.3%), *gender* (women = 52%), *age* (M = 46.4 years, SD = 15.6), and *social class* (lower class = 22.2%, middle class = 39.2%; upper class = 38.7%).

Our third and final research question explored if there is a relationship between exposure to news with negative frames about immigrants and having a negative judgment about this group and their presence in the country (framing effect). The results in Table 6 answer this research question. Exposure to news with negative framing about immigrants is a reason to disagree with the idea that foreigners' presence does not generate problems for the country. By contrast, exposure to positive framing about immigrants has no effect on the mode of evaluating the consequences of the presence of this group.

Table 6. Poisson † regression of the determinants of agreement that the presence of foreigners is not causing problems.

	Agreement Presence of Foreigners (Unstandardized Coefficients)
Men [Ref: Women]	−0.016 (0.0243)
Age: 35–49 [Ref: 18–34]	−0.035 (0.0393)
Age: 50–64	−0.235 *** (0.0391)
Age: 65+	−0.085 ** (0.0393)
SES Middle [Ref: Low]	0.151 *** (0.0394)
NSE Upper	0.409 *** (0.0386)
Political position [1 = Left; 10 = Right]	−0.139 *** (0.0058)
Economic situation: Stagnant (Ref: Making progress)	−0.161 *** (0.0294)
Economic situation: Declining	−0.316 *** (0.0429)
Low fear of crime [Ref: No afraid]	−0.118 * (0.0522)
Somewhat afraid of crime	−0.445 *** (0.0534)
High fear of crime	−0.732 *** (0.0585)
Immigrant relations	0.099 *** (0.0102)
Exposure positive frame (Ref: Not exposed to news)	−0.056 (0350)
Exposure negative frame	−0.118 ** (0358)
Intercept	2.166 *** (0.0800)
Observations	2133
Log likelihood	−4771.737
Akaike Inf. Crit.	9575.474

* $p < 0.5$; ** $p < 0.01$; *** $p < 0.001$, † The Poisson regression—and not a multiple regression model—was used due to the variable being a count data, composed of the sum of the questions in which the respondents agreed with some statements related to immigrants. The counter had a minimum value of 0 (equivalent to having no positive opinion about migrants) and a maximum value of 10 (M = 3.3; SD = 2.9). This type of variable does not have a normal distribution and does not meet the assumptions required by a multiple linear regression. For this reason, the literature recommends the use of a Poisson regression to analyze this type of data.

Other variables related to disagreeing with the idea that immigrants' presence does not generate problems include being older (50 years or older), having right-wing political positions, considering that the economy is stagnant or declining, and being afraid of becoming a crime victim. By contrast, the variables associated with agreeing that foreigners do not cause problems included belonging to medium or high-income groups and having frequent personal relations with immigrants in different aspects of social life.

4. Discussion

4.1. Key Findings and Implications

This study provides relevant empirical support for two important theoretical perspectives on mass media effects on public opinion, agenda setting and framing, applied to a central phenomenon that affects many countries around the globe and millions of human beings: the growing flows of international migration. The results demonstrate the influence of news content on the attitudes and opinions of the national audience. These conclusions are the result of a rarely implemented methodological design, which consists of using an experimental strategy in the context of a survey in a country that has experienced an accelerated and growing influx of immigrants from various parts of Latin America in a short period of time. This is important because, in the field of news framing research, past studies have used experiments similar to a laboratory condition [31,52,60,65,67,69,72], obtaining data with valuable internal validity, but with little external validity and no possibility of representing the general population or identifying the differences among the segments studied.

One of the central purposes of this study was to utilize a more robust methodological approach, implementing an explanatory analysis strategy over a representative sample of the general population in Chile. Consistent with previous studies, the results show that media content can influence the audiences in two different ways: the importance given to a subject matter, the agenda-setting effect [32,36], and the way they think about this subject, or the framing effect [34,40]. In each way, the representativeness of the data allows other relevant determinants of people's opinions to be identified. Along with exposure to news about migrants, other determining factors for considering whether immigration is one of the main issues affecting the country (agenda-setting effect) are: (a) being part of the youngest segments, (b) belonging to lower-income groups, (c) expressing conservative political positions, (d) feeling very afraid of being a victim of a crime, and (e) maintaining frequent contact with foreigners in different aspects of daily life.

The study also contributes to understanding the role of mass media on citizens' attitudes on immigrants. Results are consistent with previous literature [31,64,65,67,72], showing that people exposed to news with a negative frame of migration express significantly more intolerant attitudes toward immigrants than those exposed to positive or neutral frames. It is interesting to observe that positive frames do not show an influence on attitudes towards immigrants, something that, although contrary to what the theory would predict, is consistent with previous studies such as that of Kim and colleagues [73]. These researchers reported that news content that shows immigrants as a real or symbolic threat generates negative emotions and attitudes, but non-threatening messages also show a small negative effect on their emotions. In the same way, coefficients of both frames in our analysis were negative, but the relation of the positive frame did not reach statistical significance.

The representativeness of the sample allows us to establish that attitudes toward immigrants are not homogeneous. Attitudes range from a majority group that is highly open to immigration (83%) to a minority group that shows a strong rejection to interacting with foreigners in daily life and to sharing different spaces with them (17%). The composition of these groups is associated with variables such as age, SES, political position, and fear of being a victim of a crime. The most reactive groups towards immigrants are, on average, those with a lower socioeconomic status (less educated and with fewer economic resources), which is consistent with previous literature on xenophobia determinants. These studies highlight economic competition as a strong trigger of negative attitudes toward immigrants [58,59].

On the other hand, the association between attitudes towards migration and the political position of individuals has also been confirmed by numerous studies [60,74,75]. Greater levels of fear of crime being associated with anti-immigrant views is consistent with content analysis research that has shown the tendency of news to link immigrants with conflicting events and concepts such as illegality and criminality in Chile [61], as in many developed countries (see, e.g., [61–63]).

4.2. Limitations

Despite its valuable findings, this study has a number of limitations. First, the field work was carried out during the period of the COVID-19 pandemic. As a result, the massive influx of immigrants into the country was halted for a few months and it caused a decrease in migratory pressure in some areas of the country. Nevertheless, in general the number of foreigners living in Chile did not decrease during the pandemic (National Statistics Institute—INE, 2021). Although this situation did not affect the results of the experiment, the problems associated with field work during the pandemic meant we needed to use an online survey rather than a face-to-face approach as we had planned. This may have caused two problems: (a) less sample representativeness in terms of the characteristics of the country's population and (b) a self-selection effect which increased the interest in survey participation among people who either reject the presence of immigrants or support their presence in Chile.

5. Conclusions

This study provides evidence regarding the effect of the media on the perception of the Chilean population of migrants in the context of a country that has increased the number of immigrants in a short period of time. The negative representation of migrants shown by the media can lead to acts of xenophobia, which can further harm the precarious situation of many foreigners who have come to Chile from other Latin American countries. Such results may influence a reflection among actors in the media about the way they report on immigrants in Chile and among other stakeholders linked to the issue, such as immigration authorities and civil society organizations.

Author Contributions: Conceptualization, A.S. and N.E.; data curation, A.S. and N.E.; methodology, A.S.; formal analysis, A.S. and N.E; validation, A.S., N.E., I.P. and D.G.; writing—original draft preparation, A.S., N.E., I.P. and D.G.; writing—review and editing, A.S., N.E. and I.P.; funding acquisition, A.S., N.E., I.P. and D.G. All authors have read and agreed to the published version of the manuscript.

Funding: This project was funded by Fondo Nacional de Desarrollo Científico y Tecnológico (grant N° 1210923) and Millennium Nucleus Center for the Study of Politics, Public Opinion and Media in Chile (MEPOP, NCS2021_063).

Institutional Review Board Statement: The study was conducted in accordance with the Declaration of Singapur and received ethical approval from the Research Ethics Committee (CEI-UDP) of Universidad Diego Portales, approval number: 0001-2019.

Informed Consent Statement: Informed consent was obtained from all subjects involved in the study.

Data Availability Statement: The information from this study is in the hands of the researchers and can be made available to the journal, respecting the anonymity of the respondents, if its editors deem it necessary.

Acknowledgments: The authors wish to provide thanks for the support of the Research Department of the Adolfo Ibáñez University in the development of this research article.

Conflicts of Interest: The authors declare no conflict of interest.

Appendix A Stimuli Used in the Experiment

1. **Positive frame of migrants (newspapers).**

C 2 NACIONAL Santiago: Lunes 4 de Enero del 2021

Chile es el país americano con mayor aumento de inmigrantes

Un reciente informe de The Economist informa que nuestro país registra el mayor crecimiento de la inmigración en todo el continente, con un aumento de la población extranjera que supera el 300% en los últimos tres años.

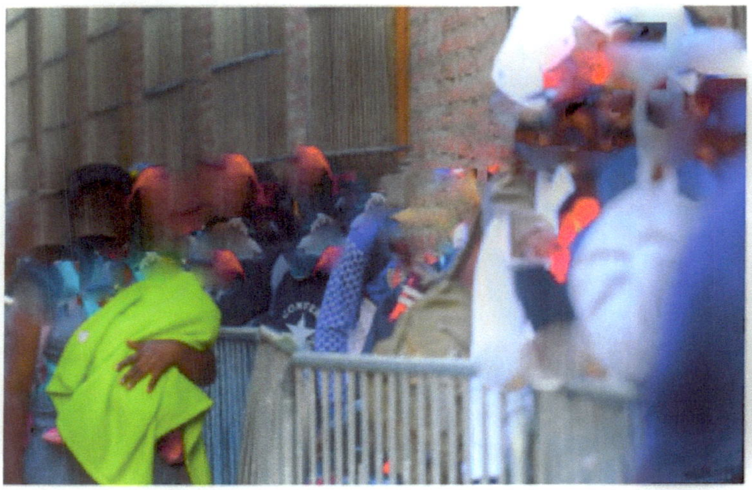

The Economista destaca la velocidad del fenómeno migratorio que vive el país, ya que al comenzar el siglo la población inmigrante en Chile no alcanzaba las 50 mil personas, en 2015 llegó a los 500 mil y actualmente supera los 1,5 millones de personas.

Según Álvaro Bellolio, director del Departamento de Extranjería, estas cifras respaldan la urgencia con la que se requiere una nueva legislación migratoria, aludiendo a la nueva Ley de Migración y Extranjería impulsada por el gobierno de Sebastián Piñera bajo el lema "ordenar la casa", que actualmente se discute en el Congreso.

Según el ministro del Interior, Rodrigo Delgado, "el objetivo es que el derecho que tienen las personas a migrar se haga de una forma regular, y que se gestione desde el país de origen para evitar al máximo que sean vulnerados los derechos de la población extranjera que queda al margen de la regulación", afirmó el ministro del Interior. Numerosos académicos y organizaciones sociales coinciden en que es necesario modernizar la regulación migratoria -la más antigua de Sudamérica, pero sin poner un énfasis restrictivo.

Harald Bauder, director del Programa de Estudios de Inmigración en la Universidad Ryerson de Toronto, afirma que el aumento de la migración internacional es un fenómeno inevitable en el contexto de la globalización, en todo el mundo. Para el experto, no sólo "resulta imposible frenar la circulación de seres humanos que buscan legítimamente una mejor vida. Particularmente para Chile, sería totalmente contraproducente", aludiendo a una serie de externalidades positivas de la migración reciente, como un mayor dinamismo en el mercado laboral, que entre 2019 y el presente ha incrementado los salarios y el Producto Interno Bruto (PIB) en torno a un 4%.

En torno los aportes de la migración, Shamshad Akhtar, presidenta de la Comisión Económica y Social para Asia y el Pacífico (CESPAP), asegura que son una pieza central en el engranaje de una economía como la nuestra, al llenar las espacios vacíos en el mercado laboral y en la disponibilidad de conocimientos. "La migración es beneficiosa para los países que se enfrentan a una reducción de la población en edad de trabajar, algo que se observa en el caso chileno. Contrario a los tradicionales mitos anti-inmigración, aquí no han generado una baja en los empleos o salarios, por el contrario, estos han crecido en la última década gracias a la presión migratoria".

En igual sentido, el informe de The Economist asegura que la migración reciente ha permitido mantener el crecimiento económico chileno en un contexto histórico especialmente complejo, así como a contrarrestar el envejecimiento poblacional que experimenta nuestra sociedad debido a su baja tasa de natalidad. Dado este diagnóstico, advierten de las negativas consecuencias que tendría para un país como el nuestro impulsar una legislación migratoria restrictiva.

Según la directora del Servicio Jesuita Migrante, Valeska Ureta, aunque en algunos medios y grupos políticos se estigmatice la migración, vinculándola con temas negativos como la falta de empleo y el delito, se trata de estereotipos sin respaldo empírico, dando como ejemolo que "sólo 0,01% de los delitos a nivel nacional es atribuible a inmigrantes, cuando representan más del 7% de la población total... ¿por qué no muestran el 99% de las experiencias exitosas de personas migrantes? Se trata muy mayoritariamente de personas que trabajan, que quieren regularizarse y vienen a impulsar el trabajo".

2. **Negative frame of migrants (newspapers).**

C 2 NACIONAL Santiago: Lunes 4 de Enero del 2021

Chile es el país americano con mayor aumento de inmigrantes

Un reciente informe de The Economist informa que nuestro país registra el mayor crecimiento de la inmigración en todo el continente, con un aumento de la población extranjera que supera el 300% en los últimos tres años.

The Economist destaca la velocidad del fenómeno migratorio que vive el país, ya que al comenzar el siglo la población inmigrante en Chile no alcanzaba las 50 mil personas, en 2015 llegó a los 500 mil y actualmente supera los 1,5 millones de personas.

Según Álvaro Bellolio, director del Departamento de Extranjería, estas cifras respaldan la urgencia con la que se requiere una nueva legislación migratoria, aludiendo a la nueva Ley de Migración y Extranjería impulsada por el gobierno de Sebastián Piñera bajo el lema "ordenar la casa", que actualmente se discute en el Congreso.

Numerosas autoridades de gobierno han salido a respaldar la nueva ley, que busca endurecer las normas asociadas al ingreso y regularización de documentos para los inmigrantes. El Ministro de Relaciones Exteriores, Andrés Allamand, en conferencia de prensa llamó al Senado a "garantizar una migración ordenada, segura y regular", ya que sólo en los últimos cuatro años ingresó 1 millón de inmigrantes, el 90% de ellos con visa de turismo, aun cuando sus reales intenciones eran establecerse en el país. Según el Canciller, enfrentamos una presión migratoria desde el exterior particularmente fuerte, asegurando que las "estimaciones apuntan incluso a que la presión migratoria podría superar las 500.000 personas" este año.

Según Bellolio, la principal diferencia de esta ley es que los extranjeros deberán "sincerar" las razones por las que vienen al país antes de entrar al país, de modo que quien ingrese como turista o por un paso ilegal no tendrá forma alguna de regularizar después su permanencia, afirmando que "quien entre de manera clandestina, no siguiendo las reglas, van a enfrentar un proceso de expulsión". Esta medida afectaría inmediatamente a los inmigrantes que han ingresado por pasos fronterizos clandestinos que, según el subsecretario del Interior Juan Francisco Galli, superaron los 5 mil entre enero y agosto de 2020, a pesar de estar en medio de la pandemia.

La nueva ley también aumenta la lista de delitos establecidos en el Código Penal por los cuales un extranjero no podrá ingresar al país, entre ellos las personas condenadas por tráfico ilícito de estupefacientes, femicidio, secuestro de menores y robo con violación. Según Bellolio se trata de un resguardo fundamental ante esta ola migratoria, ya que "poco ayuda la visión buenista de que Chile sea centro de rehabilitación de migrantes delincuentes".

3. **Positive frame of migrants (online).**

Santiago: Lunes 4 de Enero del 2021 Actualizado 10:56

D Noticias | Economía | Deportes | Espectáculos | Tendencias | Autos | Servicios | [O] | [tv] | 360°

Chile | Mundo | Tecnología | Educación | Documentos | Multimedia | Juegos | Especial Coronavirus | Pasatiempos |

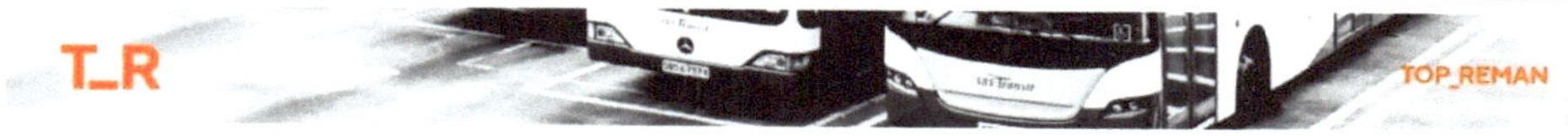

Chile es el país americano con mayor aumento de inmigrantes

Un reciente informe de The Economist informa que nuestro país registra el mayor crecimiento de la inmigración en todo el continente, con un aumento de la población extranjera que supera el 300% en los últimos tres años.

4 de Enero de 2021 | 10:50 | Redactado por Andrés V, Diario

The Economista destaca la velocidad del fenómeno migratorio que vive el país, ya que al comenzar el siglo la población inmigrante en Chile no alcanzaba las 50 mil personas, en 2015 llegó a los 500 mil y actualmente supera los 1,5 millones de personas.

Según Álvaro Bellolio, director del Departamento de Extranjería, estas cifras respaldan la urgencia con la que se requiere una nueva legislación migratoria, aludiendo a la nueva Ley de Migración y Extranjería impulsada por el gobierno de Sebastián Piñera bajo el lema "ordenar la casa", que actualmente se discute en el Congreso.

Según el ministro del Interior, Rodrigo Delgado, "el objetivo es que el derecho que tienen las personas a migrar se haga de una forma regular, y que se gestione desde el país de origen para evitar al máximo que sean vulnerados los derechos de la población extranjera que queda al margen de la regulación", afirmó el ministro del Interior. Numerosos académicos y organizaciones sociales coinciden en que es necesario modernizar la regulación migratoria -la más antigua de Sudamérica, pero sin poner un énfasis restrictivo. Harald Bauder, director del Programa de Estudios de Inmigración en la Universidad Ryerson de Toronto, afirma que el aumento de la migración internacional es un fenómeno inevitable en el contexto de la globalización, en todo el mundo. Para el experto, no sólo "resulta imposible frenar la circulación de seres humanos que buscan legítimamente una mejor vida. Particularmente para Chile, sería totalmente contraproducente", aludiendo a una serie de externalidades positivas de la migración reciente, como un mayor dinamismo en el mercado laboral, que entre 2019 y el presente ha incrementado los salarios y el Producto Interno Bruto (PIB) en torno a un 4%.

En torno los aportes de la migración, Shamshad Akhtar, presidenta de la Comisión Económica y Social para Asia y el Pacífico (CESPAP), asegura que son una pieza central en el engranaje de una economía como la nuestra, al llenar las espacios vacíos en el mercado laboral y en la disponibilidad de conocimientos. "La migración es beneficiosa para los países que se enfrentan a una reducción de la población en edad de trabajar, algo que se observa en el caso chileno. Contrario a los tradicionales mitos anti-inmigración, aquí no han generado una baja en los empleos o salarios, por el contrario, estos han crecido en la última década gracias a la presión migratoria".

RECOMENDADOS DIARIO

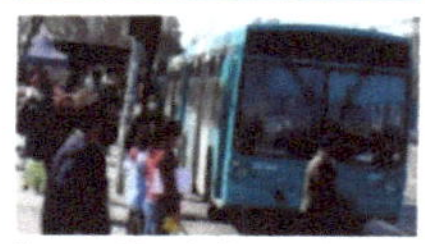

Nuevas cifras de Transantiago para 2021.

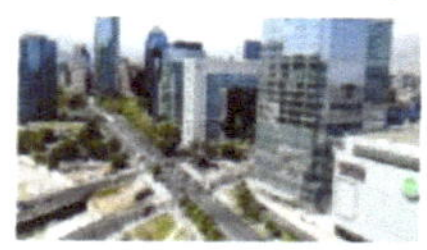

Conoce las mejores ciudades para vivir y sus proyecciones.

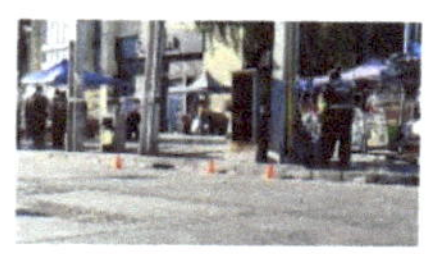

Balacera en Maipú que dejó dos fallecidos.

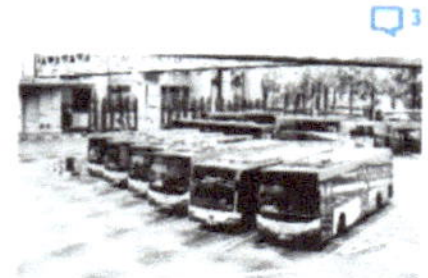

Planifica tus viajes en los nuevos buses electricos.

4. **Negative frame of migrants (online).**

Santiago: Lunes 4 de Enero del 2021 Actualizado 10:56

D Noticias | Economía | Deportes | Espectáculos | Tendencias | Autos | Servicios

Chile | Mundo | Tecnología | Educación | Documentos | Multimedia | Juegos | Especial Coronavirus | Pasatiempos

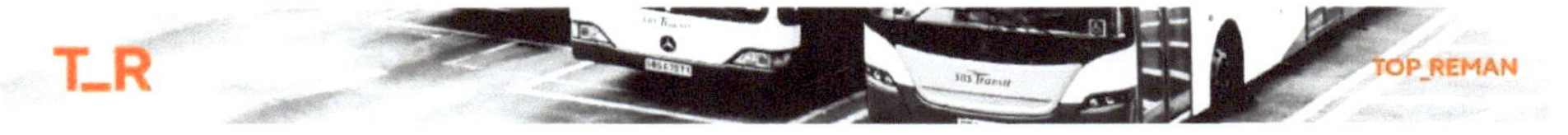

Chile es el país americano con mayor aumento de inmigrantes

Un reciente informe de The Economist informa que nuestro país registra el mayor crecimiento de la inmigración en todo el continente, con un aumento de la población extranjera que supera el 300% en los últimos tres años.

4 de Enero de 2021 | 10:50 | Redactado por Andrés V, Diario

The Economist destaca la velocidad del fenómeno migratorio que vive el país, ya que al comenzar el siglo la población inmigrante en Chile no alcanzaba las 50 mil personas, en 2015 llegó a los 500 mil y actualmente supera los 1,5 millones de personas.

Según Álvaro Bellolio, director del Departamento de Extranjería, estas cifras respaldan la urgencia con la que se requiere una nueva legislación migratoria, aludiendo a la nueva Ley de Migración y Extranjería impulsada por el gobierno de Sebastián Piñera bajo el lema "ordenar la casa", que actualmente se discute en el Congreso.

Numerosas autoridades de gobierno han salido a respaldar la nueva ley, que busca endurecer las normas asociadas al ingreso y regularización de documentos para los inmigrantes. El Ministro de Relaciones Exteriores, Andrés Allamand, en conferencia de prensa llamó al Senado a "garantizar una migración ordenada, segura y regular", ya que sólo en los últimos cuatro años ingresó 1 millón de inmigrantes, el 90% de ellos con visa de turismo, aun cuando sus reales intenciones eran establecerse en el país. Según el Canciller, enfrentamos una presión migratoria desde el exterior particularmente fuerte, asegurando que las "estimaciones apuntan incluso a que la presión migratoria podría superar las 500.000 personas" este año.

Según Bellolio, la principal diferencia de esta ley es que los extranjeros deberán "sincerar" las razones por las que vienen al país antes de entrar al país, de modo que quien ingrese como turista o por un paso ilegal no tendrá forma alguna de regularizar después su permanencia, afirmando que "quien entre de manera clandestina, no siguiendo las reglas, van a enfrentar un proceso de expulsión". Esta medida afectaría inmediatamente a los inmigrantes que han ingresado por pasos fronterizos clandestinos que, según el subsecretario del Interior Juan Francisco Galli, superaron los 5 mil entre enero y agosto de 2020, a pesar de estar en medio de la pandemia.

La nueva ley también aumenta la lista de delitos establecidos en el Código Penal por los cuales un extranjero no podrá ingresar al país, entre ellos las personas condenadas por tráfico ilícito de estupefacientes, femicidio, secuestro de menores y robo con violación. Según Bellolio se trata de un resguardo fundamental ante esta ola migratoria, ya que "poco ayuda la visión buenista de que Chile sea centro de rehabilitación de migrantes delincuentes".

RECOMENDADOS DIARIO

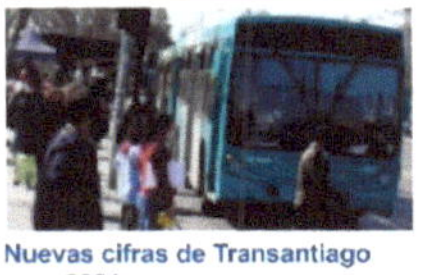

Nuevas cifras de Transantiago para 2021.

3

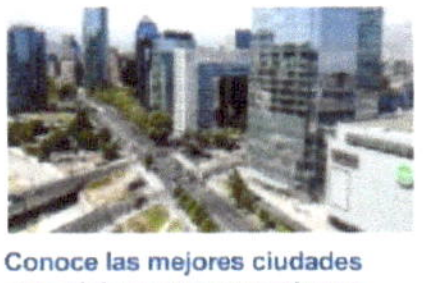

Conoce las mejores ciudades para vivir y sus proyecciones.

3

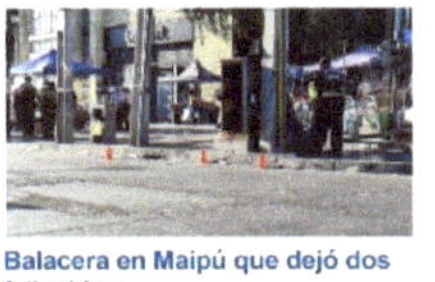

Balacera en Maipú que dejó dos fallecidos.

3

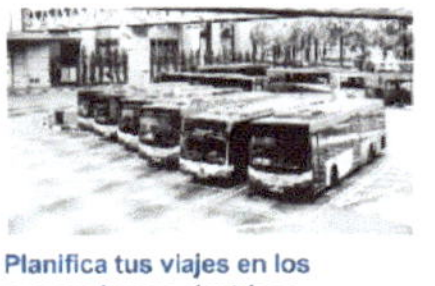

Planifica tus viajes en los nuevos buses electricos.

3

The audio of the positive and negative frames (radial format) can be downloaded from the following link: https://www.dropbox.com/sh/kftaep75cbf81e6/AAB2Z_hAo_fJp85pyC5lmlK7a?dl, (accessed on 4 May 2022).

Appendix B

On a scale from 1 to 5, where 1 means "Strongly Disagree" and 5 means "Strongly Agree", how much do you agree or disagree with the following statements?

Table A1. Questions Used to Construct the Dependent Variable on the Perception of the Presence of Immigrants in Chile (Dependent Variable to Measure the Framing Effect).

	Strongly Disagree			Strongly Agree	
The arrival of foreigners has increased the unemployment of Chilean workers.	1	2	3	4	5
The arrival of foreigners in Chile is related to the increase in crime.	1	2	3	4	5
The arrival of foreigners to Chile is a contribution to the country's culture.	1	2	3	4	5
Immigrants take on jobs that Chilean people do not want to do.	1	2	3	4	5
By accepting lower salaries, foreign workers lower the salaries of Chilean workers.	1	2	3	4	5
In general, immigrants are contributing to the development of Chile.	1	2	3	4	5
All illegal immigrants should be expelled, even if they have Chilean relatives (women, children).	1	2	3	4	5
The government should not let more immigrants enter the country until the emergency of COVID-19 ends.	1	2	3	4	5
The number of foreigners in Chile is excessive.	1	2	3	4	5
Public health should be preferred for Chilean people before migrants.	1	2	3	4	5

References

1. Cano, V.; Soffia, M. Los estudios sobre migración internacional en Chile: Apuntes y comentarios para una agenda de investigación actualizada [Studies on international migration in Chile: Notes and comments for an updated research agenda]. *Pap. Población* **2009**, *15*, 129–167. Available online: http://www.scielo.org.mx/pdf/pp/v15n61/v15n61a7.pdf (accessed on 2 April 2022).
2. Thayer, L. Expectativas de reconocimiento y estrategias de incorporación. La construcción de trayectorias degradadas en migrantes latinoamericanos residentes en la Región Metropolitana de Santiago [Recognition expectations and onboarding strategies. The construction of degraded trajectories in Latin American migrants residing in the Metropolitan Region of Santiago]. *Polis* **2013**, *12*, 259–285. Available online: https://www.redalyc.org/pdf/305/30528720012.pdf (accessed on 2 April 2022).
3. Canales, A. La inmigración contemporánea en Chile. Entre la diferenciación étnico-nacional y la desigualdad de clases [Contemporary immigration in Chile. From ethnic-national differentiation to class inequality]. *Pap. Población* **2019**, *25*, 53–72. [CrossRef]
4. Rojas, N.; Silva, C.; Amode, N.; Vásquez, J.; Orrego, C. Boletín Informative [Newsletter]. Departamento de Extranjería y Migración de Chile [Department of Foreigners and Migration of Chile]. 2016. Available online: https://www.extranjeria.gob.cl/media/2016/09/boletin-1.pdf (accessed on 5 April 2022).
5. González, L.; Hernández, A. Elementos socioestructurales y destino de los flujos migratorios venezolanos [Sociostructural elements and destination of Venezuelan migratory flows]. *Erasmus Semilleros Investig.* **2020**, *5*, 19–31.
6. Navarrete Yáñez, B. Percepciones sobre inmigración en Chile: Lecciones para una política migratoria [Perceptions of Immigration in Chile. Lessons for Immigration Policy]. *Migr. Int.* **2017**, *9*, 179–209. Available online: http://www.scielo.org.mx/scielo.php?script=sci_arttext&pid=S1665-89062017000100179 (accessed on 5 April 2022).
7. Ministerio de Desarrollo Social y Familia. Informe Final Consejo Asesor Para la Cohesión Social: Diagnóstico Para Una Aproximación a la Cohesión Social en Chile y Recomendaciones Para Fortalecer el Aporte de la Política Social [Advisory Council for Social Cohesion Final Report: Diagnosis for an Approach to Social Cohesion in Chile and Recommendations to Strengthen the Contribution of Social Policy]. 2020. Available online: https://www.desarrollosocialyfamilia.gob.cl/storage/docs/Informe_Final_Consejo_Cohesion_Social.pdf (accessed on 2 April 2022).
8. Silva, J.; Lufin, M. *Situación de Inmigración y Asentamiento de Grupos Afrocolombianos en la Región Antofagasta, con Énfasis en las mujeres [Immigration Situation and Settlement of Afro-Colombian Groups in the Antofagasta Region, with Emphasis on Women]*; DOCUMENTOS de Trabajo en Economía y Ciencia Regional, 35; Universidad Catolica del Norte: Antofagasta, Chile, 2013.

9. Méndez, L.; Cárdenas, M. Hacia la construcción de un modelo comprensivo de análisis de la "situación de inmigración" de mujeres sudamericanas en Chile [Building a Comprehensive Analytical Model of the "Immigration Situation" of South American Women in Chile]. *Psicoperspectivas* **2012**, *11*, 252–272. Available online: https://scielo.conicyt.cl/pdf/psicop/v11n1/art12.pdf (accessed on 7 April 2022).
10. Galvez, R. Iquique: Marcha contra migrantes terminó en la quema de pertenencias de extranjeros [Iquique: March against migrants ended in the burning of foreigners' belongings]. La Tercera. 26 September 2021. Available online: www.latercera.com (accessed on 20 April 2022).
11. Valenzuela-Vergara, E.M. Media representations of immigration in the Chilean press: To a different narrative of immigration? *J. Commun. Inq.* **2018**, *43*, 129–151. [CrossRef]
12. Yañez, S.; Cárdenas, M. Estrategias de aculturación, indicadores de salud mental y bienestar psicológico en un grupo de inmigrantes sudamericanos en Chile [Acculturation Strategies, Indicators of Mental Health and Psychological Well-Being in a group of South American immigrants in Chile]. *Salud Soc.* **2010**, *1*, 51–70. Available online: https://www.redalyc.org/pdf/4397/439742462006.pdf (accessed on 10 April 2022).
13. Scherman, A.; Etchegaray, N. News Frames in the Context of a Substantial Increase in Migration: Differences Between Media Platforms and Immigrants' Nationality. *Int. J. Commun.* **2021**, *15*, 5051–5073. Available online: https://ijoc.org/index.php/ijoc/article/view/16993/3608 (accessed on 4 April 2022).
14. Etchegaray, N.; Correa, T. Media Consumption and Immigration: Factors related to the Perception of Stigmatization among Immigrants. *Int. J. Commun.* **2015**, *9*, 3601–3620. Available online: https://ijoc.org/index.php/ijoc/article/viewFile/3997/1506 (accessed on 6 April 2022).
15. Couldry, N.; Hepp, A. Media Cultures in a Global Age: A transcultural approach to an expanded spectrum. In *The Handbook of Global Media Research*; Volkmer, I., Ed.; John Wiley & Sons: Hoboken, NJ, USA, 2012; pp. 92–109.
16. D'Haenens, L. ICT in Multicultural Society: The Netherlands: A Context for Sound Multiform Media Policy? *Int. Commun. Gaz.* **2003**, *65*, 401–421. Available online: https://bit.ly/3LLXQQg (accessed on 20 April 2022).
17. Hall, S. Cultural Identity and Diaspora. In *Theorizing Diaspora: A Reader*; Braziel, J., Mannur, A., Eds.; Blackwell: Oxford, UK, 2003; pp. 233–246.
18. Bailey, O.; Georgiou, M.; Harindranath, R. (Eds.) *Transnational Lives and the Media: Re-Imagining Diaspora*; Palgrave Macmillan: London, UK, 2007.
19. Georgiou, M. *Diaspora, Identity and the Media: Diasporic Transnationalism and Mediated Spacialities*; Cresskill, N.J., Ed.; Hampton Press: New York, NY, USA, 2006.
20. Gillespie, M. *Television, Ethnicity and Cultural Change*; Routledge: London, UK, 1995.
21. Berthoud, R.; Modood, T.; Smith, P. *Introduction. Ethnic Minorities in Britain: Diversity and Disadvantage*; Modood, T., National Survey of Ethnic Minorities, Eds.; Policy Studies Institute: London, UK, 1997; pp. 1–17.
22. Buckingham, D. *Youth, Identity, and Digital Media*; MIT Press: Cambridge, MA, USA, 2008.
23. Kim, Y. *Communication and Cross-Cultural Adaptation: An Integrative Theory*; Multilingual Matters: Philadelphia, PA, USA, 1998.
24. Taket, A.; Crisp, B.; Nevill, A.; Lamaro, G.; Graham, M.; Barter-Godfrey, S. (Eds.) *Theorising Social Exclusion*; Routledge: New York, NY, USA, 2009.
25. Keyes, C. Social well-being. *Soc. Psychol. Q.* **1998**, *61*, 121–140. [CrossRef]
26. Valkenburg, P.M.; Semetko, H.A.; De Vreese, C.H. The effects of news frames on readers' thoughts and recall. *Commun. Res.* **1999**, *26*, 550–569. Available online: https://bit.ly/38L6KyQ (accessed on 15 April 2022). [CrossRef]
27. Chong, D.; Druckman, J.N. A theory of framing and opinion formation in competitive elite environments. *J. Commun.* **2007**, *57*, 99–118. [CrossRef]
28. Blinder, S.; Allen, W.L. Constructing immigrants: Portrayals of migrant groups in British national newspapers, 2010–2012. *Int. Migr. Rev.* **2016**, *50*, 3–40. Available online: https://bit.ly/37XciX9 (accessed on 15 April 2022). [CrossRef]
29. Valentino, N.A.; Brader, T.; Jardina, A.E. Immigration opposition among US Whites: General ethnocentrism or media priming of attitudes about Latinos? *Political Psychol.* **2013**, *34*, 149–166. [CrossRef]
30. Muñiz, C. Encuadres Noticiosos e Inmigración: Del Análisis de los Contenidos al Estudio de los Efectos Mediáticos [News Frames and Immigration: From Content Analysis to the Study of Media Effects]. Ph.D. Thesis, Universidad de Salamanca, Salamanca, Spain, 2007. Available online: http://bit.ly/1qB9gLX (accessed on 13 April 2022).
31. Igartua, J.J.; Moral, F.; Fernández, I. Cognitive, attitudinal and emotional effects of the news frame and group cues on processing news about immigration. *J. Media Psychol.* **2011**, *23*, 174–185. [CrossRef]
32. Iyengar, S. *Is Anyone Responsible? How Television Frames Political Issues*; The University of Chicago Press: Chicago, IL. USA, 1991.
33. Bateson, G. *Steps to an Ecology of Mind: Collected Essays in Anthropology, Psychiatry, Evolution, and Epistemology*; University of Chicago Press: Chicago, IL, USA, 2000.
34. Goffman, E. *Frame analysis: Los Marcos de la Experiencia*; CIS: Madrid, Spain, 2006.
35. McCombs, M.; Valenzuela, S. *Setting the Agenda: Mass Media and Public Opinion*; John Wiley & Sons: Hoboken, NJ, USA, 2020.
36. McCombs, M.E.; Shaw, D.L.; Weaver, D.H. New directions in agenda-setting theory and research. *Mass Commun. Soc.* **2014**, *17*, 781–802. [CrossRef]
37. Semetko, H.; y Valkenburg, P. Framing European politics: A content analysis of press and television news. *J. Commun.* **2000**, *50*, 93–109. [CrossRef]

38. Checa, L. Del encuadre a los marcos estructurales: Teorías de análisis de medios y contexto socio-cultural [From framing to structural frames: Media analysis theories and socio-cultural context]. *Rev. Faro* **2013**, *1*, 3–25.
39. Reese, S.D. The framing project: A bridging model for media research revisited. *J. Commun.* **2007**, *57*, 148–154. [CrossRef]
40. Entman, R.M. Framing: Toward clarification of a fractured paradigm. *J. Commun.* **1993**, *43*, 51–58. [CrossRef]
41. Entman, R. Representation and reality in the portrayal of Blacks on network television news. *Journal. Q.* **1994**, *71*, 509–520. [CrossRef]
42. Tankard, J.W. The empirical approach to the study of Media Framing. In *Framing Public Life. Perspectives on Media and Our Understanding of the Social World*; Reese, S.D., Gandy, O.H., Grant, A.E., Eds.; Lawrence Erlbaum Associates: Mahwah, NJ, USA, 2001.
43. Lakoff, G. *Puntos de Reflexión: Manual de un Progresista [Reflection Points. Manual of a Progressive]*; Ediciones Península: Barcelona, Spain, 2008.
44. Price, V.; Tewksbury, D.; Powers, E. Switching trains of thought: The impact of news frames on readers' cognitive responses. *Commun. Res.* **1997**, *24*, 481–506. Available online: https://bit.ly/37VYfBa (accessed on 20 April 2022). [CrossRef]
45. Druckman, J.N. On the limits of framing effects: Who can frame? *J. Politics* **2001**, *63*, 1041–1066. Available online: https://bit.ly/3MLzyWH (accessed on 21 April 2022). [CrossRef]
46. Cisneros, J.D. Contaminated communities: The metaphor of "immigrant as pollutant" in media representations of immigration. *Rhetor. Public Aff.* **2008**, *11*, 569–601. [CrossRef]
47. Balabanova, E.; Balch, A. Sending and receiving: The ethical framing of intra-EU migration in the European press. *Eur. J. Commun.* **2010**, *25*, 382–397. [CrossRef]
48. Lawlor, A.; Tolley, E. Deciding who's legitimate: News media framing of immigrants and refugees. *Int. J. Commun.* **2017**, *11*, 967–991.
49. Igartua, J.J.; Cheng, L. Moderating effect of group cue while processing news on immigration: Is the framing effect a heuristic process? *J. Commun.* **2009**, *59*, 726–749. [CrossRef]
50. Roggeband, C.; Vliegenthart, R. Divergent framing: The public debate on migration in the Dutch parliament and media, 1995–2004. *West Eur. Politics* **2007**, *30*, 524–548. [CrossRef]
51. Hainmueller, J.; Hopkins, D.J. Public attitudes toward immigration. *Annu. Rev. Political Sci.* **2014**, *17*, 225–249. [CrossRef]
52. Muñiz, C.; Igartua, J.J.; Humanes, M.L.; Cheng, L.; García, M.; Gomes, D.; García, A.R.; Gomes, Á.M. *Imágenes de la Inmigración Latinoamericana en los Medios de Comunicación. Perspectivas Empíricas desde la Teoría del Encuadre [Images of Latin American Immigration in the Media. Empirical Perspectives from the Framing Theory]*; Presentation at the Conference Diálogo Internacional Comunicación y Diversidad Cultural; Universidad de Salamanca: Salamanca, Spain, 2004.
53. Kim, S.H.; Carvalho, J.P.; Davis, A.G.; Mullins, A.M. The view of the border: News framing of the definition, causes, and solutions to illegal immigration. *Mass Commun. Soc.* **2011**, *14*, 292–314. [CrossRef]
54. Lakoff, G.; Ferguson, S. *The Framing of Immigration*; The Rockridge Institute: Berkeley, CA, USA, 2006.
55. Brader, T.; Valentino, N.A.; Suhay, E. What triggers public opposition to immigration? Anxiety, group cues, and immigration threat. *Am. J. Political Sci.* **2008**, *52*, 959–978. [CrossRef]
56. National Institute of Statistics. Estimación de Personas Extranjeras Residentes Habituales en Chile al 31 de Diciembre 2020. 2021. Available online: https://bit.ly/38NAR8I (accessed on 5 April 2022).
57. CNN Chile. Desmantelan Campamento y Destruyen Pertenencias de Personas Extranjeras Durante Marcha en Iquique. 30 January 2021. Available online: https://www.cnnchile.com/pais/marcha-iquique-campamento-pertenencias-personas-extranjeros_20220130/ (accessed on 20 April 2021).
58. Costello, K.; Hodson, G. Social dominance-based threat reactions to immigrants in need of assistance. *Eur. J. Soc. Psychol.* **2011**, *41*, 220–231. [CrossRef]
59. Jackson, L.M.; Esses, V.M. Effects of perceived economic competition on people's willingness to help empower immigrants. *Group Process. Intergroup Relat.* **2000**, *3*, 419–435. [CrossRef]
60. Damstra, A.; Jacobs, L.; Boukes, M.; Vliegenthart, R. The impact of immigration news on anti-immigrant party support: Unpacking agenda-setting and issue ownership effects over time. *J. Elect. Public Opin. Parties* **2021**, *31*, 97–118. [CrossRef]
61. Doña, C. *Percepción de la Inmigración Reciente en Chile a Través del Análisis de Medios de Prensa*; Tesis Para Optar al Título de Sociólogo, (Inédito); Universidad de Chile: Santiago, Chile, 2002.
62. Chavez, M.; Whiteford, S.; Hoewe, J. Reporting on immigration: A content analysis of major US newspapers' coverage of Mexican immigration. *Norteamérica* **2010**, *5*, 111–125.
63. Farris, E.M.; Silber Mohamed, H. Picturing immigration: How the media criminalizes immigrants. *Politics Groups Identities* **2018**, *6*, 814–824. [CrossRef]
64. Greussing, E.; Boomgaarden, H.G. Shifting the refugee narrative? An automated frame analysis of Europe's 2015 refugee crisis. *J. Ethn. Migr. Stud.* **2017**, *43*, 1749–1774. [CrossRef]
65. Wright, M.; Citrin, J. Saved by the stars and stripes? Images of protest, salience of threat, and immigration attitudes. *Am. Politics Res.* **2011**, *39*, 323–343. [CrossRef]
66. Boomgaarden, H.G.; Vliegenthart, R. Explaining the rise of anti-immigrant parties: The role of news media content. *Elect. Stud.* **2007**, *26*, 404–417. [CrossRef]

67. Parrott, S.; Hoewe, J.; Fan, M.; Huffman, K. Portrayals of Immigrants and Refugees in U.S.News Media: Visual Framing and its Effect on Emotions and Attitudes. *J. Broadcasting Electron. Media* **2019**, *63*, 677–697. [CrossRef]
68. Beyer, A.; Matthes, J. Public perceptions of the media coverage of irregular immigration: Comparative insights from France, the United States, and Norway. *Am. Behav. Sci.* **2015**, *59*, 839–857. [CrossRef]
69. Muñiz, C.; Igartua, J.; de la Fuente, J.; y Otero, J. Narrando la inmigración: Análisis del tratamiento informativo y evaluación de los efectos de las noticias en España. *Rev. Mex. Cienc. Políticas Soc.* **2009**, *51*, 117–135.
70. De Vreese, C. New avenues for framing research. *Am. Behav. Sci.* **2012**, *56*, 365–375. [CrossRef]
71. Geers, S.; Bos, L.; De Vreese, C. Informed switchers? How the impact of election news exposure on vote change depends on political information efficacy. *Int. J. Commun.* **2017**, *11*, 1857–1878.
72. Joris, W.; d'Haenens, L.; Van Gorp, B.; Mertens, S. The refugee crisis in Europe: A frame analysis of European newspapers. In *Migrants, Refugees, and the Media*; Routledge: London, UK, 2018; pp. 59–80.
73. Kim, C.; Harwood, J.; Xian, J. The Negative and Positive Influences of Threat and Nonthreat Media Messages about Immigrants. *Int. J. Commun.* **2018**, *12*, 950–972.
74. Pew Research Center. In a Politically Polarized Era, Sharp Divides in Both Partisan Coalitions. 2019. Available online: https://www.pewresearch.org/politics/2019/12/17/views-on-race-and-immigration/ (accessed on 20 April 2022).
75. Moses, J. The Politics of Immigration: Introduction to a Special Isuue on US Immigration. *Eur. J. Am. Stud.* **2009**, *4*. [CrossRef]

MDPI AG
Grosspeteranlage 5
4052 Basel
Switzerland
Tel.: +41 61 683 77 34

International Journal of Environmental Research and Public Health Editorial Office
E-mail: ijerph@mdpi.com
www.mdpi.com/journal/ijerph

www.ingramcontent.com/pod-product-compliance
Lightning Source LLC
Chambersburg PA
CBHW041427210926
51850CB00013B/3370
* 9 7 8 3 7 2 5 8 4 1 2 9 5 *